# CARDIOMYOPATHIES - TYPES AND TREATMENTS

Edited by **Kaan Kırali**

**Cardiomyopathies - Types and Treatments**
http://dx.doi.org/10.5772/62816
Edited by Kaan Kırali

**Contributors**

Tatsushi Mutoh, Peter Michael Magnusson, Okechukwu Ogah, Halil Haldun Emiroglu, Nelgin Gerenli, Nimet Cindik, Coskun Celtik, Ana G. Almeida, María Ángeles Rosero Arenas, Alfonso Martínez Cornejo, Marta Bertolo Domínguez, Vicente Miranda Gozalvo, Miguel Angel Garcia Garcia, Seckin Pehlivanoglu, Hakan Altay, Christian Hamilton-Craig, Shuai Wang, Dao-Quan Peng, Bandar Al-Ghamdi, Kinji Shirota, Ryuta Kawashima, Kazumasu Sasaki, John Konhilas, Antoine Muchir, Maurilio Sampaolesi, Thomas Meyer, Carolina Galvez-Monton, Josep Lupón, Antoni Bayes-Genis, Santiago Roura, Sara Nunes, Anabela Rolo, Carlos Palmeira, Flávio Reis, Agnieszka Pawlak, Kaan Kırali, Tanıl Özer, Mustafa Mert Özgür

**Published by InTech**
Janeza Trdine 9, 51000 Rijeka, Croatia



**Publishing Process Manager** Andrea Koric
**Technical Editor** SPi Global
**Cover** InTech Design team

First published April, 2017
Printed in Croatia
Legal deposit, Croatia: National and University Library in Zagreb

Additional hard copies can be obtained from orders@intechopen.com

Cardiomyopathies - Types and Treatments, Edited by Kaan Kırali
p. cm.
Print ISBN 978-953-51-3039-0
Online ISBN 978-953-51-3040-6

For EU product safety concerns:
IN TECH d.o.o., Prolaz Marije Krucifikse Kozulić 3, 51000 Rijeka, Croatia,
info@intechopen.com or visit our website at intechopen.com.

# Meet the editor

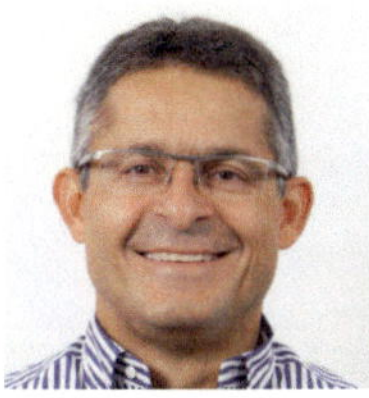

Prof Kirali received his PhD in 1997 at the Kosuyolu Heart and Research Hospital in Istanbul. He is collaborating with two cardiac centers: he is the Head of Heart Transplantation and Ventricular Assist Device department of Kosuyolu Hospital (Istanbul) and works at the CVS department of Faculty of Medicine of Sakarya University (Sakarya). Over the last 20 years, he has focused his scientific interests on the topics related to cardiovascular therapies. He is an expert in congenital cardiac surgery, coronary bypass surgery, minimal invasive cardiac surgery, valve repair, and aortic root surgery. He has been interested in heart transplantation since 2000 and in theleft ventricular assist devices in the last years. He has been also interested in preventive medicine on cardiac failure since his public health MHSc in 2000 at the Istanbul University. He published numerous SCI journal papers and book chapters and edited/reviewed many academic journals.

# Contents

# Preface

Cardiomyopathies are the basic and featured cardiac pathologies in the 21st century, which threaten public health and health care budgets. New technologies for diagnosis, new researches for genetic structure, new definitions for nature of malformations and malfunctions, new classifications for pathologic types, and new surgical approaches for curative treatment will improve survival of patients with end-stage heart failure as well as clinical status. Every cardiomyopathy type has its own pathophysiologic changes, etiologic development, structural disruption, and functional behavior but similar clinical progress: dilated (decreased left ventricular systolic function) or restrictive (preserved left ventricular systolic function) myocardial dysfunction. The main scenario is depressed left ventricular function with varying degrees of left heart failure syndrome associated without or with right heart failure syndrome. In the last decade, a third form of heart failure type has been added: post-implant right heart failure. Left ventricular assist devices are developed to maintain cardiac cycle via continued drainage intercavitar ventricular blood volume into arterial circulation, especially on the left heart. If the right heart cannot adapt to this non-physiologic function, right heart failure can develop so as to cause death. Specific cardiomyopathies have peculiar features, and each of them is a separate subject for investigation. This book includes topics on pathophysiology, general forms and also specific types of cardiomyopathies, but also introduces new research in this field. The summary of last surgical treatment approaches, point out the technologic advance in health care. This book has been created by professionals around the world, who avert readers' attention on this gigantic health problem and present latest treatment solutions.


**Prof. Dr. Kaan Kırali**
Department of Cardiovascular Surgery
Faculty of Medicine, Sakarya University
Sakarya, Turkey

Head of Cardiac Transplantation and Ventricular Assist Device Department
Kartal Koşuyolu YIEA Hospital
Istanbul, Turkey

Section 1

# Introduction

Chapter 1

# Introductory Chapter: Last Crossroad

Kaan Kırali

Additional information is available at the end of the chapter

http://dx.doi.org/10.5772/65368

Cardiomyopathy (CMP) is the heart muscle disease causing cardiac myocyte injury and myocardial dysfunction, which impair structural and/or functional ventricular filling or ejection of blood in the absence of structural or vascular heart disease. Most CMPs are complex and heterogeneous familial diseases, and the inheritance is autosomal dominant in majority of cases. The classification of these cardiac diseases has been based on morphofunctional phenotypes, but it has been changed according to molecular genetics in recent years. As we know, the traditional classification proposed by the World Health Organization (WHO) is easy to differentiate between various CMPs in a couple structural and functional phenotypes (**Table 1**), which helps us to define common treatment strategies [1]. New classification-orientated genomic and molecular science helps us to understand the complexity and heterogeneity of these diseases (**Table 2**), which may occur primary or secondary [2]. The American Heart Association (AHA) Scientific Statement proposes the definition: "Cardiomyopathies are a heterogeneous group of diseases of the myocardium associated with mechanical and/or electrical dysfunction that usually (but not invariably) exhibit inappropriate ventricular hypertrophy or dilatation and are due to a variety of causes that frequently are genetic. Cardiomyopathies either are confined to the heart (primary) or are part of generalized systemic disorders (secondary), often leading to cardiovascular death or progressive heart failure-related disability." The last classification system (MOGES) proposed by the World Heart Federation (WHF) includes all characteristics: morphofunctional phenotype (M), organ(s) involvement (O), genetic inheritance (G), etiology (E), and functional status (S) (**Table 3**) [3].

From the clinical perspective, the most important objective is diagnosis of the mechanism of the heart failure and delivery of the appropriate effective treatment. Heart failure incidence increases with age and rises from 20% in the seventh decade to more than 80% in octogenarians [4]. Advancing age or cardiac aging is another risk factor for heart failure, and it is a heterogeneous process characterized by genomic DNA damage, telomere shortening, and epigenetic modifications, which can affect protein homeostasis, mitochondrial function, and regenerative potential of stem cells adversely [5]. The hemodynamic changes are dependent on the nature of cardiomyopathies, which cause myocardial dysfunction due to mechanical or arrhythmogenic pathophysiologic mechanisms.

1. Dilated
2. Hypertrophic
3. Restrictive
4. Arrhythmogenic
5. Unclassified (mitochondrial diseases, fibroelastosis)
6. Specific
    a. Ischemic
    b. Valvular
    c. Hypertensive
    d. Inflammatory
    e. Metabolic
    f. General systemic disease
    g. Muscular dystrophies
    h. Neuromuscular disorders
    i. Sensitivity and toxic reactions
    j. Peripartum

**Table 1.** World Health Organization (WHO) classification for cardiomyopathies.

**A. Primary (predominantly involving the heart)**

**a. Genetic**

1) Hypertrophic cardiohyopathy
2) Arrhythmogenic right ventricular dysplasia
3) Glycogen storage (PRKAG2, Danon)
4) Conduction defects
5) Mitochondrial myopathies
6) Ion channel disorders (LQTS, SQTS, CVPT, Brugada, Asian SUNDS)

b. **Acquired**

1) Inflammatory (myocarditis)

2) Stress-provoked (Tako-Tsubo)

3) Peri- or postpartum

4) Tachycardia-induced

5) Infants of insulin-dependent diabetic mothers

c. **Mixt**

1) Dilated cardiomyopathy

2) Restrictive (non-hypertrophied and non-dilated)

2. **Secondary**

a. Infiltrative (amyloidosis; Gaucher disease; Hurler's disease; Hunter's disease)

b. Storage (hemochromatosis; Fabry's disease; Glycogen storage disease = type II Pompe; Niemann-Pick disease)

c. Toxicity (drugs, heavy metals, chemical agents)

d. Endomyocardial (endomyocardial fibrosis; hypereosinophilic syndrome = Löeffler's endocarditis)

e. Inflammatory = granulomatous (Sarcoidosis)

f. Endocrine (diabetes mellitus; hyperthyroidism; hypothyroidism; hyperparathyroidism; pheochromocytoma; acromegaly)

g. Cardiofacial (Noonan syndrome; Lentiginosis)

h. Neuromuscular/neurological (Friedreich's ataxia; Duchenne-Becker muscular dystrophy; Emery-Dreifuss muscular dystrophy; myotonic dystrophy; neurofibromatosis; Tuberous sclerosis)

i. Nutritional deficiencies (Beriberi, pallagra, scurvy, selenium, carnitine, kwashiorkor)

j. Autoimmune/collagen (systemic lupus erythematosis; dermatomyositis; Rheumatoid arthritis; scleroderma; polyarteritis nodosa)

k. Electrolyte imbalance

l. Consequence of cancer therapy (anthracyclines: doxorubicin (adriamycin), daunorubicin; cyclophosphamide; radiation)

**Table 2.** American Heart Association (AHA) Classification for Cardiomyopathies.

| Notation | **M** Morpho-functional phenotype | | **O** Organ/system involvement | | **G** Genetic inheritance | | **E** Etiology | | **S** Stage | |
|---|---|---|---|---|---|---|---|---|---|---|
| Characteristics | Cardiomyopathy diagnosis (DCMP, HCMP, RCMP, ARVC/D, LVNC) | | Clinical history and evaluation<br>- *organ involvement*<br>- *multidisiplinary evaluation* | | Genetic counseling with pedigree<br>*- familial (inheritance)*<br>*-nonfamilial (sporadic)*<br>clinical family screening<br>*-affected and asymptomatic*<br>*-with ECG and/or ECHO abnormalities*<br>*-healthy family members* | | Genetic testing in the proband:<br>-positive<br>-negative | | Functional status (ACC/AHA; NYHA) | |
| Subscript | D | Dilated | H | Heart | N | Family history negative | G | Genetic cause | A-D | ACC/AHA stages |
| | H | Hypertrophic | | *LV=left ventricle* | U | Family history unknown | OC | Obligate carrier | NA | Not applicable |
| | R | Restrictive | | *RV=right ventricle* | AD | Autosomal dominant | ONC | Obligate non-carrier | NU | Not used |
| | R EMF | Endomyocardial fibrosis | | *RLV=biventricular* | AR | Autosomal recessive | DN | De novo | I-IV | NYHA classes |
| | | *LV=left ventricle* | M | Muscle | XLD | X-linked dominant | Neg | Genetic test negative for the known familial mutation | | |
| | | *RV=right ventricle* | N | Nervous | XLR | X-linked recessive | N | Genetic defect not identified | | |
| | | *RLV=biventricular* | C | Cutaneous | XL | X-linked | O | No genetic test, any reason | | |
| | A | Arrhythmogenic right ventricular cardiomyopathy | E | Eye, ocular | M | Matrilineal | G-A-TTR | Genetic amyloidosis | | |
| | | *M=major* | A | Auditory | O | Family history not investigated | G-HFE | Hemochromatosis | | |
| | | *m=minor* | K | Kidney | S | Phenotpically sporadic | | | | |
| | | *c=category* | G | Gastrointestinal | | | *non-genetic etiologies:* | | | |
| | | *LV=left ventricle* | Li | Liver | | | M | Myocarditis | | |
| | | *RV=right ventricle* | Lu | Lung | | | V | Viral infection (add the virus) | | |
| | | *RLV=biventricular* | S | Skeletal | | | AI | Autoimmune/immune-mediated (suspected AI-S; proven AI-P) | | |
| | NC | Left ventricular noncompaction | O | Abscence of organ involvement | | | A | Amyloidosis (add type: A-K, A-L, A-SAA) | | |
| | E | Early | | | | | I | Infectious, non-viral | | |
| | NS | Nonspecific phenotype | | | | | T | Toxicity (add cause/drug) | | |
| | NA | Information non available | | | | | Eo | Hypereosinophilic heart disease | | |
| | O | Unaffected | | | | | O | Other | | |

**Table 3.** World Heart Federation (WHF) MOGE(S) classification for cardiomyopathies.

Cardiac contraction is a specific motion of myocardium that results in an adequate ejection (>60%) with lower dynamic change and energy consumption (15% fiber shortening) [6]. Subendocardially located cardiomyocytes create right-handed helix (smaller-radius) and subepicardially located cardiomyocytes left-handed helix (larger-radius), and this helixodical structure of the myocardium generates a torsional motion pattern caused by rotation in a clockwise direction at basal level and counter clockwise rotation at the apical level. In hypertrophic CMP, basal rotation increases and if the septum has sigmoid curvature apical rotation is more certain, and both mechanisms increase outflow tract obstruction level, decrease untwisting velocity, and cause subendocardial ischemia. In dilated CMP, the abnormal shape of the left ventricle changes fiber orientation and increasing dilatation is associated with more decreased twist.

The diagnosis of CMPs is assessed echocardiographically, but cardiovascular magnetic resonance (MR) is also powerful tool in diagnosis. Both are complementary imaging modalities. Echocardiography is superior in assessment of diastolic function and dynamic outflow tract obstruction. Cardiac MR has several advantages such as three-dimensional visualization, demonstration of relationships between the heart and thoracic structures, quantification of cardiac volumes and function, excellent resolution, tissue characterization (scar or infiltration), safely repetition [7].

## 1. Irreversible cardiomyhopaties

***Dilated CMP*** is the most common (>60%) final pathway during clinical nature of CMPs, which has more than 50% idiopathic etiology. Furthermore, some infiltrative CMP diseases may progress, as a consequence of remodeling, from one state (non-dilated) to another (dilated) during their natural clinical course. Mechanical impairment of filling or ejecting of ventricles causes significant cardiac decompensation with a clinic presentation from asymptomatic left ventricular dysfunction to severe heart failure symptoms. Annual mortality ratio changes between 10 and 50%, whereas between 1/4 and 1/3 of patients with new-onset dilated CMP presents cardiac recovery. Reverse remodeling may develop spontaneously or occur after medical or device treatment. Most patients have normal coronary circulation, and a definition for ischemic CMP needs a >70% stenosis in a major epicardial coronary artery. The main pathophysiologic mechanism is progressive systolic dysfunction dependent on four-chamber dilatation of the heart with normal left ventricular wall thickness. The annular enlargement causes significant valvular insufficiency, which makes the clinical status worse. Pulmonary hypertension with increased pulmonary vascular resistance develops gradually and diagnosis can result from cardiac catheterization. The diagnosis and management of patients with CMP are evaluated with noninvasive (echocardiography, MR imaging, multidetector computed tomography) or invasive cardiac tests (cardiac catheterization, endomyocardial biopsy). Large-scale treatment options give clinicians a wide range of follow-up of their patients. Asymptomatic patients can be followed medically, but mild-moderate symptomatic patients must be treated pharmacologically (diuretics, neurohormonal antagonists, anti-pulmonary hypertensives). Severe symptomatic conditions require invasive treatment options in a sequence: anti-arrhythmogenic devices, anti-regurgitant devices, anti-failure mechanic devices, and heart transplantation. Assessment of exercise capacity guides this treatment sequence, and 6-min walk test is the simplest valuable tool for switching to invasive treatments. The best test to gradate exercise capacity and to determine the cardiac-cause is the cardiopulmonary exercise testing, which is the most important test to determine whether to put patients on to waiting list.

***Hypertrophic CMP*** is the most common cardiomyopathy with genetic transmission and characterized by a thickened, hypertrophied left ventricle without dilatation. Hypertrophic CMP is caused by a variety of mutations encoding contractile proteins of the cardiac sarcomere. Hypertrophy is usually diffuse and involves both septum and left ventricular free wall (≥15 mm; +family history 13–14 mm; in children ≥ +2 standard deviation). Diastolic dysfunction develops due to the presence of a small left ventricular cavity; contrarily, systolic function can be preserved at the beginning of the pathology. Longstanding left ventricular outflow tract obstruction due to ventricular thickness with or without systolic anterior motion of mitral valve is the main predictor of heart failure or sudden death. Myocardial ischemia occurs due to microvascular dysfunction, which results in left ventricular scarring and remodeling. Reduced ventricular compliance causes diastolic dysfunction, which is diagnosed by exertional dyspnea. The greatest risk for adverse outcome is arrhythmogenic complication without heart failure symptoms. Atrial fibrillation is the most common (20%) rhythm disorder and cannot be tolerated well and results in embolic stroke or progressive heart failure. The lethal arrhythmia is ventricular fibrillation and has several signs: family history, unexplained syncope, hypotensive blood pressure response to exercise, abnormal ventricular tachycardia, massive left ventricular hypertrophy. The first stage treatment is the implantation of a cardioverter-defibrillator. Dual chamber pacing has limited effect. Septal myectomy or alcohol septal ablation is an alternative invasive treatment option, but heart transplantation is the final and only option for curative therapy.

***Restrictive CMP*** appears increasing in stiffness of the ventricular walls and consequently developing diastolic failure. At the beginning, the systolic function is normal, but it decreases during the progress of the disease. The most common specific etiology is amyloidosis. The pathologic changes of impairment of diastolic filling are myocardial fibrosis, infiltration or scarring of the endomyocardial surface. The first symptom is exercise intolerance, but with advancing disease, volume balance shifts to the generalized edema due to diastolic dysfunction and to the filling reduction in ventricles due to diuresis. In the late period of the restrictive CMP, ventricular dilatation can be added to the pathology and prognosis deteriorates rapidly. Treatment options are limited: anti-arrhythmogenic devices, biventricular pacing, and heart transplantation. Left ventricular assist devices (LVAD) cannot be used in this group of diseases.

***Arrhythmogenic right ventricular dysplasia*** is a rare, inherited pathology that is characterized by ventricular arrhythmias, sudden cardiac death, and right ventricular dysfunction due to myocyte loss with fatty or fibro-fatty tissue replacement of the right ventricular myocardium (and less commonly left). The pathophysiologic basis of this disease can be dependent on defective desmosomal proteins (impaired mechanical coupling between individual cells) or intracellular signaling pathways [8]. Several genes and gene loci are associated with this disease, but cardiac magnetic resonance and signal-averaged electrocardiography are more definitive diagnostic tests than endomyocardial biopsy. Genetic testing is essential for family screening, because more than 60% of patients have a pathogenic mutation. The natural progress of the pathology has four steps: asymptomatic period, arrhythmogenic period, development of the right heart failure, and finally biventricular failure. The prior clinic course is syncope or sudden death (20%) before development of heart failure, which is the late manifestation of the disease. Diagnosis must be evaluated on major and/or minor criteria, where several signs on the electrocardiography are essential for diagnosis: T wave inversion in the right precordial leads (v1–v3), right bundle branch block, Epsilon wave, and terminal activation delay. Because prevention of sudden cardiac death caused by ventricular arrhythmias is the primary goal of management, a cardioverter-defibrillator implantation is the first stage of the therapy. Beta-blocker therapy with exercise restriction should be included in the medical treatment, because exercise is the only triggered predictor for ventricular arrhythmias and sudden death. But, the curative treatment for significant heart failure is the cardiac transplantation.

## 2. Specific reversible cardiomyopathies

Secondary CMPs affects the myocardium in a multi-organ approach. There are several etiologic diseases that impair the physiologic functions of the heart and cause structural changes, which can result in chronic heart failure and/or arrhythmias [9]. Most of them are reversible, if the appropriate management is implemented.

***Ischemic CMP*** is included in dilated CMP group with the highest frequency (2/3–3/4 of all cases). Hibernating, stunning or severe ischemic myocardium make the clinical status worse temporarily, but diffuse fibrosis or necrotic and scarred myocardium results in irreversible myocardial dysfunction. In the presence of viable tissue, coronary revascularization with or without surgical correction of mechanical complications may remove this adverse remodeling. Transmural myocardial infarction, incomplete coronary revascularization, coronary bypass graft failure or inadequate myocardial protection during open-heart surgery can trigger ischemic CMP. If ischemia cannot be resolved, this pathology causes irreversible remodeling and left ventricular dilatation, therefore medical treatment is poor. Mechanical complications of coronary artery disease such as mitral regurgitation and left ventricular aneurysm can complicate the clinic course and precipitate heart failure, but surgical treatment modalities of heart failure can only extend patient-life. Left ventricular assist device or heart transplantation must be the preferred treatment in patients with end-stage heart failure. In limited cases, left ventricular reconstruction associated coronary revascularization can terminate irreversible remodeling phase and improve left ventricular function.

***Myocarditis*** is defined as inflammation of the myocardium, and it has an acute or chronic process. The pathology is characterized by inflammatory cells, interstitial edema, focal myocyte necrosis, and fibrosis, whereas autoimmune reaction can cause myocardial damage. Etiologic factors are different: infectious agents (viruses), toxins, drugs, cytotoxic chemotherapy, and hypersensitivity reactions. Viral cause (coxsackie, cytomegalovirus, HIV, etc.) is the most common reason for myocarditis, and three pathophysiological phases show pathologic course: viral, immunologic response, and cardiac remodeling phases. The most important phase is the immunologic response with a dual role. It is activated to eliminate as many virus-infected cells as possible to control the infection. Second role is the control of this response to prevent excessive tissue damage and organ dysfunction against monoclonal antibodies, which attack directly to receptors on viruses and also receptors on cardiomyocytes. This causes in subacute and chronic inflammation, which results in myocyte necrosis, fibrosis, and remodeling. Ventricular remodeling includes chamber dilatation, regional hypertrophy, and regional wall motion abnormalities. Patients with mild cardiac involvement will generally recover without long-term sequel, whereas chronic form has a lower recovery rate (30%) and the majority develops dilated CMP. The first-line therapy is supportive care; a hemodynamic support can be necessary in a small group of patients. Patients with end-stage heart failure must be treated with mechanical support using LVAD or heart transplantation.

***Sepsis-induced CMP*** occurs very common (60%) during sepsis or septic shock with high incidence of death. The myocardium is functionally and structurally injured by inflammatory cytokines and mitochondrial dysfunction [10]. It has a classical triad: affecting both ventricles and causing global ventricular dysfunction (decreasing biventricular ejection fraction), left ventricular dilatation (diastolic dysfunction with elevated left ventricular end-diastolic volume), and recovery in 7–10 days. Chemical mediators (endotoxins, cytokines, histones, and nitric oxide) decrease myofibril response to calcium, downregulate β-adrenergic receptors and induce mitochondrial dysfunction. The therapy should include antibiotics, vasopressor support, and perhaps, plasmapheresis. Inotropic catecholamines support, such as dobutamine and dopamine, is not suggested due to causing of hyperkinesis; on the contrary, β-blockade may be effective by lowering adrenergic stimulation. Levosimendan and/or intra-aortic balloon pumping can improve myocardial function and cardiac output.

***Peripartum CMP*** is a rare phenotype of dilated CMP, and congestive heart failure can develop in the third trimester of pregnancy or the first 6 months postpartum. The cause is unknown, but this cardiomyopathy develops generally in obese, multiparous women >30 years of age with preeclampsia. The pathologic etiology is increased fetomaternal transfer of cells (fetal microchimerism), which may trigger an exaggerated autoimmune response in the postpartum period [11]. Peripartum CMP can recover completely or almost completely within 6 months in a half of patients, if not, progressive cardiac failure is the prognosis requiring LVAD support or heart transplantation.

***Sympathoexcitation-induced CMP*** is also known as stress or Takotsubo CMP, or apical ballooning syndrome. It is most present in older women like an acute coronary syndrome without any angiographic findings. Increased catecholamines lead to elevation of systemic vascular resistance and systolic blood pressure, and cardiac output. During hypercontraction of the left ventricle, basal segments of the left ventricle contract more strongly than mid and apical segments, and that asynchronism increases stress in the left ventricular apex and produces a balloon-like appearance of the distal left ventricle during systole (regional dysfunction). Restriction of exercise and the use of β-adrenergic blockers return the left ventricular function to normal within a few weeks.

***Metabolic CMP*** can develop secondary to several endocrine diseases, familial storage pathologies, or nutritional deficiencies. Typical phenotype is thyroid dysfunction, where dysthyriodism (hyper- or hypothyroidism) causes a low cardiac output CMP. Thyroid hormones act as receptors and ion channels in the myocardium to improve myocardial function, and they also have a peripheral vasodilatory effect to reduce peripheral vascular resistance. Both pathologies cause heart failure by upregulation or downregulation of the previously mentioned myocardial structures. ß-adrenoreceptor blockers normalize the left ventricular mass index and systolic function after treatment, and also prevent atrial arrhythmias.

***Cirrhotic CMP*** is a chronic cardiac dysfunction without any cardiac disease and develops secondary to end-stage liver failure caused by several factors, especially by toxic effect of alcohol. The pathophysiologic changes include attenuated systolic contractile response to any strain, diastolic dysfunction, electrophysiological abnormalities, and chronotropic incompetence. The typical hemodynamic signs of alcoholic cirrhosis are hyperdynamic circulation with high cardiac output, decreased peripheral resistance and arterial pressure. Depression or desensitization of β-adrenergic receptors impairs chronotropic and inotropic responses of the heart and can be the early sign of cirrhotic CMP [12]. The second mechanism is downregulation of intracellular calcium kinetics. The third mechanism is rising of circulatory vasodilatations such as nitric oxide (peripheral), carbon monoxide (hepatic), and endocannabinoids (splanchnic), which can have adverse effect on the heart. Because CMP worsens with the progression of the underlying liver failure, liver transplantation with withdrawn of alcohol is the first-line therapy to reverse cardiac failure.

***Obesity (lipotoxic) CMP*** has hyperdynamic circulation because of increased adipose tissue metabolism, which may cause left ventricular hypertrophy and dilatation. Obesity is one of the main causes of insulin resistance and hyperglycemia, and glucotoxicity increases pathophysiologic changes. The other reasons can be an imbalance in the adiponectin-leptin ratio, cardiac lipotoxicity or steatosis, and/or non-oxidative pathway induced by excess fatty acids. All these changes cause defective intracellular signaling, chronic inflammation, intracellular dysfunction, and apoptosis [13].

***Diabetes mellitus-related CMP*** occurs due to myocardial microangiopathy or disturbed myocardial metabolism in the absence of coronary artery atherosclerosis. It has two different phenotypes: dilated left ventricular cavity with reduced ejection fraction or restrictive left ventricular cavity with reserved ejection fraction [14]. In restrictive phenotype, the left ventricle is normal sized but stiff with high resting tension due to hypertrophied cardiomyocytes with normal sarcomeres and limited collagen deposition in-between cardiomyocytes. In dilated phenotype, the left ventricle is enlarged due to damaged cardiomyocytes with loss of sarcomeres and severe collagen deposition with fibrosis. Several pathophysiologic mechanisms affect myocardial remodeling and dysfunction: hyperglycaemia, lipotoxicity, insulin resistance, microvascular advanced glycation end-products deposition, microvascular rarefaction, and autoimmunity (especially for dilated phenotype).

## Author details

Kaan Kırali

Address all correspondence to: imkbkirali@yahoo.com

1 Cardiac Transplantation and Ventricular Assist Device Department, Kartal Koşuyolu YIEA Hospital, University of Health Sciences, Istanbul, Turkey

2 Department of Cardiovascular Surgery, Faculty of Medicine, Sakarya University, Sakarya, Turkey

## References

[1] Richardson P, McKenna W, Bristow M. Report of the 1995 World Health Organization/International Society and Federation of Cardiology Task Force on the definition and classification of cardiomyopathies. Circulation 1996;93(5):841–842.

[2] Maron BJ, Towbin JA, Thiene G, Antzelevitch C, Corrado D, Arnett D, Moss AJ, Seidman CE, Young JB. Contemporary definitions and classification of the cardiomyopathies: an American Heart Association Scientific Statement from the Council on Clinical Cardiology, Heart Failure and Transplantation Committee; Quality of Care and Outcomes research and Functional genomics and Translational Biology Interdisciplinary Working Groups; and Epidemiology and Prevention. Circulation 2006;113(14):1807–1816.

[3] Arbustini E, Narula N, Tavazzi L, Serio A, Grasso M, Favalli V, Bellazzi R, Tajik JA, Bonow RO, Fuster V, Narula J. The MOGE(S) classification of cardiomyopathy for clinicians. J Am Coll Cardiol 2014;64(3):304–318.

[4] Yancy CW, Jessup M, Bozkurt B, Butler J, Fonarow GC, Geraci SA, Horwich T, Januzzi JL, Johnson MR, Kasper EK, Levy WC, Masoudi FA, McBride PE, McMurrsy JJV, Mitchell JE, Peterson PN, Riegel B, Sam F, Stevenson LW, Tang WHW, Tsai EJ, Wilkoff BL. 2013 ACCF/AHA guideline for the management of heart failure: executive summary. Circulation 2013;128(16):1810–1852.

[5] Hariharan N, Sussman MA. Cardiac aging. Getting to the stem of the problem. J Mol Cell Cardiol 2015;83:32–36.

[6] Kauer F, Geleijnse ML, van Dalen BM. Role of left ventricular twist mechanism in cardiomyopathies, dance of the helices. World J Cardiol 2015;7(8):476–482.

[7] Quarta G, Sado DM, Moon JC. Cardiomyopathies: focus on cardiovascular magnetic resonance. Br J Radiol 2011;84(S3):S296–305.

[8] Calkins H. Arrhythmogenic right ventricular dysplasia/cardiomyopathy-three decades of progress. Circ J 2015;79(5):901–903.

[9] Patel H, Madanieh R, Kosmas CE, Vatti SK, Vittorio TJ. Reversible cardiomyopathies. Clin Med Insights Cardiol 2015;9(S2):7–14.

[10] Sato R, Nasu M. A review of sepsis-induced cardiomyopathy. J Intensive Care 2015;3: 48–55.

[11] Biteker M, Kayataş K, Duman D, Turkmen M, Bozkurt B. Peripartum cardiomyopathy. Current state of knowledge, new developments and future directions. Curr Cardiol Rev 2014;10(4):317–326.

[12] Gassanov N, Caglayan E, Semmo N, Massenkeil G, Er F. Cirrhotic cardiomyopathy: a cardiologist's perspective. World J Gastroenterol 2014;20(42):15492–15498.

[13] Bahrami H, Bluemke DA, Kronmal R et al. Novel metabolic risk factors for incident heart failure and their relationship with obesity. The MESA (Multi-Ethnic Study of Atherosclerosis) study. J Am Coll Cardiol 2008;51(18):1775–1783.

[14] Seferovic PM, Paulus WJ. Clinical diabetic cardiomyopathy: a two-faced disease with restrictive and dilated phenotypes. Eur Heart J 2015;36(27):1718–1727.

Section 2

# Pathophysiologylogy

Chapter 2

# Pathophysiology in Heart Failure

Kaan Kırali, Tanıl Özer and Mustafa Mert Özgür

Additional information is available at the end of the chapter

http://dx.doi.org/10.5772/66887

**Abstract**

Heart failure syndrome is defined as the inability of the heart to deliver adequate blood to the body to meet end-organ metabolic needs and oxygenation at rest or during mild exercise. Myocardial dysfunction can be defined as systolic and/or diastolic, acute or chronic, compensated or uncompensated, or uni- or biventricular. Several counter-regulatory mechanisms are activated depending on the duration of the heart failure. Neurohormonal reflexes such as sympathetic adrenergic system, renin-angiotensin cascade, and renal and peripheral alterations attempt to restore both cardiac output and end-tissue perfusion. An adequate stroke volume cannot be ejected from the left ventricle, which shifts the whole pressure-volume relationship to the right (systolic failure). Adequate filling cannot be realized due to diastolic stiffness, which shifts the diastolic pressure-volume curve upward without affecting the systolic pressure-volume curve (diastolic failure). Left ventricular heart failure is the dominant picture of heart failure syndrome, but the right heart can develop isolated failure as well. Biventricular failure is mostly an end-stage clinical situation of the heart failure syndrome. More recently, the rise in the incidence of right ventricular failure can be seen after the implantation of a left ventricular assist device. This chapter clarifies and presents pathophysiologic alterations in heart failure syndrome.

**Keywords:** heart failure, systolic dysfunction, diastolic dysfunction, myocardial stiffness, ventricular dilatation, neurohormonal, renin-angiotensin, norepinephrine

Heart failure is an epidemic contributing considerably to the overall cost of health care in developed and also developing countries. Heart failure syndrome (HFS) is the currently accepted term describing a systemic disease affecting several organs, creating high morbidity and mortality rates due to the heart's inability to supply oxygenated blood, including metabolites, to end organs and peripheral tissues (**Table 1**) [1]. Acute event or acute refractory form of chronic heart failure can be fatal, whereas chronic prognosis is characterized by terminal congestive heart failure symptoms. The failing heart strives to balance "preload" and "afterload" for compensation of impaired contractility and to deter the development of congestion using a myriad of mechanisms.

| |
|---|
| (1) Activated feedback signals from peripheral reflex circuit |
| a. Inflammation |
| b. Anabolic blunting (proteolysis) |
| c. Insulin resistance (>50% reducing normal anabolic responses) |
| d. Oxygen radical accumulation |
| (2) Global metabolic imbalance (increased catabolic/anabolic imbalance) |
| (3) Systemic dysregulation of several hormonal pathways |
| (4) Multi-organ dysfunction (hyperbilirubinemia, uremia, anemia, hypoalbuminemia, etc.) |
| (5) Development of sarcopenia and cachexia |

**Table 1.** Heart failure syndrome as a multisystem disease.

## 1. Left heart failure

Left heart failure (LHF), with any structural and/or functional cardiac abnormalities, is a complex clinical state characterized by left ventricular pump dysfunction and related clinical symptoms (dyspnea, fatigue, exercise intolerance, etc.), including signs of volume overload (pulmonary crackles, peripheral edema, etc.) [2]. All steps of energy extraction, transfer, and utilization are affected, with metabolic failure being the important underlying pathophysiologic mechanism causing first myocardial and then systemic decompensation [3]. The pathophysiologic state perpetuates the progression of the failure, regardless of the precipitating event via several compensatory mechanisms. Compensatory mechanisms exist on every level of this scenario to restrain the clinical symptoms via correction of the global imbalance between the catabolic and anabolic status; however, they can lead to further myocardial deterioration and worsening HFS.

The most important classification of LHF is dependent on whether the left ventricular ejection fraction (LVEF) is reduced or preserved. The standard relationship between intracavitary volume and pressure values is affected in heart failure, and left ventricular pressure-volume curves change according to the failure type (**Figure 1**). In systolic LHF, an adequate stroke volume cannot be sustained due to reduced ventricular systolic contractile function, which shifts the whole pressure-volume relationships to the right. In diastolic LHF, an adequate filling cannot be realized due to diastolic stiffness (poor ventricular compliance, impaired relaxation, worsened end-diastolic pressure), which shifts the diastolic pressure-volume curve upward; however, the systolic pressure-volume curve does not change.

http://dx.doi.org/10.5772/66887

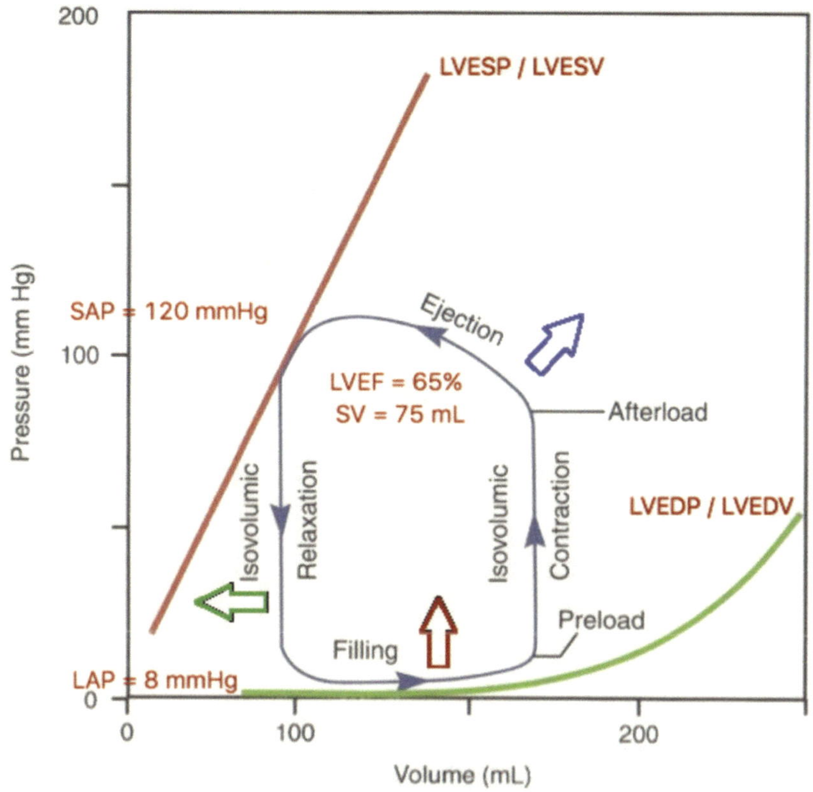


**Figure 1.** Left ventricular pressure-volume relationships: the green line represents the diastolic pressure-volume relationship, and the red line represents the end-systolic pressure-volume relationship. Both curves are shifted to the right in dilated CMP (blue arrow), to the left in hypertrophic CMP (green arrow), and only diastolic curve is shifted upward in restrictive CMP (red arrow). CMP, cardiomyopathy; LAP, left atrial pressure; LVEDP, left ventricular end-diastolic pressure; LVEDV, left ventricular end-diastolic volume; LVEF, left ventricular ejection fraction; LVESP, left ventricular end-systolic pressure; LVESV, left ventricular end-systolic volume; SAP, systolic aortic pressure; SV, stroke volume.

From asymptomatic to symptomatic stages, several counterregulatory mechanisms are activated (**Table 2**). First, inadequate stroke volume induces sympathetic nervous system activation, which increases cardiac contractile frequency and strength. This chronotropic effect leads to enhancement of total stroke volume per minute via increasing heart rate frequency, but this positive effect is reversed after tachycardia reaches a threshold of 140–150 beats/min (**Figure 2**). The next step is the augmentation of intravascular volume via neurohormonal system activation, which results in increasing intravascular volume, enlarging ventricular chambers, and improvement in myocardial fiber tension [4]. The inotropic effect via the Frank-Starling mechanism increases myocardial contraction power, but this positive effect reverses after the sarcomere length reaches the upper limit of 2.2 μm (**Figure 3**). At this stage, no physiologic mechanism can improve the contractility, stroke volume, and cardiac decompensation, and the left ventricle (LV) undergoes progressive alterations from reversible cellular to irreversible myocardial remodeling. The heart is a self-renewing organ, characterized by an increase in myocyte turnover rate during pathological stress, especially in heart failure. The turnover mechanism becomes overwhelmed by a faster loss of myocytes, and this unfavorable imbalance causes the progression of ventricular remodeling during heart failure.

| |
|---|
| (a) Activation of neurohormonal systems |
| (b) Increasing preload to help to sustain cardiac performance |
| (c) Myocardial cell regeneration and apoptosis |
| (d) Myocardial hypertrophy and/or ventricular dilatation |
| (e) Compensation of symptoms |
| (f) Irreversible myocardial remodeling |
| (g) Decompensation of clinic status |
| (h) End-stage multi-organ dysfunction |

**Table 2.** Step-by-step counterregulatory actions during ventricular failure.

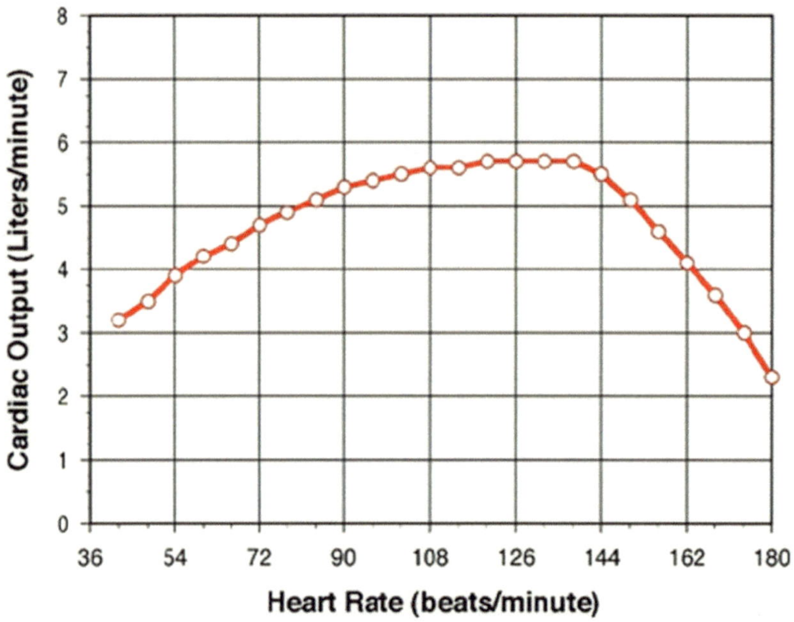


**Figure 2.** Relationship between cardiac output and heart rate (chronotropy; Bowditch effect).

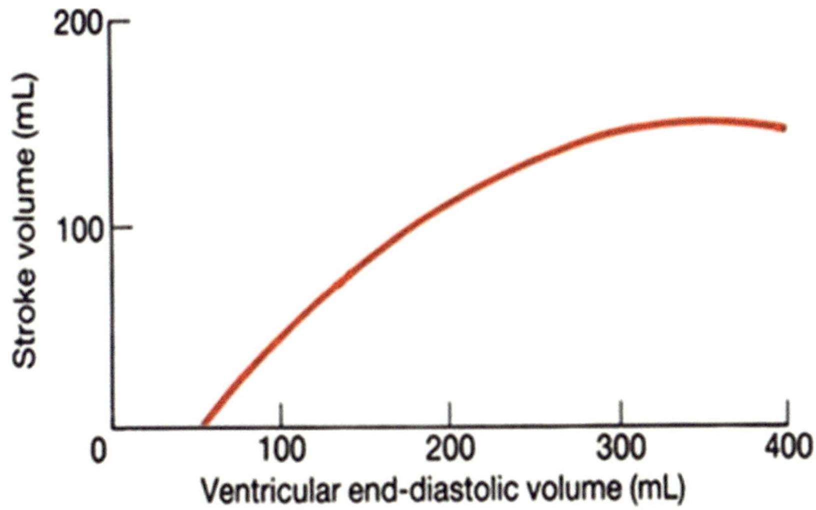


**Figure 3.** Relation between cardiac output and left ventricular filling (inotropy; Frank-Starling effect).

### 1.1. Morphological changes

Any of the cardiac pathology causing myocardial dysfunction results in abnormal myocyte growth, with a resultant cascade of gene activation stimulating cardiac remodeling. The hallmarks of cardiac remodeling are myocardial cell hypertrophy and cardiac dilatation with increased interstitial matrix formation. This compensatory mechanism to preserve contraction capability shifts to a maladaptive process after a cutoff level and contributes to the worsening of heart failure during myocardial degenerative progression. Progressive necrotic, apoptotic, or autophagic myocyte loss may contribute to worsening cardiac dysfunction and left ventricular remodeling. Changes within the extracellular matrix such as fibrillary collagen synthesis and degradation, loss of collagen struts, and collagen cross-linking characterize subsequent myocardial adaptation during cardiac remodeling. Cardiac fibroblasts are transformed into myofibroblasts and migrate into the area surrounding injured tissues to secrete collagen and restrict the injured site by scar formation (myocardial fibrosis).

Extracellular matrix requires myocytes to take appropriate position during the cardiac cycles and allows the opening of capillary vessels. Cardiac mitochondria are the main structure to generate energy, in the form of adenosine triphosphate (ATP), through oxidative phosphorylation and to continue cardiac function. Therefore, mitochondrial dysfunction is the major determinant for the development of heart failure via activation of cell death caused by excessive production of reactive oxygen radicals. In the early stage of left ventricular hypertrophy, the number of cardiac myocytes with preserved cellular organization increases; however, they are larger than normal due to the growing number of myofibrils and mitochondria, as well as the large size of the mitochondria and nuclei. Myocytes also increase autophagic activity in order to maintain ATP levels, to sustain contractile function during these demanding nutritional and energy-consuming phases. Mitophagy is a critical mitochondrial quality control mechanism in myocytes, whereas damaged mitochondria and autophagosomes are selectively sequestered and broken down. This process helps to prevent oxidative damage or myocardial stress under baseline conditions, whereas impaired or dysregulated mitophagy is a major contributor to the development and progression of heart failure [5]. Inhibiting autophagy reduces ATP levels and exacerbates remodeling, whereas enhancing autophagy mitigates remodeling and cardiac dysfunction. The hemodynamic and neurohormonal alterations cause an increase in cytosolic calcium entry, which augments myocardial contractility; on the other hand, it impairs the lusitropic effect and leads to increased myocardial energy consumption resulting in further reduction of cardiac function.

Long-standing hypertrophy disrupts cellular organization, such as enlarged nuclei with myofibril displacement. Additionally, some collagen lytic enzymes (matrix metalloproteinase) activated by neurohormonal substances can create progressive degradation of extracellular matrix. In late stages, the pathologic progress is characterized by myocytolysis, a disruption of sarcomeres and Z-bands. In the chronic phase, some components increase and cause myocyte death, creating perivascular fibrosis within intramuscular vessels. This process causes fibrillary collagen to fill the place of dead myocytes. Ultimately, the disruption of mechanical power by the damaged myocytes becomes detrimental, and the left ventricular wall becomes thinner and dilated.

### 1.2. Neuroendocrine changes

The pathophysiology of LHF is characterized by hemodynamic abnormalities resulting in autonomic nervous system imbalance and neurohormonal activation. Alterations in receptor activation cause an autonomic imbalance with increased sympathetic activity and diminished vagal activity, both of which may have profound effects on cardiac function and structure. Neurohormonal alterations act as a complex and combined compensatory mechanism to support and maintain tissue perfusion during the HFS (**Table 3**). However, these neurohormonal responses become maladaptive due to uncontrollable activation and promote progression of heart failure. The main sympathetic neurohormones are norepinephrine (noradrenaline) and angiotensin II, which act in an autocrine (myocardial synthesis) and paracrine (endocrine synthesis) manner.

#### *1.2.1. Autonomic nervous system*

Sympathetic (adrenergic) and parasympathetic (cholinergic) nerve systems are controlled by the central nervous system and are in balance in healthy individuals, where sympathetic activation is lower at rest, as well as in the normal heart [6]. Baroreceptors at the aortic arch and carotid sinuses, as well as mechanoreceptors at the cardiopulmonary tract, sense arterial wall tension and produce afferent signals resulting in a significant increase of excitatory (sympathetic) impulses via norepinephrine or inhibitory (parasympathetic) impulses via acetylcholine (**Figure 4**). Chemoreceptors at the peripheral vessels and metaboreceptors in the muscles sense acid-base balance and oxygenation of the blood and produce afferent signals resulting in a significant increase of sympathetic stimulation (the excitatory impulse). Mechanical and

http://dx.doi.org/10.5772/66887

chemical changes like hypoxia, hypotension, or acid-base imbalance are sensed by receptors, creating a feedback cascade to maintain cardiovascular homeostasis. In the case of heart failure, the first response of sympathetic nervous system activation is the increasing release and decreasing uptake of norepinephrine at the adrenergic nerve endings. In response, the parasympathetic receptor activity becomes dysfunctional by the increased sympathetic stimulation, which in turn leads to increasing systemic vascular resistance and heart rate.

| |
|---|
| (1) Sympathetic nervous system |
| (2) Renin-angiotensin system |
| (3) Neurohormonal alterations of renal function |
| (a) Arginine vasopressin |
| (b) Natriuretic peptides |
| (4) Neurohormonal alterations in the peripheral vasculature |
| (a) Vasoconstrictors |
| (i) Endothelin |
| (ii) Neuropeptide Y |
| (iii) Urotensin II |
| (iv) Thromboxane $A_2$ |
| (b) Vasodilators |
| (i) Nitric oxide |
| (ii) Bradykinin |
| (iii) Adrenomedullin |
| (iv) Prostaglandins ($PGI_2$ and $PGE_2$) |
| (v) Adipokines |
| (5) Remodeling factors |
| (a) Tumor necrosis factor |
| (b) Soluble ST2 |
| (c) Growth differentiation factor (GDF)-15 |
| (d) Gelectin-3 |
| (6) Interleukin activation |
| (7) Anabolic metabolism dysfunctions |
| (a) Insulin resistance |
| (b) Growth hormone resistance |
| (c) Anabolic steroid resistance |

**Table 3.** Neuroendocrine responses.

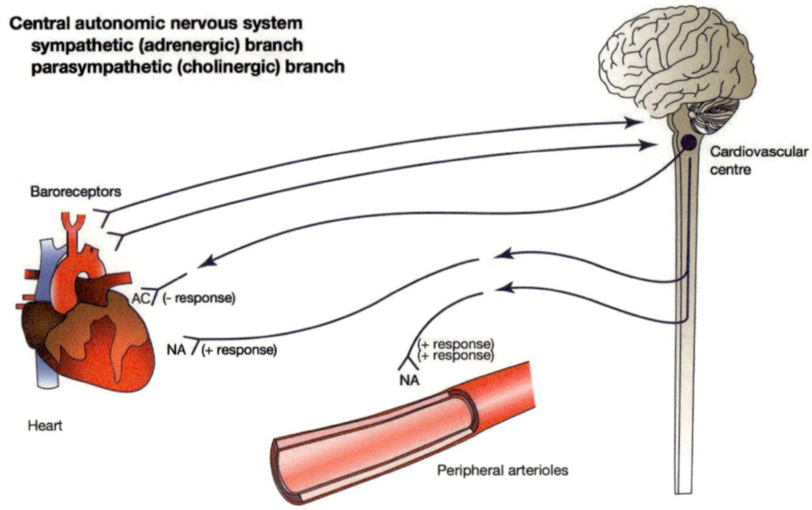


**Figure 4.** Autonomic nervous system function.

In the HFS, sympathetic stimulation affects several key organs to maintain cardiac output, especially the heart, the kidney, and the peripheral vasculature. Increased sympathetic activity (1) augments ventricular contractility and heart rate to sustain stroke volume, (2) stimulates efferent arteriole vasoconstriction and proximal tubular sodium reabsorption to improve ventricular preload, and (3) leads to systemic vasoconstriction and enhanced venous tone to increase systemic vascular resistance and blood pressure. Alternatively, alterations in autonomic function are broadly associated with both increased cardiovascular and, in many cases, all-cause mortality in humans. Norepinephrine is a potent adrenergic neurotransmitter and increases three to four times more than the normal level in HFS. This process has opposed effects: acute excretion or lower level of norepinephrine is associated with improvement of cardiac function; however, higher levels are associated with worsening of the HFS [7]. $\alpha$-Adrenergic receptors are present in vascular smooth muscle much more so than in cardiac myocytes; however, only $\alpha^1$-subtype receptors demonstrate significant density in myocardium, and their numbers increase modestly in heart failure, which leads to myocyte hypertrophy. Stimulation of these receptors in cardiac myocytes by norepinephrine induces myocyte growth and hypertrophy and reproduces fetal isoforms of contractile proteins. β-Adrenergic receptors consist of $\beta^1$ subtype and are present in more than 80% in the heart. This system plays a critical role in modulating cardiac performance, specifically inotropy, chronotropy, and lusitropy. However, chronically elevated stimulation of the sympathetic system has detrimental repercussions in HFS (cardiac β-adrenergic desensitization). Ongoing adrenergic stimulation reduces the β-adrenergic receptor, particularly $\beta^1$ concentrations in the myocardium (downregulation). This causes an increased expression of β-adrenergic receptor kinase inhibiting β-receptor (both $\beta^1$ and $\beta^2$) activation by phosphorylating them (functional desensitization).

http://dx.doi.org/10.5772/66887

*1.2.2. Renin-angiotensin-aldosterone system*

The renin-angiotensin-aldosterone system is a secondary compensatory mechanism that maintains intravascular volume and vascular resistance. This system is activated later in heart failure due to renal hypoperfusion, decreased sodium in the macula densa of the distal tubule, increased sympathetic stimulations ($\beta^1$ adrenergic activity), and diuretic therapy. The system is very sensitive and is activated with the extrication of renin from the juxtaglomerular apparatus. Renin is responsible for the conversion of angiotensinogen to angiotensin I (inactive decapeptide), and angiotensin I is then converted to angiotensin II (active octapeptide) by angiotensin-converting enzyme. The majority of angiotensin-converting enzyme (>90%) is found in tissues, with the rest located in the circulation. The activity of angiotensin-converting enzyme increases during heart failure with increased expression of myocardial form. Two opposing receptors are present; renin receptor type 1 and renin receptor type 2. Activation of type 1 receptors leads to cell growth, causing the release of norepinephrine from sympathetic nerves, either directly or indirectly. This in turn decreases lusitropy, increases afterload by inducing the release of aldosterone from the adrenal cortex indirectly and contributes to the increase of intravascular volume directly by promoting tubular reabsorption of sodium. Furthermore, this stimulates water intake by increasing thirst. The activation of type 2 receptors leads to the inhibition of cell growth, vasodilatation, and natriuresis. On the other hand, atrial natriuretic peptide (ANP) inhibits the release of renin.

Excessive production of angiotensin II can lead to fibrosis of several organs, especially the heart and kidneys, and can also induce cellular proliferation of cardiac fibroblasts and the rate of myocyte apoptosis. Aldosterone has similar actions with unfavorable effects of angiotensin II. Aldosterone provokes hypertrophy and fibrosis within the vasculature and myocardium, resulting in ventricular stiffness, endothelial cell and baroreceptor dysfunction, and the inhibition of norepinephrine uptake.

*1.2.3. Renal neuroendocrine alterations*

The most adverse outcome of HFS is increased salt and water retention by the kidneys, which results in the worsening of heart failure. Regulation of the fluid balance of the body is primarily managed by body fluid osmolality and changes in plasma volumes [8]. This is a normal pathway that is observed in non-failed hearts due to excessive intake of sodium, but it is a detrimental pathway in heart failure. Decreasing plasma volume or blood pressure is perceived as tissue hypoperfusion, which then stimulates specialized baroreceptors, and in turn activates several neurohormonal pathways that produce hypoperfusion of the tissues. Inadequate perfusion of the kidney and other organs results in adverse impulses that increase vasopressor response via angiotensin II, aldosterone, and norepinephrine production. This central response increases arginine vasopressin secretion, which regulates free water clearance and plasma osmolality. All of these responses try to prevent tissue hypoperfusion. Additionally, they can aggravate the process of heart failure and cause cardiac remodeling. Treatment modalities against any kind of heart failure syndrome can cause hyponatremia, which occurs as either depletional or delusional [9].

The natriuretic peptides provide the most important counterregulatory effect of the neurohormonal system via increasing excretion of sodium and water. Atrial (ANP) and B-type (BNP) natriuretic peptides are produced primarily in response to myocardial stretch due to pressure or volume overload: ANP from the atrial wall and BNP from the ventricular wall. Both peptides are responsible for vasodilatation, natriuresis, diuresis (inhibition of renin and aldosterone cascade), and inhibition of vascular smooth muscle proliferation. The third (C-type) natriuretic peptide released from endothelial cells results in vasodilatation and inhibits endothelin but does not promote natriuresis. These peptides increase during heart failure or decompensated situations, but they can also be used to guide heart failure therapy [10]. Both biomarkers are influenced by other factors such as obesity, arrhythmia, anemia, sepsis, pulmonary embolism, etc.

### *1.2.4. Peripheral neuroendocrine alterations*

The main goal of the body is to preserve brain and cardiac circulation throughout the HFS via decreasing blood flow to peripheral tissues and visceral organs. The increased sympathetic adrenergic stimulation of the peripheral arteries causes arteriolar vasoconstriction for the maintenance of arterial pressure and vasoconstriction of the peripheral veins to increase venous return. Counterregulatory vasodilator responses result in vasodilatation of the peripheral vasculature to prevent aggressive overload of the circulatory system. Loss of the endothelium-mediated vasodilatory responsiveness in HFS causes the inability of counterregulatory and/or control of sympathetic adrenergic activation, which subsequently exacerbates heart failure, cardiac remodeling, and symptoms.

### *1.2.5. Anabolic metabolism alterations*

Insulin is the strongest anabolic stimulatory signal via activation of transcription factor 4, which is complementary to the general amino acid control pathway. In heart failure, the anabolic efficiency of insulin decreases more than 50%. As a principal metabolic feature of heart failure, increased insulin resistance impairs functional capacity of the heart and muscles and worsens heart failure via impaired metabolic efficacy, tissue fibrosis, apoptosis, and lipotoxicity. Growth hormone or insulin-like growth factor 1 causes an anabolic signal rise; however, it cannot prevent cachexia. Anabolic steroid metabolism is also impaired in HFS.

Anabolic failure of the body occurring during long-standing heart failure appears with different clinical signs (**Table 4**). Skeletal muscle is the largest amino acid storage pool in the body, and its atrophy is the first clinical sign for cardiac cachexia (proteolysis). Adipose tissue is actively affected by different lipolytic signals, whereas insulin resistance blocks activation of lipogenic enzymes (lipolysis). Osteopenia or osteoporosis can develop in higher stages of the disease. This catabolic/anabolic imbalance leads to tissue wasting, weight loss, and ultimately cardiac cachexia (body weight loss > 6% in < 1 year), which is the worst and gravest prognosis of the HFS. Iron deficiency is another important metabolic dysfunction that occurs secondary to blood loss, malnutrition, inflammation (hepcidin dysfunction), and impaired synthesis of bioactive heme, and it impairs enzymatic electron transfer activities in the body with or without anemia.

| |
|---|
| 1. Proteolysis |
| 2. Lipolysis |
| 3. Osteolysis |
| 4. Cardiac cachexia |
| a. Hypoalbuminemia |
| b. Anemia |
| c. Impaired glucose tolerance |
| d. Inflammation |
| e. Anorexia |
| 5. Iron deficiency |
| 6. Hyperuricemia |

**Table 4.** Clinical presentation of imbalanced catabolic status in heart failure.

### 1.3. Left ventricular remodeling

Reversible or irreversible left ventricular failure (LVF) results in left ventricular remodeling via complex changes of cardiac myocytes and nonmyocyte components of the myocardium (**Table 5**) [11]. Treatment of reversible pathologies affecting the heart can reverse this process and maintain the anatomohistologic structure. Irreversible pathologies lead to progressive loss of myofilaments and contractile function, as well as alterations in excitation-contraction coupling, fatal arrhythmias, and desensitization of ß-adrenergic signaling. This type of left heart failure impacts the development of left ventricular hypertrophy, in that pressure overload or myocardial accumulation causes concentric hypertrophy with increased left ventricular wall stiffness, with or without left ventricular thickening. However, volume overload also causes eccentric hypertrophy with dilation of the left ventricular wall, with or without thinning. A progressive loss of connectivity of the collagen network causes progressive left ventricular dilatation, but it preserves the structural integrity of the heart. A change in left ventricular shape from an elliptical form to a spherical form creates increasing wall stress and mechanical energy, which results in left ventricular dilatation and wall thinning. This progressive dilatation causes pull-apart pathology of the papillary muscles resulting in significant mitral regurgitation from the inability of the valve leaflets to coapt. In addition, myocardial fibrosis results in arrhythmia and/or sudden death.

The heart anatomically consists of a single, intertwined muscle band. The muscle fibers, both inside and out, achieve maximum contractile performance by making a 60° angle from each other. This angle increases when a stretching occurs, as in heart failure, and the elliptical shape of the heart mutates into a spherical shape, which decreases stroke work and volume significantly. The oblique arrays of apical fibers create 60% LVEF with 15% fractional shortening, while transverse arrays can create just 15% LVEF. When the arrays of myocardial fibers are unbalanced from any cause, the contractile performance of the heart will be affected (**Table 6**). The enlargement of myocardial cells alters left ventricular shape and function.

Systolic dysfunction disrupts emptying of the ventricular chamber and decreases stroke volume, whereas volume overload increases left ventricular end-diastolic pressure. Diastolic dysfunction reduces the filling capacity of the LV due to myocardial stiffness, despite the relatively preserved contractile performance and ejection fraction. Each type of cardiomyopathy has one or both dysfunctional processes. Dilated cardiomyopathy is characterized by impaired systolic function, with enlargement of cardiac chambers, whereas hypertrophic cardiomyopathy is depicted by a smaller ventricular cavity due to a hypertrophic myocardium. Restrictive cardiomyopathy occurs secondarily from diastolic dysfunction and exhibits normal chamber size.

| |
|---|
| (1) Structural alterations |
| (a) Ultrastructural remodeling |
| (b) Mitochondrial remodeling |
| (c) Extracellular matrix remodeling |
| (d) Metabolic remodeling |
| (2) Electrophysiologic alterations |
| (a) Action potential remodeling |
| (b) Excitation-contraction coupling remodeling |
| (c) Repolarization remodeling |
| (3) ß-Adrenergic receptor signaling alterations |

**Table 5.** Myocardial remodeling.

| |
|---|
| (a) Myocardial infarction causes loss of contraction and subsequent to fibrosis of affected heart muscle, which breakdowns the array of myocardial fibers due to stretching of myocardial fibers |
| (b) Valvular and/or congenital heart diseases leading to biventricular volume overload derange the array of myocardial fibers due to ventricular dilatation |
| (c) Cardiomyopathies and the intrinsic disorders of the myocardium may cause a breakdown of the array of myocardial fibers due to both mechanisms |

**Table 6.** Pathophysiologic changes in different etiologies.

## 2. Right heart failure

The right ventricle (RV) is not a mirror image of the LV and has its own anatomy, circulation, physiology, and hemodynamics. The RV consists of separated inlet (receives blood from the right atrium) and outlet (funnels blood into the pulmonary artery) portions and has a crescent-shaped structure with a concave free wall and convex interventricular septum (IVS) [12]. It is relatively thin walled with the muscle mass of the RV being relatively less than that

http://dx.doi.org/10.5772/66887

of the LV (about 1/6). However, the RV can eject almost an equal stroke volume as the LV into a lower afterloaded (low pressure-low resistance) and highly compliant pulmonary circuit with a more complex contractile mechanism, but with lower stroke work than the LV (25% of the left ventricular stroke work). The dominant movements of the RV include longitudinal shortening, pressing of the free wall against the septum, contraction of the IVS, and a "wringing" action of the LV (**Table 7**). Right heart failure (RHF) is defined as persistent signs and symptoms of right ventricular dysfunction (RVD) in the absence of LVF, cardiac tamponade, ventricular arrhythmias, and/or pneumothorax.

| | |
|---|---|
| 1. Longitudinal/twisting motion (septal contraction) | 80% |
| *Interventricular septum shares fibers with both ventricles* | |
| *LV maintains 20–40% RV contractile function* | |
| 2. Transverse motion (free wall contraction) | 20% |
| 3. Traction of the RV free wall at the points of binding to the LV | |

**Table 7.** Right ventricular contractile functions.

### 2.1. Pathophysiology of right heart failure

Right-sided heart failure has been accepted as an eventual consequence of left-sided heart failure (the LV as guilty and the RV as victim), and the RV has been largely ignored as a passive conduit or a bystander chamber for several decades [13]. The International Right Heart Foundation Working Group describes a comprehensive definition of RHF: "A clinical syndrome due to an alteration of structure and/or function of the right heart circulatory system that leads to suboptimal delivery of blood flow (high or low) to the pulmonary circulation and/or elevated venous pressures—at rest or with exercise" [14]. The definition of RHF represents a dysfunction of any components that constitute the right heart circulatory system, from systemic veins (post-systemic capillaries) to the pulmonary artery (pre-pulmonary capillaries). Right ventricular failure (RVF) can develop most commonly secondarily to left-sided HFS, but some specific etiologic pathologies result in isolated right-sided HFS (**Table 8**) [15]. The well-known etiologic reasons of RVF are pulmonary arterial hypertension (PAH) with or without LHF, LVF, or implantation of a left ventricular assist device (LVAD).

Pulmonary arterial hypertension (PAH) is seen in almost all RHF scenarios and occurs as a consequence of chronic left heart pathologies, chronic lung diseases, pulmonary embolism, or any pathology affecting the distal pulmonary vascular bed. Pressure overload caused by pre- or post-capillary dynamics starts the "RVD and RVF" vicious circle (**Figure 5**). The hemodynamic definition of PAH type is critical to determine the appropriate treatment modality. Pulmonary hypertension is a common complication of LHF and the diagnosis of PAH-related hemodynamic parameters (**Table 9**). The main differentiation between pre- and post-pulmonary types is pressure gradients between both sides of the pulmonary capillaries, whereas the diastolic pressure gradient has more prognostic value due to lesser dependence of stroke volume and loading conditions [16]. The threshold level of the transpulmonary pressure gradient (TPG) to discriminate between pre- and post-capillary PHT should be 12 mmHg. The diastolic pulmonary gradient (<5 mmHg) combined with the systemic blood pressure and cardiac output is superior to the TPG for determining the differential diagnosis between pulmonary vascular disease, high output or high left heart filling state, and sepsis.

1. Pressure overload
   a. Left-sided HFS (most common cause)
   b. Primary pulmonary hypertension
   c. Pulmonary embolism
   d. RVOT obstruction and/or peripheral pulmonary stenosis
2. Volume overload
   a. Tricuspid regurgitation
   b. Pulmonary regurgitation
   c. Atrial septal defect and/or anomalous pulmonary venous return
   d. Coronary artery fistula into right chambers
   e. Carcinoid syndrome
3. Ischemia and infarction
4. Intrinsic myocardial process
5. Arrhythmogenic RV dysplasia
6. Chronic lung diseases

**Table 8.** Etiology of right heart failure.

Right ventricular failure has a specific pathophysiologic algorithm (**Figure 6**). Increased afterload due to pressure overload of the pulmonary circulation prolongs the systolic contraction of the RV. On the other hand, the RV is able to tolerate an increased preload due to volume overload. In the early phase of RVF, wall thickening and enhanced contractility are the first important responses of pressure overload, which creates an adaptive remodeling with concentric hypertrophy and preserved right ventricular function. In chronic, higher afterload states even though myocardial contractility is advanced, the right pump functions decrease proportionally, and contractile dysfunction occurs later in the process. This remodeling process is sustained by the contribution of neurohormonal, genetic, and molecular components. Meanwhile, the RV dilates to provide adequate stroke volume, but this counter effect leads to tricuspid annular dilatation, valve coaptation defect, and eventually significant tricuspid regurgitation. This process triggers a maladaptive remodeling, which causes eccentric hypertrophy and deteriorated right ventricular function. In the beginning of diastole of the LV, the RV is contracting, and the IVS moves leftward causing ventricular dyssynchrony. Ventricular dyssynchrony accelerates right heart and biventricular failure with several fatal complications such as arrhythmia, hepatorenal failure, protein-losing enteropathy, and cardiac cachexia. Myocardial ischemia or infarction of the RV is not a significant factor for heart failure as it is in LVF, because the right ventricular free wall is supplied by a single coronary artery, whereas the IVS and the rest of the RV have the benefit of left-sided collateral blood flow, which protects the RV against ischemia.

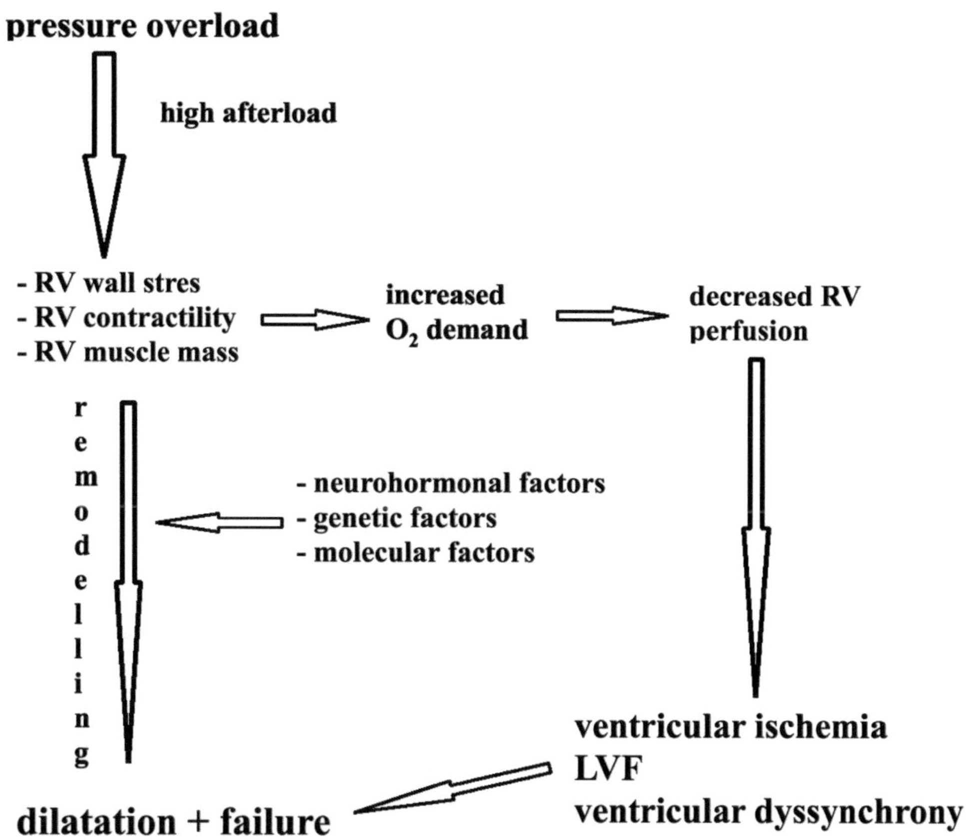


**Figure 5.** Pathophysiological changes caused by pulmonary hypertension on the right heart.

### 2.2. Transition of left heart failure to right heart failure

The main cause of RHF is PAH related to an intolerable afterload increase in pulmonary circulation due to LHF and is associated with elevated left ventricular filling pressure, severe mitral regurgitation, and impaired left atrial compliance secondary to a dilated LV. Therefore, LHF is the most common (65–80%) reason for PAH (group 2 PAH) [17]. Sudden elevation of the left heart and consequently pulmonary circulatory pressure increases endothelial permeability causing fluid infiltration into alveolar and interstitial spaces. Pulmonary edema is one of the first signs of acute left HFS, although decreased permeability in the chronic stage of LHF does not cause pulmonary congestion. Significant overloading of the pulmonary arterial vasculature leads to mechanical, neurohormonal, and molecular changes in the pulmonary vasculature system. Destructive neurohormonal changes cause the desensitization of the pulmonary vascular bed against vasodilator agents (nitric oxide, natriuretic peptides, etc.) and excretion of vasoconstrictor agents (endothelin-1, etc.). Vasoconstriction is the net response of the pulmonary vasculature system to sustain and maintain the right heart stroke volume. If this process cannot be treated or resolved, long-standing PAH will cause reactive structural changes and interstitial fibrosis in the pulmonary vasculature, specifically in the small pulmonary resistance arteries, and will result in increasing pulmonary vascular resistance (PVR) [18]. The next step of this maladaptive process is pulmonary arteriolar remodeling, which includes thickening of the alveolar-capillary membrane, medial hypertrophy, intimal and adventitial fibrosis, and luminal occlusion in small pulmonary arterioles. Arterial resistance and compliance in the lung are determined by the small pulmonary resistance vessels, in contrast to the systemic circulation determined by the aorta. The last stage after irreversible PVR is remodeling of the right heart and organs behind the RV. Maladaptive remodeling of the RV is similar to that of the LV in that there is an increase in myocardial fibrosis, dilatation, wall thinning, tricuspid insufficiency, and contractile failure (**Figure 6**) [19]. Pulmonary hypertension associated with left heart disease is a significant predictor for rehospitalization and mortality [20].

| | LVEF | RVEF | CVP (RAP) | mPAP | PCWP (LVEDP) | TPG | DPG | PVR |
|---|---|---|---|---|---|---|---|---|
| Normal | Normal | Normal | <10 mmHg | <15 mmHg | <10 mmHg | <10 mmHg | <5 mmHg | <2 WU |
| Precapillary (PVD) | Normal | Decreased | >15 mmHg | ≥25 mmHg | ≤15 mmHg | >12 mmHg | >7 mmHg | >3 WU |
| Post-capillary (LHF) | Decreased | Normal | >15 mmHg | ≥25 mmHg | >15 mmHg | ≤12 mmHg | <7 mmHg | <3 WU |
| Combined | Decreased | Decreased | >15 mmHg | ≥25 mmHg | >15 mmHg | >12 mmHg | >7 mmHg | >3 WU |
| Irreversible PAH | Decreased | Decreased | >15 mmHg | ≥25 mmHg | >15 mmHg | >15 mmHg | >10 mmHg | >6 WU |

CVP, central venous pressure; DPG, diastolic pulmonary gradient; LHF, left heart failure; LVEDP, left ventricular end-diastolic pressure; LVEF, left ventricular ejection fraction; PAH, pulmonary arterial hypertension; mPAP, mean pulmonary artery pressure; PCWP, pulmonary capillary wedge pressure; PVD, pulmonary vascular disease; PVR, pulmonary vascular resistance; Rap, right atrial pressure; RVEF, right ventricular ejection fraction; TPG, trans-pulmonary gradient.

**Table 9.** Pulmonary hypertension types.

Increased filling pressure of the right heart chambers reflects back to the systemic venous system and affects visceral and peripheral tissues. The left HFS with low systemic perfusion pressure and elevated PVR contributes to this process and aggravates organ dysfunction. The liver is the most affected organ in RHF via congestive hepatopathy. Cardiac hepatopathy is a clinical entity with signs and symptoms of elevated hepatic biomarkers approximately twice the upper limit of normal: aspartate aminotransferase > 100 U/L, alkaline phosphatase > 200 U/L, and serum bilirubin > 2 mg/dL [21]. Increased elevation of the right atrial pressure and/or severe tricuspid regurgitation implies increased hepatic venous pressure causing hepatic circulatory failure, hepatic congestion, and hepatic ischemia. In the early phase, sinusoidal congestion with hemorrhagic necrosis and hepatocyte degeneration dominates the reversible silent clinical status. Chronically elevated right heart pressures disrupt hepatic venous return and consequently hepatic arterial circulation, so that decreased hepatic oxygen and nutrient delivery results in hepatocellular necrosis, fatty changes, and fibrosis. The congested and hypoxic liver cannot work properly, and, ultimately, cardiac cirrhosis develops, which is characterized by hepatic insufficiency such as portal hypertension, coagulation abnormality, biliary malfunctions, and other metabolic dysfunctions.

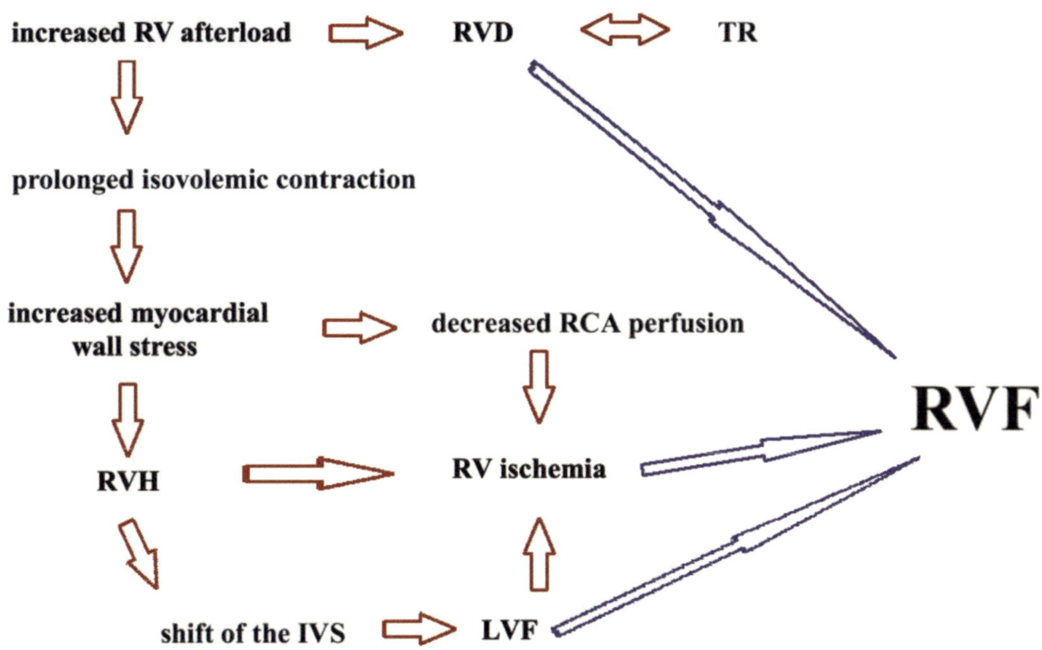


**Figure 6.** RVF pathophysiology. IVS, interventricular septum; LVF, left ventricular failure; RCA, right coronary artery; RV, right ventricle; RVD, right ventricular dysfunction; RVF, right ventricular failure; RVH, right ventricular hypertrophy; TR, tricuspid regurgitation.

## 3. Right ventricular failure after left ventricular assist device implantation

End-stage HFS requires mechanical uni- or biventricular circulatory support, but isolated LVAD implantation covers the majority (>90%) of treatments. Uni- or biventricular failure can be treated only by LVAD implantation. This therapy has several indications (**Table 10**). Currently, more LVADs have been implanted as destination therapy in advanced LVF with both advantages and disadvantages. The main intention of LVAD therapy is to provide support to the failing LV, allowing for improved stroke volume that ultimately promotes peripheral tissue perfusion. Furthermore, the LVAD improves right ventricular function due to unloading of the LV and consequently the RV [22]. The most serious complication of LVAD therapy can be a newly developed or continued deterioration of RVF as pathophysiologic sequela, which worsens postoperative mortality and morbidity, end-organ dysfunction due to severe congestion (coagulopathy, malnutrition, renal and hepatic dysfunctions, edema, ascites, etc.), hospitalization durations, and success of bridge to transplant therapy. The classification of RVF after LVAD implantation is described by The Interagency Registry for Mechanically Assisted Circulatory Support (INTERMACS) and is associated with increased perioperative mortality, prolonged length of stay, and worse survival even after cardiac transplantation (**Table 11**) [23]. The definition of serious RVF after LVAD implantation must be very clear, because it needs to be treated by heart transplantation or mechanical circulatory support (**Table 12**) [24]. Post-implant RVF can occur beyond the immediate postoperative period or later, and it significantly impacts survival after LVAD implantation because it is a progressive condition. Early post-implant RVF results in worse survival and is predicted by greater preoperative tricuspid incompetence [25]. Prolonged RVF for more than 2 weeks is associated with adverse outcomes, with the incidence of moderate or severe RVF necessitating right or biventricular ventricular assist device placement after LVAD implantation ranging between 10 and 40% [26].

1. Bridge to transplantation (BTT)
2. Bridge to candidacy for transplantation (BTC)
3. Destination therapy (DT)
4. Bridge to recovery (BTR)

**Table 10.** LVAD indications.

1. Mild
   a. Post-implant inotropes, inhaled nitric oxide, or intravenous vasodilators not continued beyond post-op Day 7 after LVAD implant
2. Moderate
   a. Post-implant inotropes, inhaled nitric oxide, or intravenous vasodilators continued beyond post-op Day 7 and up to post-op Day 14 after LVAD implant
   b. CVP or right atrial pressure >16 mm Hg
3. Severe
   a. Prolonged post-implant inotropes, inhaled nitric oxide, or intravenous vasodilators continued beyond post-op Day 14 after LVAD implant
   b. CVP or right atrial pressure >16 mmHg
   c. Need for RVAD at any time after LVAD implant

CVP, central venous pressure; INTERMACS, Interagency Registry for Mechanically Assisted Circulatory Support; LVAD, left ventricular assist device; RVAD, right ventricular assist device; RVF, right ventricular failure.

**Table 11.** INTERMACS definition of post-implant RVF (severity scale).

Right ventricular output determinants such as preload, afterload, and contractility are deranged in RVF after LVAD implantation (**Table 13**). Post-implant RVF is multifactorial and includes leftward shifting of the IVS, suboptimal RV afterload reduction, and RV myocardial dysfunction. Echocardiography is the primary imaging modality for monitoring cardiac function, filling and contraction behaviors, and device malfunctions [27].

http://dx.doi.org/10.5772/66887

| |
|---|
| 1. Need for intravenous inotrope and pulmonary vasodilator therapy > 14 days |
| 2. Need for RVAD implantation |
| 3. Hemodynamic parameters |
| a. CVP > 16 mmHg |
| b. CVP/PCWP > 2/3 |
| c. PVR > 2 Wood units |
| d. MAP < 55 mmHg |
| e. CI < 2 L/min/m$^2$ |
| f. Inotropic support > 20 U |
| g. MVS < 55% |
| h. HR > 100 / min |
| 4. Laboratory parameters |
| a. Bilirubin > 2 mg/dL |
| b. Creatinine > 2 mg/dL |
| c. AST > 80 IU/L |
| d. Albumin < 3 g/dL |
| 5. Echocardiographic parameters |
| a. TAPSE < 7.5 mm |
| b. RAD > 5 cm |
| c. RVEDD > 3.5 cm |
| d. RVEF < 30% |

AST, aspartate aminotransferase; CI, cardiac index; CVP, central venous pressure; HR, heart rate; MAP, mean arterial pressure; MVS, mixed venous oxygen saturation; PCWP, pulmonary capillary wedge pressure; PVR, pulmonary vascular resistance; RAD, right atrial diameter; RVAD, right ventricular assist device; RVEDD, right ventricular end-diastolic diameter; RVEF, right ventricular ejection fraction; RVF, right ventricular failure; TAPSE, tricuspid annular plane systolic excursion.

**Table 12.** Definition of serious RVF.

Increased preload (volume overload) causes the RV to fail due to the overstretching of the right ventricular myocardium. Improved left-sided forward flow with mechanical unloading in conjunction with perioperative transfusions of blood products suggests that increased venous return to the RV can be well tolerated. However, excessive fluid transfusions can aggravate RVF due to the effect of the Frank-Starling mechanism, exacerbation of tricuspid regurgitation, reduction of septal contribution, and ventriculo-arterial uncoupling. The main echocardiographic findings are a leftward shift of the interatrial septum, distension of the RV, worsening of tricuspid regurgitation, and plethora.

Despite the benefit of the LVAD decompressing the LV and reducing pulmonary overload significantly, it is not successful in every situation due to irreversibility of PAH, which is the main determinant for irreducible afterload. Reverse remodeling of the pulmonary vasculature can potentially occur with continued unloading, and, unlike heart transplantation, elevated PVR is not able to predict post-implant RVF. The second reason is continuity of preoperative significant mitral regurgitation due to untouched strategy, which cannot be improved and results pulmonary congestion though implantation of LVAD postoperatively. Because the RV has a very different myocardial structure than the left side and is very sensitive to acute change in afterload, any limited or huge failure of afterload decreasing causes significant post-implant RVF due to ineffectiveness of Frank-Starling mechanism on the right heart.

Improvement of right ventricular contractility after LVAD implantation is a predictor for positive outcomes; however, if the right ventricular systolic function does not improve, there are several risk-scoring algorithms that can be used to help predict the need for biventricular support [28]. Excessive leftward shift of the IVS due to volume overload and/or aggressive LV decompression may decrease septal contribution to right ventricular contraction causing mechanical dyssynchrony and elevation of right ventricular work. The main echocardiographic findings of post-implant RVF are decreased tricuspid annular plane systolic excursion (TAPSE < 7.5 mm), reduced right ventricular fractional area change (RVFAC < 35%), increased RV/LV ratio (>0.75), and septal akinesia. Severe unloading of the LV affects left ventricular contraction, depending on it right ventricular systolic function. In normal heart, the left ventricular contraction supplies roughly one half and septal contraction one quarter of the right ventricular ejection function. Prevention and treatment of RVF can be provided with the maintenance of the ejection function of the LV.

| |
|---|
| 1. Preload |
| a. Increased left ventricular output and venous return (approximately 100%) |
| b. Excessive administration of blood products and fluids |
| 2. Afterload |
| a. Maintenance of pulmonary arterial hypertension |
| b. Respiratory problems |
| 3. Contractility |
| a. Overstretched cardiac myofibrils (decreasing stroke volume) |
| b. Aggravated annular dilatation and tricuspid regurgitation |
| c. Impaired ventricular interdependence (left ventricular failure) |
| d. Dyssynchronism of interventricular septum (noncontractible and/or leftward shift of the septum) |

**Table 13.** Determinants leading to RVF after LVAD.

## Author details

Kaan Kırali[1, 2*], Tanıl Özer[1] and Mustafa Mert Özgür[1]

*Address all correspondence to: imkbkirali@yahoo.com

1 Department of Cardiac Transplantation and Ventricular Assist Device, Kartal Koşuyolu YIEA Hospital, Istanbul, Turkey

2 Department of Cardiovascular Surgery, Faculty of Medicine, Sakarya University, Sakarya, Turkey

http://dx.doi.org/10.5772/66887

## References


[1] Warriner D, Sheridan P, Lawford P. Heart failure: Not a single organ disease but a multisystem syndrome. Br J Hosp Med 2015;76(6):330–336.

[2] King M, Kingery J, Casey B. Diagnosis and evaluation of heart failure. Am Fam Physician 2012;85(12):1161–1168.

[3] Doehner W, Frenneaux M, Anker SD. Metabolic impairment in heart failure. J Am Coll Cardiol 2014;64(13):1388–1400.

[4] Gaggin HG, Januzzi JL Jr. Biomarkers and diagnostics in heart failure. Biochim Biophys Acta 2013;1832(12):2442–2450.

[5] Shires ES, Gustafsson AB. Mitophagy and heart failure. J Mol Med 2015;93(3):253–262.

[6] Florea VG, Cohn JN. The autonomic nervous system and heart failure. Circ Res 2014;114:1815–1826.

[7] Joyner MJ. Preclinical and clinical evaluation of autonomic function in humans. J Physiol 2016;594(12):4009–4013.

[8] Waldreus N, Hahn RG, Jaarsma T. Thirst in heart failure: A systematic literature review. Eur Heart J 2013;15(2):141–149.

[9] Verbrugge FH, Steels P, Grieten L, Nijst P, Tang WHW, Mullens W. Hyponatremia in acute decompensated heart failure: Depletion versus dilution. J Am Coll Cardiol 2015;65(5):480–492.

[10] Troughton R, Felker GM, Januzzi JL Jr. Natriuretic peptide-guided heart failure management. Eur Heart J 2014;35:16–24.

[11] Gloschat CR, Koppel AC, Aras KK, Brennan JA, Holzem KM, Efimow IR. Arrhythmogenic and metabolic remodelling of failing human heart. J Physiol 2016;594(14):3963–3980.

[12] Kevin LG, Barnard M. Right ventricular failure. Contin Educ Anaesth Crit Care Pain 2007;7(3):89–94.

[13] Ryan JJ, Tedford RJ. Diagnosis and treating the failing right heart. Curr Open Cardiol 2015;30(3):292–300

[14] Mehra MR, Park MH, Landzberg MJ, Lala A, Waxman AB. Right heart failure: Toward a common language. Pulm Circ 2013;3(4):963–967. [Consensus statement from the International Right Heart Foundation Working Group includes a comprehensive definition of right heart failure.]

[15] Gerges M, Gerges C, Pistritto AM, Lang MB, Trip P, Jakowitsch J, Binder T, Lang IM. Pulmonary hypertension in heart failure. Epidemiology, right ventricular function, and survival. Am J Respir Crit Care Med 2015;192(10):1234–1246.

[16] Naeije R, Vachiery JL, Yerly P, Vanderpool R. The transpulmonary pressure gradient for the diagnosis of pulmonary vascular disease. Eur Respir J 2013;41(1):217–223.

[17] Rosenkranz S, Gibbs JSR, Wachter R, De Marco T, Vonk-Noordegraaf A, Vachiery JL. Left ventricular heart failure and pulmonary hypertension. Eur Heart J 2016;37(12):942–954.

[18] Vanderpool RR, Naeije R. Progress in pulmonary hypertension with left heart failure. beyond new definitions and acronyms. Am J Respir Crit Care Med 2015;192(10):1152–1154.

[19] Borgdorff MAJ, Dickinson MG, Berger RMF, Bartelds B. Right ventricular failure due to chronic pressure load: What have we learned in animal models since the NIH working group statement? Heart Fail Rev 2015;20(4):475–491.

[20] Dzudie A, Kengne AP, Thienemann F, Sliwa K. Predictors of hospitalisations for heart failure and mortality in patients with pulmonary hypertension associated with left heart disease: A systematic review. BMJ Open 2014;4(7):e004843.

[21] Megalla S, Holtzmann D, Aranow WS, Nazari R, Korenfeld S, Schwarcz A, Goldberg Y, Spevack DM. Predictors of cardiac hepatopathy in patients with right heart failure. Med Sci Monit 2011;17(10):537–541.

[22] Morgan JA, Paone G, Nemeh HW, Murthy R, Williams CT, Lanfear DE, Tita C, Brewer RJ. Impact of continuous-flow left ventricular assist device support on right ventricular function. J Heart Lung Transplant 2013;32:398–403.

[23] Lampert BC, Teuteberg JJ. Right ventricular failure after left ventricular assist devices. J Heart Lung Transplant 2015;34:1123–1130.

[24] Koprivanac M, Kelava M, Siric F, Cruz VB, Moazami N, Mihaljevic T. Predictors of right ventricular failure after left ventricular assist device implantation. Croat Med J 2014;55(6):587–595.

[25] Baumwol J, MacDonald PS, Keogh AM, Kotlyar E, Spratt P, JanszP Hawyard CS. Right heart failure and "failure to thrive" after left ventricular assist device: Clinical predictors and outcomes. J Heart Lung Transplant 2011;30(8):888–895.

[26] Fida N, Loebe M, Estep JD, Guha A. Predictors and management of right heart failure after left ventricular assist device implantation. Methodist DeBakey Cardiovasc J 2015;11(1):18–23.

[27] Argiriou M, Kolokotron SM, Sakellaridis T, Argiriou O, Charitos C, Zarogoulidis P, Katsikogiannis N, Kougioumtzi I, Machairiotis N, Tsiouda T, Tsakiridis K, Zarogoulidis K. Right heart failure post left ventricular assist device implantation. J Thorac Dis 2014;6(S1):S52–S59.

[28] Atluri P, Goldstone AB, Fairman AS, MacArthur JW, Shudo Y, Cohen JE, Acker AL, Hiesinger W, Howard JL, Acker MA, Woo YJ. Predicting right ventricular failure in the modern, continuous flow left ventricular assist device era. Ann Thorac Surg 2013;96(3):857–863.

Chapter 3

# Heart Failure with Preserved Ejection Fraction

Hakan Altay and Seckin Pehlivanoglu

Additional information is available at the end of the chapter

http://dx.doi.org/10.5772/66758

**Abstract**

Heart failure with preserved ejection fraction (HFpEF) is now recognized as a major and growing public health problem worldwide. This heart failure subtype disproportionately affects women and the elderly and is commonly associated with other cardiovascular comorbidities, such as hypertension, diabetes and chronic kidney disease. There are uncertainties and debates regarding the definition, diagnosis and pathophysiology with the consequence that all outcome trials performed so far cannot yield an effective treatment as in heart failure with reduced ejection fraction (HFrEF). Here we present an overview of epidemiology, pathophysiology, diagnosis and therapeutic approaches emerging from large outcome clinical trials.

**Keywords:** heart failure, ejection fraction, diastolic, diagnosis, treatment

## 1. Introduction

Heart failure (HF) is a clinical syndrome of dyspnea, fatigue and fluid retention secondary to impaired cardiac function [1]. Cardiac function may be impaired structurally or functionally with resultant decreased ejection or filling capacity both of which can reduce cardiac output and/or increase intracardiac pressures at rest or during exercise. Systolic dysfunction leading to reduced left ventricular ejection fraction (LVEF) (LVEF < 40%) had long been believed to be the predominant cause of heart failure. However, HF remains to be a growing health problem in the community despite recent improvements in the management of HF with reduced ejection fraction (HFrEF). Another subset of heart failure which occurs in the setting of normal or near normal left ventricular ejection fraction (LVEF > 50%) has been evolving for the last two decades. This distinct HF subtype has been called HF with preserved ejection fraction (HFpEF). Once included in HFpEF, the newly defined HF with midrange EF (HFmrEF) comprises the HF patients with EF between 40 and 50% [2]. HFmrEF will be discussed in the context of HFPEF because most of the trials and epidemiological studies to date have included patients with EF > 40%.

Current data indicate that at least half of the HF population has a normal or near-normal LVEF [3]. Even more striking is the finding that the percent of patients with HFpEF appears to be increasing in relation to the percent that have HFrEF [4]. One of the reasons for this shift in the ratio between HFpEF and HFrEF is related to the greater availability of therapeutic interventions that limit myocardial damage (particularly, in the setting of an acute myocardial infarction), hence reducing incidence of HFrEF. Another important reason for this increase in prevalence of HFpEF is increasing number of obese and elderly patients. It is also worth mentioning that there is an increased number of patients with possible misdiagnosis of HFpEF who have otherwise alternative causes for their symptoms such as obesity, lung disease and myocardial ischemia [5].

In the past, HFpEF was thought to be a benign condition, but now it is well known that it causes substantial morbidity and mortality [6]. Despite being an enormous and dreadful problem of this era, there has been little progress in developing effective treatments that will alter the natural history of the condition. Contemporary medicine can offer nothing but only diuretic for treatment. This is partly due to an incomplete understanding of the disease and partly due to the huge diversity of clinical phenotype.

## 2. Epidemiology

Over 90% of patients with HFpEF are aged ≥60 years at the time of diagnosis making it obvious that this is a disease of elderly [7]. The prevalence in the community has varied from 1.1% to 5.5% of the general population [8]. This wide variation is primarily attributed to the different cutoff values of normal EF in different studies. Moreover, the prevalence has been found to vary with age and gender. A large community-based study found that the prevalence of HFpEF increased from 0% in males to 1% in females in the age group of 25–49 years to 4–6% in males and 8–10% in females above 80 years, indicating a dramatic rise in the prevalence with increasing age but additionally a higher prevalence among females as compared to age-matched males [9]. The demographic characteristics present in patients with HFpEF differ significantly from those in patients with HFREF. Compared with those with HFrEF, patients with HFpEF are older, more often female, more often have hypertensive heart disease and less often have ischemic heart disease [10]. There is a similar prevalence of DM but remarkably higher prevalence of obesity in patients with HFpEF compared to HFrEF. Atrial fibrillation (AF) is also more prevalent in HFpEF [11]. HFpEF patients also have a higher burden of both cardiovascular and non-cardiovascular comorbid diseases. **Table 1** summarizes various comorbidities usually seen in association with HFpEF. Comorbid conditions especially renal insufficiency and atrial fibrillation may be less common in randomized controlled trials than hospital-based registries due to exclusion criteria.

Whether overall mortality rates differ between patients with HFpEF and HFrEF is not clear. Some community-based epidemiological studies have shown that the annual mortality rate is

| Comorbid conditions | Frequency |
|---|---|
| Hypertension | 60–80% |
| Ischemic heart disease | 35–70% |
| Diabetes | 20–45% |
| Atrial fibrillation | 15–40% |
| COPD | 31% |
| Renal insufficiency | 26% |

COPD: Chronic obstructive pulmonary disease.

**Table 1.** Comorbid conditions seen in association with HFPEF.

same and approaches 15% for both groups of patients [4]. Conversely, data from randomized clinical trials suggest that patients with HFpEF have a lower annual mortality (approaching 5%) than patients with HFrEF. The lower mortality rate detected in the randomized trials can be explained by strict exclusion of comorbid diseases [12]. When the data from I-PRESERVE (The Irbesartan in Heart Failure With Preserved Ejection Fraction Study) trial was analyzed with respect to mode of death in HFpEF, it was seen that cardiovascular (CV) diseases (60%) are the leading cause of death including sudden cardiac death (26%), HF (15%), myocardial infarction (5%) and stroke (9%) followed by non-CV causes (30%) and unknown (10%) [13]. Compared with HFrEF [14], HFpEF patients have more non-cardiovascular (30% vs. 15%), fewer sudden (26% vs. 40%) and fewer heart failure deaths (15% vs. 35%). In parallel with I-PRESERVE trial results, the cause-specific mortality estimates show that the non-cardiovascular causes of death constitute nearly 30 to 50% of all deaths in HFpEF patients while only 15–18% in HFrEF patients [15]. The older age and high burden of comorbidities can explain the higher non-cardiovascular mortality in HFpEF patients. Large HFpEF trials showed that the patients with HFpEF have lower hospitalization rates than those with HFrEF [16]. Furthermore, HFrEF patients have nearly 1% absolute higher in-hospital mortality rate than HFpEF patients [17].

## 3. Pathophysiology

In contrast to HFrEF patients who have main abnormalities in systolic function, left ventricular dilation and eccentric remodeling, patients with HFpEF have main abnormalities in diastolic function, normal left ventricular size and concentric hypertrophy. Normal LVEF does not imply normal cardiac output. In HFrEF, decreased cardiac output can be explained more easily with reduced ejection fraction and subsequent reduced stroke volume. HFpEF patients also exhibit a low cardiac output that is comparable to that seen in HFrEF patients. The pathophysiological abnormality leading to decreased cardiac output in HFpEF is more complex and since HFpEF is a heterogeneous clinical diagnosis, it encompasses a variety of underlying pathophysiological processes.

HFpEF is caused by the complex interplay of multiple impairments in ventricular diastolic function, adverse cardiac remodeling, stiffening of the ventricles, pulmonary hypertension, atrial dysfunction and abnormal ventricular-vascular coupling related to stiffening of the vasculature and hence decreased vascular compliance, endothelial dysfunction, impaired vasodilatation and coronary ischemia, impaired renal handling of salt and fluid and impairment of heart rate (HR) reserve [18]. Left ventricular diastolic dysfunction is the result of myocardial hypertrophy, fibrosis and/or altered myocyte calcium handling (delayed calcium uptake by the myocyte sarcoplasmic reticulum and calcium efflux from the myocyte) [19]. The pathophysiology of diastolic dysfunction includes delayed relaxation, impaired LV filling and/or increased stiffness. A slowing of the normal diastolic relaxation of the ventricle can in turn increase the left ventricular and left atrial pressures [20].

There are a number of causes, which lead to HFpEF. Age seems to be the dominant risk factor for HFpEF. Heart failure with preserved EF is exclusively a disease of elderly. As one ages, there is an increased collagen deposition with a reduction in the amount of elastin, which can lead to increased stiffness of the heart and blood vessels leading to ultimate HFpEF. Chronic hypertension, which is highly prevalent in HFpEF, leads to left ventricular hypertrophy and increased connective tissue content, both of which decrease cardiac compliance. Due to decreased compliance, in HFpEF LV functions on a steeper diastolic pressure-volume relationship compared with the normal ventricle. This leads to decreased LV end-diastolic volumes and a compensatory rise in LV filling pressure to maintain cardiac output. This high LV filling pressures lead to fluid accumulation in the lungs, which cause dyspnea, which is the common symptom of heart failure. As well as leading to symptoms of dyspnea, elevation in LV filling pressures produces secondary pulmonary hypertension and atrial remodeling that can predispose a patient to the development of right ventricular (RV) dysfunction and atrial fibrillation, respectively. Although epicardial coronary artery disease causing ischemic heart disease is less common in patients with HFpEF compared to HFrEF, subendocardial ischemia related to increased left ventricular diastolic pressures in a left ventricle with concentric remodeling is more common in patients with HFpEF. Multiple studies have shown an association between endothelial dysfunction and HFpEF and endothelial dysfunction was suggested to be as a prominent determinant of HFpEF [21]. Vascular stiffness is also an important contributor to pathophysiological process that leads to HFpEF. As a result of ventricular-arterial uncoupling, cardiac output decreases. Regardless of EF, ultimate decrease in cardiac output causes activation of neurohormonal mechanisms that lead to activation of vasoconstriction, salt and water retention and increased diastolic filling pressures [22]. HFpEF patients display neurohormonal profiles similar to HFrEF, with elevated circulating neurohormones, such as natriuretic peptides and norepinephrine [23].

Chronotropic incompetence (CI) is a potential pathophysiological factor in HFpEF, contributing to reduced exercise capacity. The increase in heart rate as a result of an activity or exercise is one of the two main contributors of increased cardiac output to meet the excess need of energy consumption. Moreover, the increase in HR is the strongest contributor to the ability to perform sustained aerobic exercise [24]. Phan et al. have shown that CI can be seen in patients with HFpEF during maximal exercise [25]. In this study, the prevalence of CI was 35% in HFpEF subjects. Chronotropic incompetence may be a significant contributor to severe, symptomatic exercise intolerance, which is the most common symptom in HFpEF. Atrial fibrillation (AF) is also common in patients with diastolic dysfunction and contributes

http://dx.doi.org/10.5772/66758

to the pathophysiology of HFpEF. AF eliminates the late diastolic atrial contribution to LV filling, upon which patients with diastolic dysfunction are dependent and is poorly tolerated leading to both pulmonary edema and decreased cardiac output.

## 4. Diagnosis

The diagnosis of HFpEF is more challenging than the diagnosis of HFrEF. Part of the challenge is the fact that the HFpEF is a heterogeneous clinical entity, whose manifestations and outcomes remain difficult to be predicted. In essence, it's a diagnosis of exclusion. According to the recent ESC 2016 HF guideline [2], for the diagnosis of HFpEF, three essential criteria should be met. **Table 2** shows these criteria for diagnosis of HFpEF. As in HFrEF, HFpEF is a clinical diagnosis. Symptoms are often nonspecific and do not, therefore, help discriminate between HFpEF and HFrEF. Exercise dyspnea may be the only symptom with no detectable sign especially in the early stages of HFpEF. Exercise dyspnea is particularly difficult to interpret in elderly and in obese, comprising most of the HFrEF population. Objective evidence of reduced exercise capacity provided by cardiometabolic exercise testing with measurement of peak exercise oxygen consumption ($VO_{2max}$) or by the 6 min walking test can be used for judgment of exercise dyspnea in the context of HF symptom. Signs of congestive HF such as lung crepitations, pulmonary edema, jugular venous distention and ankle edema may not always be present, especially in the early stages. The "presence of signs or symptoms of congestive heart failure" as the first criterium for the diagnosis of HFpEF is therefore put instead of the "presence of signs and symptoms of congestive heart failure" [2].

Once a clinical diagnosis of HF has been made, the presence of HFpEF can be established by confirming a normal or near-normal LVEF, often by an echocardiogram. Echocardiography is an essential tool in evaluating patients with unexplained dyspnea. Bearing in mind that HFpEF is a diagnosis of exclusion, echocardiography should first provide information about the left ventricular systolic performance (commonly assessed using ejection fraction), valvular disease and pericardial disease. After exclusion of other possible explanations for HF, echocardiography should provide evidence of structural heart disease such as left ventricular hypertrophy, left atrial enlargement and pulmonary hypertension. Diastolic dysfunction can also be diagnosed further using the Doppler echocardiography (based on mitral inflow

| |
|---|
| 1) Symptoms and/or signs of congestive heart failure |
| 2) Non-dilated left ventricle (LV end-diastolic volume index (LVEDVI) < 97 mL/m²) with preserved ejection fraction (≥50%) |
| 3) a) Elevated levels of natriuretic peptides<br>b) At least one additional criterion<br>i) Relevant structural heart disease (LVH and/or LAD)<br>ii) Diastolic dysfunction |

BNP, B-type natriuretic peptide; HFPEF, heart failure with preserved ejection fraction; LAD, left atrial dilation; LV, left ventricular; LVH, left ventricular hypertrophy.
a Signs may not be present in the early stages of HF (especially in HFpEF) and in patients treated with diuretics.
b BNP > 35 pg/ml and/or NT-proBNP > 125 pg/mL.

**Table 2.** Criteria for the diagnosis of HFPEF.

velocities). It is graded based on the ratio of the early, E, to late diastolic, inflow velocity, A (mild, moderate and severe) [26]. Grade I is abnormal relaxation pattern (E < A), grade II is pseudonormal pattern (E > A), grade III is restrictive pattern (E >> A) and grade IV is irreversible restrictive pattern [27]. The pseudonormal stage (grade II), which refers to a situation when filling pressures are elevated but the mitral inflow pattern appears normal, is creating a state of confusion. Assessment of pulmonary vein flow (PVF) velocity waveforms provide information complementary to that obtained from transmitral flow (TMF) patterns. Therefore, PVF pattern can be used to differentiate a normal from a pseudonormal TMF pattern. Grade III and grade IV diastolic dysfunctions are called restrictive filling dynamics. These are both severe forms of diastolic dysfunction and patients tend to have advanced HF symptoms at this stage.

Elevated LV filling pressures are the main and essential physiologic consequence of diastolic dysfunction. In the presence of symptoms and/or signs of HF and normal or near-normal EF, high LV filling pressures help a lot to put the diagnosis of HFpEF. Pulsed-Doppler-derived TMF is largely influenced by preload. Left ventricular filling pressures can also be estimated by myocardial tissue-Doppler-derived early diastolic annular velocity, designated E′ which is, to a large extent, regarded as a preload-independent index of diastolic performance. The use of tissue Doppler imaging-derived indices that correct for the influence of myocardial relaxation on the load-dependent early diastolic mitral flow E/E′ ratio (i.e., the ratio of mitral inflow, E, to early diastolic annular velocity, E′) as a means of estimating LV filling pressure is more reliable. Therefore, noninvasive diagnostic evidence of diastolic LV dysfunction is preferably derived from myocardial TD. If myocardial TD yields values E/E′ > 15, it puts diagnosis of high LV filling pressure. When the ratio is lower than 8, LV filling pressures are considered low. If TD yields an E/E′ ratio suggestive of LV diastolic dysfunction but not diagnostic (15 > E/E′ > 8), then additional echo variables are required for diagnostic evidence of LV diastolic dysfunction, which include Doppler flow profile of mitral valve or pulmonary veins, measurement of LV mass index (LVMi) or left atrium volume index (LAVi), electrocardiographic evidence of atrial fibrillation, or high levels of BNP or NT-proBNP. No single echocardiography variable is sufficiently accurate to be used in isolation to make a diagnosis of LV diastolic dysfunction. Therefore, a comprehensive echocardiography examination incorporating all relevant two- dimensional and Doppler data is recommended [2]. Invasive method of measuring filling pressure is more precise and yields higher diagnostic performance but not practical. Invasive diagnostic evidence of diastolic LV dysfunction can be obtained by LV end-diastolic pressure (LVEDP) or pulmonary capillary wedge pressure (PCWP). Filling pressures are considered elevated when the mean PCWP is >12 mm Hg or when the LVEDP is >16 mm Hg.

It is noteworthy that diastolic dysfunction is not always present in HFpEF, being observed by echocardiography in only two-thirds of patients at rest [28]. However, many patients with HFpEF display elevated LV filling pressures only during the stress of exercise, indicating an earlier stage of disease [29]. In such patients, the diagnosis of HFpEF could only be made using exercise hemodynamic evaluation using supine bicycle diastolic stress test. After stress, an increase in E/E′ and tricuspid regurgitation (TR) velocity indicating a high pulmonary artery systolic pressure can truly put the diagnosis of HFpEF [2].

Biomarkers have been recently used in the diagnostic workup of HF. BNP is synthesized and released upon LV wall stretch from increased pressure or volume. The plasma levels of BNP are raised in HF regardless of EF. However, natriuretic peptides (NPs) are less elevated in HFpEF compared to HFrEF. NPs are an important aid for the diagnosis of HF, especially in the non-acute setting when echocardiography is not immediately available. In the Breathing Not Properly study, BNP levels at the time of emergency admission were significantly elevated in HFpEF, when compared to other causes of dyspnea (median 413 vs. 34 pg/ml, $p < 0.001$) but significantly lower than in patients with HFrEF (median 413 vs. 821 pg/ml, $p < 0.001$) [30]. Many patients with HFpEF display elevated filling pressures only during exercise. This intermittent nature of pressure elevation is likely to explain the reduced BNP level observed in patients with HFpEF [31].

## 5. Challenges in the diagnosis of HFpEF

Diagnosis of HFpEF is more difficult than the diagnosis of HFREF because it is largely one of the exclusions, i.e., potential noncardiac causes of patients' symptoms (lung disease, anemia, chronic kidney disease, or obesity) that must first be eliminated. For most patients with a diagnosis of heart failure but preserved left ventricular systolic function based on symptoms and signs of HF which are highly nonspecific and normal EF, the diagnosis of HFpEF is rarely needed [5]. Before ascribing symptoms to HFpEF for which there is no evidence-based treatment, we should thoroughly investigate patient for other possible treatable causes of dyspnea with calculation of body mass index, pulmonary function testing, exercise electrocardiography and probably stress echocardiography.

The diagnostic criteria put forward for HFpEF has some important pitfalls. In HFpEF, exertional dyspnea is frequently the earliest symptom due to increased LV filling pressures ensuing some degree of pulmonary congestion. Since many patients with HFPEF present with dyspnea and no signs of fluid overload, exertional dyspnea was considered sufficient clinical evidence to suggest the presence of clinical heart failure in the recent guidelines [2]. Keeping in mind that dyspnea is a ubiquitous complaint especially in elderly and obese who represent a large proportion of HFpEF patients and other comorbid conditions such as chronic obstructive pulmonary disease and renal insufficiency which are usually present concomitant with HFpEF, dyspnea cannot be a reliable diagnostic criteria without objective evidence of reduced exercise performance provided by metabolic exercise testing. Meanwhile, because early signs and symptoms of HFpEF such as exercise dyspnea may also be the presenting symptoms of other alternative conditions or diseases, delayed diagnosis has also been a matter.

Diastolic dysfunction as assessed noninvasively by echocardiography is highly prevalent in elderly population who has no symptoms attributable to HF. This condition suggests some controversy regarding the accuracy of noninvasive measures of diastolic function by echocardiography [32]. Assessment should take into consideration patients' ages and heart rates (mitral E, E/A ratio and annular e′ decrease with increasing heart rate). Specifically, in older individuals without histories of cardiovascular disease, caution should be exercised before concluding that grade I diastolic dysfunction is present. Because the majority of subjects aged over 60 years without histories of cardiovascular disease have E/A ratios, <1 and E deceleration time (EDT) > 200 ms, such values in the absence of further indicators of LV dysfunction (e.g., LV hypertrophy and LA enlargement), can be considered normal for age. In other words, echocardiogram suggesting diastolic dysfunction on the basis of an abnormal E/A ratio is not diagnostic and represents insufficient investigation. Second, the echocardiographic markers of diastolic dysfunction may be absent in a significant proportion of patients diagnosed with HFpEF.

Natriuretic peptides could give inconclusive results in a number of situations. In normal individuals, the concentration of NT-proBNP rises with age and is higher in women than in men [33]. Therefore, age-stratified cutoff points for NT-proBNP (≥450 for ages < 50 years, ≥900 for 50–75 years and ≥1800 pg/mL for >75 years) were shown to perform the best diagnostic performance for rule in acute HF setting [34]. Beyond HF, a number of cardiopulmonary disorders are also associated with elevated BNP or NT-proBNP values: acute coronary syndrome, myocarditis, valvular heart disease, hypertrophic cardiomyopathy, cardiotoxic drugs, atrial fibrillation, or flutter and right ventricular dysfunction in the setting of significant pulmonary disease (pulmonary hypertension, pulmonary embolism). Other conditions that are associated with higher BNP or NT-proBNP levels may be related to comorbidities such as advanced age, renal dysfunction, stroke, sepsis and other high output states. It should be kept in mind that plasma levels of BNP rise independently of LV filling pressures once glomerular filtration rate falls below 60 mL/min because renal dysfunction is highly prevalent in HFpEF population. AF also confounds the utility of BNP for diagnosing HFpEF [35, 36].

## 6. Treatment

Prevention of HFpEF through treatment of risk factors (e.g., hypertension, diabetes and coronary artery disease) especially at early stages is effective and still the most important part of management of HFpEF since specific treatments are yet to be discovered [37]. Hypertension antedates the development of HFpEF in nearly 90% of the cases and it confers a two- to threefold increased risk of developing HFpEF [38]. Therefore, strict control of hypertension will inevitably prevent development of HFpEF. Improving cardiorespiratory fitness among low-fit sedentary individuals by exercise training could be another preventive approach against HFpEF. And, targeting obesity in the early childhood will also prevent development of HFpEF in the future.

As a non-pharmacologic therapy, exercise training has clearly been shown to benefit cardiorespiratory health in patients with HFrEF. Recent studies have addressed the effects of exercise training in patients with HFpEF. Although the effects on HF-related mortality and hospitalizations were not studied, these reports showed that moderate supervised exercise program had positive effects on the quality of life, exercise tolerance but not left ventricular EF [39, 40]. No pharmacologic therapy has been shown to be effective in improving outcomes in patients with heart failure with HFpEF. There is no single explanation for the negative results of past HFpEF trials. Potential contributors include an incomplete understanding of HFpEF pathophysiology, inadequate diagnostic criteria, recruitment of patients without true HF or at early stages of the syndrome, poor matching of therapeutic mechanisms and primary pathophysiological processes, suboptimal study designs, inadequate statistical power, or patient heterogeneity [41]. Another possible explanation is the fact that non-cardiovascular mortality is higher in HFpEF than HFrEF highlighting one of the difficulties in the development of an effective therapeutic strategy in the overall patients with HFpEF.

The treatment recommendations from the American Heart Association have set four goals in the management of these patients: (a) control of hypertension, (b) control of heart rate especially in the patients with atrial fibrillation, (c) control of pulmonary and peripheral edema and (d) prevention of myocardial ischemia [1]. 2013 ACC/AHA Guideline on HF had only two class I recommendations for HFpEF treatment. One of them is the use of diuretics in order to reduce volume overload and improve dyspnea. The second one is the control of blood pressure. The guideline also recommends revascularization in patients whom symptoms or demonstrable ischemia are thought to contribute HF symptoms as class II recommendation. Management of AF is another class II recommendation of the American guideline. The guideline does not underscore rhythm control or rate control in HFpEF since there was no specific trial comparing these two strategies in HFpEF until now. The recent 2016 European Society of Cardiology (ESC) Guideline could not make any further recommendations on top of 2013 American guideline in this regard except recommending screening patients with HFpEF for both cardiovascular and non-cardiovascular comorbidities, which then should be treated accordingly [2].

**Table 3** summarizes the major clinical trials that have evaluated the efficacy of various therapeutic drugs in patients with HFpEF. The renin-angiotensin-aldosterone system (RAAS) is involved in many of the pathophysiological processes associated with this disease (including hypertension, left ventricular hypertrophy, myocardial fibrosis and vascular dysfunction) and inhibitors of this system can prevent neurohormonal activation and prevent ventricular remodeling [22]. RAAS blockers have been long time investigated whether they could be effective therapeutic option for these patients. Three large trials have evaluated inhibitors of the RAAS in patients with HFpEF but none of them proved to be beneficial. The Candesartan in Heart Failure: Assessment of Reduction in Mortality and Morbidity (CHARM)-preserved trial evaluated the effect of candesartan on elderly patients with HFpEF [42]. Candesartan showed no significant reduction of cardiovascular death but showed significant reduction in HF hospitalization. The Perindopril in Elderly People with Chronic Heart Failure (PEP-CHF) trial was a randomized placebo-controlled trial which evaluated the effect of perindopril on patients with HFpEF [43]. At the end of the study, perindopril showed no significant effect on mortality, but showed significant benefit in unplanned HF hospitalization in 1 year. The Irbesartan in Heart Failure with Preserved Ejection Fraction Study (I-PRESERVE) investigated the effect of the angiotensin-receptor blocker irbesartan on mortality and cardiovascular morbidity in patients with HFpEF [44]. Treatment with irbesartan did not reduce the risk of death or hospitalization for cardiovascular causes among HFpEF patients nor did it improve any of the secondary clinical outcomes, including disease-specific quality of life.

The Study of the Effects of Nebivolol Intervention on Outcomes and Rehospitalization in Seniors (SENIORS) with Heart Failure, which consist of both HFrEF and HFpEF patients,

| Trial | Year | Intervention | No. of subjects | Key inclusion criteria | Key exclusion criteria | Outcome(s) | Findings |
|---|---|---|---|---|---|---|---|
| CHARM-preserved | 2003 | Candesartan versus placebo | 3023 | Age > 18 years<br>LVEF > 40%<br>NYHA class II–IV | Persistent systolic or diastolic hypertension | Hospitalization<br>Mortality | No effect on mortality<br>Slight reduction in HF hospitalization |
| PEP-CHF | 2006 | Perindopril versus placebo | 846 | >40% | | Rehospitalization at 1 year<br>Mortality | No effect on mortality<br>Decreased 1 year rehospitalization and increased exercise capacity |
| SENIORS | 2006 | Nebivolol versus placebo | 752 | >35% | | CV-related hospitalization<br>Mortality | No effect on mortality or hospitalization in patients with EF > 40% |
| I-PRESERVE | 2008 | Irbesartan versus placebo | 4128 | Age > 60 years<br>LVEF > 45%<br>NYHA class II–IV and HF hospitalization < 6 months or NYHA class III/IV and abnormal CXR, ECG, or echocardiogram | AF with resting heart rate > 120 beats/min<br>Cor pulmonale<br>Clinically significant pulmonary disease<br>Significant valvular disease<br>Hb < 11 g/dl<br>BP > 160/95 mm Hg despite therapy | Mortality<br>Hospitalization | No effect on mortality or CV hospitalization |
| ALDO-DHF | 2013 | Spironolactone versus placebo | 422 | Age > 50<br>LVEF > 50%<br>NYHA class II or III<br>Echo evidence of diastolic dysfunction (grade ≥I)<br>Atrial fibrillation at presentation, maximum exercise capacity (peak $VO_2$) < 25 mL/kg/min | Significant CAD<br>Significant pulmonary disease<br>GFR < 30 ml/min<br>MI or CABG in past 3 months | Improvement in diastolic function (E/e′)<br>And maximal exercise capacity ($VO_2$) | Improved diastolic function<br>Induced reverse remodeling<br>Improved neuroendocrine activation but not improve heart failure symptoms or quality of life and slightly reduced 6 min walk distance |

http://dx.doi.org/10.5772/66758

| Trial | Year | Intervention | No. of subjects | Key inclusion criteria | Key exclusion criteria | Outcome(s) | Findings |
|---|---|---|---|---|---|---|---|
| TOPCAT | 2014 | Spironolactone versus placebo | 3445 | Age > 50<br>LVEF > 45%<br>≥1 HF hospitalization in the previous 12 months or<br>BNP ≥100 pg/mL or NT-proBNP ≥360 pg/mL<br>Controlled systolic blood pressure asystolic blood pressure < 140 mm Hg or 140 to 160 mm Hg if on ≥3 antihypertensive medications | COPD<br>Infiltrative of hypertrophic CMP<br>Significant valve disease<br>AF with resting heart rate >90 beats/min<br>GFR < 30 ml/min<br>MI or CABG in past 3 months<br>PCI in past 30 days | Death from cardiovascular causes<br>Aborted cardiac arrest<br>Hospitalization for HF | No effect on cardiovascular death<br>Reduced HF hospitalization<br>Induced an increase in serum creatinine and potassium levels |
| PARAMOUNT | 2012 | LCZ 696 versus valsartan | 301 | Age > 40 years<br>EF > 45%,<br>NYHA class II and III,<br>Elevations of NT-proBNP > 400 pg/ml | LVEF < 45%<br>Isolated right heart failure owing to pulmonary disease<br>Dyspnea from non cardiac causes<br>GFR < 30 ml/min<br>Primary valvular or myocardial diseases<br>Coronary or cerebrovascular diseases needing revascularization within 3 months | Reduction in NT-proBNP at 12 weeks<br>NYHA functional class and LA dimension at 36 weeks | Reduced natriuretic peptides at 12 weeks<br>Improved NYHA class and improved left atrial dimensions at 36 weeks |

| Trial | Year | Intervention | No. of subjects | Key inclusion criteria | Key exclusion criteria | Outcome(s) | Findings |
|---|---|---|---|---|---|---|---|
| RELAX HF | 2013 | versus placebo | **216** | LVEF > 45%<br>NYHA II–IV<br>Previous hospitalization for HF<br>Increased pro NT-pro BNPİ or invasively measured high filling pressure<br>Peak $VO_2$ < 60% | Any obstacle for exercise testing<br>Need for nitrate therapy<br>Primary pulmonary Arteriopathy<br>Primary valve disease<br>Other causes of dyspnea | Exercise capacity<br>Clinical status | No effect on exercise capacity or clinical status |

All abbreviations are explained in the text of the manuscript.

**Table 3.** Major clinical trials in patients with HFPEF.

showed that a beta1-blocker with nitric oxide-potentiating vasodilatory effect, nebivolol, reduces hospitalization in older HF patients with preserved and reduced EF but had no effect on mortality [45]. Preserved EF was considered as EF > 35% which constitutes 35% of the overall study population. The proportion of patients with truly preserved EF (>50%) was very small. Therefore, although the overall study suggests a modest benefit of nebivolol, the results can't be extrapolated to true HFpEF patients.

The mineralocorticoid receptor antagonists spironolactone and eplerenone have been shown to reduce total and cardiovascular mortality across the spectrum of HFrEF and in patients with acute myocardial infarction complicated by left ventricular dysfunction and heart failure [46–48]. By reducing cardiac fibrosis and hypertrophy, aldosterone antagonists have the potential to be beneficial in heart failure with preserved ejection fraction (HFpEF) [49]. In the Aldosterone Receptor Blockade in Diastolic Heart Failure (Aldo-DHF) trial, the effect of spironolactone on diastolic function and exercise capacity in patients with HFpEF was tested [50]. The left ventricular end-diastolic filling, left ventricular remodeling (LV mass index decreased but LA diameter not changed) and neurohumoral activation (NT pro-BNP decreased) were improved with spironolactone, demonstrating aldosterone effect on improving diastolic function and reversing cardiac remodeling. However, spironolactone had no effect on functional exercise capacity in this trial. Upon positive findings with spironolactone on diastolic function and cardiac remodeling, the Treatment of Preserved Cardiac Function Heart Failure with an Aldosterone Antagonist (TOPCAT) trial was planned to investigate whether treatment with spironolactone would reduce morbidity and mortality in patients with HFpEF [51]. The TOPCAT trial found that, compared to placebo, spironolactone did not reduce the composite of cardiovascular death, aborted cardiac arrest or heart failure hospitalization in patients with HFpEF but reduced the individual component of heart failure hospitalization. However, there was a significant interaction between treatment effect and patient recruitment strategy (natriuretic peptides vs. hospitalization with HF). In patients recruited based on previous hospitalization, spironolactone had no effect on outcome, whereas in patients recruited based on high BNP, spironolactone showed a benefit. This difference highlights the importance of patient selection criteria and recruitment of patients with true HFpEF for future trials. The efficacy of eplerenone on 6 min walking distance was evaluated in a single-center, randomized study. It was found that after 24 weeks of eplerenone treatment, there was no change in 6 min walk distance [52]. Another randomized, clinical study evaluated the effect of eplerenone on the primary outcome comprising of death from cardiovascular causes, nonfatal reinfarction, hospitalization for unstable angina, or decompensation of heart failure [53]. Eplerenone was found to have no significant effect on the primary outcome.

Phosphodiesterase-5 (PDE-5) metabolizes the nitric oxide and natriuretic peptide systems' second messenger cyclic guanosine monophosphate and thus may limit beneficial nitric oxide and natriuretic peptide actions in the heart, vasculature and kidneys. Phosphodiesterase type 5 inhibitors (PDE5I) increase cGMP levels by blocking their catabolism. PDE5I may reduce ventricular-vascular stiffening, antagonize maladaptive chamber remodeling, improve endothelial function, reduce pulmonary vascular resistance and enhance renal responsiveness to natriuretic peptides [54, 55]. Phosphodiesterase type 5 inhibitor, sildenafil, was proved to improve hemodynamic parameters in HFrEF patients [56]. The Phosphodiesterase-5

Inhibition to Improve Clinical Status and Exercise Capacity in Heart Failure with Preserved Ejection Fraction (RELAX) trial was conducted to investigate the effect of the PDE-5 inhibitor, on exercise capacity in HFpEF [57]. At the end of 24 weeks, long-term PDE-5 inhibition in HFpEF had no effect on maximal or submaximal exercise capacity, clinical status, quality of life, left ventricular remodeling, diastolic function parameters, or pulmonary artery systolic pressure.

It is known that in both the failing heart and in case of ischemia, the late sodium current is increased, leading to an Na+ accumulation in cardiac myocytes [58]. The increased Na+ concentration reverses the mode direction of the Na+/Ca2+exchanger, contributing to a Ca2+ overload in the cell. Increased diastolic Ca2+ impairs relaxation leading to diastolic dysfunction. By inhibiting the late Na+ channel, ranolazine is theoretically expected to prevent (or reduce) sodium accumulation in the myocyte. This should improve calcium extrusion through the Na+/Ca2+ exchanger and thereby improve relaxation of the myocardium. The Ranolazine for the Treatment of Diastolic Heart Failure (RALI-DHF) study was designed to evaluate the effect of ranolazine versus placebo on hemodynamics, measures of diastolic dysfunction and biomarkers in 20 patients with HFpEF [59]. After 30 min of infusion, significant decreases from baseline were observed in LVEDP and PCWP in the ranolazine group, but not in the placebo group. However, ranolazine had no effect on invasively determined relaxation parameters and the noninvasive E/E′ ratio.

In the recent PARADIGM-HF trial, the patients taking LCZ 696 showed steep reduction in the primary endpoint of CV death/heart failure hospitalization [60]. McMurray et al. noted that a subgroup of patients in the reduced EF spectrum's high end, i.e., LVEF approaching 40%, also benefits to the same extent as the overall study group [61]. Solomon et al. conducted prospective comparison of Angiotensin Receptor Neprilysin Inhibitor (ARNi) with Angiotensin Receptor Blocker (ARB) on Management of heart failure with preserved ejection fraction, PARAMOUNT trial, a double-blind randomized trial in 301 patients with heart failure with HFpEF, which compared LCZ696 with valsartan [62]. The primary endpoint, the decline in NT-proBNP, was significantly greater in the LCZ696 group than in the valsartan group. After 36 weeks, both left atrial volume and dimension, which reflect left ventricular filling pressure, also declined more with LCZ696 and there was greater improvement in the New York Heart Association (NYHA) functional class with LCZ696 than with valsartan.

These encouraging results with LCZ696 have provided the rationale for a large outcomes trial in HFpEF. Prospective Comparison of ARNI with ARB Global Outcomes in Heart Failure with Preserved Ejection Fraction (PARAGON-HF) will use a similar overall study design to that of PARAMOUNT to determine whether LCZ696 can reduce cardiovascular death or total HF hospitalizations in patients with HFpEF. PARAGON-HF will enroll 4,300 patients with HFpEF until the end of 2016.

## 7. Future perspectives

Diagnosis of HFpEF should only be made after complete workup and if noninvasive diagnostic data comprising of LA dilation, diastolic dysfunction and high natriuretic peptide levels,

http://dx.doi.org/10.5772/66758

or invasively measured high LVEDP or PCWP proves indisputably the presence of high LV filling pressure. Only when more specific diagnostic criteria have emerged over time and started to be used in the clinical trials for patient recruitment, we will see improvements in outcome for this common and growing form of cardiac disease. The strategy of a tailored "precision" approach considering both the comorbidities concomitant with HFpEF and underlying pathophysiologic mechanism of reduced cardiac and vascular reserve will lead to improvement in prognosis of HFpEF.

## Author details

Hakan Altay* and Seckin Pehlivanoglu

*Address all correspondence to: sakaltay@yahoo.com

Cardiology Department, Faculty of Medicine, Baskent University, Istanbul Hospital, Turkey

## References

[1] Yancy CW, Jessup M, Wright RS, et al. ACCF/AHA guideline for the management of heart failure: a report of the American College of Cardiology Foundation/American Heart Association Task Force on practice guidelines. *Circulation*. 2013;128(16):e240–e327.

[2] Ponikowski P, Voors AA, Anker SD, Bueno H, Cleland JG, Coats AJ, Falk V, González-Juanatey JR, Harjola VP, Jankowska EA, Jessup M, Linde C, Nihoyannopoulos P, Parissis JT, Pieske B, Riley JP, Rosano GM, Ruilope LM, Ruschitzka F, Rutten FH, van der Meer P; Authors/Task Force Members; Document Reviewers. 2016 ESC guidelines for the diagnosis and treatment of acute and chronic heart failure: the task force for the diagnosis and treatment of acute and chronic heart failure of the European Society of Cardiology (ESC). Developed with the special contribution of the Heart Failure Association (HFA) of the ESC. *Eur J Heart Fail*. 2016;18(8):891–975.

[3] Senni M, Tribouilloy CM, Rodeheffer RJ, Jacobsen SJ, Evans JM, Bailey KR, Redfield MM. Congestive heart failure in the community: a study of all incident cases in Olmsted county, Minnesota, in 1991. *Circulation*. 1998;98:2282–2289.

[4] Owan TE, Hodge DO, Herges RM, Jacobsen SJ, Roger VL, Redfield MM. Trends in prevalence and outcome of heart failure with preserved ejection fraction. *N Engl J Med*. 2006;355:251–259.

[5] Caruana L, Petrie MC, Davie AP, McMurray JJ. Do patients with suspected heart failure and preserved left ventricular systolic function suffer from "diastolic heart failure" or from misdiagnosis? A prospective descriptive study. *BMJ*. 2000;321:215–219.

[6] Bhatia RS, Tu JV, Lee DS, Austin PC, Fang J, Haouzi A, Gong Y, Liu PP. Outcome of heart failure with preserved ejection fraction in a population- based study. *N Engl J Med*. 2006;355:260–269.

[7] Bursi F., et al. Systolic and diastolic heart failure in the community. *JAMA*. 2006; 296:2209–2216.

[8] Owan TE, Hodge DO, Davie AP, et al. Epidemiology of chronic heart failure. *Prog Cardiovasc Dis*. 2005;47:320–332.

[9] Ceia F, Fonseca C, Mota T, Morais H, Matias F, de Sousa A, et al. Prevalence of chronic heart failure in southwestern Europe: the EPICA study. *Eur J Heart Fail*. 2002;4:531–539. This study reports the prevalence of HFpEF in Portuguese reporting a higher prevalence than HFrEF.

[10] Hogg K, Swedberg K, McMurray JJ. Heart failure with preserved left ventricular systolic function; epidemiology, clinical characteristics and prognosis. *J Am Coll Cardiol*. 2004;43:317–327.

[11] Lenzen MJ, Scholte op Reimer WJ, Boersma E, et al. Differences between patients with a preserved and a depressed left ventricular function: a report from the EuroHeart Failure Survey. *Eur Heart J*. 2004;25:1214–1220.

[12] Solomon SD, Wang D, Finn P, Skali H, Zornoff L, McMurray JJV, Swedberg K, Yusuf S, Granger CB, Michelson EL, Pocock S, Pfeffer MA. Effect of candesartan on cause-specific mortality in heart failure patients: the Candesartan in Heart Failure Assessment of Reduction in Mortality and Morbidity (CHARM) program. *Circulation*. 2004;110:2180–2183.

[13] Zile MR, Gaasch WH, Anand IS, et al. Mode of death in patients with heart failure and a preserved ejection fraction: results from the Irbesartan in heart failure with preserved ejection fraction study (I-Preserve) trial. *Circulation*. 2010;121:1393–1405.

[14] Poole-Wilson PA, Uretsky BF, Thygesen K, Cleland JGF, Massie BM, Rydén L. Mode of death in heart failure: findings from the ATLAS trial. *Heart*. 2003;89:42–48.

[15] Hamaguchi S, Kinugawa S, Sobirin MA, Goto D, Tsuchihashi-Makaya M, Yamada S, et al. Mode of death in patients with heart failure and reduced versus preserved ejection fraction: report from the registry of hospitalized heart failure patients. *Circ J*. 2012;76(7):1662–1669.

[16] Campbell RT, Jhund PS, Castagno D, Hawkins NM, Petrie MC, McMurray JJ. What have we learned about patients with heart failure and preserved ejection fraction from DIG-PEF, CHARM-preserved and I-PRESERVE? *J'Coll Cardiol*. 2012;60(23):2349–2356.

[17] Yancy CW, Lopatin M, Stevenson LW, De Marco T, Fonarow GC. Clinical presentation, management and in-hospital outcomes of patients admitted with acute decompensated heart failure with pre-served systolic function: a report from the Acute Decompensated Heart Failure National Registry (ADHERE) database. *J Am Coll Cardiol*. 2006;47(1):76–84.

[18] Kass DA, Bronzwaer JG, Paulus WJ. What mechanisms underlie diastolic dysfunction in heart failure? *Circ Res*. 2004;94:1533–1542.

[19] Borlaug BA, Kass DA. Mechanisms of diastolic dysfunction in heart failure. *Trends Cardiovasc Med*. 2006;16:273–279.

[20] Oxenham HC, Young AA, Cowan BR, et al. Age related changes in myocardial relaxation using three dimensional tagged magnetic resonance imaging. *J Cardiovasc Magn Reson*. 2003;5:421–430.

[21] Paulus WJ, Tschope C. A novel paradigm for heart failure with preserved ejection fraction: comorbidities drive myocardial dysfunction and remodeling through coronary microvascular endothelial inflammation. *J Am Coll Cardiol*. 2013;62:263–271.

[22] Hogg K, McMurray J. Neurohumoral pathways in heart failure with preserved systolic function. *Prog Cardiovasc Dis*. 2005;47:357–366.

[23] Kitzman DW, Little WC, Brubaker PH, et al. Pathophysiological characterization of isolated diastolic heart failure in comparison to systolic heart failure. *JAMA*. 2002;288:2144–2150.

[24] Higginbotham MB, Morris KG, Williams RS, McHale PA, Coleman RD, Cobb FR. Regulation of stroke volume during submaximal and maximal upright exercise in normal man. *Circ Res*. 1986;58:281–291.

[25] Phan TT, Shivu GN, Abozuia K, et al. Impaired heart rate recovery and chronotropic incompetence in patients with heart failure with pre- served ejection fraction. *Circ Heart Fail*. 2010;3:29–34.

[26] Nagueh SF, Appleton CP, Gillebert TC, et al. Recommendations for the evaluation of left ventricular diastolic function by echocardiography. *J Am Soc Echocardiogr*. 2009;22(2):107–133.

[27] Murata K. Predictive significance of evaluation of left ventricular diastolic function in patients with heart failure. *Rinsho Byoki*. 2010;58:792–798.

[28] Shah AM, et al. Cardiac structure and function in heart failure with preserved ejection fraction: baseline findings from the echocardiographic study of the treatment of preserved cardiac function heart failure with an aldosterone antagonist trial. *Circ Heart Fail*. 2014;7:104–115.

[29] Borlaug BA, Nishimura RA, Sorajja P, Lam CS, Redfield MM. Exercise hemodynamics enhance diagnosis of early heart failure with preserved ejection fraction. *Circ Heart Fail*.2010;3:588–595.

[30] Maisel AS, McCord J, Nowak RM, et al. Bedside B type natriuretic peptide in the emergency diagnosis of heart failure with reduced or preserved ejection fraction. Results from the Breathing Not Properly Multinational Study. *J Am Coll Cardiol*. 2003;41:2010–2017.

[31] Anjan VY, et al. Prevalence, clinical phenotype and outcomes associated with normal B-type natriuretic peptide levels in heart failure with preserved ejection fraction. *Am J Cardiol*. 2012;110:870–876.

[32] Tschöpe C, Paulus WJ. Doppler echocardiography yields dubious estimates of left ventricular diastolic pressures. *Circulation*. 2009;120:810–820.

[33] McDonagh TA, Holmer S, Raymond I, Luchner A, Hildebrant P, Dargie HJ. NT-proBNP and the diagnosis of heart failure: a pooled analysis of three European epidemiological studies. *Eur J Heart Fail*. 2004;6:269–273.

[34] Januzzi JL, van Kimmenade R, Lainchbury J, et al. NT-proBNP testing for diagnosis and short-term prognosis in acute destabilized heart failure: an international pooled analysis of 1256 patients: The International Collaborative of NT-proBNP Study. *Eur Heart J*. 2006;27:330–337.

[35] Tsutamoto T, Wada A, Sakai H, Ishikawa C, Tanaka T, Hayashi M, Fujii M, Yamamoto T, Dohke T, Ohnishi M, Takashima H, Kinoshita M, Horie M. Relationship between renal function and plasma brain natriuretic peptide in patients with heart failure. *J Am Coll Cardiol*. 2006;47:582–586.

[36] Knudsen CW, Omland T, Clopton P, et al. Impact of atrial fibrillation on the diagnostic performance of Btype natriuretic peptide concentration in dyspneic patients: an analysis from the breathing not properly multinational study. *J Am Coll Cardiol*. 2005;46(5):838–844.

[37] Schocken DD, Benjamin EJ, Fonarow GC, Krumholz HM, Levy D, Mensah GA, Narula J, Shor ES, Young JB, Hong Y. Prevention of heart failure: a scientific statement from the American Heart Association Councils on Epidemiology and Prevention, Clinical Cardiology, Cardiovascular Nursing and High Blood Pressure Research; Quality of Care and Outcomes Research Interdisciplinary Working Group; and Functional Genomics and Translational Biology Interdisciplinary Working Group. *Circulation*. 2008;117:2544–2565.

[38] Chobanian AV, Bakris GL, Black HR, Cushman WC, Green LA, Izzo Jr JL, et al. The seventh report of the joint national committee on prevention, detection, evaluation and treatment of high blood pressure: the JNC 7 report. *JAMA*. 2003;289:2560–2572.

[39] Kitzman DW, Brubaker PH, Morgan TM, Stewart KP, Little WC. Exercise training in older patients with heart failure and preserved ejection fraction: a randomized, controlled, single-blind trial. *Circ Heart Fail*. 2010;3:659–667.

[40] Kitzman DW, Brubaker PH, Herrington DM, Morgan TM, Stewart KP, Hundley WG, et al. Effect of endurance exercise training on endothelial function and arterial stiffness in older patients with heart failure and preserved ejection fraction: a randomized, controlled, single-blind trial. *J Am Coll Cardiol*. 2013;62:584–592.

[41] Paulus WJ, van Ballegoij JJ. Treatment of heart failure with normal ejection fraction: an inconvenient truth! *J Am Coll Cardiol*. 2010;55:526–537.

[42] Yusuf S, Pfeffer MA, Swedberg K, et al. Effects of candesartan in patients with chronic heart failure and preserved left-ventricular ejection fraction: the CHARM-preserved trial. *Lancet*. 2003;362:777–781.

[43] Cleland JG, Tendera M, Adamus J, Freemantle N, Polonski L, Taylor J. The perindopril in elderly people with chronic heart failure (PEP-CHF) study. *Eur Heart J*. 2006;27:2338–2345.

[44] Massie BM, Carson PE, McMurray JJ, Komajda M, McKelvie R, Zile MR anderson S, Donovan M, Iverson E, Staiger C, Ptaszynska A; I-PRESERVE Investigators. Irbesartan in patients with heart failure and preserved ejection fraction. *N Engl J Med*. 2008;359(23):2456–2467.

[45] Flather MD, Shibata MC, Coats AJ, Van Veldhuisen DJ, Parkhomenko A, Borbola J, et al. Randomized trial to determine the effect of nebivolol on mortality and cardiovascular hospital admission in elderly patients with heart failure (SENIORS). *Eur Heart J*. 2005;26:215–225.

[46] Pitt B, Zannad F, Remme WJ, et al.; Randomized Aldactone Evaluation Study Investigators. The effect of spironolactone on morbidity and mortality in patients with severe heart failure. *N Engl J Med*. 1999;341(10):709–717.

[47] Zannad F, McMurray JJ, Krum H, et al.; EMPHASIS-HF Study Group. Eplerenone in patients with systolic heart failure and mild symptoms. *N Engl J Med*. 2011;364(1):11–21.

[48] Pitt B, Remme W, Zannad F, et al.; Eplerenone Post-Acute Myocardial Infarction Heart Failure Efficacy and Survival Study Investigators. Eplerenone, a selective aldosterone blocker, in patients with left ventricular dysfunction after myocardial infarction. *N Engl J Med*. 2003;348(14):1309–1321.

[49] Lacolley P, Safar ME, Lucet B, Ledudal K, Labat C, Benetos A. Prevention of aortic and cardiac fibrosis by spironolactone in old normotensive rats. *J Am Coll Cardiol*. 2001;37:662–667.

[50] Edelmann F, Schmidt AG, Gelbrich G, et al. Rationale and design of the "Aldosterone Receptor Blockade in Diastolic Heart Failure" trial: a double-blind, randomized, placebo-controlled, parallel group study to determine the effects of spironolactone on exercise capacity and diastolic function in patients with symptomatic diastolic heart failure (Aldo-DHF). *Eur J Heart Fail*. 2010;12(8):874–882.

[51] Pitt B, Pfeffer MA, Assmann SF, Boineau R, Anand IS, Claggett B, Clausell N, Desai AS, Diaz R, Fleg JL, Gordeev I, Harty B, Heitner JF, Kenwood CT, Lewis EF, O'Meara E, Probstfield JL, Shaburishvili T, Shah SJ, Solomon SD, Sweitzer MK, Yang S, McKinlay SM. Spironolactone for heart failure with preserved ejection fraction. *N Engl J Med*. 2014;370:1383–1392.

[52] Deswal A, Richardson P, Bozkurt B, Mann DL. Results of the randomized aldosterone antagonism in heart failure with preserved ejection fraction trial (RAAM-PEF). *J Card Fail*. 2011;17:634–642.

[53] Kampourides K, Tziakas D, Chalikias G, et al. Usefulness of matrix metalloproteinase-9 plasma levels to identify patients with preserved left ventricular systolic function after acute myocardial infarction who could benefit from eplerenone. *Am J Cardiol*. 2012;110:1085–1091.

[54] Vlachopoulos C, Hirata K, O'Rourke MF. Effect of on arterial stiffness and wave reflection. *Vasc Med*. 2003;8:243–248.

[55] Katz SD, Balidemaj K, Homma S, Wu H, Wang J, Maybaum S. Acute type 5 phosphodiesterase inhibition with enhances flow-mediated vasodilation in patients with chronic heart failure. *J Am Coll Cardiol*. 2000;36:845–851.

[56] Lewis GD, Shah R, Shahzad K, et al. improves exercise capacity and quality of life in patients with systolic heart failure and secondary pulmonary hypertension. *Circulation*. 2007;116(14):1555–1562.

[57] Redfield MM, Chen HH, Borlaug BA, Semigran MJ, Lee KL, Lewis G, LeWinter MM, Rouleau JL, Bull DA, Mann DL, Deswal A, Stevenson LW, Givertz MM, Ofili EO, O'Connor CM, Felker GM, Goldsmith SR, Bart BA, McNulty SE, Ibarra JC, Lin G, Oh JK, Patel MR, Kim RJ, Tracy RP, Velazquez EJ, Anstrom KJ, Hernandez AF, Mascette AM, Braunwald E; RELAX Trial. Effect of phosphodiesterase-5 inhibition on exercise capacity and clinical status in heart failure with preserved ejection fraction: a randomized clinical trial. *JAMA*. 2013;309(12):1268–1277

[58] Valdivia CR, Chu WW, Pu J, et al. Increased late sodium current in myocytes from a canine heart failure model and from failing human heart. *J Mol Cell Cardiol*. 2005;38:475–483.

[59] Acobshagen C, Belardinelli L, Hasenfuss G, Maier LS. Ranolazine for the treatment of heart failure with preserved ejection fraction: background, aims and design of the RALI-DHF study. *Clin Cardiol*. 2011;34:426–432.

[60] McMurray JJ, Packer M, Desai AS, Gong J, Lefkowitz MP, Rizkala AR, Rouleau JL, Shi VC, Solomon SD, Swedberg K, Zile MR; PARADIGM-HF Investigators and Committees. Angiotensin-neprilysin inhibition versus enalapril in heart failure. *N Engl J Med*. 2014;371:993–1004.

[61] Solomon S, Packer M, Zile M, et al. The angiotensin receptor neprilysin inhibitor LCZ696 is effective across the spectrum of ejection fraction in heart failure with reduced ejection fraction. *J Card Fail*. 2015;21:S45.

[62] Solomon SD, Zile M, Pieske B, et al.; for the Prospective comparison of ARNI with ARB on Management Of heart failUre with preserved ejectioN fracTion (PARAMOUNT) Investigators. The angiotensin receptor neprilysin inhibitor LCZ696 in heart failure with preserved ejection fraction: a phase 2 double-blind randomized controlled trial. *Lancet*. 2012;380:1387–1395.

Chapter 4

# Left Ventricular Noncompaction

Ana G. Almeida

Additional information is available at the end of the chapter

http://dx.doi.org/10.5772/66291

**Abstract**

Left ventricular noncompaction (LVNC) is accepted as an unclassified (the American Heart Association) or a genetic cardiomyopathy (the European Society of Cardiology), but some argue that this phenotype may be a morphologic trait shared by different cardiomyopathies. This chapter covers the state of the art on the pathology, underlying mechanisms, its clinical manifestations, and diagnosis and treatment modalities of LVNC. LVNC may be defined as follows: an inner non-compacted layer with prominent left ventricular trabeculae and deep intertrabecular recesses and a thin outer compacted layer. Mechanisms are still debatable, with the hypothesis of compaction arrest during embryogenesis as the most accepted theory. Genetic data support LVNC as a distinct cardiomyopathy, although evidence for LVNC as a shared morphological trait is not ruled out, since LVNC may be associated with other cardiomyopathies, congenital heart diseases and in some cases may be acquired. Diagnosis is based on imaging and may be confirmed by the use of genetics. Clinical picture and prognosis and the management options are discussed.

**Keywords:** cardiomyopathy, Noncompaction, Echocardiography, cardiovascular magnetic resonance, prognosis

## 1. Introduction

Left ventricular noncompaction (LVNC) is a myocardial disorder that has been thought to occur due to the failure of left ventricle (LV) compaction during embryogenesis, leading to distinct morphological characteristics in the ventricular chamber [1]. In its first description, about 80 years ago, LVNC occurred in association with complex congenital heart diseases. More recently, an isolated form of LVNC was described [2], followed by many other reports. The involvement of the right ventricle in the noncompaction process has been increasingly identified, and the condition is now included among the cardiomyopathies, but currently there is an intense debate whether LVNC is a distinct entity or a trait common to several cardiac conditions [3].

## 2. Anatomy and pathology

Left ventricular noncompaction (LVNC) is defined by essential markers: an inner noncompacted layer with prominent left ventricular (LV) trabeculae and deep intertrabecular recesses, and a thin compacted layer. There is a spectrum of morphologic variability, ranging from hearts with different degrees of noncompaction extension and amount, and right ventricular involvement.

From hearts obtained from autopsies or transplantation, LVNC diagnosis is based on the presence of a two-layered ventricular wall, comprising a thinner compact epicardial layer and an inner noncompacted layer, with prominent trabeculations associated with deep, intertrabecular recesses that communicate with the ventricular cavity but not with the coronary circulation [2, 3].

Noncompacted areas are commonly located at the LV apex and mid-apical wall segments, but typically spares the interventricular septum. When associated with hypertrophic cardiomyopathy phenotype (HCM), the hypertrophied septum coexists with the LVNC phenotype. Other described associations include dilated cardiomyopathy (DCM) and, more rarely, restrictive cardiomyopathy (RCM) or arrhythmogenic right ventricular cardiomyopathy (ARVC). Besides the relationship of LVNC with other cardiomyopathies, which may share the same genetic basis, there has been considerable controversy regarding the differentiation from normal LV trabeculation, which seems to occur in some normal asymptomatic individuals as found in analysis from the MESA study [4].

Histopathology has shown continuity between the endothelium of inter-trabecular recesses and that of the endocardium, distinguishing LVNC from persistent sinusoids. Other findings have included loosely organised myocytes and endocardial and subendocardial replacement fibrosis suggestive of ischaemic necrosis, which has been demonstrated by imaging techniques *in vivo* [5].

LV dilatation and ischemia are frequently present, and thrombus formation in the recesses may occur, which may be associated with possible thromboembolic events.

## 3. Aetiology and mechanisms

There are several etiologic hypotheses for LVNC. It may occur as an isolated disease (isolated LVNC) or in association with genetic diseases and congenital defects, as observed more commonly in infancy. The condition may also be sporadic and acquired, in physiological or pathologic conditions, and may also be permanent or transient. Thus, LVNC can originate during embryonic development or be acquired later in life.

http://dx.doi.org/10.5772/66291

The theory that supports the embryogenic hypothesis has been based in observational foetal studies showing the coexistence of LVNC with heart block and congenital heart diseases and from experimental studies on LVNC [6]. In humans, the embryonic myocardium is composed of a loose meshwork of interwoven fibres separated by deep recesses, which communicate with the LV cavity, allowing an increase in the myocardial surface area and the exchange diffusion from the cavity. From the 5th–8th weeks of embryogenesis, LV trabecular compaction occurs simultaneously with the invasion of the myocardium by the coronary vasculature coming from the epicardium. The LV compaction progresses from the heart base to the apex and from the epicardium to the endocardium [1]. LVNC is thus thought to result from the arrest of trabecular compaction during this phase of embryogenesis. A second embryogenic hypothesis suggests that LVNC results from the inhibition of the regression of embryonic structures that would maintain the looseness of cells or of cell bundles [7].

On the other hand, evidence supports the hypothesis that the pathogenetic mechanisms leading to noncompaction may occur in adult life, ending in acquired forms of LVNC and supporting a non-embryogenic theory. This is the case of young athletes, pregnant women, patients with sickle cell disease, and renal failure, which may present the phenotype of LVNC. In athletes, the phenotype seems to relate to intensive training, but in a small proportion of 0.9% has been found to develop ultimately LV dysfunction suggestive of a LVNC cardiomyopathy [8]. In pregnancy, an important proportion of women, described as up to 25% were found to develop LVNC phenotype de novo, which was reversible. This pattern was not shown to be associated with deleterious clinical events and has been proposed to result from a response to increased loading conditions [9]. Also, in sickle cell disease, this pattern has been found and hypothesised to result from chronic anaemia and increased preload, resulting in a stimulus for hypertrabeculation [10].

## 4. Genetics

The LVNC trait may be familial, inherited, or non-familial, sporadic. Non-familial forms are diagnosed when LVNC is proven absent in relatives. As presented above, sporadic LVNC can be acquired and may be transient, as in highly trained athletes, sickle cell anaemia patients, and pregnancy. Many familial cases identified to date are associated with mutations in the same genes that cause other types of cardiomyopathies but may also occur isolated.

In fact, several studies suggest that noncompaction of the LV myocardium is a genetically heterogeneous disorder [11], with a familial and a sporadic form. Studies of the familial form have shown that LVNC may be transmitted as an autosomal dominant inheritance with incomplete penetrance, as an autosomal recessive, and as X-linked traits. Sporadic cases of LVNC and *de novo* mutations have also been recognised. To date, several disease *loci* have been identified.

The Barth syndrome was the first recognised genetic LVNC, characterised by dilated cardiomyopathy associated with LVNC. It is an X-linked disease with mutations in the G4.5 gene, located at Xq28, which encodes the tafazzins (a family of proteins) with acetyltransferase functions in the mitochondria. This mutation was also identified in an X-linked severe neonatal LVNC, allelic with the Barth syndrome.

Another mutation, located in the $\alpha$-dystrobrevin gene, was identified subsequently in patients with LVNC and associated with congenital heart diseases. [12]; $\alpha$-dystrobrevin is a cytoskeletal protein component of the dystrophin associated glycoprotein complex, which links the extracellular matrix to the dystrophin cytoskeleton of the muscle fibre. This mutation was associated with a significant phenotypic variability with variable severity.

Mutations in the Z-line protein Cypher/ZASP have been identified in association with LVNC and dilated cardiomyopathy. This protein appears to play an important role in the maintenance of the normal myocyte architecture of cardiac and skeletal muscle.

Another LVNC phenotype has been reported in association with a mutation in the Lamin A/C protein, which has been linked to dilated cardiomyopathy, conduction system diseases, and muscular dystrophy.

Recently, LVNC has been linked to sarcomere gene mutations, causing hypertrophic cardiomyopathy. In a study of 247 families with cardiomyopathy, a mutation in the $\alpha$-cardiac actin gene, essential for cell maintenance, was associated with LVNC, apical hypertrophic cardiomyopathy, and septal defects. Moreover, in a large study of patients with phenotype of LVNC, nine heterozygous mutations were identified in a proportion of the probands in genes encoding $\alpha$-myosin heavy chain (MYH7), β-cardiac actin (ACTC), and cardiac troponin T (TNNT2), with 100% penetrance in the family members [13]. Another study identified a mutation in the sarcomeric TPM1 gene, at 15q22.1, in a family with LVNC and a history of sudden death.

Some studies have suggested that the phenotype for isolated LVNC may appear during adult life in patients with muscular dystrophy and with myocarditis. Nevertheless, these cases were not followed serially clinically and with an imaging modality, and the significance of the LV hypertrabeculation described is still unclear.

Although, many genes associated with LVNC are associated with additional phenotypes, like hypertrophic or dilated cardiomyopathies or congenital heart defects, several mutations were described in association with isolated LVNC. For instance, mutations in gene MIB1 were identified in two families with LVNC and autosomal dominant inheritance [14]. Recently, an important role in trabeculation for endocardial expression of a Notch ligand, Fkbp1a, was reported, [15] which was confirmed in a mouse model, suggesting its direct involvement in the LVNC phenotype.

A large number of genes have been identified in relation with the LVNC phenotype in association with other cardiomyopathies, congenital and acquired heart diseases, as well as part of syndromes; specific genetic mutations have been related with the LVNC phenotype, and there is a need for large databases and systematic follow-up with clinical and imaging to obtain definite conclusions on the clinical and prognostic significance of LVNC phenotype in relation with the genotype.

The role of modifying genes or epigenetics and load changes may influence the relationship of genotype-phenotype and contribute to explain the phenotype variability.

## 5. Epidemiology

LVNC has been considered rare, and its incidence and prevalence are uncertain, but is commonly diagnosed, due to increased awareness and more accurate imaging methods.

LVNC has been described to occur in infants (0.81 per 100,000 infants/year), children (0.12 cases per 100,000 children/year), and adults (prevalence suggested as 0.014% of patients referred for echocardiography and 0.05% among all adult echocardiograms in a large institution) [16, 17]. In a large population of patients with LV ejection fraction <45%, the prevalence was 3.7% [18]. However, LVNC can occur as an isolated myocardial trait or be associated with cardiomyopathies (hypertrophic, restrictive, dilated, and arrhythmogenic), congenital heart diseases, and complex syndromes affecting multiple organs and tissues, including mitochondrial diseases caused by mutations in both nuclear and mitochondrial genes, leading to increased uncertainty on the prevalence.

In fact, given the variability of clinical presentation, the prevalence of LVNC is largely unknown.

## 6. Clinical manifestations

Heart failure, ventricular and atrial arrhythmias, and systemic embolic events comprise the typical complications in patients with LVNC and may occur at any age. However, the initial presentation is variable and the patient may be asymptomatic (frequently diagnosed during a family screening) or present any of the clinical features and complications, including sudden death.

In its severe neonatal form, LVNC may manifest as heart failure or ventricular arrhythmias, which may lead to sudden death [2]. Studies of older children and adults have reported a high incidence of severe manifestations [7, 17, 19–22] such as LV dysfunction, thromboembolic events, which probably originate in the deep intertrabecular recesses, arrhythmias, and sudden death. Other studies, however, have found a much lower incidence of complications, suggesting subclinical or milder cases [23]. **Table 1** presents clinical findings from published studies.

There is no agreement so far on the natural history and outcomes in LVNC because most studies are retrospective, populations are limited and use distinct study methods.

Heart failure seems to occur frequently, as over 50% of symptomatic patients, and most researchers also report ventricular arrhythmias, cardiovascular deaths, and sudden cardiac death. A recent registry of a large population of adult patients with LVNC found heart failure in 74%, LV systolic dysfunction in 88%, strokes in 10%, and syncope episodes in 9%, [20] suggesting the need for long term surveillance of LVNC patients. Other series have found a more benign prognosis [23]. A recent published series describe a mean freedom from death or transplantation of 97% at 46 months in adults with LVNC.

| Author | Chin | Ichida | Oechslin | Murphy | Lofiego | Aras | Stanton | Greutmann |
|---|---|---|---|---|---|---|---|---|
| Patients (N) | 8 | 27 | 34 | 45 | 65 | 67 | 30 | 132 |
| Population | Paediatric | Paediatric | Adult | Adult | Adult | Adult | Adult | >14 years-old |
| Follow-up | ≤5 years | ≤17 years | 44 months | 46 months | 46 months | 30 months | 2.5 years | 2.7 years |
| Family history (%) | 50 | 44 | 18 | 51 | 31 | 33 | – | 23 |
| Embolic events (%) | 38 | 0 | 21 | 4 | 5 | 9 | 0 | 4 |
| Ventricular tachycardia (%) | 38 | 0 | 41 | 20 | 6 | 36 | 27 | 4 |
| Heart failure (%) | 63 | 30 | 68 | 67 | 34 | 34 | – | 13 |
| CV death or transplantation (%) | 0 | 11 | 47 | 2 | 24 | 15 | 10 | 23 |
| Sudden death (%) | 13 | 0 | 18 | 2 | 5 | 9 | 10 | 9 |

LVNC, left ventricle noncowmpaction; CV, cardiovascular.

**Table 1.** LVNC clinical characteristics and outcomes.

Predictors of death and heart transplantation have been difficult to assess due to the variability of the phenotype and the variable underlying pathophysiological scenarios. However, the presence of heart failure, history of sustained ventricular tachycardia or systemic thromboembolism seem to be associated with an unfavourable prognosis among other phenotypes with distinct outcomes [21, 22]. In a recent study, mortality did not differ significantly between patients with isolated LVNC and control patients with dilated cardiomyopathy, [24] suggesting that LV dysfunction rather than the phenotype itself is the risk-increasing mechanism. However, this finding has not been confirmed by others [17].

## 7. Diagnosis

Cardiac imaging is essential for establishing the diagnosis of LVNC, not only to detect the characteristic features and application of the diagnostic criteria, but to assess the systolic and diastolic function, valve regurgitation, pulmonary hypertension, the presence of thrombus in the ventricular recesses. However, there is still a lack of agreement from the medical community regarding the best technique and the most reliable diagnostic criterion. **Table 2** summarises the most frequently used imaging criteria for LVNC diagnosis.

### 7.1. Echocardiography

Cardiac ultrasound is a first-line technique for diagnosing LVNC, since it is a bedside modality, uses no radiation and is readily available. This modality allows the detection, location,

| Jenni et al. [25] | Stlöberger et al. [26] | Petersen et al. [30] | Jacquier et al. [31] |
|---|---|---|---|
| Echo | Echo | CMR | CMR |
| - Ratio noncompacted/ compacted >2.0 | - Three trabeculations protruding from the LV wall, apically to the papillary muscles, visible in one image plane | - Ratio noncompacted/ compacted >2.3 | - Trabecular LV mass >20% of global LV mass, |
| - Intratrabecular recesses filled by blood flow from the LV cavity | - Intertrabecular spaces perfused from the ventricular cavity on colour Doppler imaging | - Acquisition: long-axis end-diastolic images | - Acquisition: end-diastolic images |
| - Acquisition: short-axis; end-systolic images | - Trabeculations with the same echogenicity as the myocardium and synchronous with LV<br>- Acquisition: oblique views to differentiate false chords, aberrant bands, trabeculations | | |

LV, left ventricle.

**Table 2.** The most frequently used diagnostic criteria in left ventricle noncompaction.

and confirmation of this condition. The first criterion was proposed by Chin et al. [2], who recommended the assessment of the ratio of X/Y dimensions in diastole—where X is the distance from the epicardial surface to the trough of the trabecular recesses, and Y the distance from the epicardial surface to the peak of the trabeculation. An X/Y ratio of up to 0.5 would be required for the diagnosis. The more widely used criterion, however, was proposed by Jenni et al. in which the ratio of noncompacted and compacted myocardium, measured from end systolic short-axis images. If the ratio is >2, the criterion for LVNC is considered fulfilled [25] (**Figures 1** and **2**). Additionally, observation and quantification of the apical trabeculations are available by echocardiography, although sometimes challenging, and permit the use of the LVNC criterion proposed by Stöllberger et al. [26].

The inherent limitation of echocardiography in evaluating the LV apex and, often, other LV walls poses a diagnostic issue. If the image quality is poor, LVNC can be confused with apical cardiomyopathy, thrombus or fibroelastosis. The use of contrast echocardiography, which permits the visualisation of the trabeculations and the recesses that communicate with the cavity, may help in clarifying the diagnosis [27]. Additional information with prognostic impact may be derived from the evaluation of LV systolic and diastolic function, mitral regurgitation, pulmonary hypertension. Systolic dysfunction is frequently present in LVNC. It has been hypothesised that microvascular disease with impaired coronary flow reserve and myocardial necrosis, as well as a primary myocardial disease, is responsible for the functional abnormalities [5], although in other cases a DCM may be associated, The presence of thrombus in the ventricular recesses, although rare, has been described.

More recently, speckle tracking has revealed abnormal LV rotation and twist, and these findings are promising for diagnosis even in patients with normal ejection fraction [28]. Three-dimension echocardiography has been proposed as an alternative for detecting LVNC due to

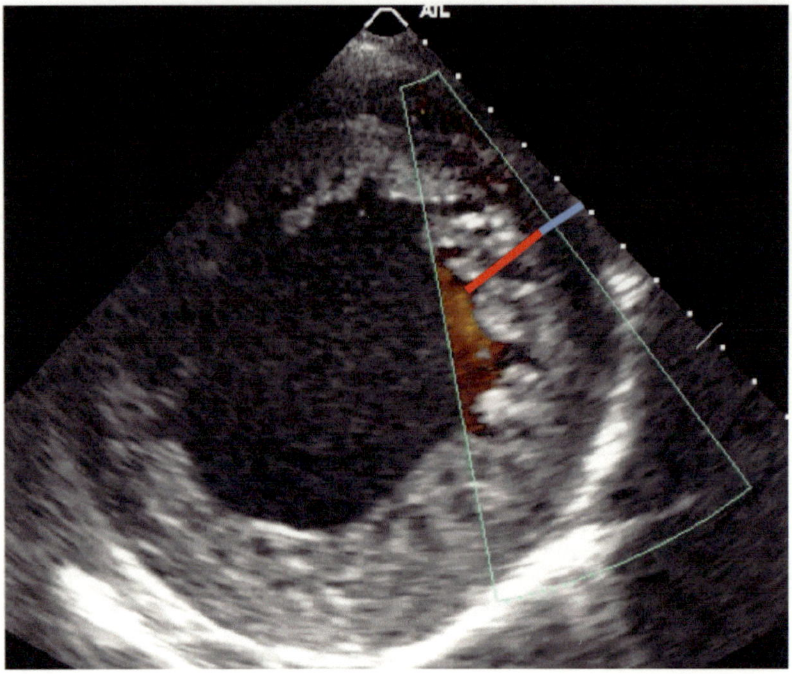

**Figure 1.** A systolic short-axis image from an echocardiogram of a 27-year-old patient with LVNC, showing the ratio measurement of compacted layer (blue line) to noncompacted layer (red line) of >2; Doppler colour shows the blood flow in the recesses.

the lower dependence on the observer for image acquisition and higher reproducibility [29]. However, the image quality and resolution may be compromised in comparison with the conventional 2D, remaining uncertain its real value.

### 7.2. Cardiovascular magnetic resonance (CMR)

CMR is a non-ionising high-resolution technique without acoustic limitations, which reveals a wider extent of disease, particularly at the LV apex and the poorly observed segments, which are often problematic with echocardiography.

This modality confirms the presence of the anatomic features of LVNC, as well as an accurate and reproducible measurement of the noncompacted and compacted myocardial layers (**Figures 3** and **4**). The diagnosis is supported if the end-diastolic thickness of the noncompacted layer is ≥2.3 times the compacted one, as proposed by Petersen et al. [30]. This criterion yielded >43% of positive subjects in MESA study, although this population included only asymptomatic individuals, with low pretest probability of disease [4].

CMR confirmation of trabeculated LV mass >20% of global LV mass fulfils the criterion proposed by Jacquier et al. [31] although the feasibility and reproducibility of this methodology have been debated.

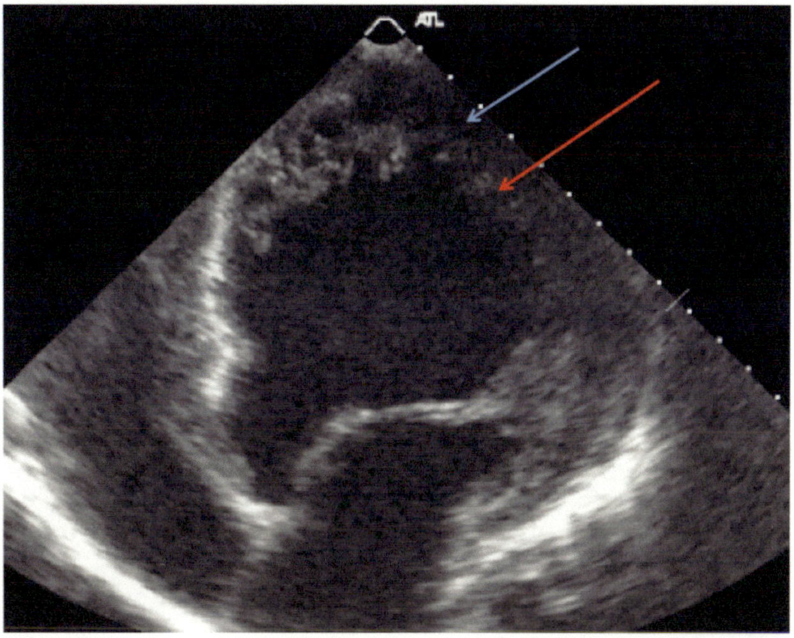


**Figure 2.** A diastolic four-chamber image from an echocardiogram of a patient with LVNC. Blue arrow—compacted layer; red arrow—noncompacted layer.

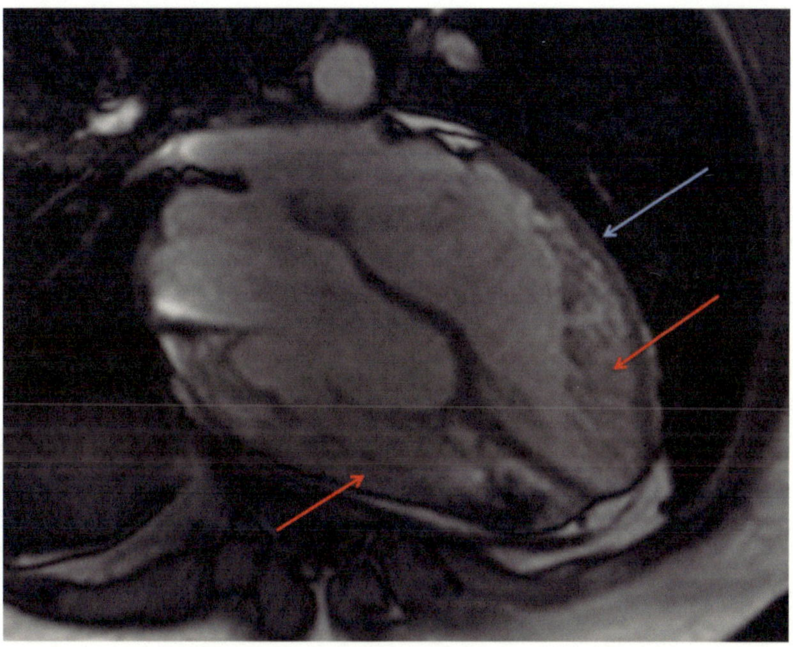

**Figure 3.** A diastolic four-chamber view from a magnetic resonance cine study of a 23-year-old patient with LVNC, showing biventricular noncompaction. Blue arrow—compacted layer; red arrows—noncompacted layers.

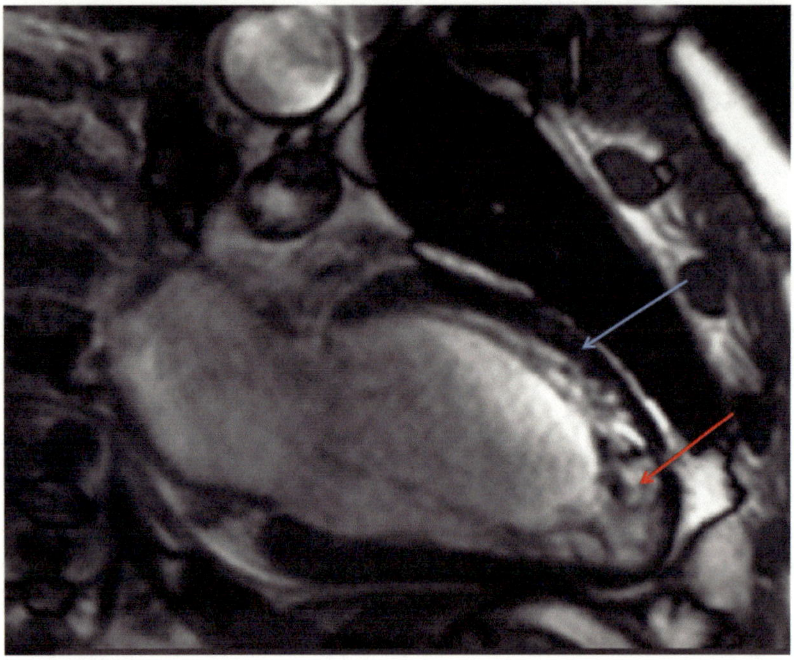

**Figure 4.** A diastolic two-chamber view from a magnetic resonance cine study of a patient with LVNC and arrhythmia. Blue arrow—compacted layer; red arrows—noncompacted layer.

Fractal analysis was also used to quantify LV trabeculae. In a study of 30 patients of Captur et al., the combination of end-diastolic measurements at basal, mid, and apical segments was found to be the best selector of LVNC cases from the normal population [32].

The combined use of echocardiography and CMR may contribute to lessening the risk of over diagnosing LVNC, which can occur with the isolated use of ultrasound, and overcome the limitations on reproducibility of echocardiography [33], but such an approach has not yet been validated.

Reliable evaluation of LV function is an additional advantage offered by CMR. Involvement of the right ventricle remains controversial because echocardiography presents inherent difficulties in analysing this chamber, but CMR has been increasingly detecting biventricular LVNC, although no specific criteria have been proposed so far.

Late gadolinium enhancement (LGE) CMR, as a surrogate marker of fibrosis, has been detected in patients with LVNC and confirmed by histology. A recent study suggests that the presence and amount of LGE is associated with more severe clinical [34]. Abnormal T2-weighting myocardial intensity and perfusion defects have been described as additional information obtained from CMR but its usefulness is not established so far.

### 7.3. Cardiac computed tomography

This modality has been proposed as an alternative to patients that have acoustic limitations to echocardiography and contra-indications for CMR, due to the high spatial resolution provided by this technique [35].

### 7.4. Electrocardiogram

Electrocardiogram (ECG) may be normal. ECG changes, when present, are non-specific and include LV hypertrophy and repolarisation abnormalities. Left bundle branch block is common, especially in patients with LV dysfunction. Wolff–Parkinson–White has been frequently detected in paediatric patients [36].

## 8. Management and prognosis

The true significance of noncompaction still remains a matter of debate, due to the genetic heterogeneity, the overlapping phenotype with other cardiomyopathies sharing the same genetic background, the high prevalence in neuromuscular diseases. These findings suggest that other factors may play a role in the development of LVNC disease [37]. Another important challenge is the clear differentiation of the LVNC phenotype from the normal heart, since this is associated with the risk of overdiagnosis.

There are no specific guidelines for management of LVNC since evidence supporting the management is limited. First of all, management includes confirmation of the diagnosis by echocardiography or CMR.

Guidelines suggest that familial LVNC should be diagnosed by echocardiographic screening of family members [38]. Echocardiographic screening is recommended for family members, given that the symptoms are variable and the risks include heart failure and sudden cardiac death.

According to current guidelines, mutation-specific genetic testing is recommended for family members and appropriate relatives, following the identification of an LVNC causative mutation in the index case. Moreover, this testing may be useful for patients where the cardiologist has established a clinical diagnosis of LV noncompaction based on examination of the patient's clinical manifestations (namely with increased pre-test probability or left ventricular dysfunction [39]) and family history, electrocardiographic and echocardiographic phenotype or when associated with another cardiomyopathy or congenital heart disease. Following genetic and imaging assessment, the possibility of an early diagnosis of LVNC increases, ensuring appropriate monitoring and prophylactic measures.

According to recent American Heart Association/American College of Cardiology Scientific Statement on Eligibility and Disqualification Recommendations for Competitive Athletes With Cardiovascular Abnormalities, "until more clinical information is available, participation in competitive sports may be considered for asymptomatic patients with a diagnosis of LVNC and normal systolic function, without important ventricular tachyarrhythmias on ambulatory monitoring or exercise testing, and specifically with no prior history of unexplained syncope (Class IIb; Level of Evidence C)" [40].

The main therapeutic objectives are the prevention and treatment of complications, using conventional measures. Thromboembolism, heart failure, and arrhythmias constitute the typical clinical features of LVNC to be addressed.

Anticoagulation for prevention of thromboembolism is probably only indicated in cases of LV dilatation and dysfunction, or when a previous history of embolic events is present, although to date no data are available to support these options. For symptomatic ventricular arrhythmias, particularly the ones associated with LV and for heart failure, the treatment should follow current guidelines. In patients with severe LV dysfunction, ICD implantation and CRT therapy are measures to improve heart failure and prevent sudden death. In some cases, heart transplantation may be the option for patients with refractory heart failure [41].

## 9. Conclusion

The pathogenesis and diagnosis of LVNC remains a challenge. The disease may be secondary to genetic mutations that induce the myocardial pathology. However, phenotypes are heterogeneous, are frequently shared with other cardiomyopathy, suggesting the influence of additional modifiers or a common aetiology.

The detection of new genetic mutations and the evaluation of its relationship with phenotypes may shed light on the pathogenesis of this condition, which may have an impact on follow-up and management.

The current awareness of the disease and the availability of high-resolution imaging, namely CMR, have increased the number of diagnosed patients. There is, however, a risk of overdiagnoses. The genotype and phenotype heterogeneity suggests the need for multicentre studies involving large populations, allowing more

robust conclusions regarding all the important areas of LVNC including the clinical ground, genetics, pathogenesis, diagnosis, and management.

## Acknowledgements

Funding source: Cardiovascular Centre of Lisbon University.

## Author details

Ana G. Almeida

Address all correspondence to: anagalmeida@gmail.com; amalmeida@medicina.ulisboa.pt

Faculty of Medicine of Lisbon University, University Hospital Santa Maria/CHLN/Academic Centre of Lisbon University, Cardiovascular Centre of Lisbon University (FCT), Lisbon, Portugal.

## References

[1] Sedmera D, Pexieder T, Vuillemin M, et al. Developmental patterning of the myocardium. Anat Rec. 2000;258:319–37.

[2] Chin TK, Perloff JK, Williams RG, et al. Isolated noncompaction of left ventricular myocardium. A study of eight cases. Circulation. 1990;82:507–13.

[3] Arbustini E, Weidemann F, Hall JL. Left ventricular noncompaction: a distinct cardiomyopathy or a trait shared by different cardiac diseases? J Am Coll Cardiol. 2014;64:1840–50.

[4] Zemrak F, Ahlman MA, Captur G, Mohiddin SA, Kawel-Boehm N, Prince MR, Moon JC, Hundley WG, Lima JA, Bluemke DA, Petersen SE. The relationship of left ventricular trabeculation to ventricular function and structure over a 9.5-year follow-up: the MESA study. J Am Coll Cardiol. 2014 ;64:1971–80.

[5] Jenni R, Wyss CA, Oechslin EN, et al. Isolated ventricular noncompaction is associated with coronary microcirculatory dysfunction. J Am Coll Cardiol. 2002;39:450–4.

[6] Vinograd CA, Srivastava S, Panesar LE. Fetal diagnosis of left-ventricular noncompaction cardiomyopathy in identical twins with discordant congenital heart disease. Pediatr Cardiol. 2013;34:1503–7.

[7] Oechslin EN, Attenhofer Jost CH, Rojas JR, et al. Long-term follow-up of 34 adults with isolated left ventricular noncompaction: a distinct cardiomyopathy with poor prognosis. J Am Coll Cardiol 2000;36:493–500.

[8] Gati S, Chandra N, Bennett RL, et al. Increased left ventricular trabeculation in highly trained athletes: do we need more stringent criteria for the diagnosis of left ventricular non-compaction in athletes? Heart. 2013;99:401–8.

[9] Gati S, Papadakis M, Papamichael ND, et al. Reversible de novo left ventricular trabeculations in pregnant women: implications for the diagnosis of left ventricular noncompaction in low-risk populations. Circulation. 2014;130:475–83.

[10] Gati S, Papadakis M, Van Niekerk N, et al. Increased left ventricular trabeculation in individuals with sickle cell anaemia: physiology or pathology? Int J Cardiol. 2013;168:1658–60.

[11] Oechslin E, Jenni R. Left ventricular non-compaction revisited: a distinct phenotype with genetic heterogeneity? Eur Heart J. 2011;32:1446–56.

[12] Ichida F, Tsubata S, Bowles KR, et al. Novel gene mutations in patients with left ventricular noncompaction or Barth syndrome. Circulation. 2001;103:1256–63.

[13] Klaassen S, Probst S, Oechslin E, et al. Mutations in sarcomere protein genes in left ventricular noncompaction. Circulation. 2008;117:2893–90.

[14] Luxan G, Casanova JC, Martinez-Poveda B, et al. Mutations in the NOTCH pathway regulator MIB1 cause left ventricular noncompaction cardiomyopathy. Nat Med. 2013;19:193–201.

[15] Chen H, Zhang W, Sun X, et al. Fkbp1a controls ventricular myocardium trabeculation and compaction by regulating endocardial Notch1 activity. Development. 2013;140:1946–57.

[16] Ritter M, Oechslin E, Sütsch G, Attenhofer C, Schneider J, Jenni R. Isolated noncompaction of the myocardium in adults. Mayo Clin Proc. 1997; 72:26–31.

[17] Aras D, Tufekcioglu O, Ergun K, et al. Clinical features of isolated ventricular noncompaction in adults long-term clinical course, echocardiographic properties, and predictors of left ventricular failure. J Card Fail. 2006;12:726–33.

[18] Sandhu R, Finkelhor RS, Gunawardena DR, Bahler RC. Prevalence and characteristics of left ventricular noncompaction in a community hospital cohort of patients with systolic dysfunction. Echocardiography. 2008;25:8–12.

[19] Ichida F, Hamamichi Y, Miyawaki T, et al. Clinical features of isolated noncompaction of the ventricular myocardium: long-term clinical course, hemodynamic properties, and genetic background. J Am Coll Cardiol. 1999;34:233–40.

[20] Habib G, Charron P, Eicher JC, et al. Isolated left ventricular non-compaction in adults: clinical and echocardiographic features in 105 patients. Results from a French registry. Eur J Heart Fail. 2011;13:177–85.

[21] Lofiego C, Biagini E, Pasquale F, et al. Wide spectrum of presentation and variable outcomes of isolated left ventricular noncompaction. Heart. 2007;93:65–71.

[22] Greutmann M, Mah ML, Silversides CK, et al. Predictors of adverse outcome in adolescents and adults with isolated left ventricular noncompaction. Am J Cardiol. 2012;109:276–81.

[23] Murphy RT, Thaman R, Blanes JG, et al. Natural history and familial characteristics of isolated left ventricular noncompaction. Eur Heart J. 2005;26:187–92.

[24] Stanton C, Bruce C, Connolly H, et al. Isolated left ventricular noncompaction syndrome. Am J Cardiol. 2009;104:1135–8.

[25] Jenni R, Oechslin E, Schneider J, et al. Echocardiographic and pathoanatomical characteristics of isolated left ventricular non-compaction: a step towards classification as a distinct cardiomyopathy. Heart. 2001;86:666–71.

[26] Stöllberger C, Finsterer J, Blazek G. Left ventricular hypertrabeculation, noncompaction and association with additional cardiac abnormalities and neuromuscular disorders. Am J Cardiol. 2002;90:899–902.

[27] Chow CM, Lim KD, Wu L, et al. Images in cardiovascular medicine. Isolated left ventricular noncompaction enhanced by echocontrast agent. Circulation. 2007;116:e90–1.

[28] Bellavia D, Michelena HI, Martinez M, et al. Speckle myocardial imaging modalities for early detection of myocardial impairment in isolated left ventricular non-compaction. Heart. 2010;96:440–7.

[29] Caselli S, Autore C, Serdoz A, et al. Three-dimensional echocardiographic characterization of patients with left ventricular noncompaction. J Am Soc Echocardiogr. 2012;25:203–9.

[30] Petersen SE, Selvanayagam JB, Wiesmann F, et al. Left ventricular non-compaction: insights from cardiovascular magnetic resonance imaging. J Am Coll Cardiol. 2005;46:101–5.

[31] Jacquier A, Thuny F, Jop B, et al. Measurement of trabeculated left ventricular mass using cardiac magnetic resonance imaging in the diagnosis of left ventricular non-compaction. Eur Heart J. 2010;31:1098–104.

[32] Captur G, Muthurangu V, Cook C, et al. Quantification of left ventricular trabeculae using fractal nalysis. J Cardiovasc Magn Reson. 2013;15:36.

[33] Stöllberger C, Gerecke B, Engberding R, et al. Interobserver agreement of the echocardiographic diagnosis of LV hypertrabeculation/noncompaction. J Am Coll Cardiol Img. 2015;8:1252–1257.

[34] Nucifora G, Aquaro GD, Pingitore A, et al. Myocardial fibrosis in isolated left ventricular noncompaction and its relation to disease severity. Eur J Heart Fail. 2011;13:170–6.

[35] Sidhu MS, Uthamalingam, Ahmed SW, et al. Defining left ventricular noncompaction using cardiac computed tomography. J Thorac Imaging. 2014;29:60–6.

[36] Petersen SE. Left ventricular noncompaction. A clinically useful diagnostic label? JACC Cardiovasc Imaging. 2015;8:947–8.

[37] Almeida AG, Pinto FJ. Non-compaction cardiomyopathy. Heart. 2013;99:1535–1542.

[38] Hershberger RE, Lindenfeld J, Mestroni L, et al. Genetic evaluation of cardiomyopathy—a Heart Failure Society of America practice guideline. J Card Fail. 2009;15:83–97.

[39] Aung N, Zemrak F, Mohiddin SA, Petersen SB. LV noncompaction cardiomyopathy or just a lot of trabeculations? JACC Cardiovasc Imaging. 2016 Aug 20.

[40] Maron BJ, Udelson JE, Bonow RO, et al. Eligibility and disqualification recommendations for competitive athletes with cardiovascular abnormalities: Task Force 3: hypertrophic cardiomyopathy, arrhythmogenic right ventricular cardiomyopathy and other cardiomyopathies, and myocarditis: a scientific statement from the American Heart Association and American College of Cardiology. J Am Coll Cardiol. 2015;66:2362–71.

[41] Arbustini E, Favalli V, Narula N, Serio A, Grasso M. Left ventricular noncompaction: a distinct genetic cardiomyopathy? J Am Coll Cardiol. 2016;68:949–66.

Section 3

# Non-specific Cardiomyopathies

Chapter 5

# Inherited Cardiomyopathies: From Genotype to Phenotype

Marissa Lopez-Pier, Yulia Lipovka,
Eleni Constantopoulos and John P. Konhilas

Additional information is available at the end of the chapter

http://dx.doi.org/10.5772/65393

**Abstract**

The heart undergoes extensive morphological, metabolic, and energetic remodeling in response to inherited, or familial, hypertrophic cardiomyopathies (FHC). Myocyte contractile perturbations downstream of $Ca^{2+}$, the so-called sarcomere-controlled mechanisms, may represent the earliest indicators of this remodeling. We can now state that the *dynamics* of cardiac contraction and relaxation during the progression of FHC are governed by downstream mechanisms, particularly the *kinetics* and *energetics* of actin and myosin interaction to drive the trajectory of pathological cardiac remodeling. This notion is unambiguously supported by elegant studies above linking inheritable FHC-causing mutations to cardiomyopathies, known to disturb contractile function and alter the energy landscape of the heart. Although studies examining the biophysical properties of cardiac myocytes with FHC-causing mutations have yielded a cellular and molecular understanding of myofilament function, this knowledge has had limited translational success. This is driven by a critical failure in elucidating an integrated and sequential link among the changing energy landscape, myofilament function, and initiated signaling pathways in response to FHC. Similarly, there continues to be a major gap in understanding the cellular and molecular mechanisms contributing to sex differences in FHC development and progression. The primary reason for this gap is a lack of a "unifying" or "central" hypothesis that integrates signaling cascades, energetics, sex and FHC.

**Keywords:** hypertrophic cardiomyopathy, sex differences, contractility, sarcomere, mutations

## 1. Introduction to inherited cardiomyopathies

Cardiomyopathies are a major underlying cause of heart failure (HF) and often have a significant heritable component. Although the origin of the inherited trigger can be traced to a single mutation in a sarcomeric gene, the development and progression of a cardiomyopathic phenotype depends on a complex interaction between initiated cellular signaling pathways, environmental stressors, and individual genotype (including sex/gender). Inherited, or familial, cardiomyopathy (FHC) is a disease of the cardiac sarcomere and can be classified as either a hypertrophic (HCM), dilated (DCM), or restrictive (RCM) cardiomyopathy. Inherited cardiomyopathies, FHC, are relatively common in the general population with a penetrance of 1:500 [1].

Although subjects with an identified genotype are at risk for sudden cardiac death (SCD) or HF, it is clinically heterogeneous with severe, mild, or no symptoms. For example, subjects with severe left ventricular (LV) hypertrophy defined as LV thickness >30 mm are at increased risk for SCD [2]. However, subjects with inherited hypertrophic cardiomyopathy (HCM) may present with little LV hypertrophy but yet still be at risk for SCD and HF. Unlike subjects with non-inherited LV hypertrophy, HCM patients may present with cardiac dysfunction that is not proportional to LV thickness [3–5].

HCM is highly progressive and often transitions to DCM. As the name suggests, DCM is characterized by a dilated LV hypertrophy accompanied by worsening cardiac function [6]. Although primary DCM is less common than HCM, DCM is the most genetically heterogeneous [6]. This is best illustrated by findings that DCM can be linked to genes that are also linked to HCM mutations further highlighting the complex nature of FHC.

HCM with abnormal LV diastolic filling associated with intracellular or interstitial infiltration and/or fibrosis in the absence of LV dilation has been described as a RCM. The prevalence of primary RCM is not known, but RCM is less common than both HCM and DCM with poorer clinical outcomes [5]. Again, co-existent HCM and RCM in the same family illustrates the importance of elucidating the pathogenesis that is not entirely based on genotype. Our ability to develop novel approaches or therapies for FHC will depend on a clear understanding of the genotype-to-phenotype interrelationship and potentially translate into personalized treatment options. Since the primary genetic defect in HCM, DCM, and RCM impacts the biophysics of the cardiac sarcomere, we discuss the genotype-phenotype relationship for inherited cardiomyopathies focusing on cardiomyocyte kinetics and energetics in a sex dimorphic manner.

## 2. Genotype to phenotype

Approximately 100 genes are genetically linked to FHC with most gene mutations encoding for sarcomeric proteins including β-myosin heavy chain (β-MYHC), cardiac troponin T (cTnT), cardiac myosin binding protein C (cMyBP-C), α-tropomyosin (α-Tm), cardiac troponin I (cTnI), myosin regulatory light chain (RLC), and titin [6–8]. FHC follows an autosomal dominant pattern of inheritance and rarely arises from de novo mutations; although founder mutations are less common, some have been traced to a common ancestor in certain populations and countries [7]. The first identified HCM-causing mutation is a missense in the thick filament gene (*MYH7*) encoding β-MyHC [9]. Since the initial discovery, hundreds of *MYH7* mutations have been genetically linked to HCM and account for 30–40% of all inherited FHCs.

Mutations in *MYBPC3*, a thick filament gene encoding cMyBP-C, is genetically linked to 40–50% distinct HCM-causing mutations, making *MYH7* and *MYBPC3* the most common genes underlying FHC-based disease [3, 10]. Despite the predominance of these gene mutations in HCM, *MYH7* mutations typically result in amino acid substitutions whereas *MYBPC3* variants disrupt the reading frame, leading to a truncated cMyBP-C protein and, often, haploinsufficiency [3]. Considering the role of β-MyHC in cardiomyocyte force generation, a missense mutation within a known critical domain of the *MYH7* gene can be more directly linked to a contractile deficit, usually through a gain-of-function and increased energy cost [11–13]. On the other hand, haploinsufficiency leads to loss of protein or accumulation of truncated protein making it difficult to mechanistically link the mutation to a biophysical effect. In general, patients with *MYBPC3* mutations present with less severe or delayed-onset HCM compared to patients with *MYH7* mutations [3, 6, 10]. Further illustrating profound genetic heterogeneity in FHC-causing mutations, *MYH7* and *MYBPC3* mutations have been linked to inherited DCM as well, even when the mutation is within the same functional domain [2, 6].

Less frequent FHC-causing mutations exist in other thick filament proteins as well. A third thick filament gene linked to FHC, although at a much lower prevalence, is *MLC2*, which encodes for myosin regulatory light chain (RLC). RLC associates with β-MYHC to impact the kinetics of actin-myosin interaction and contractile dynamics [14, 15]. Clinical presentation in patients with *MLC2* mutations is similar to other patients with thick filament mutations, including the phenotypic diversity. Mutations in thin filament proteins (cTnT, α-Tm, and cTnI) have been linked to both HCM, DCM, and RCM [2]. Interestingly, mutations in *TNNT2* (cTnT) and *TPM1* (α-Tm) are potentially more dangerous but with a variable penetrance [4]. For example, subjects are characterized as having "mild hypertrophy" and "less fibrosis", with a significant percentage of SCD patients displaying little to no phenotype [4].

From the above summary, it is clear that a clinical phenotype cannot be categorically assigned to a particular FHC genotype. Still, as a disease of the sarcomere, the prevailing assumption is that FHC-causing mutations perturb the biophysics of muscle contraction. As more sophisticated techniques are available to precisely locate the origins of biophysical abnormalities, investigators remain tasked with detailing the interrelationship between genetic aberrations and basic cardiac sarcomere biology.

## 3. Sarcomere contractile dynamics

Force generation in a sarcomere is produced by cyclic interactions between myosin and actin, process that is energetically driven by ATP hydrolysis. The myosin-actin interaction is regulated by the tropomyosin and troponin complex; calcium ($Ca^{2+}$) binding to the troponin complex initiates a macromolecular rearrangement on the thin filament and permits myosin binding to actin [2, 14]. Contractile perturbations downstream of $Ca^{2+}$ cycling, the so-called sarcomere-controlled mechanisms, represent the earliest indicators of HF [16]. We can now state the *dynamics* of cardiac contraction and relaxation during the progression of HF are governed by downstream mechanisms, particularly the *kinetics* and *energetics* of the cross-bridge cycle to drive the trajectory of pathological cardiac remodeling [17]. This notion is unambiguously supported by elegant studies above linking inheritable FHC-causing mutations to cardiomyopathies, known to disturb contractile function and alter the energy landscape of the heart.

The ability to maintain contractile force at a given cytosolic $Ca^{2+}$ concentration ($Ca^{2+}$-sensitive tension development) provides an index of cardiac contractility and is often used to characterize the impact of FHC-causing mutations on contractile function [18–21]. While $Ca^{2+}$-sensitive tension development indexes contractility, the rate of cross-bridge (actin-myosin interaction) binding and unbinding can impart knowledge regarding the amount of force that can be extracted from ATP [22].

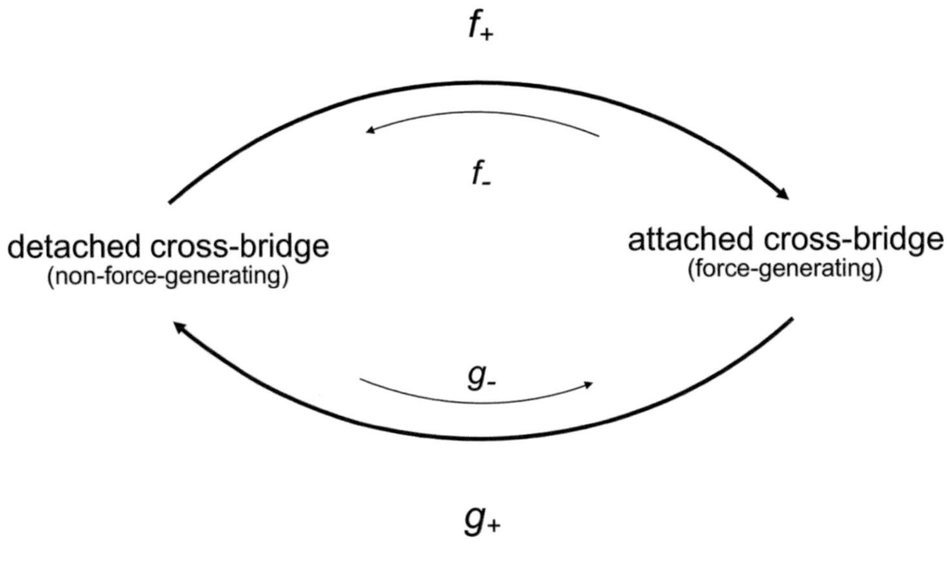


**Figure 1.** Two-state model of cross-bridge kinetics states that the rate of cross-bridge transition from non-force-generating (detached) to force-generating (attached) is described by f. Similarly, the rate of cross-bridge transition from force generating (attached) to non-force-generating (attached) is described by g. The reverse rate constants, noted as $f_-$ and $g_-$, are very small. $k_{tr}$ can be defined by $f_+ + g_+$.

The time course of $Ca^{2+}$-activated tension development following mechanical perturbation (release-restretch protocol) reveals information regarding the kinetics of cycling cross-bridges. Specifically, the rate constant for this time course ($k_{tr}$) describes the isometric cross-bridge turnover rate, i.e., the sum of the apparent rates of cross-bridges entering and leaving force-generating states using a two-state model system of cross-bridge kinetics [23, 24]. This maneuver can be applied to the muscle at the end of a contraction to measure apparent rate of tension redevelopment ($k_{tr}$). The recovery of tension toward the isometric steady-state level fitted to a single exponential yields the rate constant $k_{tr}$. We and others define the rate constant $k_{tr}$ according to the two-state model system. Cross-bridge kinetics of the two-state system can be described by rate constants, *f* and *g*, characterizing the making and breaking of cross-bridges [24, 25]. Using this two-state model, $k_{tr}$ can be defined by $f_+ + g_+$ (**Figure 1**).

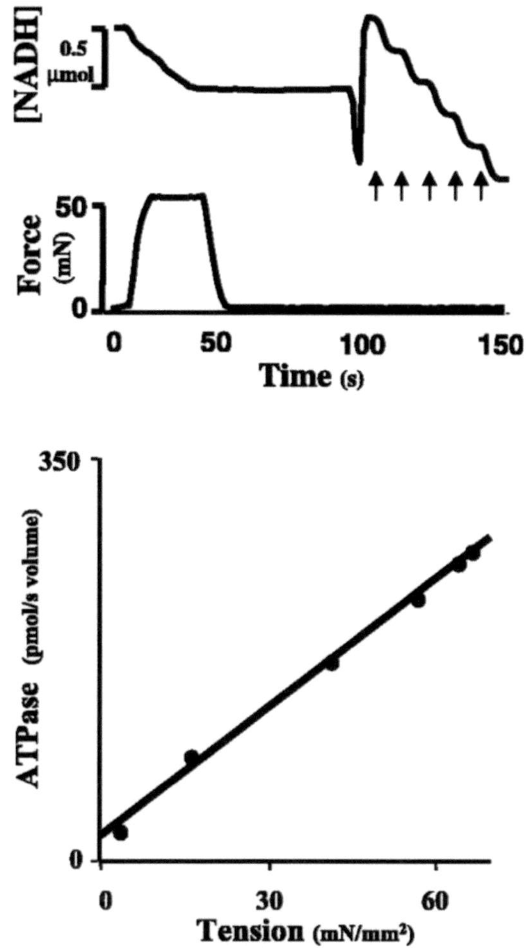


**Figure 2.** The rate of NADH absorbance is proportional to ATP consumption during isometric steady-state force development (**top panel**). The ATPase rate is plotted against force (**bottom panel**). The slope of this relationship represents the energetic cost (ATPase) of tension generation. Using a two-state model of cross-bridge kinetics, the slope of this line represents the rate of cross-bridge detachment and thus a measure of g. This figure was adapted with permission from Rundell et al. [117].

We have also exploited an apparatus to simultaneously measure force and ATP utilization [26, 27]. Briefly, the bath used for the ATPase assay allows transmission of near-UV light for the measurement of NADH absorbance. The ATPase activity of demembranated cardiac muscle strips or trabecula is measured on-line by means of an enzyme-coupled assay [26, 27]. Formation of ADP by the muscle is stoichiometrically coupled first to the synthesis of pyruvate and ATP from phosphoenolpyruvate, a reaction that is catalyzed by the enzyme pyruvate kinase, and subsequently to synthesis of lactate, a reaction that is catalyzed by the enzyme lactate dehydrogenase and during which NADH is oxidized to $NAD^+$. The breakdown of NADH is determined photometrically by measuring the absorbance of 340 nm near-UV light that is projected through the bath just beneath the preparation. Once the steady-state tension is reached, the first time derivative of this signal, which is proportional to the rate of ATP consumption in the assay bath, is determined off-line by linear regression of the sampled data using custom-designed software (**Figure 2**). The rate of ATP consumption, normalized to fiber volume, is plotted against force (**Figure 2**). This slope reflects the tension cost of contraction [26, 28]. Using the two-state model, this value approximates the rate of detachment (g). The combined measurements of $k_{tr}$ and tension cost can give determinations of cross-bridge attachment (f) and detachment (g) [26].

## 4. ATP shuttling in the cardiac sarcomere

The hypertrophic heart has long been characterized as energy starved [12], and central to this energy remodeling is an alteration in the production, use, and delivery of ATP. Given the physical barriers to rapid diffusion within the myocyte, the cardiomyocyte utilizes key enzymes and a phosphotransferase system to optimize efficient transfer of phosphoryl groups to ADP [29]. Speaking directly to its significance, disturbances in the creatine kinase (CK)/ adenylate kinase (AK) phosphotransfer system are observed early in CVD and are stronger predictors of heart failure mortality than functional status [30]. The molecular underpinnings of the metabolic derangements reside in changes in the mediators of ATP generation, utilization, and delivery. As seen in Eq. (1) creatine kinase (CK) reversibly and rapidly converts ADP and phosphocreatine (PCr) to ATP and creatine (Cr) [31].

$$ADP + PCr \xrightarrow{CK} ATP + Cr \tag{1}$$

In parallel reactions [Eqs. (1) and (2)], a network of adenylate kinase (AK) enzymes mediates a complementary intracellular phosphotransfer promoting high-energy Pi transfer from ADP to ATP (leaving an increasing AMP pool) via distinct AK isoforms with different cellular localizations [32, 33].

$$ADP + ADP \xrightarrow{AK} ATP + AMP \tag{2}$$

The diseased heart will preferentially recruit phosphotransferase reactions to keep a constant pool of ATP. As cardiac disease ensues, total Cr and PCr decreases and results in elevated ADP and AMP even if ATP is maintained [11]. Further along the disease process, CK activity is reduced leading to a gradual decrease in cellular ATP [34]. Considering the relatively high rate of ATP synthesis in the heart [12], a gradual decrease in ATP can cause disproportionate energetic deficiencies [30, 35]. Such changes in energetics limit contractile reserve and the ability to power myocellular ATPases necessary to support contractile function. Given the physical barriers to rapid diffusion within the myocyte, physical association of CK, AK, and other key enzymes in the phosphotransferase system optimizes efficient transfer of phosphoryl groups to ADP [29]. These phosphotransfer microdomains are localized to sarcomeric myofibrils and act as hubs for energetic "sensing" [32, 36]. During acute or chronic ATP supply–demand imbalance, like the one that occurs during cardiac disease, AK amplifies the amount of AMP within these microdomains to preserve ATP levels for contraction [33].

## 5. Biophysical impact of inherited cardiomyopathies

### 5.1. Mutations in β-MyHC

The R403Q point mutation in β-MyHC is the first identified mutation leading to HCM with a heritable component [9]. The R403Q mutation resides in the actin-binding domain and *in vitro* analysis of R403Q myosin kinetics yields inconsistent results such as reduced [37] or enhanced [38] actin filament velocity and reduced [39] or enhanced [40] actin-activated ATPase. On the other hand, human myofibril or multicellular R403Q samples consistently show accelerated tension generation and increased ATP hydrolysis rates [20, 41]. In a recent study, we demonstrated that R403Q male fibers develop tension at an increased energy cost of contraction than WT fibers. This is consistent with a previous study that directly measured cross-bridge kinetics in cardiac myofibrils isolated from a patient carrying the R403Q mutation [41]. In addition, R403Q male cardiac trabeculae show an elevated $k_{tr}$ at submaximal tension, again consistent with the kinetics of human R403Q-expressing myofibrils [41]. These observations show that less mechanical energy can be extracted from ATP suggesting an increase in the energy cost of tension generation in R403Q fibers.

Yet, the role that $Ca^{2+}$-sensitive tension development as an index of cardiac contractility plays in the progression of HCM is unclear. Studies consistently show that $Ca^{2+}$-sensitive tension development of cardiac fibers is not different between young (6–20 weeks) WT and R403Q hearts [42–44] even though previous studies show that intact hearts from male mice expressing the R403Q mutation show greater contractility compared to controls [45, 46]. We previously showed that cardiac trabeculae from 10-month-old male R403Q trabeculae were not different from wild-type fibers [21]. At the very least, the presence of the R403Q mutation alters myofilament function and ATP utilization at the level of the sarcomere.

### 5.2. Mutations in cMyBP-C

Historically, cMyBP-C has been viewed as a modifier of contraction through its direct interaction with myosin. In fact, genetic deletion of cMyBP-C in a murine model results in reduced systolic and diastolic parameters, reduced tension at submaximal activation, and cardiac hypertrophy [47]. Representative of a gain-of-function, myocytes lacking cMyBP-C generate more power and display increased rates of force redevelopment at the submaximal activation [48]. Interestingly, permeabilized myocytes taken from humans harboring *MYBPC3* mutations with evidence of reduced protein expression by haploinsufficiency show reduced maximal force without a change in the kinetics of actin-myosin cycling [49].

In contrast, human samples heterozygous for a missense mutation in *MYBPC3* are more sensitive to activating $Ca^{2+}$, which may be representative of enhanced contractility [50]. Again, the genetic heterogeneity of *MYBPC3* mutations mirrors the specific impact of each mutation on sarcomeric function. For example, loss of cMyBP-C protein as a result of *MYBPC3* mutations does not necessarily result in "loss-of-function". More recent studies have confirmed that cMyBP-C also interacts with actin to potentially tuning thin filament activation directly while simultaneously maintaining a functional interaction with myosin [51]. The implication for cMyBP-C is a complex regulatory role that imparts novel structural and functional mechanisms during the contractile cycle.

### 5.3. Mutations in RLC

The myosin regulatory light chain (RLC), also called as the ventricular light chain, is encoded by the *MLC2* gene. The RLC protein forms a non-covalent association with myosin and contains an EF-hand motif implicating functional regulation of myosin and subsequent tension generation [52]. Within this EF-hand "hot spot", the first FHC-causing mutations in the *MLC2* gene were identified, confirming an integral role for the RLC in contractile function [53]. To study the biophysical impact of *MLC2* mutations, mice expressing an E22K RLC transgene were engineered [15, 18]. Hearts from E22K mice display midventricular obstruction due to papillary and septal hypertrophy similar to human counterparts. However, mechanical properties of E22K sarcomeres remain unresolved.

Initial studies using glycerinated cardiac muscle fibers illustrate an increase in $Ca^{2+}$-sensitivity and $Ca^{2+}$-activated ATPase of myofibrillar samples from E22K transgenic mice than WT littermate and non-transgenic counterparts [15]. Follow-up studies by the same group report no impact of the E22K RLC mutation on $Ca^{2+}$-sensitivity of tension and a decrease in maximal ATPase [18]. Inconsistencies in biophysical results from E22K hearts are not surprising, considering the crucial role of RLC phosphorylation in the regulation of myosin mechanics [52, 54]. It is now appreciated that mutations in the *MLC2* gene may impact phosphorylation-dependent changes in force production [54].

### 5.4. Mutations in cTnT

Along the thin filament, a contractile unit consists of a repeating complex of 7 actin monomers, 1 troponin complex, and 1 $\alpha$-Tm coil-coil dimer [2]. The heterotrimeric cardiac troponin complex is comprised of cTnI, cTnT, and the $Ca^{2+}$-binding troponin subunit, cardiac troponin C (cTnC). Myofilament activation hinges on complex molecular interactions between thin filament proteins where $Ca^{2+}$-binding to cTnC activates the myofilament, changes the position of $\alpha$-Tm, and removes allosteric inhibition, allowing actin-myosin interaction. Transmission through the contractile unit following $Ca^{2+}$ binding is exquisitely controlled by precise movements of multiple proteins, perhaps predicting a potentially more dangerous phenotype and variable penetrance in patients with FHC mutations residing in thin filament proteins [4].

http://dx.doi.org/10.5772/65393

Missense or splice-site mutations in the *TNNT2* gene result in point mutations or truncated variants resulting in FHC [2, 19]. Unlike *MYBPC3* mutations, truncated cTnT proteins are incorporated into the sarcomere, and early studies in transgenic mice expressing a truncated cTnT modeled after the human condition indicate mild to no cardiac hypertrophy, significant diastolic dysfunction and die more frequently with an increasing allelic expression similar to the human phenotype [55]. Interestingly, cardiac fibers expressing a similar truncated cTnT develop less force at maximum activation [56]. The truncated form of cTnT presumably disrupts the cTnT-cTnI-α-Tm binding domain, but the exact molecular mechanism that leads to the observed phenotype remains unresolved.

Early mapping of cTnT-related FHC alleles intimated the significance of another critical region within the cTnT-α-Tm binding domain [19]. Several FHC-causing substitutions have been identified at residue 92, including R92Q, R92L, and R92W [2]. Hearts taken from mice expressing R92 point mutations are typically smaller, hypercontractile with severe diastolic dysfunction, again, similar to findings in patients with FHC [2, 19, 57]. On the other hand, biophysical studies are inconsistent and depend on experimental approach and the level of molecular resolution. Still, key characteristics can be attributed to R92 mutations, including increased force and actin-myosin cycling at lower $Ca^{2+}$ and less efficient use of ATP to generate force [57–59]. Nevertheless, these biophysical data do not fully explain the phenotypic heterogeneity of cTnT-related FHC arising from genotype-similar patients. Interestingly, a recent work demonstrates significant interplay between cTnT R92 mutations and MyHC isoform [57]. The suggestion from these recent data is that multiple levels of myofilament regulation exist and that specific cTnT FHC mutations cannot be used as surrogates for mutations comprising the functional domain. Clearly, FHC disease progression is a complex integration of myofilament function, cross-bridge kinetics, and cellular signaling, all of which can be modified by environmental and genetic factors such as sex/gender.

## 6. Sex disparities in FHC

Being male predisposes carriers of FHC-causing mutations to pathological cardiac remodeling [60]. In females, the sharp rise in FHC morbidity and mortality closely aligns with the pre- to post-menopausal transition [60–64]. Despite the longstanding knowledge that pre-menopausal women are protected from developing FHC, our fundamental understanding of the shift in FHC risk with menopause remains inadequate and impedes our ability to develop sex-specific therapeutic strategies to combat FHC and its complications.

The loss of estrogen during menopause positions 17β-estradiol (E2), the predominant naturally occurring estrogen, to play a unique role in cardioprotection. E2 signaling through classical estrogen receptors (ER), ERα and ERβ, and a third, membrane bound and G-protein coupled estrogen receptor (GPER) is initiated by environmental, genetic, and non-genetic cues to impact gene expression and cellular signaling [65–67]. E2-dependent signaling is complex and multiple molecular, and cellular mechanisms have been suggested to underlie protection against CVD [65, 66]. As part of these investigations, studies that utilized gonadectomized rodents subjected to different cardiac pathological stimuli typically demonstrate a benefit of estrogen replacement [68–72]. Unfortunately, the prospective Women's Health Initiative (WHI) and Heart and Estrogen/Progestin Replacement Study (HERS I and II) studies show an increased CVD and stroke risk with estrogen replacement in menopausal women [73, 74].

Our group has spent the past 15 years studying a murine model of HCM, which expresses an autosomal-dominant R403Q mutation in $\alpha$-myosin heavy chain and exemplifies this sex dimorphism such that R403Q male mice develop progressive left-ventricular dilation, impaired cardiac function, and a number of pathologic indicators well before R403Q female mice [21, 65, 75–80]. The trajectory of HCM due the R403Q FHC model differs between the sexes in an age-dependent manner. As illustrated in **Figure 3**, adolescent (2 month old) males display cardiac hypertrophy whereas females do not; males progress to a worsening phenotype characterized by ventricular dilation by 8 month of age while females maintain ventricular morphometry with mild hypertrophy [27, 75].

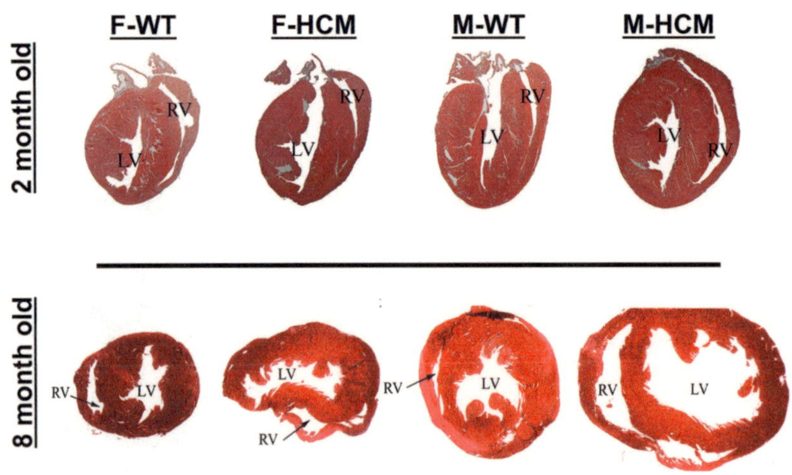


**Figure 3. Cardiac morphometry of R403Q female and male mice. Top panel**: Representative H&E stained longitudinal heart sections from R403Q female and male mice at 2 months of age. **Bottom panel**: Representative H&E stained short axis heart sections from R403Q female and male mice at 8 months of age. This figure was partly adapted with permission from [27].

The biophysical properties of cardiac sarcomeres expressing the R403Q mutation, as for cTnT mutations, depend on the experimental approach. In vitro analysis of R403Q myosin kinetics yields inconsistent results such as reduced [37] or enhanced [38] actin filament velocity and reduced [39] or enhanced [40] actin-activated ATPase. On the other hand, human myofibril or multicellular R403Q samples consistently show accelerated tension generation and increased ATP hydrolysis rates [20, 41]. We and others have reported both age- and sex-dependent effects on $Ca^{2+}$-sensitivity of tension and the rates of actin and myosin interaction, or $k_{tr}$. [21, 42, 43]. We further demonstrated that R403Q males show increased cycling (entering and exiting) of cross-bridges at a given force. Furthermore, we find a strong interaction between sex and the R403Q mutation with regard to tension cost. Coupled with measures of $k_{tr}$, this indicates higher "off" rate and more inefficient use of ATP at a given force in R403Q males with the opposite effect in R403Q females [27].

What is clear from these studies on the biophysics of the R403Q FHC mutation is that male and female myofilament function is perturbed and potentially under energy stress presumably initiated by the FHC mutation. The underlying mechanisms dictating very distinct disease trajectories in males and females are not completely elucidated by these studies necessitating alternative approaches.

### 6.1. Role of estrogen in FHC

Sex differences are primarily determined by hormonal status. When considering the effect of sex hormones on the progression of FHC, it is imperative to place a special focus on 17β-estradiol (E2) signaling. Estradiol is the main circulating sex hormone in pre-menopausal women. It is mainly synthesized in ovarian follicles, and to a smaller extent in adipose tissue, liver, breast, and neural tissues [81]. It regulates a number of physiological processes including metabolism, cell growth and proliferation, reproduction, and development [82]. It is generally agreed that estrogen plays a protective role in the myocardium and most of the cardio-protective effects have been attributed to E2. For the rest of this discussion, when we mention estrogen (E2), we are referring specifically to 17β-estradiol.

### 6.2. Estrogen signaling pathways

Estrogen exerts its physiological effects through interaction with intracellular estrogen receptors (ERs). The first described estrogen receptors, also known as classical estrogen receptors, are ER$\alpha$ and ERβ. They are members of the nuclear hormone receptor family (NHR), contain a DNA-binding domain, and share a high degree of homology [83]. In addition, another estrogen receptor has been recently described. GPER1, a membrane-bound G-protein coupled estrogen receptor, formerly known as GPR30, is a seven trans-membrane domain protein that mediates some of the non-transcriptional activity of estrogen [84].

Estrogen signaling pathways fall into two main categories: genomic (also known as classical) and non-genomic signaling. During genomic signaling, classical estrogen receptors act as transcription factors. After binding to estrogen, they undergo a conformational change that leads to the formation of homodimers (ER$\alpha$/ER$\alpha$ and ERβ/ERβ) or heterodimers (ER$\alpha$/ERβ). Receptor-dimers then bind to estrogen response elements (ERE), located near promoter regions of genes, and regulate gene transcription [83]. Estrogen signaling can also be initiated at the non-transcriptional level. Estrogen receptors interact with intracellular proteins triggering signal transduction cascades, often mediated by chain-reaction phosphorylation events. The vast array of estrogen non-transcriptional signaling pathways is mediated by ER$\alpha$, ERβ, and GPER1 [84, 85].

### 6.3. Molecular mechanisms of estrogen-mediated cardio-protection

It is most widely accepted that the overall effect of cardiac estrogen signaling has a beneficial outcome on cardiac health. Not only does estrogen mediate cardioprotection, but it is also involved in the regulation of physiological processes in the heart. ER$\alpha$ expression, for example, is required to maintain physiological glucose uptake and proper mitochondrial function in the murine heart [86, 87]. Acute E2 injections enhance cardiovascular reflexes and autonomic tone in ovariectomy (OVX) mice [88]. Estrogen receptors interact with AMP-activated protein kinase in neonatal rat cardiomyocytes (NRCM), and potentially mediate its activity [89].

More importantly, there is increasing evidence suggesting that estrogen attenuates the progression of cardiac hypertrophy and prevents HF [70, 90]. The molecular mechanisms behind estrogen effects on cardiomyocyte survival are still under study. However, there are many pieces of evidence pointing to specific molecular pathways bridging estrogen signaling and increased tolerance to hypertrophic stimuli such as those arise from FHC. Some of these findings are explored below.

Estrogen has been shown to reverse agonist-induced cardiomyocyte hypertrophy. In NRCM, E2-treatment counteracts angiotensin II (Ang II)-induced increase in cell surface area, protein synthesis, skeletal muscle actin expression, nuclear translocation, and transcriptional activity of the hypertrophic transcription factor NFAT [85]. An E2-dependent increase in SIRT1 expression levels and AMPK activity protects the cardiomyocyte from Ang II-induced injury [91]. E2 reduces cardiomyocyte apoptosis *in vivo* and *in vitro* through the activation of PI3K/Akt signaling [92]. E2 treatment of OVX mice hearts and NRCM inhibits calcineurin activity and increases its degradation [93, 94]. E2 also limits undesirable extracellular matrix (ECM) remodeling through the modulation of ECM protein expression [95]. The majority of the effects discussed above are mediated by signaling through the classical estrogen receptors.

Limited mechanistic insights are available on E2 cardiac signaling mediated through ER$\alpha$. Selective ER$\alpha$ agonism attenuates cardiac hypertrophy, increasing cardiac output, left ventricular stroke volume, and cardiac $\alpha$-MyHC expression [96–98]. Signaling through ER$\beta$ has been studied in more depth and has been shown to counteract the development of cardiac hypertrophy by reducing the expression of hypertrophic markers, attenuating fibrosis, apoptosis and inflammation [99–101]. ER$\beta$ regulates a network of miRNAs, modulates p38 and ERK signaling, and affects calcineurin expression [102, 103]. In fibroblasts, ER$\beta$ blocks TGF$\beta$1 synthesis that signals for the production of fibronectin, vimetin, collagens I and III [104].

At least three different mechanisms by which ER$\beta$ modulates hypertrophic gene expression in cardiomyocytes have been described. First, E2 signaling through ER$\beta$ induces PI3K activation that upregulates MCIP1 transcription [94]. MCIP1 blocks the Ang II-induced increase in calcineurin activity, preventing NFAT translocation to the nucleus and inhibiting the transcription of hypertrophic genes [105]. Second, ER$\beta$ signaling can reverse Ang II-induced inhibitory phosphorylation of glycogen synthase kinase-3$\beta$ (GSK3B) by Akt. This prevents GATA4 transcription factor activation and also leads to decrease in hypertrophic mRNA expression [106]. The third mechanism involves regulation of histone deacetylases (HDAC). ER$\beta$ suppress the production and activation of the pro-hypertrophic HDAC2, while promoting the retention of anti-hypertrophic HDAC in the nucleus to inhibit hypertrophic gene expression [106].

Taking into account the complex and multifaceted nature of cardiac estrogen signaling, it is critical to inquire whether the cardioprotective effect of E2 signaling is sex dependent. In the context of cardiac hypertrophy, females show a better response to E2 than males [100], but that does not necessarily mean that E2 signaling is not beneficial for the male heart. It has been shown that E2 treatment of male rats subjected to chronic volume overload attenuates ventricular remodeling and disease progression [107]. It also improves survival in male mice with TNF$\alpha$ overexpression-induced cardiomyopathy [108]. At the cellular level, E2 stimulation of c-kit-expressing cardiac progenitor cells confers cardioprotection against cardiac injury. When co-cultured, ER$\alpha$ stimulation of c-kit + cells enhances the survival of post-infarct male myocytes [109].

In summary, estrogen signaling plays an important role in preventing cardiac remodeling that occurs during hypertrophy and subsequent heart failure. The exact extent to which the different estrogen-targeted pathways contribute to that is still under study. Better understanding of the mechanisms behind estrogen cardioprotection will help to fully understand the sex differences behind the development of FHC, and therefore lead to better and more specialized therapeutic options.

### 6.4. Menopause models of estrogen depletion

One obstacle that has stalled translational progression of studies into menopausal hypersensitivity to FHC is the lack of appropriate rodent models mirroring progressive ovarian failure, i.e., one that moves from perimenopause into menopause, similar to humans. Most studies have used the surgical removal of ovaries (ovariectomy) as a model of menopause, yet only 10% of women enter menopause surgically. Our studies have utilized an ovary-intact mouse model of menopause, using the chemical 4-vinylcyclohexene diepoxide (VCD) [110]. Repeated short term daily dosing with VCD selectively targets primordial follicles of the ovaries, accelerating the natural process of follicular atresia, and inducing gradual ovarian failure. This model preserves the important "perimenopause" transitional period and androgen-secreting capacity of residual ovarian tissue, analogous to menopausal women [111, 112]. Preserving endogenous androgens in estrogen-deplete females is particularly critical when studying sex differences in FHC [113]. Although androgen levels drop during menopause, the loss of estrogen in menopause elevates the androgen to estrogen ratio and represents an independent risk factor for FHC [114, 115]. We have used this model to demonstrate that during perimenopause, females were protected from hypertension and adverse cardiac remodeling. However after menopause, hypertension and pathological remodeling, indicative of worse clinical outcomes, is a hallmark of this increase in FHC susceptibility during menopause [116]. Importantly, the worsening phenotype in menopausal females is prevented by estrogen.

## 7. Conclusions

The assertion that FHC is a complex disease is underscored by the difficulty in attributing a single cause to the disease such as aberrant biophysical function of the myofilament. What is evident from studies of FHC is that although the primary defect may reside in the sarcomere, the development of an HCM, DCM, or RCM phenotype depends on the interaction of the initiated signaling pathways, environmental stressors, and individual genotype (including sex/gender). For example, pathways downstream of $Ca^{2+}$ activation such as $Ca^{2+}$-sensitivity or actin-myosin cycling kinetics represent functional parameter that is the summation of multiple signals.

Despite an increasing appreciation of sex dimorphisms in the pathophysiology of FHC, many inconsistencies plague the cellular and molecular mechanisms underlying these sex differences. Taken together, there is a clear necessity in elucidating the cellular and molecular actions of estrogen and how this relates to the sex dimorphisms in FHC. Finally, although murine models of FHC do not exactly mimic the human *genotype*, they have proven as useful tools to elucidate the mechanisms underlying the FHC *phenotype*.

## Acknowledgements

This work was supported by National Institutes of Health grant (HL098256), by a National Mentored Research Science Development Award (K01 AR052840), and Independent Scientist Award (K02 HL105799) from the NIH awarded to J.P. Konhilas, the Interdisciplinary Training in Cardiovascular Research (HL007249), and the Cardiovascular Biomedical Engineering Training Grant (HL007955). Support was received from the Sarver Heart Center at the University of Arizona and the Steven M. Gootter Foundation.

## Author details

Marissa Lopez-Pier[1,3], Yulia Lipovka[2,3], Eleni Constantopoulos[2,3] and John P. Konhilas[2,3*]

*Address all correspondence to: konhilas@arizona.edu

1 Department of Biomedical Engineering, University of Arizona, Tucson, Arizona

2 Department of Physiology, University of Arizona, Tucson, Arizona

3 Sarver Molecular Cardiovascular Research Program, University of Arizona, Tucson, Arizona

## References

[1] Maron BJ. Hypertrophic cardiomyopathy: a systematic review. JAMA 287: 1308-1320, 2002.

[2] Tardiff JC. Thin filament mutations: developing an integrative approach to a complex disorder. Circ Res 108: 765-782, 2011.

[3] Behrens-Gawlik V, Mearini G, Gedicke-Hornung C, Richard P, and Carrier L. MYBPC3 in hypertrophic cardiomyopathy: from mutation identification to RNA-based correction. Pflugers Arch 466: 215-223, 2014.

[4] Keren A, Syrris P, and McKenna WJ. Hypertrophic cardiomyopathy: the genetic determinants of clinical disease expression. Nat Clin Pract Cardiovasc Med 5: 158-168, 2008.

[5] Sen-Chowdhry S, Syrris P, and McKenna WJ. Genetics of restrictive cardiomyopathy. Heart Fail Clin 6: 179-186, 2010.

[6] McNally EM, Barefield DY, and Puckelwartz MJ. The genetic landscape of cardiomyopathy and its role in heart failure. Cell Metab 21: 174-182, 2015.

[7] Claes GR, van Tienen FH, Lindsey P, Krapels IP, Helderman-van den Enden AT, Hoos MB, Barrois YE, Janssen JW, Paulussen AD, Sels JW, Kuijpers SH, van Tintelen JP, van den Berg MP, Heesen WF, Garcia-Pavia P, Perrot A, Christiaans I, Salemink S, Marcelis CL, Smeets HJ, Brunner HG, Volders PG, and van den Wijngaard A. Hypertrophic remodelling in cardiac regulatory myosin light chain (MYL2) founder mutation carriers. Eur Heart J 37: 1815-1822, 2016.

[8] Kensler RW, Shaffer JF, and Harris SP. Binding of the N-terminal fragment C0-C2 of cardiac MyBP-C to cardiac F-actin. J Struct Biol 174: 44-51, 2011.

[9] Geisterfer-Lowrance AA, Kass S, Tanigawa G, Vosberg HP, McKenna W, Seidman CE, and Seidman JG. A molecular basis for familial hypertrophic cardiomyopathy: a beta cardiac myosin heavy chain gene missense mutation. Cell 62: 999-1006, 1990.

[10] Maron BJ, Niimura H, Casey SA, Soper MK, Wright GB, Seidman JG, and Seidman CE. Development of left ventricular hypertrophy in adults in hypertrophic cardiomyopathy caused by cardiac myosin-binding protein C gene mutations. J Am Coll Cardiol 38: 315-321, 2001.

[11] Ingwall JS. ATP and the Heart. Boston: Kluwer Academic Publishers, 2002.

[12] Ingwall JS. Energy metabolism in heart failure and remodelling. Cardiovasc Res 81: 412-419, 2009.

[13] Walsh R, Rutland C, Thomas R, and Loughna S. Cardiomyopathy: a systematic review of disease-causing mutations in myosin heavy chain 7 and their phenotypic manifestations. Cardiology 115: 49-60, 2010.

[14] Scruggs SB and Solaro RJ. The significance of regulatory light chain phosphorylation in cardiac physiology. Arch Biochem Biophys 510: 129-134, 2011.

[15] Szczesna-Cordary D, Guzman G, Zhao J, Hernandez O, Wei J, and Diaz-Perez Z. The E22K mutation of myosin RLC that causes familial hypertrophic cardiomyopathy

increases calcium sensitivity of force and ATPase in transgenic mice. J Cell Sci 118: 3675-3683, 2005.

[16] Yar S, Monasky MM, and Solaro RJ. Maladaptive modifications in myofilament proteins and triggers in the progression to heart failure and sudden death. Pflugers Arch 466: 1189-1197, 2014.

[17] Stehle R and Iorga B. Kinetics of cardiac sarcomeric processes and rate-limiting steps in contraction and relaxation. J Mol Cell Cardiol 48: 843-850, 2010.

[18] Szczesna-Cordary D, Jones M, Moore JR, Watt J, Kerrick WG, Xu Y, Wang Y, Wagg C, and Lopaschuk GD. Myosin regulatory light chain E22K mutation results in decreased cardiac intracellular calcium and force transients. FASEB J 21: 3974-3985, 2007.

[19] Tardiff JC, Hewett TE, Palmer BM, Olsson C, Factor SM, Moore RL, Robbins J, and Leinwand LA. Cardiac troponin T mutations result in allele-specific phenotypes in a mouse model for hypertrophic cardiomyopathy. J Clin Invest 104: 469-481, 1999.

[20] Witjas-Paalberends ER, Ferrara C, Scellini B, Piroddi N, Montag J, Tesi C, Stienen GJ, Michels M, Ho CY, Kraft T, Poggesi C, and van der Velden J. Faster cross-bridge detachment and increased tension cost in human hypertrophic cardiomyopathy with the R403Q MYH7 mutation. J Physiol 592: 3257-3272, 2014.

[21] McKee LA, Chen H, Regan JA, Behunin SM, Walker JW, Walker JS, and Konhilas JP. Sexually dimorphic myofilament function and cardiac troponin I phosphospecies distribution in hypertrophic cardiomyopathy mice. Arch Biochem Biophys 535: 39-48, 2013.

[22] Tesi C, Colomo F, Nencini S, Piroddi N, and Poggesi C. The effect of inorganic phosphate on force generation in single myofibrils from rabbit skeletal muscle. Biophys J 78: 3081-3092, 2000.

[23] Hill TL, Eisenberg E, and Greene L. Theoretical model for the cooperative equilibrium binding of myosin subfragment 1 to the actin-troponin-tropomyosin complex. Proc Natl Acad Sci U S A 77: 3186-3190, 1980.

[24] Huxley AF. Muscle structure and theories of contraction. Prog Biophys 7: 255-318, 1957.

[25] Podolsky RJ, Nolan AC, and Zaveler SA. Cross-bridge properties derived from muscle isotonic velocity transients. Proc Natl Acad Sci U S A 64: 504-511, 1969.

[26] de Tombe PP and Stienen GJ. Impact of temperature on cross-bridge cycling kinetics in rat myocardium. J Physiol 584: 591-600, 2007.

[27] Birch CL, Behunin SM, Lopez-Pier MA, Danilo C, Lipovka Y, Saripalli C, Granzier H, and Konhilas JP. Sex dimorphisms of crossbridge cycling kinetics in transgenic hypertrophic cardiomyopathy mice. Am J Physiol Heart Circ Physiol 311: H125-136, 2016.

[28] de Tombe PP and Stienen GJ. Protein kinase A does not alter economy of force maintenance in skinned rat cardiac trabeculae. Circ Res 76: 734-741, 1995.

[29] Ingwall JS and Shen W. On energy circuits in the failing myocardium. Eur J Heart Fail 12: 1268-1270, 2010.

[30] Neubauer S. The failing heart—an engine out of fuel. N Engl J Med 356: 1140-1151, 2007.

[31] Nascimben L, Ingwall JS, Pauletto P, Friedrich J, Gwathmey JK, Saks V, Pessina AC, and Allen PD. Creatine kinase system in failing and nonfailing human myocardium. Circulation 94: 1894-1901, 1996.

[32] Aksentijevic D, Lygate CA, Makinen K, Zervou S, Sebag-Montefiore L, Medway D, Barnes H, Schneider JE, and Neubauer S. High-energy phosphotransfer in the failing mouse heart: role of adenylate kinase and glycolytic enzymes. Eur J Heart Fail 12: 1282-1289, 2010.

[33] Dzeja P and Terzic A. Adenylate kinase and AMP signaling networks: metabolic monitoring, signal communication and body energy sensing. Int J Mol Sci 10: 1729-1772, 2009.

[34] Weiss RG, Gerstenblith G, and Bottomley PA. ATP flux through creatine kinase in the normal, stressed, and failing human heart. Proc Natl Acad Sci U S A 102: 808-813, 2005.

[35] Shen W, Asai K, Uechi M, Mathier MA, Shannon RP, Vatner SF, and Ingwall JS. Progressive loss of myocardial ATP due to a loss of total purines during the development of heart failure in dogs: a compensatory role for the parallel loss of creatine. Circulation 100: 2113-2118, 1999.

[36] Koons S and Cooke R. Function of creatine kinase localization in muscle contraction. Adv Exp Med Biol 194: 129-137, 1986.

[37] Cuda G, Fananapazir L, Epstein ND, and Sellers JR. The in vitro motility activity of beta-cardiac myosin depends on the nature of the beta-myosin heavy chain gene mutation in hypertrophic cardiomyopathy. J Muscle Res Cell Motil 18: 275-283, 1997.

[38] Palmiter KA, Tyska MJ, Haeberle JR, Alpert NR, Fananapazir L, and Warshaw DM. R403Q and L908V mutant beta-cardiac myosin from patients with familial hypertrophic cardiomyopathy exhibit enhanced mechanical performance at the single molecule level. J Muscle Res Cell Motil 21: 609-620, 2000.

[39] Sweeney HL, Straceski AJ, Leinwand LA, Tikunov BA, and Faust L. Heterologous expression of a cardiomyopathic myosin that is defective in its actin interaction. J Biol Chem 269: 1603-1605, 1994.

[40] Yamashita H, Tyska MJ, Warshaw DM, Lowey S, and Trybus KM. Functional consequences of mutations in the smooth muscle myosin heavy chain at sites implicated in familial hypertrophic cardiomyopathy. J Biol Chem 275: 28045-28052, 2000.

[41] Belus A, Piroddi N, Scellini B, Tesi C, D'Amati G, Girolami F, Yacoub M, Cecchi F, Olivotto I, and Poggesi C. The familial hypertrophic cardiomyopathy-associated myosin mutation R403Q accelerates tension generation and relaxation of human cardiac myofibrils. J Physiol 586: 3639-3644, 2008.

[42] Palmer BM, Fishbaugher DE, Schmitt JP, Wang Y, Alpert NR, Seidman CE, Seidman JG, VanBuren P, and Maughan DW. Differential cross-bridge kinetics of FHC myosin mutations R403Q and R453C in heterozygous mouse myocardium. Am J Physiol Heart Circ Physiol 287: H91-99, 2004.

[43] Palmer BM, Wang Y, Teekakirikul P, Hinson JT, Fatkin D, Strouse S, Vanburen P, Seidman CE, Seidman JG, and Maughan DW. Myofilament mechanical performance is enhanced by R403Q myosin in mouse myocardium independent of sex. Am J Physiol Heart Circ Physiol 294: H1939-1947, 2008.

[44] Blanchard E, Seidman C, Seidman JG, LeWinter M, and Maughan D. Altered cross-bridge kinetics in the alphaMHC403/+ mouse model of familial hypertrophic cardiomyopathy. Circ Res 84: 475-483, 1999.

[45] Semsarian C, Ahmad I, Giewat M, Georgakopoulos D, Schmitt JP, McConnell BK, Reiken S, Mende U, Marks AR, Kass DA, Seidman CE, and Seidman JG. The L-type calcium channel inhibitor diltiazem prevents cardiomyopathy in a mouse model. J Clin Invest 109: 1013-1020, 2002.

[46] Georgakopoulos D, Christe ME, Giewat M, Seidman CM, Seidman JG, and Kass DA. The pathogenesis of familial hypertrophic cardiomyopathy: early and evolving effects from an alpha-cardiac myosin heavy chain missense mutation. Nat Med 5: 327-330, 1999.

[47] Harris SP, Bartley CR, Hacker TA, McDonald KS, Douglas PS, Greaser ML, Powers PA, and Moss RL. Hypertrophic cardiomyopathy in cardiac myosin binding protein-C knockout mice. Circ Res 90: 594-601, 2002.

[48] Korte FS, McDonald KS, Harris SP, and Moss RL. Loaded shortening, power output, and rate of force redevelopment are increased with knockout of cardiac myosin binding protein-C. Circ Res 93: 752-758, 2003.

[49] van Dijk SJ, Boontje NM, Heymans MW, Ten Cate FJ, Michels M, Dos Remedios C, Dooijes D, van Slegtenhorst MA, van der Velden J, and Stienen GJ. Preserved cross-bridge kinetics in human hypertrophic cardiomyopathy patients with MYBPC3 mutations. Pflugers Arch 466: 1619-1633, 2014.

[50] Sequeira V, Witjas-Paalberends ER, Kuster DW, and van der Velden J. Cardiac myosin-binding protein C: hypertrophic cardiomyopathy mutations and structure-function relationships. Pflugers Arch 466: 201-206, 2014.

[51] van Dijk SJ, Bezold KL, and Harris SP. Earning stripes: myosin binding protein-C interactions with actin. Pflugers Arch 466: 445-450, 2014.

[52] Declercq JP, Evrard C, Lamzin V, and Parello J. Crystal structure of the EF-hand parvalbumin at atomic resolution (0.91 Å) and at low temperature (100 K). Evidence for conformational multistates within the hydrophobic core. Protein Sci 8: 2194-2204, 1999.

[53] Flavigny J, Richard P, Isnard R, Carrier L, Charron P, Bonne G, Forissier JF, Desnos M, Dubourg O, Komajda M, Schwartz K, and Hainque B. Identification of two novel mutations in the ventricular regulatory myosin light chain gene (MYL2) associated with familial and classical forms of hypertrophic cardiomyopathy. J Mol Med 76: 208-214, 1998.

[54] Karabina A, Kazmierczak K, Szczesna-Cordary D, and Moore JR. Myosin regulatory light chain phosphorylation enhances cardiac beta-myosin in vitro motility under load. Arch Biochem Biophys 580: 14-21, 2015.

[55] Tardiff JC, Factor SM, Tompkins BD, Hewett TE, Palmer BM, Moore RL, Schwartz S, Robbins J, and Leinwand LA. A truncated cardiac troponin T molecule in transgenic mice suggests multiple cellular mechanisms for familial hypertrophic cardiomyopathy. J Clin Invest 101: 2800-2811., 1998.

[56] Watkins H, Seidman CE, Seidman JG, Feng HS, and Sweeney HL. Expression and functional assessment of a truncated cardiac troponin T that causes hypertrophic cardiomyopathy. Evidence for a dominant negative action. J Clin Invest 98: 2456-2461, 1996.

[57] Ford SJ, Mamidi R, Jimenez J, Tardiff JC, and Chandra M. Effects of R92 mutations in mouse cardiac troponin T are influenced by changes in myosin heavy chain isoform. J Mol Cell Cardiol 53: 542-551, 2012.

[58] Chandra M, Tschirgi ML, and Tardiff JC. Increase in tension-dependent ATP consumption induced by cardiac troponin T mutation. Am J Physiol Heart Circ Physiol 289: H2112-2119, 2005.

[59] Javadpour MM, Tardiff JC, Pinz I, and Ingwall JS. Decreased energetics in murine hearts bearing the R92Q mutation in cardiac troponin T. J Clin Invest 112: 768-775, 2003.

[60] Helms AS and Day SM. Hypertrophic cardiomyopathy: single gene disease or complex trait? Eur Heart J, 2015.

[61] Lima R, Wofford M, and Reckelhoff JF. Hypertension in postmenopausal women. Curr Hypertens Rep 14: 254-260, 2012.

[62] Rosano GM, Vitale C, Marazzi G, and Volterrani M. Menopause and cardiovascular disease: the evidence. Climacteric 10 Suppl 1: 19-24, 2007.

[63] Dubey RK, Oparil S, Imthurn B, and Jackson EK. Sex hormones and hypertension. Cardiovasc Res 53: 688-708, 2002.

[64] Olivotto I, Maron MS, Adabag AS, Casey SA, Vargiu D, Link MS, Udelson JE, Cecchi F, and Maron BJ. Gender-related differences in the clinical presentation and outcome of hypertrophic cardiomyopathy. J Am Coll Cardiol 46: 480-487, 2005.

[65] Konhilas JP and Leinwand LA. The effects of biological sex and diet on the development of heart failure. Circulation 116: 2747-2759, 2007.

[66] Yang XP and Reckelhoff JF. Estrogen, hormonal replacement therapy and cardiovascular disease. Curr Opin Nephrol Hypertens 20: 133-138, 2011.

[67] Thomas P, Pang Y, Filardo EJ, and Dong J. Identity of an estrogen membrane receptor coupled to a G protein in human breast cancer cells. Endocrinology 146: 624-632, 2005.

[68] Widder J, Pelzer T, von Poser-Klein C, Hu K, Jazbutyte V, Fritzemeier KH, Hegele-Hartung C, Neyses L, and Bauersachs J. Improvement of endothelial dysfunction by selective estrogen receptor-alpha stimulation in ovariectomized SHR. Hypertension 42: 991-996, 2003.

[69] Cavasin MA, Sankey SS, Yu AL, Menon S, and Yang XP. Estrogen and testosterone have opposing effects on chronic cardiac remodeling and function in mice with myocardial infarction. Am J Physiol Heart Circ Physiol 284: H1560-1569, 2003.

[70] van Eickels M, Grohe C, Cleutjens JP, Janssen BJ, Wellens HJ, and Doevendans PA. 17beta-estradiol attenuates the development of pressure-overload hypertrophy. Circulation 104: 1419-1423, 2001.

[71] Sharkey LC, Holycross BJ, Park S, Shiry LJ, Hoepf TM, McCune SA, and Radin MJ. Effect of ovariectomy and estrogen replacement on cardiovascular disease in heart failure-prone SHHF/Mcc- fa cp rats. J Mol Cell Cardiol 31: 1527-1537, 1999.

[72] de Jager T, Pelzer T, Muller-Botz S, Imam A, Muck J, and Neyses L. Mechanisms of estrogen receptor action in the myocardium. Rapid gene activation via the ERK1/2 pathway and serum response elements. J Biol Chem 276: 27873-27880, 2001.

[73] Grady D, Applegate W, Bush T, Furberg C, Riggs B, and Hulley SB. Heart and Estrogen/progestin Replacement Study (HERS): design, methods, and baseline characteristics. Control Clin Trials 19: 314-335, 1998.

[74] Rossouw JE, Anderson GL, Prentice RL, LaCroix AZ, Kooperberg C, Stefanick ML, Jackson RD, Beresford SA, Howard BV, Johnson KC, Kotchen JM, and Ockene J. Risks and benefits of estrogen plus progestin in healthy postmenopausal women: principal results from the Women's Health Initiative randomized controlled trial. JAMA 288: 321-333, 2002.

[75] Vikstrom KL, Factor SM, and Leinwand LA. Mice expressing mutant myosin heavy chains are a model for familial hypertrophic cardiomyopathy. Mol Med 2: 556-567, 1996.

[76] Stauffer BL, Konhilas JP, Luczak ED, and Leinwand LA. Soy diet worsens heart disease in mice. J Clin Invest 116: 209-216, 2006.

[77] Konhilas JP, Watson PA, Maass A, Boucek DM, Horn T, Stauffer BL, Luckey SW, Rosenberg P, and Leinwand LA. Exercise can prevent and reverse the severity of hypertrophic cardiomyopathy. Circ Res 98: 540-548, 2006.

[78] Geisterfer-Lowrance AA, Christe M, Conner DA, Ingwall JS, Schoen FJ, Seidman CE, and Seidman JG. A mouse model of familial hypertrophic cardiomyopathy. Science 272: 731-734, 1996.

[79] Haines CD, Harvey PA, Luczak ED, Barthel KK, Konhilas JP, Watson PA, Stauffer BL, and Leinwand LA. Estrogenic compounds are not always cardioprotective and can be lethal in males with genetic heart disease. Endocrinology 153: 4470-4479, 2012.

[80] Konhilas JP. What we know and do not know about sex and cardiac disease. J Biomed Biotechnol 2010: 562051, 2010.

[81] Simpson ER. Sources of estrogen and their importance. J Steroid Biochem Mol Biol 86: 225-230, 2003.

[82] Thomas MP and Potter BV. The structural biology of oestrogen metabolism. J Steroid Biochem Mol Biol 137: 27-49, 2013.

[83] Lipovka Y and Konhilas JP. The complex nature of estrogen signaling in breast cancer: enemy or ally. Biosci Rep, 2016.

[84] Revankar CM, Cimino DF, Sklar LA, Arterburn JB, and Prossnitz ER. A transmembrane intracellular estrogen receptor mediates rapid cell signaling. Science 307: 1625-1630, 2005.

[85] Pedram A, Razandi M, and Levin ER. Nature of functional estrogen receptors at the plasma membrane. Mol Endocrinol 20: 1996-2009, 2006.

[86] Arias-Loza PA, Kreissl MC, Kneitz S, Kaiser FR, Israel I, Hu K, Frantz S, Bayer B, Fritzemeier KH, Korach KS, and Pelzer T. The estrogen receptor-alpha is required and sufficient to maintain physiological glucose uptake in the mouse heart. Hypertension 60: 1070-1077, 2012.

[87] Rattanasopa C, Phungphong S, Wattanapermpool J, and Bupha-Intr T. Significant role of estrogen in maintaining cardiac mitochondrial functions. J Steroid Biochem Mol Biol 147: 1-9, 2015.

[88] Saleh TM, Connell BJ, and Saleh MC. Acute injection of 17beta-estradiol enhances cardiovascular reflexes and autonomic tone in ovariectomized female rats. Auton Neurosci 84: 78-88, 2000.

[89] Lipovka Y and Konhilas JP. AMP-activated protein kinase signalling in cancer and cardiac hypertrophy. Cardiovasc Pharm Open Access 4, 2015.

[90] Satoh M, Matter CM, Ogita H, Takeshita K, Wang CY, Dorn GW, 2nd, and Liao JK. Inhibition of apoptosis-regulated signaling kinase-1 and prevention of congestive heart failure by estrogen. Circulation 115: 3197-3204, 2007.

[91] Shen T, Ding L, Ruan Y, Qin W, Lin Y, Xi C, Lu Y, Dou L, Zhu Y, Cao Y, Man Y, Bian Y, Wang S, Xiao C, and Li J. SIRT1 functions as an important regulator of estrogen-mediated cardiomyocyte protection in angiotensin II-induced heart hypertrophy. Oxid Med Cell Longev 2014: 713894, 2014.

[92] Patten RD, Pourati I, Aronovitz MJ, Baur J, Celestin F, Chen X, Michael A, Haq S, Nuedling S, Grohe C, Force T, Mendelsohn ME, and Karas RH. 17beta-estradiol reduces cardiomyocyte apoptosis in vivo and in vitro via activation of phospho-inositide-3 kinase/Akt signaling. Circ Res 95: 692-699, 2004.

[93] Donaldson C, Eder S, Baker C, Aronovitz MJ, Weiss AD, Hall-Porter M, Wang F, Ackerman A, Karas RH, Molkentin JD, and Patten RD. Estrogen attenuates left ventricular and cardiomyocyte hypertrophy by an estrogen receptor-dependent pathway that increases calcineurin degradation. Circ Res 104: 265-275, 211p following 275, 2009.

[94] Pedram A, Razandi M, Aitkenhead M, and Levin ER. Estrogen inhibits cardiomyocyte hypertrophy in vitro. Antagonism of calcineurin-related hypertrophy through induction of MCIP1. J Biol Chem 280: 26339-26348, 2005.

[95] Voloshenyuk TG and Gardner JD. Estrogen improves TIMP-MMP balance and collagen distribution in volume-overloaded hearts of ovariectomized females. Am J Physiol Regul Integr Comp Physiol 299: R683-693, 2010.

[96] Pelzer T, Loza PA, Hu K, Bayer B, Dienesch C, Calvillo L, Couse JF, Korach KS, Neyses L, and Ertl G. Increased mortality and aggravation of heart failure in estrogen receptor-beta knockout mice after myocardial infarction. Circulation 111: 1492-1498, 2005.

[97] Bolego C, Rossoni G, Fadini GP, Vegeto E, Pinna C, Albiero M, Boscaro E, Agostini C, Avogaro A, Gaion RM, and Cignarella A. Selective estrogen receptor-alpha agonist provides widespread heart and vascular protection with enhanced endothelial progenitor cell mobilization in the absence of uterotrophic action. FASEB J 24: 2262-2272, 2010.

[98] Westphal C, Schubert C, Prelle K, Penkalla A, Fliegner D, Petrov G, and Regitz-Zagrosek V. Effects of estrogen, an ERalpha agonist and raloxifene on pressure overload induced cardiac hypertrophy. PLoS One 7: e50802, 2012.

[99] Babiker FA, Lips D, Meyer R, Delvaux E, Zandberg P, Janssen B, van Eys G, Grohe C, and Doevendans PA. Estrogen receptor beta protects the murine heart against left ventricular hypertrophy. Arterioscler Thromb Vasc Biol 26: 1524-1530, 2006.

[100] Fliegner D, Schubert C, Penkalla A, Witt H, Kararigas G, Dworatzek E, Staub E, Martus P, Ruiz Noppinger P, Kintscher U, Gustafsson JA, and Regitz-Zagrosek V. Female sex and estrogen receptor-beta attenuate cardiac remodeling and apoptosis in pressure overload. Am J Physiol Regul Integr Comp Physiol 298: R1597-1606, 2010.

[101] Kararigas G, Fliegner D, Gustafsson JA, and Regitz-Zagrosek V. Role of the estrogen/estrogen-receptor-beta axis in the genomic response to pressure overload-induced hypertrophy. Physiol Genom 43: 438-446, 2011.

[102] Queiros AM, Eschen C, Fliegner D, Kararigas G, Dworatzek E, Westphal C, Sanchez Ruderisch H, and Regitz-Zagrosek V. Sex- and estrogen-dependent regulation of a miRNA network in the healthy and hypertrophied heart. Int J Cardiol 169: 331-338, 2013.

[103] Gurgen D, Hegner B, Kusch A, Catar R, Chaykovska L, Hoff U, Gross V, Slowinski T, da Costa Goncalves AC, Kintscher U, Gustafsson JA, Luft FC, and Dragun D. Estrogen receptor-beta signals left ventricular hypertrophy sex differences in normotensive deoxycorticosterone acetate-salt mice. Hypertension 57: 648-654, 2011.

[104] Pedram A, Razandi M, O'Mahony F, Lubahn D, and Levin ER. Estrogen receptor-beta prevents cardiac fibrosis. Mol Endocrinol 24: 2152-2165, 2010.

[105] Pedram A, Razandi M, Lubahn D, Liu J, Vannan M, and Levin ER. Estrogen inhibits cardiac hypertrophy: role of estrogen receptor-beta to inhibit calcineurin. Endocrinology 149: 3361-3369, 2008.

[106] Pedram A, Razandi M, Narayanan R, Dalton JT, McKinsey TA, and Levin ER. Estrogen regulates histone deacetylases to prevent cardiac hypertrophy. Mol Biol Cell 24: 3805-3818, 2013.

[107] Gardner JD, Murray DB, Voloshenyuk TG, Brower GL, Bradley JM, and Janicki JS. Estrogen attenuates chronic volume overload induced structural and functional remodeling in male rat hearts. Am J Physiol Heart Circ Physiol 298: H497-504, 2010.

[108] Kadokami T, McTiernan CF, Higuichi Y, Frye CS, Kubota T, and Feldman AM. 17 Beta-estradiol improves survival in male mice with cardiomyopathy induced by cardiac-specific tumor necrosis factor-alpha overexpression. J Interferon Cytokine Res 25: 254-260, 2005.

[109] Brinckmann M, Kaschina E, Altarche-Xifro W, Curato C, Timm M, Grzesiak A, Dong J, Kappert K, Kintscher U, Unger T, and Li J. Estrogen receptor alpha supports cardiomyocytes indirectly through post-infarct cardiac c-kit + cells. J Mol Cell Cardiol 47: 66-75, 2009.

[110] Brinckmann M, Kaschina E, Altarche-Xifro W, Curato C, Timm M, Grzesiak A, Dong J, Kappert K, Kintscher U, Unger T, and Li J. Estrogen receptor alpha supports cardiomyocytes indirectly through post-infarct cardiac c-kit+ cells. J Mol Cell Cardiol 47: 66-75, 2009.

[111] Rivera Z, Christian PJ, Marion SL, Brooks HL, and Hoyer PB. Steroidogenic capacity of residual ovarian tissue in 4-vinylcyclohexene diepoxide-treated mice. Biol Reprod 80: 328-336, 2009.

[112] Mayer LP, Devine PJ, Dyer CA, and Hoyer PB. The follicle-deplete mouse ovary produces androgen. Biol Reprod 71: 130-138, 2004.

[113] Morris PD and Channer KS. Testosterone and cardiovascular disease in men. Asian J Androl 14: 428-435, 2012.

[114] Erickson GF, Magoffin DA, Dyer CA, and Hofeditz C. The ovarian androgen producing cells: a review of structure/function relationships. Endocr Rev 6: 371-399, 1985.

[115] Liu Y, Ding J, Bush TL, Longenecker JC, Nieto FJ, Golden SH, and Szklo M. Relative androgen excess and increased cardiovascular risk after menopause: a hypothesized relation. Am J Epidemiol 154: 489-494, 2001.

[116] Pollow DP, Jr., Romero-Aleshire MJ, Sanchez JN, Konhilas JP, and Brooks HL. ANG II-induced hypertension in the VCD mouse model of menopause is prevented by estrogen replacement during perimenopause. Am J Physiol Regul Integr Comp Physiol 309: R1546-1552, 2015.

[117] Rundell VL, Geenen DL, Buttrick PM, and de Tombe PP. Depressed cardiac tension cost in experimental diabetes is due to altered myosin heavy chain isoform expression. Am J Physiol Heart Circ Physiol 287: H408-413, 2004.

# Chapter 6

# Idiopathic Dilated Cardiomyopathy: Molecular Basis and Distilling Complexity to Advance

Santiago Roura, Carolina Gálvez-Montón,
Josep Lupón and Antoni Bayes-Genis

Additional information is available at the end of the chapter

http://dx.doi.org/10.5772/64996

**Abstract**

Cardiomyopathies are heterogeneous diseases of the myocardium associated with abnormal findings of chamber size, wall thickness, and/or functional contractility. In particular, dilated cardiomyopathy (DCM) is mainly characterized by ventricular chamber enlargement with systolic dysfunction and normal left ventricular (LV) wall thickness. Although DCM is thought to be induced mainly by genetic or environmental factors, in the majority of cases, the cause is unknown. With an estimated prevalence of 1:2500 and an incidence of 1:18,000 per year in adults, DCM is the most frequent indication for heart transplantation, which represents an enormous cost burden on healthcare systems. These figures warrant greater accuracy in patient diagnosis and prognosis and further insight into the underlying basis of DCM. Here, we discuss past and recent findings on the molecular mechanisms involved in DCM. Dilated cardiomyopathy has been linked to the overactivation of extracellular signal-regulated kinase (ERK1/2), which in turn is related to activation of low-density lipoprotein receptor–related protein-1 (LRP-1). Moreover, a redistribution of LRP-1 into cholesterol-enriched plasma membrane domains (lipid rafts) and alterations in cardiac DNA methylation have been reported in failing hearts. In conclusion, more comprehensive analyses of myocardial lipid rafts and epigenetic mechanisms may advance our understanding of DCM causes and progression. In turn, this understanding may promote the development of innovative treatments.

**Keywords:** dilated cardiomyopathy, heart failure, lipid rafts, LRP-1, molecular basis, cardiac muscle, vasculature

## 1. Introduction

Cardiomyopathies are heterogeneous diseases of the myocardium associated with abnormal findings of chamber size, wall thickness, and/or functional contractility [1]. Currently, cardiomyopathy is classified based on the dominant pathophysiology or by aetiological/pathogenetic factors. This system defines four distinct categories of cardiomyopathy: dilated, hypertrophic, restrictive, and arrhythmogenic (**Figure 1**) [2]. In particular, dilated cardiomyopathy (DCM) is mainly characterized by ventricular chamber enlargement or dilatation with systolic dysfunction and normal left ventricular (LV) wall thickness. In general, these abnormalities lead to progressive heart failure, a decline in LV contractile function, abnormalities in ventricular and supraventricular rhythm and conduction, thromboembolism, and finally, sudden or heart failure-related death [3]. Indeed, DCM is a common, largely irreversible cause of myocardial damage. It is thought to be induced by genetic or environmental factors that may manifest clinically over a wide range of ages (most commonly in the third or fourth decade, but also in young children). Dilated cardiomyopathy affects both sexes and all ethnic groups; it is typically identified when patients exhibit severe limiting symptoms and incapacity [4].

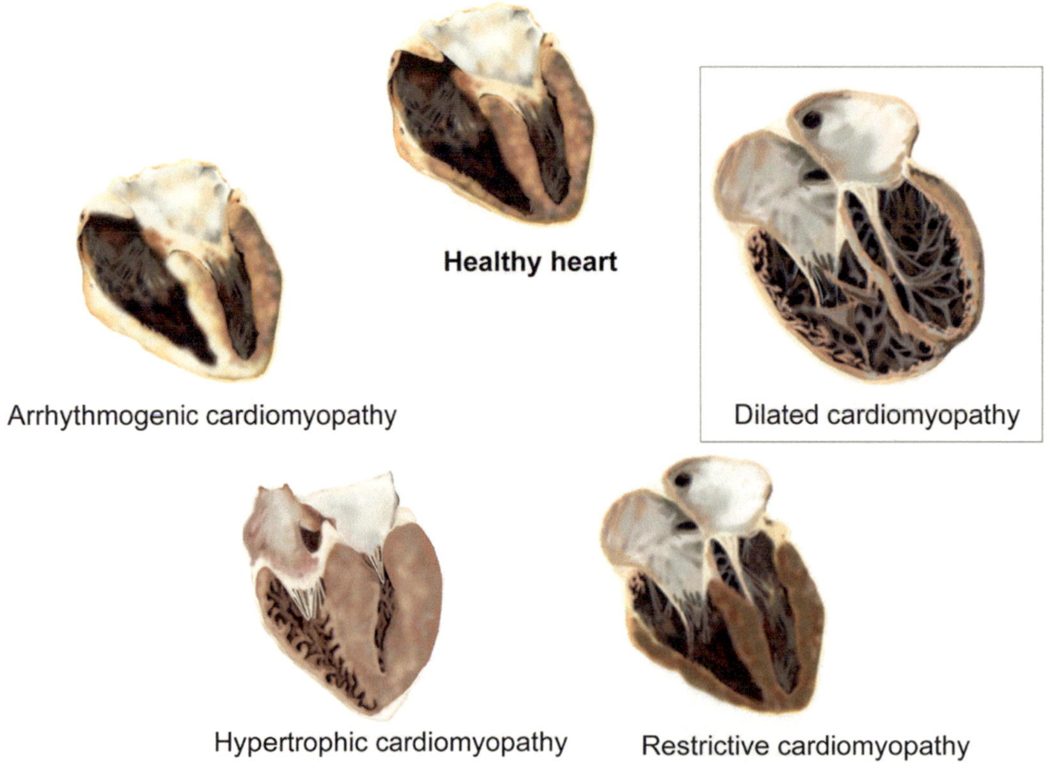


**Figure 1.** Heterogeneous diseases of the myocardium. The different types of cardiomyopathies fall into four principal categories, based on the muscle disorder involved. This chapter is confined to dilated cardiomyopathy.

http://dx.doi.org/10.5772/64996

This chapter summarizes the most important traits (aetiology, diagnosis, treatment, and pathophysiology) that characterize DCM. We focus on studies that provided novel insights into the underlying molecular basis of this extremely complex human disorder. In a sense, we will present new pieces of an intriguing puzzle, with the aim of bringing some order into the chaos of the molecular reality.

## 2. Dilated cardiomyopathy: characteristic features

Dilated cardiomyopathy has an estimated prevalence of 1:2500, an incidence of 1:15,000–18,000 per year in adults, and an estimated prevalence of 2:3 among children with unknown diseases [4, 5]. The clinical course of DCM can be progressive; one study reported that about 35% of individuals died within 5 years after diagnosis [1]. The origin of death is divided evenly between sudden death and pump failure. To date, prolonged survival has been achieved with neurohormone blockers (angiotensin-converting enzyme inhibitors and β-adrenoceptor antagonists) and devices (cardiac resynchronization and implanted defibrillators). Nevertheless, the only definitive treatment is heart transplantation, which is hampered in many instances by the limited number of heart donors and by graft rejection over time. Therefore, DCM is the most frequent indication for heart transplantation, which results in an enormous cost burden for healthcare systems throughout the world. Diagnosis is typically based on patient history and the presence of LV dilatation and impaired ejection fraction, with or without regurgitation; these signs are detected with echocardiography, cardiac magnetic resonance imaging, or both.

At the histological level, the main pathological derangements observed in explanted diseased hearts are patchy interstitial fibrosis surrounding myocardial filaments, marked lipid deposition, cardiac muscle atrophy, and lipid accumulation [6–8]. Moreover, further investigations of both patient samples and animal disease models have shown that DCM hearts exhibit marked vascular alterations [9, 10]. In most cases, the causal mechanism of disease is poorly understood. This reality has induced some authors to argue that heart disease in DCM arises from an obscure origin, and this viewpoint has given rise to the term 'idiopathic' DCM. Recently, relevant advances have been made in our understanding of the causes of this disease. The main causes include familial and genetic disorders, infectious and toxicity-related processes, autoimmunity, and inflammation [4].

Frequently, DCM has been defined as the result of an extremely complex genetic architecture that involves disruptions in a variety of myocardial proteins, which are provoked by rare variants in some genes; moreover, many of these genes are also involved in other cardiomyopathies, such as muscular dystrophy or syndromic diseases [11]. In brief, numerous DCM-associated genes have been identified. This information has provided a better understanding of disease pathogenesis, and it has promoted advances in mutation analytical techniques to facilitate the recognition of subjects and progeny that carry these mutations [12]. Alterations in more than 50 loci and genes have been identified, which mostly encode either cardiac myocyte-specific proteins or structural, nuclear membrane, and calcium metabolism proteins.

However, it is estimated that genetic disorders account for only 20–35% of DCM cases [12, 13]. Some researchers have predicted that genetic associations may have been missed due to the limited nature of previous studies; accordingly, they point to a need for more comprehensive studies in much larger cohorts of families that are rigorously phenotyped [11]. In addition, some cases of DCM are believed to be related to autoimmune and inflammatory processes [14–16]; metabolic, nutritional, and endocrine deficiencies; or heart muscle damage following exposure to viruses, exogenous drugs, or toxins (e.g., chronic alcohol consumption) [2]. Peripartum cardiomyopathy also represents a subset of LV systolic dysfunction. In the latter cases, initial symptoms of heart failure occur during the late stages of pregnancy [17]. Although there may be a variety of causes for DCM, the clinical presentation of this disease seems to be uniform, both in humans and in animal models that have been used to dissect DCM development, progression, and treatment [10].

Standard treatment of DCM involves neurohormonal inhibition of the renin-angiotensin-aldosterone system (i.e., angiotensin-converting enzyme inhibitors, angiotensin II receptor type 1 blockers, or mineralocorticoid receptor blockers) or blocking the sympathetic nervous system with β-blockers. In patients, it is crucial to focus on improving cardiac function and reducing mechanical stress. Although progress has been made in arrhythmia therapy and in sudden death prevention, many impediments for improving patient outcomes remain unresolved [4]. Innovative therapies, such as stem cell-based applications, are also being investigated [18].

## 3. Dilated cardiomyopathy affects both cardiac muscle and the vasculature

Dilated cardiomyopathy is associated with pronounced remodelling of one or both ventricles, which results in large changes in the shapes of ventricles and in the architecture of myocardial fibres. As mentioned previously, the main microscopic hallmarks of failing hearts are marked collagen deposition, patchy interstitial fibrosis, degenerated cardiac muscle cells, and sparse blood vessels. At the ultrastructural level, remodelling comprises mitochondrial abnormalities, T-tubular dilatation, and intracellular lipid droplet accumulation [10]. Because the mitochondrion is the main site of ATP production and cardiac myocytes are particularly sensitive to the supply of energy, deficits in mitochondrial function have been linked to DCM [19]. Additionally, altered levels of connexin-43 and modulation of its phosphorylation state can induce electromechanical uncoupling between neighbouring cardiac muscle cells [20].

A number of studies have indicated that programmed cell death or apoptosis contributes actively to human end-stage heart failure. Indeed, cell death occurs in myocardial ischemia-reperfusion [21], ischemia-reperfusion injury [22], and fatal myocarditis [23]. However, the role of apoptosis in the DCM myocardium remains controversial, due to some limitations in the techniques that have been used to measure apoptosis [24–26]. A positive Terminal deoxynucleotidyl transferase dUTP nick end labeling (TUNEL) signal seems to require fragmentation of only 10% of all DNA; as a result, the level of apoptosis may be highly overestimated [24]. Furthermore, cells that are apoptotic, necrotic, undergoing DNA repair, or living can emit

http://dx.doi.org/10.5772/64996

equivalent signals in the TUNEL assay [27], which renders the use of this method even more questionable. Consequently, although some authors have reported putative increases in apoptotic markers with different methodologies, including caspase-3 activity, DNA fragmentation (TUNEL), and electron microscopy [28], others have failed to detect changes in apoptosis. For instance, Bott-Flügel *et al.* did not detect any correlations between caspase-3 activity, the induction of DNA fragmentation, and haemodynamic or echocardiographic variables in patients with end-stage heart failure, including DCM. Moreover, they did not find significant differences in caspase-3 activation between DCM and control myocardium [26]. **Figure 2** shows that only slight amounts of caspase-3 mRNA and protein were detected in LV samples from patients (unpublished results). These findings suggest that cardiac muscle cells might trigger apoptotic self-destruction, without completing the process. Hence, DCM is characterized by marked abnormalities in the function and integrity of cardiac muscle.

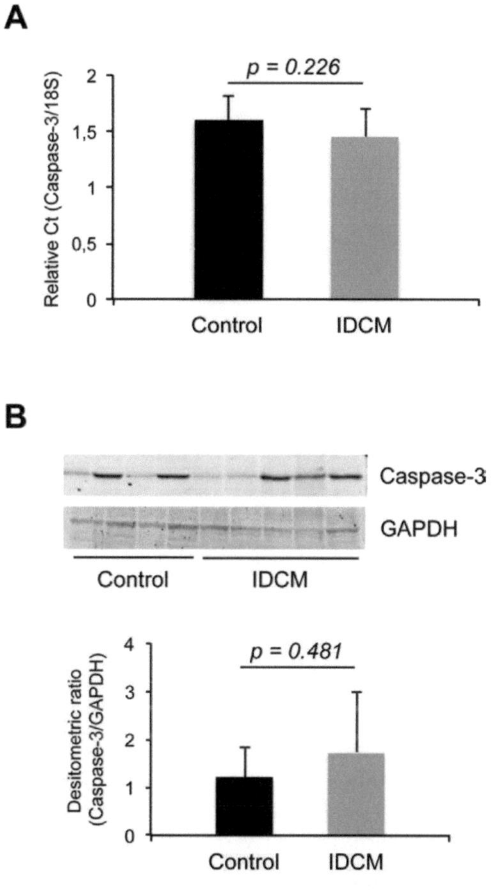


**Figure 2.** Comparative analysis of apoptosis in left ventricle samples collected from human explanted DCM hearts and control hearts from non-cardiac decedents. Representative caspase-3 gene (**A**) and protein (**B**) expression levels by quantitative RT-PCR and Western blotting, respectively.

Cardiac endothelial dysfunction was also associated with disease progression and a poor prognosis in patients with DCM. In the late 1940s, preliminary observations showed a correlation between heart weight and the total cross-sectional size of the main coronary vessels [29]. Since then, a number of studies have recognized that cardiac vasculature is a key regulator of the integrity and function of the myocardium. In an attempt to take this a step further, Brutsaert *et al.* studied the mechanical properties of the mammalian ventricular myocardium before and after damaging the endocardial surface [30]. Those authors speculated that the endocardium could affect myocardial performance by either forming an electrochemical barrier, releasing a chemical substance or messenger, or both. They subsequently demonstrated that nitric oxide synthase activity regulated the contractile responsiveness of ventricular myocytes [31]. Perhaps more significantly, additional studies in Langendorff-perfused and post-infarcted rat hearts confirmed that endothelial damage led to progressive myocardial dysfunction and that, conversely, protecting the associated vasculature preserved global myocardial homeostasis [32, 33].

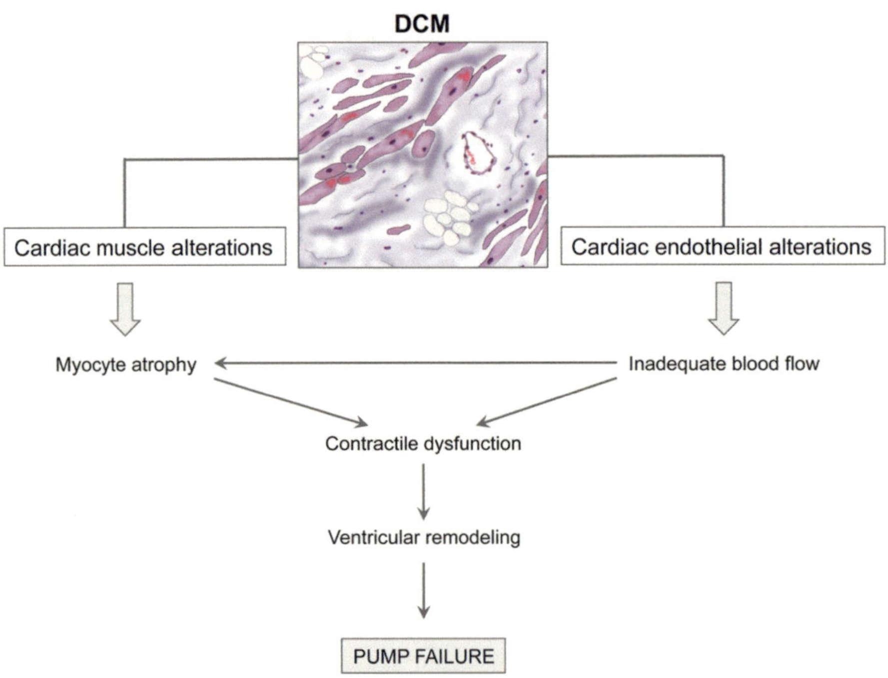


**Figure 3.** Foundation of DCM as a two-hit heart disease. The integrity and function of both cardiac muscle and vasculature are adversely compromised in DCM, which leads to LV remodelling and pump failure.

Advances in medical imaging techniques have become crucial for performing more comprehensive analyses of vascular derangements in DCM. Angiography revealed that a mismatch between artery size and LV mass in patients with DCM contributed to myocardial hypoperfusion [34–37]. Computed tomography measurements of DCM cardiac vasculature on a multislice scanner have also clearly shown side branch paucity and shortened, thinned epicardial arteries [9]. Therefore, the epicardial coronary arteries in patients with DCM are not adequately sized for the enlarged LV mass. Notably, a variety of studies described significantly reduced, sparse microvasculature in diseased myocardium samples [9, 38, 39]. In this context, numerous studies in patients with DCM have reported that the circulating levels of distinct bone marrow-derived cell populations are peripherally increased after vascular damage [40]. Although there is a correlation between the circulating levels of these progenitor cells and the progression and clinical outcomes of DCM, the clinical usefulness of this overrepresentation awaits further validation.

Collectively, these findings led to a re-examination of the pathophysiology of DCM. In 2009, Roura and Bayes-Genis [10] reviewed the extensive data from animal models and patients and concluded that DCM is a two-hit disease, where both cardiac muscle and endothelial alterations contribute equally to contractile deficiency and pump failure (**Figure 3**).

## 4. Molecular basis of dilated cardiomyopathy: past and new actors

Molecularly, in humans, DCM has been related to intramyocardial accumulation of $\alpha$-2 macroglobulin ($\alpha$-2M) [41] and increased activation of extracellular signal-regulated kinase (ERK1/2) [42]. In a mouse model of DCM, the disease was generated by a mutation in the lamin A/C gene [43, 44]. In these mice, chemically suppressing ERK1/2 activation prevented LV dilatation and greatly restored the cardiac ejection fraction.

The $\alpha$-2M protein is a highly abundant plasma protease inhibitor, which has been shown to activate various tyrosine kinases and mitogen-activated protein kinases [45]. Moreover, $\alpha$-2M was one of the first molecules to be described as a ligand of low-density lipoprotein (LDL) receptor-related protein 1 (LRP-1) [46]. A recent review described LRP-1 as a multifunctional receptor of the LDL-receptor family that mediates the clearance of a variety of structurally diverse extracellular molecules [47]. Moreover, LRP-1 plays key roles in various biological processes by interacting with multiple intracellular signalling pathways [48, 49]. As a result, LRP-1 tyrosine phosphorylation can be activated in response to diverse extracellular molecules, such as platelet-derived growth factor [50–52]. In particular, ERK1/2 activation is recognized as one of the main LRP-1 molecular relays [53–55]. In the following pages, we present and discuss novel data demonstrating that, together with the pivotal role of LRP-1 in the vascular wall and in the aetiology of atherosclerosis [56], LRP-1 is redistributed and overactivated within some specialized plasma membrane domains, termed lipid rafts, in DCM myocardium.

The decreased capillary density found in patients with DCM was shown to arise from impairments in myocardial endothelial cell survival and insufficient revascularization. These processes involve several intracellular signalling pathways, including those mediated by vascular endothelial (VE)-cadherin/β-catenin, angiopoietins, and vascular endothelial growth factors (VEGFs). In particular, VE-cadherin, β-catenin, angiopoietin-2, VEGF-A, VEGF-B, and VEGF receptor-1 (VEGFR-1) expression levels were downregulated in DCM [9, 57, 58]. Roura *et al.* [9] further demonstrated that reduced expression of β-catenin, an important angiogenic regulator [59], occurred exclusively in myocardial vascular cells in failing hearts.

Remarkably, different DNA methylation patterns have been detected in genes that regulate pathways related to heart disease and in genes with unknown functions in DCM. For example, variations in DNA methylation were observed in lymphocyte antigen 75, tyrosine kinase-type cell surface receptor HER3, homeobox B13, and adenosine receptor A2A [60]. These validated targets are most likely involved in modifying DCM rather than independently causing disease. Furthermore, other authors found differentially methylated gene promoters and a depletion of mitochondrial DNA that resulted in a thymidine kinase deficiency in DCM hearts [61, 62]. Indeed, investigating epigenetic mechanisms represents an attractive approach for finding novel mechanisms of disease.

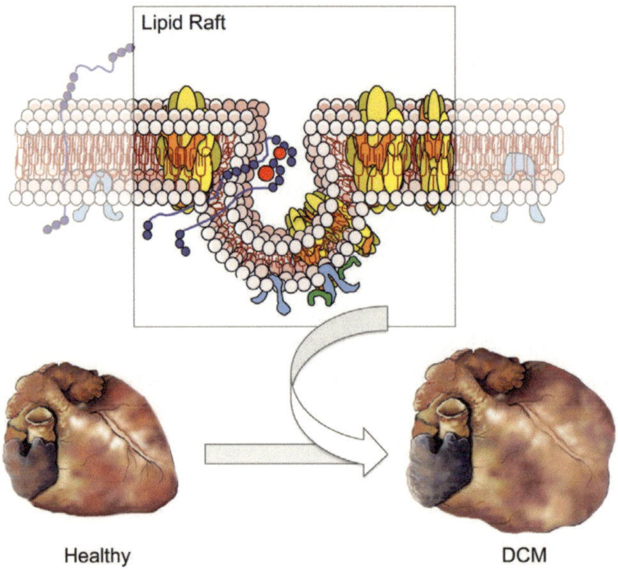


**Figure 4.** Potential impact of lipid raft–associated signalling on DCM. Schematic illustration of a lipid raft domain in a portion of the cell surface. Proteins potentially involved in disease progression are either packed into or excluded from these specialized plasma membrane areas.

For more than 40 years, the Singer and Nicolson model of the cell membrane, where proteins are viewed as icebergs floating in a sea of lipids, has provided a solid foundation for studying cell membrane properties [63]. This enduring model was subsequently reinterpreted with the discovery of localized, highly cholesterol- and glycosphingolipid-enriched plasma membrane areas, referred to as 'lipid rafts' [64]. Many proteins, particularly those involved in cell signalling and cytokine presentation, were found to be densely packed together in these specialized surface domains [65]. Accordingly, lipid rafts facilitate interactions between protein receptors and mediators by maintaining them tightly packed together in one location. Interestingly, LRP-1 was reported to be associated with lipid rafts [66, 67].

As previously mentioned, recent research has given us new molecular aspects of the disease. Particularly, in patients with DCM, LRP-1 was seen redistributed and further activated, through tyrosine phosphorylation, within lipid rafts enriched in caveolin-3 and flotillin-1 [68]. Of note, these observations suggested that movement of LRP-1 within these specialized membrane domains contribute to the overactivation of ERK1/2-mediated signalling described in DCM. However, further confirmatory exploration is warranted to determine whether this overactive signalling leads to the characteristic promotion of extracellular matrix metalloproteinase activity and subsequent LV remodelling (**Figure 4**) [69, 70].

To investigate this novel regulatory impact of lipid rafts on DCM, Roura *et al*. extracted lipid rafts from failing myocardium and detected elevated amounts of the mobilizing cytokine, stromal cell-derived factor (SDF)-1 [71]. In that same study, the authors showed that deficiencies in ILK and ERK1/2 signalling impeded SDF-1-mediated migration of circulating progenitor cells. As a result, impaired cell migration compromised endothelial maintenance and recovery, which contributed to the marked vascular derangements observed in diseased myocardium [72].

Taken together, these observations support the growing body of data that led to the recognition of myocardial lipid rafts and their associated proteins as modulators of cardiac performance and as novel therapeutic targets [73–75].

## 5. Conclusions

Heart failure has become an increasingly common disorder worldwide, and it is associated with substantial morbidity and mortality. Many causes of heart failure are easily identified in clinical practice, including abnormal heart valves, inherited cardiomyopathies, severe coronary artery disease, or hypertensive heart disease. However, the precise mechanisms that govern the progression of heart failure and ventricular remodelling in DCM remain obscure. Some authors have appropriately pointed out that, for both clinicians and researchers, attempting to discover the underlying genetic and environmental causes linked to complex human diseases, such as DCM, is like facing a drawer filled with thousands of puzzle pieces mixed together from an unknown number of jigsaw puzzles [76, 77]. The question remains, how can they begin to solve it?

There is a growing body of data that describes the multifaceted genetic diversity involved in DCM and the alterations in both cardiac muscle and vasculature that contribute to the disease. However, several crucial issues remain to be addressed. For example, it is not clear whether the marked vascular deficiencies observed in patients with DCM develop secondary to heart remodelling, or whether they directly contribute to myocardial alterations and to the temporal evolution of LV dilatation. Accordingly, researchers are providing novel mechanistic insights that might bring some order to this 'disordered' collection of data. For example, they have shown that lipid rafts participate in the mechanism underlying the spatial regulation of LRP-1-mediated ERK1/2 activity. Undoubtedly, further work is needed to increase our comprehension of the causes underlying this 'obscure' disease. To that end, the current state of knowledge summarized in the present review provides a starting point for addressing the remaining questions in the pathophysiology of this disease. Moreover, we highlight new avenues for discovering potentially effective treatments.

## Funding sources

This work was supported by grants from the Ministerio de Educación y Ciencia (SAF2014-59892), Fundació La MARATÓ de TV3 (201502 and 201516), Fundació Daniel Bravo Andreu, Sociedad Española de Cardiología, Societat Catalana de Cardiologia, Generalitat de Catalunya (SGR 2014), and Acadèmia de Ciències Mèdiques i de la Salut de Catalunya i de Balears. This work was also funded by the Red de Terapia Celular - TerCel (RD12/0019/0029), Red de Investigación Cardiovascular - RIC (RD12/0042/0047), and Fondo de Investigación Sanitaria, Instituto de Salud Carlos III (FIS PI14/01682) projects as part of the Plan Nacional de I+D+I and cofounded by ISCIII-Sudirección General de Evaluación y el Fondo Europeo de Desarrollo Regional (FEDER).

## Author details

Santiago Roura[1,2*], Carolina Gálvez-Montón[1], Josep Lupón[3,4] and Antoni Bayes-Genis[1,3,4]

*Address all correspondence to: sroura@igtp.cat

1 ICREC Research Program, Germans Trias i Pujol Health Science Research Institute, Badalona, Spain

2 Center of Regenerative Medicine in Barcelona, Barcelona,Spain

3 Cardiology Service, Germans Trias i Pujol University Hospital, Badalona, Spain

4 Department of Medicine, Autonomous University of Barcelona, Barcelona, Spain

## References

[1] Towbin JA, Bowles NE: The failing heart. Nature. 2002;415:227-233.

[2] Maron BJ, Towbin JA, Thiene G, Antzelevitch C, Corrado D, Arnett D, Moss AJ, Seidman CE, Young JB; American Heart Association; Council on Clinical Cardiology, Heart Failure and Transplantation Committee; Quality of Care and Outcomes Research and Functional Genomics and Translational Biology Interdisciplinary Working Groups; Council on Epidemiology and Prevention. Contemporary definitions and classification

of the cardiomyopathies: an American Heart Association Scientific Statement from the Council on Clinical Cardiology, Heart Failure and Transplantation Committee; Quality of Care and Outcomes Research and Functional Genomics and Translational Biology Interdisciplinary Working Groups; and Council on Epidemiology and Prevention. Circulation. 2006;113:1807-1816.

[3] Towbin JA, Lorts A: Arrhythmias and dilated cardiomyopathy common pathogenetic pathways? J Am Coll Cardiol. 2011;57:2169-2171.

[4] Jefferies JL, Towbin JA: Dilated cardiomyopathy. Lancet. 2010;375:752-762.

[5] Towbin JA, Lowe AM, Colan SD, Sleeper LA, Orav EJ, Clunie S, Messere J, Cox GF, Lurie PR, Hsu D, Canter C, Wilkinson JD, Lipshultz SE: Incidence, causes, and outcomes of dilated cardiomyopathy in children. JAMA. 2006;296:1867-1876.

[6] Marijianowski MM, Teeling P, Mann J, Becker A: Dilated cardiomyopathy is associated with an increase in the type I/type III collagen ratio: a quantitative assessment. J Am Col Cardiol. 1995;25:1263–1272.

[7] Gunja-Smith Z, Gunja-Smith Z, Morales AR, Romanelli R, Woessner JF Jr: Remodeling of human myocardial collagen in idiopathic dilated cardiomyopathy. Role of metallo-proteinases and pyridinoline cross-links. Am J Pathol. 1996;148:1639-1648.

[8] Pauschinger M, Knopf D, Petschauer S, Doerner A, Poller W, Schwimmbeck PL, Kühl U, Schultheiss HP: Dilated cardiomyopathy is associated with significant changes in collagen type I/III ratio. Circulation. 1999;99:2750-2756.

[9] Roura S, Planas F, Prat-Vidal C, Leta R, Soler-Botija C, Carreras F, Llach A, Hove-Madsen L, Pons Lladó G, Farré J, Cinca J, Bayes-Genis A: Idiopathic dilated cardiomy-opathy exhibits defective vascularization and vessel formation. Eur J Heart Fail. 2007;9:995-1002.

[10] Roura S, Bayes-Genis A: Vascular dysfunction in idiopathic dilated cardiomyopathy. Nat Rev Cardiol. 2009;6:590-598.

[11] Hershberger RE, Hedges DJ, Morales A: Dilated cardiomyopathy: the complexity of a diverse genetic architecture. Nat Rev Cardiol. 2013;10:531-547.

[12] Jacoby D, McKenna WJ: Genetics of inherited cardiomyopathy. Eur Heart J. 2012;33:296-304.

[13] Seidman JG, Seidman C: The genetic basis for cardiomyopathy: from mutation identification to mechanistic paradigms. Cell. 2001;104:557-567.

[14] Lappé JM, Pelfrey CM, Tang WH: Recent insights into the role of autoimmunity in idiopathic dilated cardiomyopathy. J Card Fail. 2008;14:521-530.

[15] Jahns R, Boivin V, Schwarzbach V, Ertl G, Lohse MJ: Pathological autoantibodies in cardiomyopathy. Autoimmunity. 2008;41:454-461.

[16] Kaya Z, Katus HA: Role of autoimmunity in dilated cardiomyopathy. Basic Res Cardiol. 2010;105:7-8.

[17] Bachelier-Walenta K, Hilfiker-Kleiner D, Sliwa K: Peripartum cardiomyopathy: update 2012. Curr Opin Crit Care. 2013;19:397-403.

[18] Roura S, Gálvez-Montón C, Bayes-Genis A: Umbilical cord blood-derived mesenchymal stem cells: new therapeutic weapons for idiopathic dilated cardiomyopathy? Int J Cardiol. 2014;177:809-818.

[19] Limongelli G, Masarone D, D'Alessandro R, Elliott PM: Mitochondrial diseases and the heart: an overview of molecular basis, diagnosis, treatment and clinical course. Future Cardiol. 2012;8:71-88.

[20] Ai X, Pogwizd SM: Connexin 43 downregulation and dephosphorylation in nonischemic heart failure is associated with enhanced colocalized protein phosphatase type 2A. Circ Res. 2005;96:54-63.

[21] Gottlieb RA, Engler RL: Apoptosis in myocardial ischemia-reperfusion. Ann N Y Acad Sci. 1999;874:412-426.

[22] Saraste A, Pulkki K, Kallajoki M, Henriksen K, Parvinen M, Voipio-Pulkki LM: Apoptosis in human acute myocardial infarction. Circulation. 1997;95:320-323.

[23] Kytö V, Saraste A, Saukko P, Henn V, Pulkki K, Vuorinen T, Voipio-Pulkki LM: Apoptotic cardiomyocyte death in fatal myocarditis. Am J Cardiol. 2004;94:746-750.

[24] Schaper J, Lorenz-Meyer S, Suzuki K: The role of apoptosis in dilated cardiomyopathy. Herz. 1999;24:219-224.

[25] Westphal E, Rohrbach S, Buerke M, Behr H, Darmer D, Silber RE, Werdan K, Loppnow H: Altered interleukin-1 receptor antagonist and interleukin-18 mRNA expression in myocardial tissues of patients with dilatated cardiomyopathy. Mol Med. 2008;14:55-63.

[26] Bott-Flügel L, Weig HJ, Uhlein H, Nabauer M, Laugwitz KL, Seyfarth M: Quantitative analysis of apoptotic markers in human end-stage heart failure. Eur J Heart Fail. 2008;10:129-132.

[27] Kanoh M, Takemura G, Misao J, Hayakawa Y, Aoyama T, Nishigaki K, Noda T, Fujiwara T, Fukuda K, Minatoguchi S, Fujiwara H: Significance of myocytes with positive DNA in situ nick end-labeling (TUNEL) in hearts with dilated cardiomyopathy: not apoptosis but DNA repair. Circulation. 1999;99:2757-2764.

[28] Narula J, Haider N, Virmani R, DiSalvo TG, Kolodgie FD, Hajjar RJ, Schmidt U, Semigran MJ, Dec GW, Khaw BA: Apoptosis in myocytes in end-stage heart failure. N Engl J Med. 1996;335:1182-1189.

[29] Harrison CV, Wood P: Hypertensive and ischaemic heart disease; a comparative clinical and pathological study. Br Heart J. 1949;11:205-229.

[30] Brutsaert DL, Meulemans AL, Sipido KR, Sys SU: Effects of damaging the endocardial surface on the mechanical performance of isolated cardiac muscle. Circ Res. 1988;62:358-366.

[31] Ungureanu-Longrois D, Balligand JL, Okada I, Simmons WW, Kobzik L, Lowenstein CJ, Kunkel SL, Michel T, Kelly RA, Smith TW: Contractile responsiveness of ventricular myocytes to isoproterenol is regulated by induction of nitric oxide synthase activity in cardiac microvascular endothelial cells in heterotypic primary culture. Circ Res. 1995;77:486-493.

[32] Qi XL, Nguyen TL, Andries L, Sys SU, Rouleau JL: Vascular endothelial dysfunction contributes to myocardial depression in ischemia-reperfusion in the rat. Can J Physiol Pharmacol. 1998;76:35-45.

[33] Qi XL, Stewart DJ, Gosselin H, Azad A, Picard P, Andries L, Sys SU, Brutsaert DL, Rouleau JL: Improvement of endocardial and vascular endothelial function on myocardial performance by captopril treatment in postinfarct rat hearts. Circulation. 1999;100:1338-1345.

[34] MacAlpin RN, Abbasi AS, Grollman JH Jr, Eber L: Human coronary artery size during life. A cinearteriographic study. Radiology. 1973;108:567-576.

[35] Dodge JT Jr, Brown BG, Bolson EL, Dodge HT: Lumen diameter of normal human coronary arteries. Influence of age, sex, anatomic variation, and left ventricular hypertrophy or dilation. Circulation. 1992;86:232-246.

[36] Mosseri M, Zolti E, Rozenman Y, Lotan C, Ershov T, Izak T, Admon D, Gotsman MS: The diameter of the epicardial coronary arteries in patients with dilated cardiomyopathy. Int J Cardiol. 1997;62:133-141.

[37] Mela T, Meyer TE, Pape LA, Chung ES, Aurigemma GP, Weiner BH: Coronary arterial dimension-to-left ventricular mass ratio in idiopathic dilated cardiomyopathy. Am J Cardiol. 1999;83:1277-1280, A9.

[38] Abraham D, Hofbauer R, Schäfer R, Blumer R, Paulus P, Miksovsky A, Traxler H, Kocher A, Aharinejad S: Selective downregulation of VEGF-A(165), VEGF-R(1), and decreased capillary density in patients with dilative but not ischemic cardiomyopathy. Circ Res. 2000;87:644-647.

[39] Schäfer R, Abraham D, Paulus P, Blumer R, Grimm M, Wojta J, Aharinejad S: Impaired VE-cadherin/beta-catenin expression mediates endothelial cell degeneration in dilated cardiomyopathy. Circulation. 2003;108:1585-1591.

[40] Roura S, Gálvez-Montón C, Fernández MA, Lupón J, Bayes-Genis A: Circulating endothelial progenitor cells: Potential biomarkers for idiopathic dilated cardiomyopathy. J Cardiovasc Transl Res. 2016;9:80-84.

[41] Sharma S, Adrogue JV, Golfman L, Uray I, Lemm J, Youker K, Noon GP, Frazier OH, Taegtmeyer H: Intramyocardial lipid accumulation in the failing human heart resembles the lipotoxic rat heart. FASEB J. 2004;18:1692-1700.

[42] Haq S, Choukroun G, Lim H, Tymitz KM, del Monte F, Gwathmey J, Grazette L, Michael A, Hajjar R, Force T, Molkentin JD: Differential activation of signal transduction pathways in human hearts with hypertrophy versus advanced heart failure. Circulation. 2001;103:670-677.

[43] Muchir A, Shan J, Bonne G, Lehnart SE, Worman HJ: Inhibition of extracellular signal-regulated kinase signaling to prevent cardiomyopathy caused by mutation in the gene encoding A-type lamins. Hum Mol Genet. 2009;18:241-247.

[44] Wu W, Muchir A, Shan J, Bonne G, Worman HJ: Mitogen-activated protein kinase inhibitors improve heart function and prevent fibrosis in cardiomyopathy caused by mutation in lamin A/C gene. Circulation. 2011;123:53-61.

[45] Herz J, Strickland DK: LRP: a multifunctional scavenger and signaling receptor. J. Clin Invest. 2001;108:779-784.

[46] Cáceres LC, Bonacci GR, Sánchez MC, Chiabrando GA: Activated $\alpha(2)$ macroglobulin induces matrix metalloproteinase 9 expression by low-density lipoprotein receptor-related protein 1 through MAPK-ERK1/2 and NF-kB activation in macrophage-derived cell lines. J Cell Biochem. 2010;111:607-617.

[47] Huang W, Dolmer K, Liao X, Gettins PG: NMR solution structure of the receptor binding domain of human alpha(2)-macroglobulin. J Biol Chem. 2000;275:1089-1094.

[48] Lillis AP, Van Duyn LB, Murphy-Ullrich JE, Strickland DK: LDL receptor-related protein 1: unique tissue-specific functions revealed by selective gene knockout studies. Physiol Rev. 2008;88:887-918.

[49] Franchini M, Montagnana M: Low-density lipoprotein receptor-related protein 1: new functions for an old molecule. Clin Chem Lab Med. 2011;49:967-970.

[50] Boucher P, Liu P, Gotthardt M, Hiesberger T, Anderson RG, Herz J: Platelet-derived growth factor mediates tyrosine phosphorylation of the cytoplasmic domain of the low density lipoprotein receptor-related protein in caveolae. J Biol Chem. 2002;277:15507-15513.

[51] Loukinova E, Ranganathan S, Kuznetsov S, Gorlatova N, Migliorini MM, Loukinov D, Ulery PG, Mikhailenko I, Lawrence DA, Strickland DK: Platelet-derived growth factor (PDGF)-induced tyrosine phosphorylation of the low density lipoprotein receptor-related protein (LRP). Evidence for integrated co-receptor function between LRP and the PDGF. J Biol Chem. 2002;18:15499-15506.

[52] van der Geer P: Phosphorylation of LRP-1: regulation of transport and signal transduction. Trends Cardiovasc Med. 2002;12:160-165.

[53] Langlois B, Perrot G, Schneider C, Henriet P, Emonard H, Martiny L, Dedieu S: LRP-1 promotes cancer cell invasion by supporting ERK and inhibiting JNK signaling pathways. PLoS One. 2010;5:e11584.

[54] Muratoglu SC, Mikhailenko I, Newton C, Migliorini M, Strickland DK: Low density lipoprotein receptor-related protein 1 (LRP1) forms a signaling complex with platelet-derived growth factor receptor-beta in endosomes and regulates activation of the MAPK pathway. J Biol Chem. 2010;285:14308-14317.

[55] Geetha N, Mihaly J, Stockenhuber A, Blasi F, Uhrin P, Binder BR, Freissmuth M, Breuss JM: Signal integration and coincidence detection in the mitogen-activated protein kinase/extracellular signal-regulated kinase (ERK) cascade: concomitant activation of receptor tyrosine kinases and of LRP-1 leads to sustained ERK phosphorylation via down-regulation of dual specificity phosphatases (DUSP1 and -6). J. Biol. Chem. 2011;286:25663-25674.

[56] Llorente-Cortés V, Badimon L: LDL receptor-related protein and the vascular wall: implications for atherothrombosis. Arterioscler Thromb Vasc Biol. 2005;25:497-504.

[57] Abraham D, Hofbauer R, Schäfer R, Blumer R, Paulus P, Miksovsky A, Traxler H, Kocher A, Aharinejad S: Selective downregulation of VEGF-A(165), VEGF-R(1), and decreased capillary density in patients with dilative but not ischemic cardiomyopathy. Circ Res. 2000;87:644-647.

[58] Schäfer R, Abraham D, Paulus P, Blumer R, Grimm M, Wojta J, Aharinejad S: Impaired VE-cadherin/beta-catenin expression mediates endothelial cell degeneration in dilated cardiomyopathy. Circulation. 2003;108:1585-1591.

[59] Reis M, Liebner S: Wnt signaling in the vasculature. Exp Cell Res. 2013;319:1317-1323.

[60] Haas J, Frese KS, Park YJ, Keller A, Vogel B, Lindroth AM, Weichenhan D, Franke J, Fischer S, Bauer A, Marquart S, Sedaghat-Hamedani F, Kayvanpour E, Köhler D, Wolf NM, Hassel S, Nietsch R, Wieland T, Ehlermann P, Schultz JH, Dösch A, Mereles D, Hardt S, Backs J, Hoheisel JD, Plass C, Katus HA, Meder B: Alterations in cardiac DNA methylation in human dilated cardiomyopathy. EMBO Mol Med. 2013;5:413-429.

[61] Koczor CA, Lee EK, Torres RA, Boyd A, Vega JD, Uppal K, Yuan F, Fields EJ, Samarel AM, Lewis W: Detection of differentially methylated gene promoters in failing and nonfailing human left ventricle myocardium using computation analysis. Physiol Genomics. 2013;45:597-605.

[62] Koczor CA, Torres RA, Fields EJ, Boyd A, He S, Patel N, Lee EK, Samarel AM, Lewis W: Thymidine kinase and mtDNA depletion in human cardiomyopathy: epigenetic and translational evidence for energy starvation. Physiol Genomics. 2013;45:590-596.

[63] Singer SJ, Nicolson GL: The fluid mosaic model of the structure of cell membranes. Science. 1972;175:720-731.

[64] Sonnino S, Prinetti A: Membrane domains and the "lipid raft" concept. Curr Med Chem. 2013;20:4-21.

[65] Chiantia S, London E: Sphingolipids and membrane domains: recent advances. Handb Exp Pharmacol. 2013;215:33-55.

[66] Simons K, Ikonen E: Functional rafts in cell membranes. Nature. 1997;387:569-572.

[67] Parton RG, Simons: The multiple faces of caveolae. Nat. Rev. Mol. Cell. Biol. 2007;8:185-194.

[68] Roura S, Cal R, Gálvez-Montón C, Revuelta-Lopez E, Nasarre L, Badimon L, Bayes-Genis A, Llorente-Cortés V: Inverse relationship between raft LRP1 localization and non-raft ERK1,2/MMP9 activation in idiopathic dilated cardiomyopathy: potential impact in ventricular remodeling. Int J Cardiol. 2014;176:805-814.

[69] Fedak PW, Moravec CS, McCarthy PM, Altamentova SM, Wong AP, Skrtic M, Verma S, Weisel RD, Li RK. Altered expression of disintegrin metalloproteinases and their inhibitor in human dilated cardiomyopathy. Circulation. 2006;113:238-245.

[70] Sivakumar P, Gupta S, Sarkar S, Sen S: Upregulation of lysyl oxidase and MMPs during cardiac remodeling in human dilated cardiomyopathy. Mol Cell Biochem. 2008;307:159-167.

[71] Roura S, Gálvez-Montón C, Pujal JM, Casani L, Fernández MA, Astier L, Gastelurrutia P, Domingo M, Prat-Vidal C, Soler-Botija C, Llucià-Valldeperas A, Llorente-Cortés V, Bayes-Genis A: New insights into lipid raft function regulating myocardial vascularization competency in human idiopathic dilated cardiomyopathy. Atherosclerosis. 2013;230:354-364.

[72] Roura S, Gálvez-Montón C, Bayes-Genis A. The challenges for cardiac vascular precursor cell therapy: lessons from a very elusive precursor. J Vasc Res. 2013;50:304-323.

[73] Insel PA, Patel HH: Membrane rafts and caveolae in cardiovascular signaling. Curr Opin Nephrol Hypertens. 2009;18:50-56.

[74] Tsutsumi YM, Kawaraguchi Y, Horikawa YT, Niesman IR, Kidd MW, Chin-Lee B, Head BP, Patel PM, Roth DM, Patel HH: Role of caveolin-3 and glucose transporter-4 in isoflurane-induced delayed cardiac protection. Anesthesiology. 2010;112:1136-1145.

[75] Gazzerro E, Bonetto A, Minetti C. Caveolinopathies: translational implications of caveolin-3 in skeletal and cardiac muscle disorders. Handb Clin Neurol. 2011;101:135-142.

[76] Hunter DJ: Gene-environment interactions in human diseases. Nat Rev Genet. 2005;6:287-298.

[77] Craig J: Complex diseases: Research and applications. Nature Education. 2008;1:1.

Chapter 7

# Cardiomyopathy Caused by Mutations in Nuclear A-Type Lamin Gene

Gisèle Bonne and Antoine Muchir

Additional information is available at the end of the chapter

http://dx.doi.org/10.5772/65315

**Abstract**

Heart disease is a major cause of morbidity and premature mortality. Cardiomyopathy is an anatomic and pathologic condition associated with muscle and electrical dysfunction of the heart, often leading to heart failure–related disability. Dilated cardiomyopathy caused by mutations in A-type lamin gene (i.e., *LMNA* cardiomyopathy) is characterized by an increase in both myocardial mass and volume. The ventricular walls become thin and stretched, compromising cardiac contractility and ultimately resulting in poor left ventricular function. Despite current strategies to aggressively manage "*LMNA* cardiomyopathy," the disorder remains a common cause of heart failure with decreased ejection fraction, and a prevalent diagnosis in individuals is referred for cardiac transplantation. Despite progress in reducing "*LMNA* cardiomyopathy"–related mortality, hospitalizations remain very frequent and rates of readmission continue to rise. It appears important and necessary to further increase our knowledge on the pathophysiology of "*LMNA* cardiomyopathy" to unveil novel molecular/cellular mechanisms to target future therapeutic approaches.

**Keywords:** Dilated cardiomyopathy, Genetics, *LMNA*, A-type lamins, Nuclear lamina

## 1. Introduction

Cardiomyopathy, a major cause of morbidity and premature mortality in developed countries, is an anatomic and pathologic condition associated with muscle and electrical dysfunction of the heart, often leading to heart failure-related disability, which is a staggering clinical and public health problem. The mechanical component of the heart is liable for pumping blood throughout the body. The electric component, as for it, produces a rhythm for the blood to be pumped correctly. Hence, both components are tightly connected and regulated. Most common symptoms of dilated cardiomyopathy are shortness of breath, leg swelling, decreased exercise tolerance, fatigue, dizziness, coughing or wheezing, weight gain, and palpitation. Given the diversity in severity of symptoms in dilated cardiomyopathy, the disease is not always diagnosed. Cardiomyopathies are a clinically heterogeneous group of cardiac muscle disorders [1]. Cardiomyopathies have historically been broken down into several major phenotypic categories. Dilated cardiomyopathy, the most common form, is a condition where the heart muscle becomes enlarged and weakened, resulting in poor left ventricular function. Despite current strategies to aggressively manage dilated cardiomyopathy, the disorder remains a common cause of heart failure with a decrease below 45% of ejection fraction and a referring for cardiac transplantation. Notwithstanding progress in reducing heart failure-related mortality, hospitalizations for heart failure remain very frequent and rates of readmissions continue to rise. It appears important and necessary to increase our knowledge on the pathophysiology of cardiomyopathies to unveil novel molecular/cellular mechanisms for future therapeutic approaches.

## 2. Inherited cardiomyopathies

While the most common cardiomyopathies are secondary to acquired conditions, many are inherited. Genetic mutations have been identified in 25–35% of patients presenting dilated cardiomyopathy. These mutations affect genes that encode components of a wide variety of cellular compartments and pathways, including the nuclear envelope (e.g., *LMNA*, *EMD*), the contractile apparatus (e.g., *MYH7*, *ACTC1*, *TPM1*, *TTN*), the force transduction apparatus (e.g., *MLP*, *DES*, *TNNT2*), and calcium handling (e.g., *SERCA*). The cardiac cell is composed of a complex network of proteins linking the sarcomere to the sarcolemma and the extracellular matrix, providing structural support for subcellular structures and transmitting mechanical signals within and between cells (**Figure 1**). Mutations in genes encoding proteins of the sarcolemma are disrupting the anchoring and hence abrogate the transmission of the force

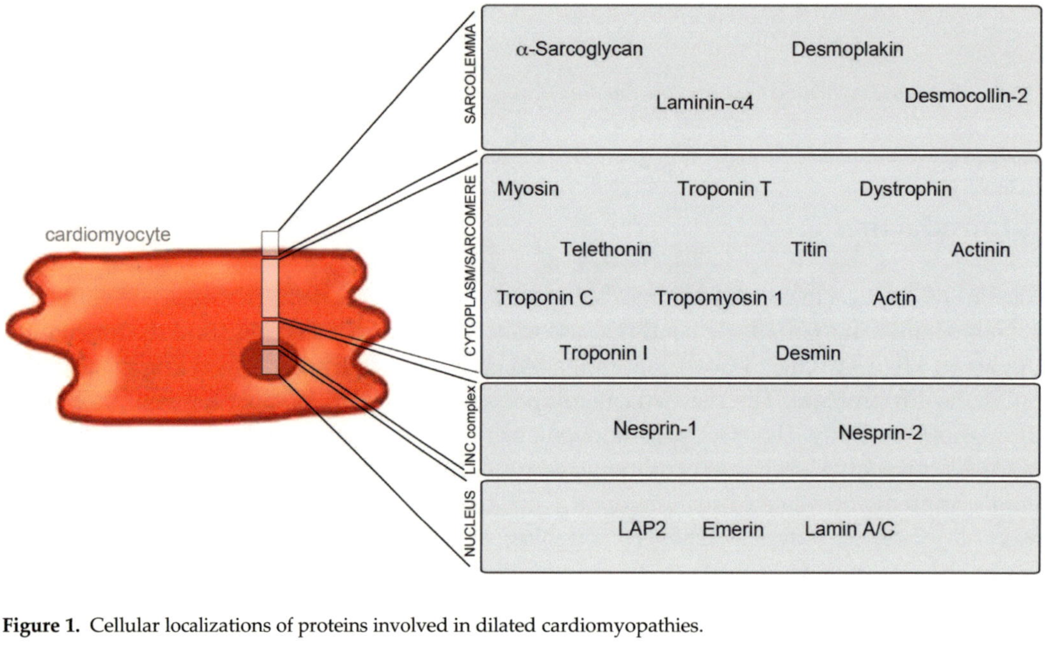


**Figure 1.** Cellular localizations of proteins involved in dilated cardiomyopathies.

generated by muscle contraction. Muscle contraction is due to the interaction between an actin filament and myosin heavy chain. Mutations in genes encoding contractile elements were identified as the cause of dilated cardiomyopathy. Functional units of striated muscle are called sarcomeres. Because the generated power of muscle contraction is transmitted to adjacent sarcomeres through the Z-disk, mutations in genes encoding proteins of the Z-disk causes also dilated cardiomyopathy. Part of hereditary dilated cardiomyopathies is caused by mutations in the genes encoding proteins of the nuclear envelope. Hence, disruption of the links from the sarcolemma to the sarcomere and nucleus could have a "domino effect," which leads to the disruption of systolic function and to the development of dilated cardiomyopathy.

## 3. *LMNA* cardiomyopathy

Among the causing genes of dilated cardiomyopathy, it has been estimated that mutations in *LMNA*, encoding nuclear lamin A/C [2], accounts for about 5–10% of familial dilated cardiomyopathy, thus representing one of the major causative genes. Affected patients often exhibit early conduction defects before left ventricle dysfunction and dilatation occur [3]. "*LMNA* cardiomyopathy" usually presents in early to mid-adulthood with symptomatic conduction system disease or arrhythmias or with symptomatic dilated cardiomyopathy (**Figure 2A**). "*LMNA* cardiomyopathy" has an intrusive clinical progression with higher rates of aggressive arrhythmias and faster course toward heart failure than most other cardiac diseases. Given the increased awareness among physicians, cardiologists are now facing difficult queries regarding patient management. These queries concern the use of defibrillators in order to avoid sudden death from aggressive ventricular arrhythmias and pharmacological interventions to improve heart failure symptoms. Once dilated cardiomyopathy is detected clinically, the management for "*LMNA* cardiomyopathy" follows the standard of care for heart failure. It is unclear whether early institution of these therapeutic agents prior to detectable cardiac dysfunction can modify the aggressive nature of "*LMNA* cardiomyopathy." There is no definitive treatment for the progressive cardiac dilatation and loss of contractility in "*LMNA* cardiomyopathy" short of heart transplantation [4].

## 4. A-type nuclear lamins

The *LMNA* gene, on chromosome 1q21.2-21.3, encodes nuclear A-type lamins. Lamin A and lamin C, the major somatic A-type lamins, arise via alternative splicing of pre-mRNA [5] (**Figure 3A**). Lamin A is primarily synthesized as a precursor, the prelamin A. Prelamin A has a particular C-terminal amino acid tail, which undergoes several enzymatic reactions to produce mature lamin A. Two other genes, *LMNB1* and *LMNB2*, encode lamins B1 and B2, respectively. Lamins are class V intermediate filament proteins that polymerize to form the nuclear lamina (**Figure 3B**), a fibrous network underlining the inner nuclear membrane of most eukaryotic cells (**Figure 3C**) [6–8]. The nuclear lamina is bounded to the inner nuclear membrane via interactions with integral proteins and to the chromatin. It has also been shown that lamin A/C can also interact with the cytoskeleton, through the linker of nucleoskeleton and cytoskeleton ("LINC") complex [9]. One function of the lamina is to provide structural

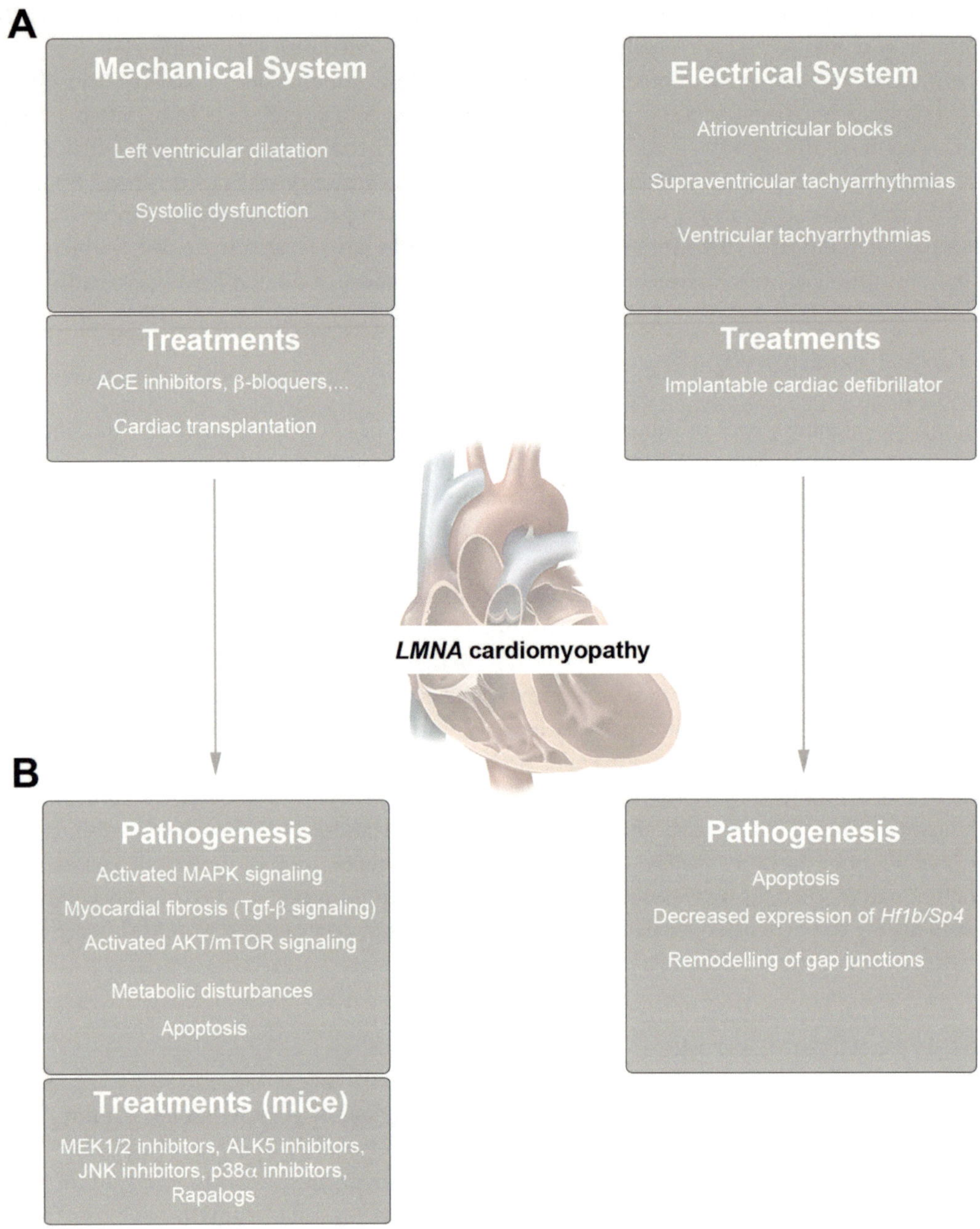


**Figure 2.** Cardiac symptoms of "*LMNA* cardiomyopathy (A) and pathological mechanisms (B).

support to the nucleus. Nuclear lamins have also been implicated in processes such as chromatin organization, gene regulation, DNA replication, and RNA splicing [10]. However, the specific mechanistic roles of lamins in these processes, particularly in a cell- or tissue-type–specific context, remain obscure.

http://dx.doi.org/10.5772/65315

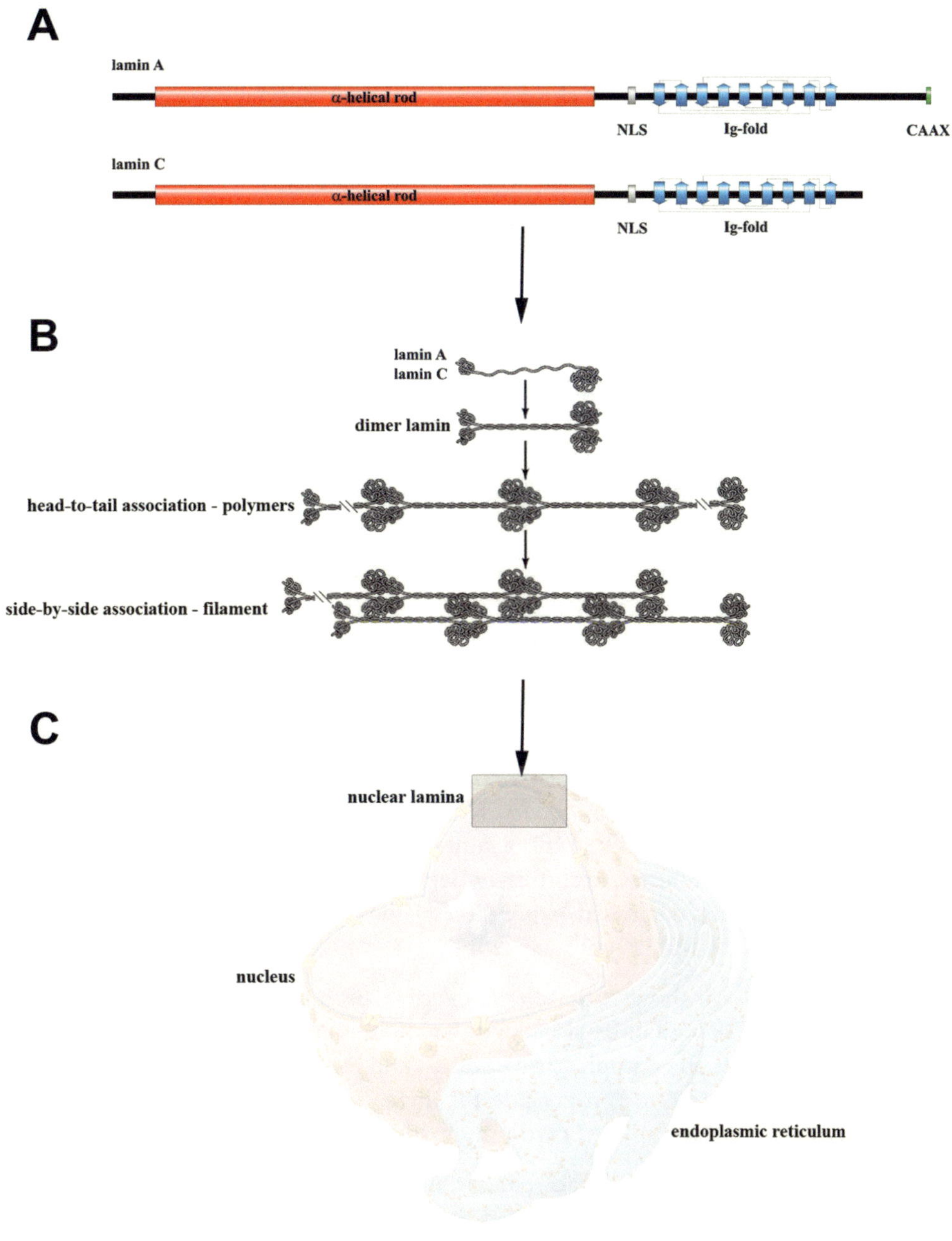


**Figure 3.** Nuclear lamins: structure (A), organization (B), and cellular localization (C). Modified from [10].

## 5. Pathogenesis

Identification of disease-causing mutations in the heart has contributed to the delineation of "*LMNA* cardiomyopathy." However, much work remains in elucidating the specific cellular mechanisms of the disease. Several hypotheses have been proposed attempting to link the pathophysiology of "*LMNA* cardiomyopathy" to known or emerging functions of lamin A/C. Among these functions include those based on that lamin A/C likely have in maintaining the mechanical integrity of cells subject to external and internal cues and signal transduction (i.e., the mechanical stress hypothesis). The "mechanical stress hypothesis" is attractive when trying to explain striated muscle diseases. It is based on the premise that the striated muscles are constantly subjected to mechanical forces and that mutations in "nucleocytoskeletal" support elements make them susceptible to damage from recurrent stress. Mouse models have been extremely helpful in deciphering crucial mechanisms, which could partially explain the pathogenesis of the disease. The development of $Lmna^{-/-}$ mice by Sullivan and colleagues was the first animal model of the disease [11]. Since, other models (knock-in and transgenic) have been created to study the cardiac dysfunction caused by *LMNA* mutation [12–15]. We and others reported an aberrant cardiac activation of signaling pathways in "*LMNA* cardiomyopathy" [16, 17] in mice and human, which participate to the development of contractile dysfunction (mitogen-activated protein kinase (MAPK) signaling, AKT/mTOR signaling, TGF-β signaling, etc.) [16, 18, 19] and electrical disturbances (connexin 43 remodeling, apoptosis, Hf1b expression) (**Figure 2B**).

*MAPK signaling*—One of the most prevalent and best-characterized responses to mechanical stress is the phosphorylation of proteins, which could be mediated by mitogen-activated protein kinase (MAPK) signaling pathway. Genes encoding proteins in MAPK signaling pathway demonstrated significantly altered expression in hearts of *Lmna* H222P mice by transcriptomic analysis [16]. We demonstrated an aberrant activation of ERK1/2, JNK, and p38$\alpha$ signaling, three main branches of MAPK signaling pathway involved in cellular mechanotransduction, in hearts from *Lmna* H222P mice, as early as 4 weeks of age [16, 17]. Our work proved that the activation of MAPK signaling pathway preceded the cardiac dysfunction of *Lmna* H222P mice and that it is a consequence of alterations in lamin A/C and not secondary to nonspecific effects. Accordingly, lamin A/C-deficient fibroblasts subjected to cyclic strain respond with decreased expression of the mechanosensitive genes, which are downstream targets of the MAPK pathway [20].

*AKT/mTOR signaling*—We showed that the *Lmna* pH222P mutation results in aberrant activation of the AKT/mTOR signaling cascade, downstream of the MAPK pathway [18]. Given that activated mTOR inhibits autophagic responses and reduces tolerance to energy deficits, the heart is therefore unable to compensate for increased energy demand and, over time, develops muscle damage and dilated cardiomyopathy.

*TGF-β signaling*—Cardiac fibrosis exacerbates the clinical progression of heart failure. We showed that *Lmna* H222P mice had elevated expression of TGF-β signaling as early as 12 weeks of age, which is a time that preceded development of both cardiac fibrosis and the onset of overt cardiac dysfunction [13, 19]. Our observations indicate that TGF-β is a mediator of the cardiomyopathy that develops as a result of *LMNA* mutations.

*Connexin 43 remodeling*—Gap junction communications describe the electrical coupling of cells through specialized cell contacts called gap junctions. In adult heart, connexin 43 is expressed in the atrial and ventricular working (contractile) myocardium. The working cardiomyocytes of the ventricle are extensively interconnected by clusters of connexin 43 located at the intercalated disks. The intercalated disks of working ventricular myocardium have a step-like configuration, with the gap junctions situated predominantly in the "horizontal" facing segments of these steps rather than the vertical segments [21, 22]. Features of gap junction organization encourage preferential propagation of the impulse in the longitudinal axis, thus contributing to the normal pattern of anisotropic spread of the impulse of healthy ventricular myocardium. The most striking form of structural remodeling connexin 43 is typically scattered in disordered fashion over the lateral surfaces in the heart from *Lmna* N195K mice (i.e., lateralization) [12].

*Apoptosis*—Apoptosis in all metazoan cells is mediated by caspases, a multigene family of cysteine proteases that hydrolyzes peptide bonds carboxyl to aspartic acid residues. Once activated, caspases cut cellular proteins, leading to the apoptotic demise of the cell. During the past few years, there has been accumulating evidence in both human and animal models suggesting that apoptosis may be an important mode of cell death during heart failure [23]. Myocyte apoptosis has been reported in the atrioventricular tissue from $Lmna^{+/-}$ mice [24], which could account for the evolution of electrophysiologic dysfunction.

*Hf1b/Sp4*—This transcription factor has been described as important for the development of the cardiac conduction system [25]. Mounkes and colleagues found that expression and localization of Hf1b/Sp4 were altered in the heart from *Lmna* N195K mice [12]. Strikingly, this study reported that Hf1b/Sp4 was not found in the ventricles and was strongly expressed in the atria in the heart from *Lmna* N195K mice, which mirror the localization in control animals. This finding needs further analysis.

The exact mechanisms by which defects in nuclear lamins cause dysregulated signaling remain to be elucidated.

## 6. Treatments

Advances in molecular techniques have improved the understanding of mechanisms responsible for cardiac dysfunction in "*LMNA* cardiomyopathy." It is clear that mutations in nuclear lamin A/C in cardiomyocytes can perturb cardiac function. Alterations in cardiomyocyte function initiate cascades of cellular responses that attempt to compensate for these insults. However, persistent responses at the cellular level lead to organ-wide alterations, which correlated with sudden cardiac death and heart failure. Although there exists no treatment to directly address the causes of "*LMNA* cardiomyopathy," basic studies of the processes that mediate cellular responses to cardiac stress have allowed the development of innovative treatments that address the reduction of symptoms that include drugs that decrease blood pressure (ACE inhibitors, angiotensin II receptor blockers, beta-blockers) and heart rate (beta-blockers, calcium channel blockers, digoxin) to reduce the strain on the ventricular walls. Utilization of animal and cellular models to further dissect the mechanisms of "*LMNA* cardiomyopathy" and demonstrate efficacy of drugs that specifically target disease-causing pathways holds promise that further reduction in the mortality associated with "*LMNA* cardiomyopathy" can be achieved [17–19, 26, 27].

## 7. Conclusion

In the past decade, there has been an extraordinary burst of researches on lamin A/C and the nuclear lamina, which has been accelerated by attempts to explain the pathogenesis of "*LMNA* cardiomyopathy." One important unanswered question is how mutations in genes expressed in most differentiated somatic cells lead to human disease affecting the cardiac tissue. Within the next several years, we will likely have more clues to answer this question, and these answers will hopefully lead to new ways to treat or prevent "*LMNA* cardiomyopathy."

## Author details

Gisèle Bonne and Antoine Muchir*

*Address all correspondence to: a.muchir@institut-myologie.org

Center of Research in Myology, Paris, France

## References

[1] Maron BJ, Towbin JA, Thiene G, Antzelevitch C, Corrado D, Arnett D, Moss AJ, Seidman CE, Young JB: Contemporary definitions and classification of the cardiomyopathies: an American Heart Association Scientific Statement from the Council on Clinical Cardiology, Heart Failure and Transplantation Committee; Quality of Care and Outcomes Research and Functional Genomics and Translational Biology Interdisciplinary Working Groups; and Council on Epidemiology and Prevention. Circulation. 2006;**113**:1807–1816. DOI: 10.1161/CIRCULATIONAHA.106.174287

[2] Fatkin D, MacRae C, Sasaki T, Wolff MR, Porcu M, Frenneaux M, Atherton J, Vidaillet HJ Jr, Spudich S, De Girolami U, Seidman JG, Seidman C, Muntoni F, Müehle G, Johnson W, McDonough B: Missense mutation in the rod domain of he lamin A/C gene as cause of dilated cardiomyopathy and conduction-system disease. N Engl J Med. 1999;**341**:1715–1724. DOI: 10.1056/NEJM199912023412302

[3] Meune C, Van Berlo JH, Anselme F, Bonne G, Pinto YM, Duboc D: Primary prevention of sudden death in patients with lamin A/C gene mutations. N Engl J Med. 2006;**354**:209–210. DOI: 10.1056/NEJMc052632

[4] Ben Yaou R, Gueneau L, Demay L, Stora S, Chikaoui K, Richard P, Bonne G: Heart involvement in lamin A/C related diseases. Arch Mal Coeur Vaiss. 2006;**99**:848–855.

[5] Lin F, Worman HJ: Structural organization of the human gene encoding nuclear lamin A and nuclear lamin C. J Biol Chem. 1993;**268**:16321–16326.

[6] Fisher DZ, Chaudhary N, Blobel G: cDNA sequencing of nuclear lamins A and C reveals primary and secondary structural homology to intermediate filament proteins. Proc Natl Acad Sci U S A 1986;**83**:6450–6454.

[7] McKeon FD, Kirschner MW, Caput D: Homologies in both primary and secondary structure between nuclear envelope and intermediate filament proteins. Nature 1986;**319**:463–468. DOI: 10.1038/319463a0

[8] Aebi U, Cohn J, Buhle L, Gerace L: The nuclear lamina is a meshwork of intermediate-type filaments. Nature 1986;**323**:560–564. DOI: 10.1038/323560a0

[9] Stewart CL, Roux KJ, Burke B: Blurring the boundary: the nuclear envelope extends its reach. Science 2007;**318**:1408–1412. DOI: 10.1126/science.1142034

[10] Dechat T, Pfleghaar K, Sengupta K, Shimi T, Shumaker DK, Solimando L, Goldman RD: Nuclear lamins: major factors in the structural organization and function of the nucleus and chromatin. Genes Dev. 2008;**22**:832–853. DOI: 10.1101/gad.1652708

[11] Sullivan T, Escalante-Alcade D, Bhatt H, Anver M, Bhat N, Nagashima K, Stewart CL, Burke B: Loss of A-type lamin expression compromises nuclear envelope integrity leading to muscular dystrophy. J Cell Biol. 1999;**147**:913–920.

[12] Mounkes LC, Kozlov SV, Rottman JN, Stewart CL: Expression of an LMNA-N195K variant of A-type lamins results in cardiac conduction defects and death in mice. Hum Mol Genet. 2005;**14**:2167–2180. DOI: 10.1093/hmg/ddi221

[13] Arimura T, Helbling-Leclerc A, Massart C, Varnous S, Niel F, Lacène E, Fromes Y, Toussaint M, Mura AM, Keller DI, Amthor H, Isnard R, Malissen M, Schwartz K, Bonne G: Mouse model carrying H222P-Lmna mutation develops muscular dystrophy and dilated cardiomyopathy similar to human striated muscle laminopathies. Hum Mol Genet. 2005;**14**:155–169. DOI: 10.1093/hmg/ddi017

[14] Wang Y, Herron AJ, Worman HJ: Pathology and nuclear abnormalities in hearts of transgenic mice expressing M371K lamin A encoded by an LMNA mutation causing Emery-Dreifuss muscular dystrophy. Hum Mol Genet. 2006;**15**:2479–2489. DOI: 10.1093/hmg/ddl170

[15] Cattin ME, Bertrand AT, Schlossarek S, Le Bihan MC, Jensen SS, Neuber C, Crocini C, Maron S, Lainé J, Mougenot N, Varnous S, Fromes Y, Hansen A, Eschenhagen T, Decostre V, Carrier L, Bonne G: Heterozygous Lmna delK32 mice develop dilated cardiomyopathy through a combined pathomechanism of haploinsufficiency and peptide toxicity. Hum Mol Genet. 2013;**22**:3152–3164. DOI: 10.1093/hmg/ddt172

[16] Muchir A, Pavlidis P, Decostre V, Herron AJ, Arimura T, Bonne G, Worman HJ: Activation of MAPK pathways links *LMNA* mutations to cardiomyopathy in Emery-Dreifuss muscular dystrophy. J Clin Invest. 2007;**117**:1282–1293. DOI: 10.1172/JCI29042

[17] Muchir A, Reilly SA, Wu W, Iwata S, Homma S, Bonne G, Worman HJ: Treatment with selumetinib preserves cardiac function and improves survival in cardiomyopathy caused

by mutation in the lamin A/C gene. Cardiovasc Res. 2012;**93**:311–319. DOI: 10.1093/cvr/cvr301

[18] Choi JC, Muchir A, Wu W, Iwata S, Homma S, Morrow JP, Worman HJ: Temsirolimus activates autophagy and ameliorates cardiomyopathy caused by lamin A/C gene mutation. Sci Transl Med. 2012;**4**:144ra102. DOI: 10.1126/scitranslmed.3003875

[19] Chatzifrangkeskou M, Le Dour C, Wu W, Morrow JP, Joseph LC, Beuvin M, Sera F, Homma S, Vignier N, Mougenot N, Bonne G, Lipson KE, Worman HJ, Muchir A: ERK1/2 directly acts on CTGF/CCN2 expression to mediate myocardial fibrosis in cardiomyopathy caused by mutation in the lamin A/C gene. Hum Mol Genet. 2016;ddw090. DOI: 10.1093/hmg/ddw090

[20] Lammerding J, Schulze PC, Takahashi T, Kozlov S, Sullivan T, Kamm RD, Stewart CL, Lee RT: Lamin A/C deficiency causes defective nuclear mechanics and mechanotransduction. J Clin Invest. 2004;**113**:370–378. DOI: 10.1172/JCI19670

[21] Severs NJ: Gap junction shape and orientation at the cardiac intercalated disk. Circ Res. 1989;**65**:1458–1461.

[22] Severs NJ: The cardiac gap junction and intercalated disc. Int J Cardiol. 1990;**26**:137–173.

[23] Kang PM, Izumo S: Apoptosis and heart failure: a critical review of the literature. Circ Res. 2000;**86**:1107–1113.

[24] Wolf CM, Wang L, Alcalai R, Pizard A, Burgon PG, Ahmad F, Sherwood M, Branco DM, Wakimoto H, Fishman GI, See V, Stewart CL, Conner DA, Berul CI, Seidman CE, Seidman JG: Lamin A/C haploinsufficiency causes dilated cardiomyopathy and apoptosis-triggered cardiac conduction system disease. J Mol Cell Cardiol. 2008;**44**:293–303. DOI: 10.1016/j.yjmcc.2007.11.008

[25] Nguyen-Tran VT, Kubalak SW, Minamisawa S, Fiset C, Wollert KC, Brown AB, Ruiz-Lozano P, Barrere-Lemaire S, Kondo R, Norman LW, Gourdie RG, Rahme MM, Feld GK, Clark RB, Giles WR, Chien KR: A novel genetic pathway for sudden cardiac death via defects in the transition between ventricular and conduction system cell lineages. Cell 2000;**102**:671–682.

[26] Muchir A, Shan J, Bonne G, Lehnart SE, Worman HJ: Inhibition of extracellular signal-regulated kinase signaling to prevent cardiomyopathy caused by mutation in the gene encoding A-type lamins. Hum Mol Genet. 2009;**18**:241–247. DOI: 10.1093/hmg/ddn343

[27] Wu W, Muchir A, Shan J, Bonne G, Worman HJ: Mitogen activated protein kinase inhibitors improve heart function and prevent fibrosis in cardiomyopathy caused by lamin A/C gene mutation. Circulation 2011;**123**:53–61. DOI: 10.1161/CIRCULATIONAHA.110.970673

Chapter 8

# Arrhythmogenic Right Ventricular Cardiomyopathy/ Dysplasia

Bandar Al-Ghamdi

Additional information is available at the end of the chapter

http://dx.doi.org/10.5772/65316

**Abstract**

Arrhythmogenic right ventricular cardiomyopathy/dysplasia (ARVC/D) is a rare disease characterized by progressive fibrofatty replacement of the myocardium, primarily involving the right ventricle (RV). The structural changes in the ventricular myocardium form a substrate for ventricular arrhythmia ranging from premature ventricular complexes to ventricular tachycardia typically of RV origin and may result in RV failure and progress to congestive heart failure at a later stage. ARVC/D is a recognized cause of sudden cardiac death in young people, but it may occur at any age. With the discovery of underlying pathogenic mutations involved in the disease development and insight from long-term follow-up of ARVC/D patients, ARVC/D is an inherited cardiomyopathy. Mutations in at least eight genes have been involved in ARVC/D genesis in 30–50% of patients. Most of these genes are involved in the function of desmosomes, which are structures that attach heart muscle cells to one another. Desmosomes provide strength to the myocardium and play a role in signaling between neighboring cells. Mutations in the genes responsible for ARVC/D often impair the normal desmosomal function. There has been significant advancement in the diagnosis and management of ARVC/D in the past few decades. This chapter provides an overview of ARVC/D pathophysiology, clinical presentations, diagnosis, and management.

**Keywords:** cardiomyopathy, arrhythmia, right ventricle, sudden cardiac death, heart failure

## 1. Introduction

Arrhythmogenic right ventricular cardiomyopathy/dysplasia (ARVC/D) is a rare disease characterized by progressive fibrofatty replacement of the myocardium, primarily involving the right ventricle (RV) [1–4].

The typical age of presentation is between the second and the fourth decade of life. The structural changes in the ventricular myocardium form a substrate for ventricular arrhythmia ranging from premature ventricular complexes (PVCs) to ventricular tachycardia (VT), typically of RV origin and may result in RV failure, and progress to congestive heart failure at a later stage. ARVC/D is a recognized cause of sudden cardiac death (SCD) in young individuals, but it may occur at any age [4].

ARVC/D was first described by Frank et al. [1], and the first clinical profile of the disease was published in 1982 [2]. It was described as a disease in which "the right ventricular musculature is partially or totally absent and is replaced by fatty and fibrous tissue [2]." With the discovery of underlying pathogenic mutations involved in the disease development and insight from long-term follow-up of ARVC/D patients, the ARVC/D is currently considered to be an inherited cardiomyopathy [4–6]. However, the presence of sporadic cases of ARVC/D increased the possibility of nongenetic causes.

Mutations in at least eight genes have been involved in the ARVC/D genesis in 30–50% patients. Most of these genes are involved in the function of desmosomes, which are structures that attach heart muscle to one another. Desmosomes provide strength to the myocardium and also play a role in signaling between neighboring cells. Mutations in the genes responsible for ARVC/D often impair the normal desmosomal function. This results in cells of the myocardium detaching from one another and dying (apoptosis). They are then replaced with fibrous and fibrofatty tissue. The apoptosis occurs predominantly when the heart muscle is placed under stress (such as during vigorous exercise). Most of these gene code for desmosome proteins—plakoglobin (JUP), desmoplakin (DSP), plakophilin-2 (PKP2), the desmoglein-2 (DSG2), and desmocollin-2 (DSC2)—and other genes that code for nondesmosomal protein (e.g., RYR2 and TMEM43) have also been associated with ARVC/D [7]. Additionally, an autosomal recessive variant of ARVC/D has been described. The first disease-causing gene, encoding the desmosomal protein plakoglobin (JUP), was identified in patients with Naxos disease and is an autosomal recessive variant of ARVC/D. It was first reported from the Greek island of Naxos and is associated with palmoplantar keratoderma and wooly hair [8]. Another recessive mutation of DSP has been reported and associated with Carvajal syndrome, another cardio-cutaneous disease [9].

In the past few decades, there has been a significant improvement in our understanding of this disease pathogenesis, natural course, diagnosis, and management.

This chapter provides an overview of ARVC/D pathophysiology, clinical presentations, diagnosis, and management.

## 2. Epidemiology

The estimated prevalence of ARVC/D in the general population ranges from 1 in 2000 to 1 in 5000 individuals; men are more frequently affected than women, with an approximate ratio of 3:1 [10, 11].

http://dx.doi.org/10.5772/65316

The median age at onset of the disease is about 30 years, whereas it rarely manifests before the age of 12 or after the age of 60 years [12, 13]. ARVC/D is a leading cause of sudden cardiac death (SCD) accounting for 11–22% of cases of SCD in the young athlete patient population 8 [13–15]. However, this varies based on the geographic area as it accounts for approximately 22% of SCD cases in athletes in northern Italy [5] and about 17% of SCD in young people in the United States [16]. The genes involved and different mode of inheritance may explain the ARVC/D ethnic variations [17]. The most prevalent mode of inheritance of ARVC/D is an autosomal dominant; however, autosomal recessive form has also been described such as Naxos disease. This disease was first described in Naxos Island, Greece, and it is associated with cutaneous manifestations such as palmoplantar keratosis [8]. Although there are no genetic studies in ARVC/D Chinese patients, some studies showed a lower familial incidence of premature SCD among these patients [18].

## 3. Molecular genetics

ARVC/D is a genetically determined cardiac disease because one or more first-degree relatives also display signs of the disease in 30–50% of cases [2, 19].

A large majority of mutations in ARVC/D patients have been found in genes encoding different components of the cardiac desmosome, i.e., plakophilin 2 (PKP2), desmocollin 2 (DSC2), desmoglein 2 (DSG2), desmoplakin (DSP), and plakoglobin (JUP), suggesting that ARVC/D is primarily a disease of disturbed desmosomal function. However, mutations in other genes (nondesmosomal genes) have also been reported in ARVC/D, including transmembrane protein 43 (TMEM43), desmin (DES), and titin (TTN), indicating genetic heterogeneity. Several ARVC/D cases were found to be caused by multiple mutations in the same gene (compound heterozygosity) or mutations in different genes (digenic inheritance), which could result in an earlier onset and increased disease severity [7] (**Figure 1**).

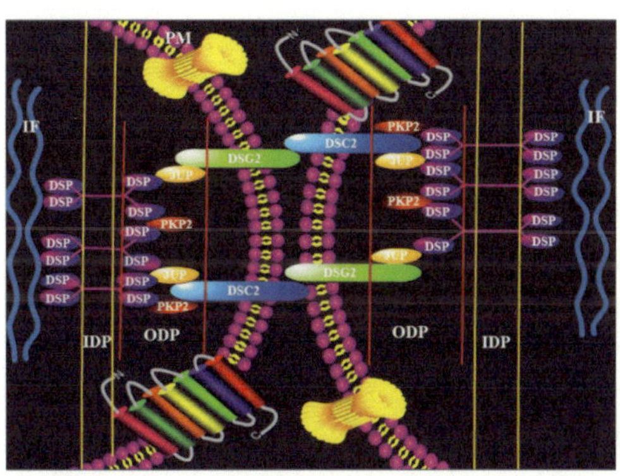


**Figure 1.** The structural schematic diagram of desmosome. IDP, inner dense plaque; ODP, outer dense plaque; PM, plasma membrane; DSG2, desmoglein-2; DSC2, desmocollin-2; JUP, plakoglobin; PKP2, plakophilin-2; DSP, desmoplakin; IF, intermediate filaments. Adapted with permission from Que et al. [186].

The ARVC/D is inherited predominantly as an autosomal dominant (the classical form), and as autosomal recessive (nonclassical form) such as Naxos disease and Carvajal syndrome [8, 9].

**Table 1** summarizes ARVC/D genes and corresponding phenotypes.

| ARVC/D subtype | Location (chromosome/locus) | Inheritance | Gene/locus (encoded protein) |
|---|---|---|---|
| **ARVC/D 1** | 14q24.3 | AD | TGFβ3 |
| **ARVC/D 2** | 1q43 | AD | RyR2 |
| **ARVC/D 3** | 14q12-q22 | AD | – |
| **ARVC/D 4** | 2q32.1-q32.3 | AD | – |
| **ARVC/D 5** | 3p25.1 | AD | TMEM43 |
| **A\RVC/D 6** | 10p14-p12 | – | – |
| **ARVC/D 7** | 10q22.3 | AD | DES |
| **ARVC/D 8** | 6p24.3 | AD | DSP |
| **ARVC/D 9** | 12p11.21 | AD | PKP2 |
| **ARVC/D 10** | 18q12.1 | AD | DSG2 |
| **ARVC/D 11** | 18q12.1 | AR/AD | DSC2 |
| **ARVC/D 12** | 17q21.2 | AD | JUP |
| **Naxos disease** | 17q21.2 | AR | JUP |
| **ARVC/D 13** | 10q21.3 | AD | CTNNA3 |

**Abbreviations:** AD: autosomal-dominant; AR: autosomal-recessive; ARVC/D: arrhythmogenic right ventricular cardiomyopathy/dysplasia; CTNNA3: catenin Alpha; DSC2: desmocollin-2; DSG2: desmoglein-2; DES: desmin; DSP: desmoplakin; JUP: junction plakoglobin; PKP2: plakophilin-2; RyR2: Ryanodine receptor 2; TGF: transforming growth factor; TMEM43: transmembrane protein 43.

**Table 1.** Arrhythmogenic ventricular cardiomyopathy/dysplasia genetics from OMIM®and Online Mendelian Inheritance in Man®.

### 3.1. Desmosomal ARVC/D

#### *3.1.1. Autosomal dominant disease*

##### *3.1.1.1. Plakophilin-2*

Plakophilin-2 is a protein that in humans is encoded by the PKP2 gene [20]. Plakophilin 2 is expressed in cardiac muscle as well as skin, where it functions to link cadherins to intermediate filaments in the cytoskeleton. In cardiac muscle, plakophilin-2 is found in desmosome structures located within intercalated discs [21]. In 2004, Syrris et al. [22] was the first to show that mutations in PKP2 are a major cause of ARVC/D. The disease was incompletely penetrant in most mutation carriers as confirmed by subsequent studies [23–26]. It is estimated that up to 70% of all mutations associated with ARVC/D are within the PKP2 gene [27, 28]. This finding is consistent with this chapter author's experience of ARVC/D patients in Saudi Arabia [29]. Specific and sensitive markers of PKP2 and plakoglobin mutation carriers in ARVC/D have been identified to include T-wave inversions, right ventricular wall motion abnormalities, and ventricular extrasystoles [30]. Investigations looking at the clinical and genetic characterization of ARVC/D to understand the penetrance associated with PKP2 mutations, as well as other genes encoding desmosomal proteins, in disease progression and outcome, are of major interest [31–40]. PKP2 mutations were also found to coexist with sodium channelopathies in patients with Brugada syndrome [41, 42].

*3.1.1.2. Desmoplakin*

Desmoplakin is a protein in humans that is encoded by the DSP gene [43, 44]. Desmoplakin is a critical component of desmosome structures in cardiac muscle and epidermal cells, which function to maintain the structural integrity at adjacent cell contacts. In cardiac muscle, desmoplakin is localized to intercalated discs, which mechanically couple cardiac cells to function in a coordinated syncytial structure. Mutations in this gene are the cause of several cardiomyopathies, including dilated cardiomyopathy (DCM) [9, 45], and ARVC/D [46–50]. Mutations in DSP have also been associated with striate palmoplantar keratoderma [9, 48, 51]. Carvajal syndrome results from an autosomal recessive mutation in DSP gene [45] (see below).

*3.1.1.3. Desmoglein-2*

Desmoglein-2 is a protein that in humans is encoded by the DSG2 gene [52]. Desmoglein-2 is highly expressed in cardiomyocytes and epithelial cells. Desmoglein-2 is localized to desmosome structures at regions of cell-cell contact and functions to structurally adhere adjacent cells together. In cardiac muscle, these regions are specialized regions known as intercalated discs. Mutations in desmoglein-2 have been associated with ARVC/D [53] and familial dilated cardiomyopathy [54].

*3.1.1.4. Desmocollin-2*

Desmocollin-2 is a protein that in humans is encoded by the DSC2 gene [55]. Desmocollin-2 is a cadherin-type protein that functions to link adjacent cells together in desmosomes. Desmocollin-2 is widely expressed and is the only desmocollin isoform expressed in cardiac muscle, where it localizes to intercalated discs. Mutations in DSC2 have been causally linked to ARVC/D.

Syrri et al. [56] reported 4 DSC2 mutations in 77 probands who were negative for other mutations. Disease expression was variable, and most mutation carriers had LV involvement. Other studies show the same findings [33, 34, 57, 58].

*3.1.1.5. Plakoglobin*

The first dominant mutation in plakoglobin was described in a German family [59]. Affected individuals carried an insertion of an extra serine residue at position 39 in the N-terminus of plakoglobin (S39_K40insS) [59]. None of the individuals affected by the S39_K40insS mutation showed apparent cutaneous abnormalities, in contrast to abnormalities seen in patients with Naxos disease.

*3.1.2. Autosomal recessive*

*3.1.2.1. Plakoglobin*

Plakoglobin, also known as junction plakoglobin or gamma-catenin, is a protein that in humans is encoded by the JUP gene. Plakoglobin is a cytoplasmic component of desmosomes and adherens junctions structures located within intercalated discs of cardiac muscle that function to anchor sarcomeres and join adjacent cells in cardiac muscle. It is the first gene that was identified as a cause of ARVC/D by Protonotarios et al. [60] in 1986. The mutations in JUP specifically cause an autosomal recessive form of the disease referred to as Naxos disease. It was first described in patients originating from the Hellenic island of Naxos. Naxos disease is characterized phenotypically by cutaneous manifestations such as wooly hair plus palmar and plantar erythema that progresses to keratosis with physical activity involving the palms and soles of the feet [7, 36–38, 61–63]. Noninvasive cardiac screening identified T-wave inversion, abnormalities in RV wall motion, and frequent ventricular extrasystoles as sensitive and specific markers of a JUP mutation [30].

*3.1.2.2 Desmoplakin*

Carvajal syndrome is a variety of Naxos disease presenting at a younger age with more pronounced left ventricular involvement has been described in families from India and Ecuador [34, 35, 45, 64]. It results from an autosomal recessive mutation of a frameshift (7901delG) in DSP that results in a combination of above conditions, including dilated cardiomyopathy, keratoderma, and wooly hair [45]

**3.2. Nondesmosomal ARVC/D**

*3.2.1. Cardiac ryanodine receptor (RyR2)*

The RyR2 receptor is responsible for calcium release from the sarcoplasmic reticulum. Mutations in the cardiac ryanodine receptor RyR2 have been described in only one Italian ARVC/D family [65].

Mutations in the human RYR2 gene have been associated with three inherited cardiac diseases: arrhythmogenic right ventricular cardiomyopathy type 2 (ARVC/D2)[65, 66], catecholaminergic polymorphic ventricular tachycardia (CPVT) [67,68], and familial polymorphic ventricular tachycardia (FPVT) [69, 70].

*3.2.2. Transforming growth factor beta-3 (TGFβ3)*

The TGF-β superfamily of cytokines consists of proteins that regulate different physiological processes, such as embryonic development, chemotaxis, homeostasis, cell cycle control, and wound healing [71]. The gene has been mapped to chromosome 14. With the screening of the promoter and untranslated regions, a mutation of the TGFβ3 gene was found in all clinically affected members of a large family with ARVC/D [72]. TGFβs stimulate mesenchymal cells to

http://dx.doi.org/10.5772/65316

proliferate and to produce extracellular matrix components [73]. It is, therefore, possible that enhanced TGFβ3 activity can lead to myocardial fibrosis.

### 3.2.3. *Transmembrane protein 43 (TMEM43)*

Transmembrane protein 43 (also called luma) is a protein that is encoded by the TMEM43 gene in humans [74]. TMEM43 may have an important role in maintaining a nuclear envelope structure by organizing protein complexes at the inner nuclear membrane.

A high-risk form of ARVC/D with a fully penetrant, and sex influenced inheritance has been identified in 15 unrelated families in a genetically isolated population in Newfoundland, Canada. The underlying mutation for this form of the disease was a missense mutation in the TMEM43 gene [75]. The TMEM43 gene contains the response element for PPAR gamma, which is an adipogenic transcription factor. The dysregulation of the adipogenic pathway regulated by PPAR gamma as a result of TMEM43 gene mutation may explain the fibrofatty replacement of myocardium in patients with ARVC/D [75]. Several other studies also show that mutations in TMEM43 are associated with ARCV/D [75–78].

### 3.2.4. *Others*

Only isolated reports showed causal mutations in other nondesmosomal genes, such as desmin (DES), titin (TTN), Lamin A/C (LMNA), phospholamban (PLN) and αT-catenin (CTNNA3), sometimes with a clinical phenotype similar but not identical to ARVC/D, as to be considered phenocopies or overlap syndromes [79].

## 4. Pathophysiology

The structural abnormalities in ARVC/D result from the fibrofatty infiltration of the RV myocardium, which leads to progressive RV dilatation and dysfunction (**Figure 2**). The gross

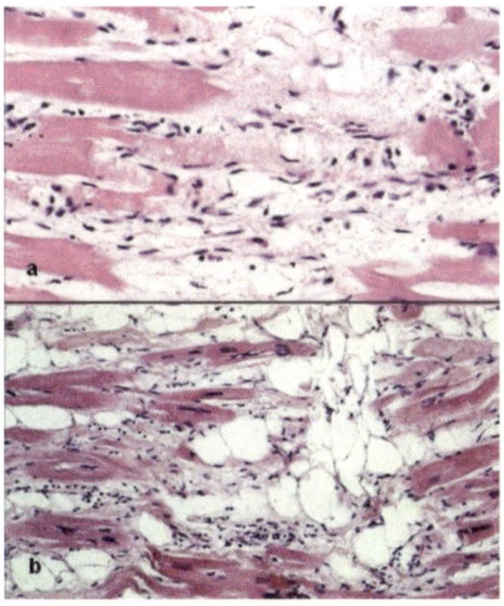


**Figure 2.** Typical histological features of ARVC/D. (a) Ongoing myocyte death and (b) early fibrosis and adipocytes infiltration. Adapted with permission from Thiene et al. [187].

pathognomonic features of ARVC/D consist of RV aneurysms, whether single or multiple, located in the so-called "triangle of dysplasia" which involve RV inflow, apex and outflow tract [4]. The left ventricle (LV) is less commonly involved, and the septum is relatively spared.

### 4.1. Early hypothesis

Basso et al. [4] suggested that the mechanism for myocardial loss and myocardial atrophy appeared to be the consequence of acquired injury (myocyte death) and repair (fibrofatty replacement), mediated by patchy myocarditis. The presence of apoptosis (programmed cell death) is confirmed in ARVC/D [80]. Inflammation, enhanced fibrosis, and loss of function are based on pathological reports of inflammatory infiltrates detected in the heart specimen collected from ARVC/D patients [81]. More recent studies showed that myocarditis might mimic ARVC/D, or it may be superimposed on existing disease in the affected heart muscle [82]. Another proposed mechanism was transdifferentiation of myocardium. This hypothesis assumes that myocardial cells can change from cardiac muscle to adipose tissue [83]. However, it was based on an observation in one patient only.

### 4.2. Current hypothesis

#### *4.2.1. Abnormal cell-cell adhesion (desmosomal disease)*

Our current understanding of ARCV/D indicates that it is a desmosomal disease. Desmosomes mediate cell-cell adhesion and provide cells with mechanical strength [84, 85]. They are present in tissues with mechanical stress like myocardium and epidermis. Desmosomes consist of three families of proteins: the armadillo proteins (junction plakoglobin and plakophilin), cadherins (desmocollins and desmogleins), and plakins (desmoplakin) [86]. Electron microscopy studies have demonstrated intercalated disc remodeling, which raised the hypothesis of an abnormal cell-cell adhesion in disease pathogenesis even before the discovery of desmosomal genes in ARVC/D [87, 88]. Reduced cell-cell adhesion was demonstrated using monolayers of neonatal rat ventricular myocytes in which PKP2 was silenced and subjected to a defined mechanical intervention [89]. However, when expressing mutant forms of either PKP2 or JUP, cells exhibited abnormal signaling in response to mechanical stress, but showed a preserved intercellular adhesion, which raised a question mark about the primary role of cell-cell adhesion in ARVC/D pathogenesis [90]. At the same time, the reduced junctional signal for JUP appears to have a significant role in the disease pathogenesis as demonstrated by Asimaki et al. [91] in myocardial samples from ARVC/D patients. This may indicate a possible role of intracellular signaling rather than adhesion, as suggested by other groups [92, 93].

#### *4.2.2. Abnormal intercellular junction proteins and intracellular signaling*

Suppression of the canonical Wnt/β-catenin signaling pathway is another proposed mechanism in the pathogenesis of ARVC/D. Plakoglobin (γ-catenin), a protein with functional similarities to catenin, can localize both to the plasma membrane and the nucleus [94]. Garcia-Gras et al. [92] demonstrated that disruption of desmoplakin frees plakoglobin from the plasma membrane allowing it to translocate to the nucleus and suppress canonical Wnt/-catenin signaling. Wnt/β-catenin signaling can inhibit adipogenesis by preventing mesodermal precursors from differentiating into adipocytes [95]. Suppression of Wnt/β-catenin signaling by plakoglobin nuclear localization could, therefore, promote the differentiation of adipose tissue in the cardiac myocardium in patients with ARVC/D [92] (**Figure 3**).

Recently, the Hippo/YAP signaling pathway has been associated with ARVC/D pathogenesis. The YAP interacts with β-catenin to drive Wnt-related gene expression in the nucleus. Chen et al. [96] demonstrated aberrant activation of the Hippo kinase cascade resulting in phosphorylation and cytoplasmic retention of YAP in ARVC/D myocardial samples, mouse models and pkp2 knockdown HL-1 myocytes.

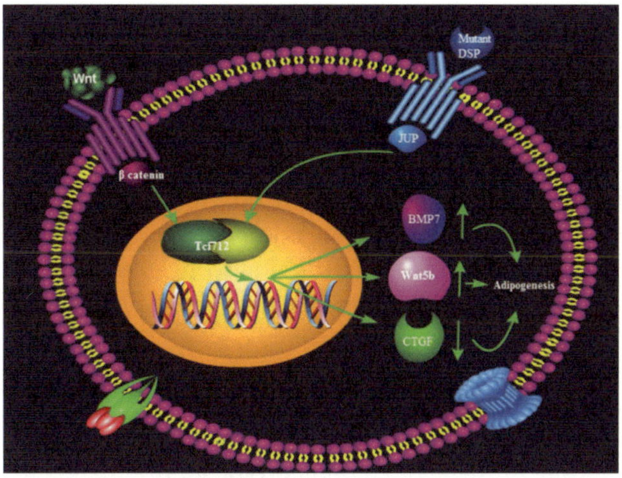


**Figure 3.** The suppression of the Wnt/β-catenin signal pathway. Mutant DSP frees JUP from the plasma membrane, allowing it to translocate to the nucleus. Nucleus location of JUP might be the initiator of the suppression of Wnt signaling. Plakoglobin competes against β-catenin for binding with Tcf712 (transcriptional factor 712), further leading to a series of consequences, increased expression of BMP7 and noncanonical Wnt5b and reduction of CTGF. Bone morphogenic protein 7 and Wnt5b are well-known promoters of adipogenesis as opposed to CTGF, which is inhibitor of adipogenesis. Ultimately, the pathological morphology of ARVC/D developed. Adapted with permission from Que et al. [186].

### *4.2.3. Gap junction and ion channel remodeling*

At the cellular level, the functional triad of desmosomes, gap junctions and sodium channels is essential for normal function. The change in the composition of one component of this triad may affect the function and integrity of the others [97]. Impairment in mechanical coupling as expressed with diminished expression of connexin-43 at the intercellular junction was demonstrated in most of ARVC/D cases [98, 99].

Furthermore, in the ARVC/D experimental model, reduced cardiac sodium current was found [100–104]. These findings led researchers to hypothesize that life-threatening ventricular arrhythmias could occur in patients with ARVC/D even preceding the structural abnormalities due to electrical uncoupling and reduced sodium current, but this has yet to be proven.

Furthermore, animal studies using high-throughput drug screening identified as SB216763 showed an ability to restore the subcellular distribution of JUP, connexin-43 and Nav1.5 and of SAP97, a protein known to mediate the forward trafficking of Nav1.5 and Kir2.1. The SB216763 is already known as an activator of the canonical Wnt signaling pathway. This might be the beginning to move from experimental models to a target gene therapy [104].

## 5. Clinical presentation

In its initially described classical form of ARVC/D, the RV is primarily affected with possible LV involvement in a later stage. However, two additional patterns of disease have been identified by clinicogenetic characterization of families. These are the left dominant phenotype, with early and predominant LV manifestations, and the biventricular phenotype with equal involvement of both ventricles. Immunohistochemical studies at a molecular level indicated that ARVC/D is a global biventricular disease [95]. However, histologically and functionally overt manifestations of the disease usually start in the RV. There is no clear explanation for this finding, but the possible mechanism is that RV is less able to withstand pressure (over)load in the presence of impaired function of mechanical junctions due to their thin wall. The rare variant of the disease with cutaneous manifestations (palmoplantar keratoderma and wooly hair) has its features that will be discussed briefly later on.

### 5.1. Classic form of ARVC/D

ARVC/D patients typically present with monomorphic VT originating from the RV. However, rarely, sudden death at young age, or RV failure may be the first presentation. Patients' symptoms may include palpitations, shortness of breath, dizziness, and syncope or near syncope. Based on clinicopathologic and patients' follow-up studies, four different disease phases have been described for the classical form of ARVC/D, i.e., primarily affecting the RV (**Table 2**):

1. Concealed phase or early ARVC/D is characterized by the absence of obvious clinical changes, however, subtle RV structural changes may be found. Generally, these patients are asymptomatic but still at risk of SCD especially during heavy exercise.

2. The overt phase of the disease is characterized by the presence of patient's symptoms such as palpitations, syncope and ventricular arrhythmias ranging from isolated PVCs to sustained VT and ventricular fibrillation (VF).

3. The third phase is characterized by RV failure as manifest by RV dilatation and the reduced RV systolic function due to progressive loss of myocardium, with the preserved LV function.

4. Biventricular failure phase is characterized by LV involvement, which usually occurs at a late stage. This phase may mimic DCM and may require cardiac transplantation.

| Phase | Characteristics |
|---|---|
| **Concealed** | No symptoms<br>Subtle structural changes |
| **Overt** | Ventricular arrhythmias (PVCs/VT of LBBB morphology)<br>RV structural abnormalities |
| **RV failure** | Symptoms and signs of RV failure<br>Preserved LV function |
| **Biventricular failure** | Symptoms and signs of LV failure<br>LV structural changes |

**Table 2.** Clinicopathologic phases of ARVC/D.

## 5.2. Nonclassic form of ARVC/D

### *5.2.1. ARVC/D with cutaneous manifestations (cardiocutanous disease)*

#### *5.2.1.1. Naxos disease*

Naxos disease is a recessively inherited stereotype association of arrhythmogenic cardiomyopathy with a cutaneous phenotype, characterized by peculiar wooly hair and palmoplantar keratoderma [60]. It is a homozygous recessive JUP mutation. The cardiac manifestations of the disease are identical to ARVC/D in both clinical and histological studies [5, 105]. Since 1995, according to the classification of World Health Organization, Naxos disease has been considered as the recessive form of ARVC/D [106].

As mentioned earlier, the disease was first described by Protonotarios et al. [60] in families originating from the Greek island of Naxos. Later on the affected families were detected in other Greek Aegean islands, and other countries [106–108]. The typical clinical presentation of the disease includes appearance of wooly hair appears from birth, whereas palmoplantar keratoderma develops during the first year of life when infants start to use their hands and feet [109]. The cardiomyopathy clinically manifests by adolescence and shows 100% penetrance [110]. Patients with Naxos disease is typically present with syncope and/or ventricular tachycardia of LBBB configuration. As with classic ARVC/D, sudden death may be the first manifestation of the disease. About one-third of patients become symptomatic before the 30th year of life, and a few clinical findings of an early heart disease can be detected during childhood in some cases [108]. They have ECG abnormalities, RV structural alterations, and LV involvement. In one series of 26 patients followed for 10 years, 62% had structural progression of RV abnormalities and 27% developed heart failure due to LV involvement [110]. Naxos ARVC/D is a rather progressive heart disease with adverse prognosis, especially in young. The annual disease-related and sudden death mortality have been estimated at 3% and 2.3%, respectively [110]. The risk factors for sudden death based on a long-term study of an unselected population of patients with Naxos disease include the history of syncope, the appearance of symptoms and severely progressed disease to the right ventricle before the age of 35 years, and the involvement of the left ventricle [110].

#### *5.2.1.2. Carvajal syndrome*

Carvajal syndrome with the same cutaneous manifestations as Naxos disease but with predominantly LV involvement has been described in families from India and Ecuador [45, 111]. It is associated with a DSP gene mutation and is also a recessive disease. The cardiomyopathy is clinically manifested during childhood leading more frequently to a dilated cardiomyopathy and heart failure. In Carvajal syndrome, the heart disease is clinically manifested earlier during childhood [45, 111]. A significant proportion of patients developed heart failure at an early stage of the disease, and most of them died during adolescence. In a single case, gross cardiac pathologic examination showed aneurysms of the RV outflow tract, apex and posterior wall and involvement of the LV. In histologic examination, findings similar to ARVC/D pathology were found with areas of extensive myocardial loss and replacement fibrosis, particularly in subepicardial layers; however, there was no fatty infiltration [112].

### *5.2.2. Left-dominant arrhythmogenic cardiomyopathy (LDAC)*

Patients with LDAC (also may refer to as left-sided ARVC/D or arrhythmogenic left ventricular cardiomyopathy) have fibrofatty changes, which predominantly involve the LV [113–117]. LDAC is characterized by ECG changes in the form of (infero)lateral T-wave inversion, arrhythmias of the LV origin. ARVC/D is distinguished from DCM by a propensity towards arrhythmia exceeding the degree of ventricular dysfunction [117]. Patients with LDAC may present with arrhythmias or chest pain, shortness of breath, syncope or presyncope at ages ranging from adolescence to over 80 years. In cardiac MRI, about one-third of patients show an LV ejection fraction less than 50% [117]. Furthermore, MRI with late gadolinium enhancement (LGE) of the LV demonstrated late enhancement extending through the outer one-third of the LV myocardium to the right side of the septum [117]. Some patients with LDAC have desmosomal gene mutations similar to ARVC/D (desmoplakin, plakophilin-2, and desmoglein-2) [64].

## 6. Diagnosis

The diagnosis of ARVC/D might be challenging in patients with early stages of the disease. The establishment of ARVC/D Task Force diagnostic criteria in 1994 and its modification in 2010 have improved the clinical diagnosis of the disease [118, 119]. The current Task Force criteria are the essential standard for classification of individuals suspected of ARVC/D. The Task Force criteria included six different categories: (1) global and regional dysfunction and structural alterations, (2) tissue characterization, (3) depolarization abnormalities, (4) repolarization abnormalities, (5) arrhythmias, and (6) family history, including pathogenic mutations. The diagnostic criteria within each category are further classified as major or minor according to their specificity for the disease. To fulfill ARVC/D diagnosis, it is required to have either two major or one major plus two minor or four minor criteria. The diagnosis of ARVC/D is regarded as definite with two major or one major and two minor criteria or four minor criteria from different categories; borderline with one major and one minor or three minor

http://dx.doi.org/10.5772/65316

criteria from different categories; and possible with one major or two minor criteria from different categories. **Table 3** presents an overview of the 2010 modified Task Force criteria.

| **The Revised Task Force Criteria for ARVC/D** | |
|---|---|
| **I. Global or regional dysfunction and structural alterations**[1] | |
| **Major** | **Minor** |
| **By 2D echo:** | **By 2D echo:** |
| • **Regional RV akinesia, dyskinesia, or aneurysm and 1 of the following (end diastole):** | • **Regional RV akinesia or dyskinesia and 1 of the following (end diastole):** |
| -PLAX RVOT ≥32 mm (corrected for body size [PLAX/BSA] ≥19 mm/m$^2$) | -PLAX RVOT ≥29 to <32 mm (corrected for body size [PLAX/BSA] ≥16 to <19 mm/m$^2$) |
| -PSAX RVOT ≥36 mm (corrected for body size [PSAX/BSA] ≥21 mm/m$^2$) | -PSAX RVOT ≥32 to <36 mm (corrected for body size [PSAX/BSA] ≥18 to <21 mm/m$^2$) |
| or | or |
| -fractional area change ≤33% | -fractional area change >33% to ≤40% |
| **By MRI:** | **By MRI:** |
| • **Regional RV akinesia or dyskinesia or dyssynchronous RV contraction and 1 of the following:** | • **Regional RV akinesia or dyskinesia or dyssynchronous RV contraction and 1 of the following:** |
| -Ratio of RV end-diastolic volume to BSA ≥110 mL/m$^2$ (male) or ≥100 mL/m$^2$ (female) | -Ratio of RV end-diastolic volume to BSA ≥100 to <110 mL/m$^2$ (male) or ≥90 to <100 mL/m$^2$ (female) |
| or | or |
| -RV ejection fraction ≤40% | -RV ejection fraction >40% to ≤45% |
| **By RV angiography:** | |
| Regional RV akinesia, dyskinesia, or aneurysm | |
| **II. Tissue characterization of wall** | |
| **Major** | **Minor** |
| • Residual myocytes<60% by morphometric analysis (or <50% if estimated), with fibrous replacement of the RV free wall myocardium in ≥1 sample, with or without fatty replacement | • Residual myocytes 60% to 75% by morphometric analysis (or 50% to 65% if estimated), with fibrous replacement of the RV free wall myocardium in ≥1 sample, with or without fatty replacement of tissue on endomyocardial biopsy |

of tissue on endomyocardial biopsy

**III. Repolarization abnormalities**

| Major | Minor |
|---|---|
| • Inverted T waves in right precordial leads ($V_1$, $V_2$, and $V_3$) or beyond in individuals >14 years of age (in the absence of complete right bundle-branch block QRS ≥120 ms) | • Inverted T waves in leads $V_1$ and $V_2$ in individuals >14 years of age (in the absence of complete right bundle-branch block) or in $V_4$, $V_5$, or $V_6$<br>• Inverted T waves in leads $V_1$, $V_2$, $V_3$, and $V_4$ in individuals >14 years of age in the presence of complete right bundle-branch block |

**IV. Depolarization/conduction abnormalities**

| Major | Minor |
|---|---|
| • Epsilon wave (reproducible low-amplitude signals between end of QRS complex to onset of the T wave) in the right precordial leads ($V_1$ to $V_3$) | • Late potentials by SAECG in ≥1 of 3 parameters in the absence of a QRS duration of ≥110 ms on the standard ECG<br>• Filtered QRS duration (fQRS) ≥114 ms<br>• Duration of terminal QRS <40 μV (low-amplitude signal duration) ≥38 ms<br>• Root-mean-square voltage of terminal 40 ms ≤20 μV<br>• Terminal activation duration of QRS ≥55 ms measured from the nadir of the S wave to the end of the QRS, including R′, in $V_1$, $V_2$, or $V_3$, in the absence of complete right bundle-branch block |

**V. Arrhythmias**

| Major | Minor |
|---|---|
| • **Nonsustain**ed or sustained ventricular tachycardia of left bundle-branch morphology with superior axis (negative or indeterminate QRS in leads II, III, and aVF and positive in lead aVL) | • Nonsustained or sustained ventricular tachycardia of RV outflow configuration, left bundle-branch block morphology with inferior axis (positive QRS in leads II, III, and aVF and negative in lead aVL) or of unknown axis<br>• >500 ventricular extrasystoles per 24 hours (Holter) |

**VI. Family history**

| Major | Minor |
|---|---|

- ARVC/D confirmed in a first-degree relative who meets current Task Force criteria
- ARVC/D confirmed pathologically at autopsy or surgery in a first-degree relative
- Identification of a pathogenic mutation[2] categorized as associated or probably associated with ARVC/D in the patient under evaluation
- History of ARVC/D in a first-degree relative in whom it is not possible or practical to determine whether the family member meets current Task Force criteria
- Premature sudden death (<35 years of age) due to suspected ARVC/D in a first-degree relative
- ARVC/D confirmed pathologically or by current Task Force Criteria in second-degree relative

- **Abbreviations:** PLAX indicates parasternal long-axis view; RVOT, RV outflow tract; BSA, body surface area; PSAX, parasternal short-axis view; aVF, augmented voltage unipolar left foot lead; and aVL, augmented voltage unipolar left arm lead.
- **Diagnostic terminology for original criteria:** This diagnosis is fulfilled by the presence of 2 major, or 1 major plus 2 minor criteria or 4 minor criteria from different groups. Diagnostic terminology for revised criteria: definite diagnosis: 2 major or 1 major and 2 minor criteria or 4 minor from different categories; borderline: 1 major and 1 minor or 3 minor criteria from different categories; possible: 1 major or 2 minor criteria from different categories.

[1] Hypokinesis is not included in this or subsequent definitions of RV regional wall motion abnormalities for the proposed modified criteria.
[2] A pathogenic mutation is a DNA alteration associated with ARVC/D that alters or is expected to alter the encoded protein, is unobserved or rare in a large non–ARVC/D control population, and either alters or is predicted to alter the structure or function of the protein or has demonstrated linkage to the disease phenotype in a conclusive pedigree.
Modified from Marcus FI et al. Diagnosis of arrhythmogenic right ventricular cardiomyopathy/dysplasia: proposed modification of the task force criteria. Circulation. 2010;121(13):1533-41. DOI:10.1161/CIRCULATIONAHA.108.840827. Eur Heart J. 2010 Apr;31(7):806-14. DOI:10.1093/eurheartj/ehq025.)

**Table 3.** The 2010 revised Task Force criteria for the diagnosis of ARVC/D.

Evaluation of patients with suspected ARVC/D should include: a detailed medical history including a detailed family history, physical examination, 12-lead electrocardiogram (ECG), signal-averaged ECG (SAECG), 24-hours Holter monitoring, exercise testing, echocardiography (including RV functional evaluation and quantitative wall motion analysis), and when appropriate a more detailed analysis of the RV function by cardiac magnetic resonance imaging (MRI). Invasive tests with RV endomyocardial biopsy and RV angiogram are also useful for diagnostic purposes. Electrophysiology studies might be helpful in the evaluation of the VT site of origin and ablation of VT when indicated.

A brief description of diagnostic tests based on the Task Force criteria will be outlined below.

### 6.1. Global and regional dysfunction and structural alterations

Various imaging modalities have been used to evaluate RV (and LV) size and function, including echocardiography, cardiac MRI, computed tomography scan (CT scan) and/or RV angiography. According to the Task Force criteria, major criteria are defined as the presence of akinetic or dyskinetic areas in the RV combined with severe dilatation of the RV or RV ejection fraction 40% or lower [119]. In RV angiography the finding of only regional akinesia, dyskinesia or an aneurysm is considered to be sufficient for qualification as a major criterion. RV angiography has historically been considered the most sensitive method to visualize RV structural abnormalities, with a high specificity of 90% [120]. Compared to angiography, echocardiography is noninvasive, widely available, low in cost, and easy to perform and interpret, and has played a crucial role in imaging structural and functional abnormalities of the RV (**Figure 4**). It serves as the first-line imaging technique for evaluating patients suspected of ARVC/D and in family screening. There are numerous reports of the use of echocardiography to aid in the diagnosis of ARVC/D. These studies have found that the presence of right ventricular dysfunction by two-dimensional echocardiography has a high specificity and predictive value for ARVC/D [121–123]. The development of new echocardiographic techniques such as three-dimensional right ventricular (3D-RV), strain and tissue Doppler, and tissue deformation imaging, may improve the diagnostic, and prognostic performance of echocardiography in these patients, which help in minimizing the number of false-negative echocardiographic results and improve the sensitivity and specificity of this test [124]. Cardiac MRI has a significant role in the diagnosis of ARVC/D. It has the advantage of assessing the RV (and LV) function, size, global or regional wall motion abnormalities, and quantification of myocardial wall thinning and hypertrophy. The disadvantages of this technique are the lack of wide availability, and the need for interpretation by an expert specialized radiologist to prevent misdiagnosis. Incorrect interpretation of cardiac MRI is the most common cause of over diagnosis and physicians should be reluctant to diagnose ARVC/D when structural abnormalities are present only on MRI [125] (**Figure 5**). Quantitative analysis showed that RV end-diastolic diameter and outflow tract area were significantly higher and RV ejection fractions lower in ARVC/D patients when compared to controls. Although CMRI is a potentially useful test because it can distinguish fat from muscle, the sensitivity and specificity of CMRI detection of RV intramyocardial fat in the diagnosis of ARVC/D are variable, ranging from 22 to 100% [126–130]. Identifying fat can be challenging because of the thin RV wall; therefore, it is difficult to distinguish pathologic adipose infiltration from adjacent epicardial fat and it is not included in the Task Force diagnostic criteria.

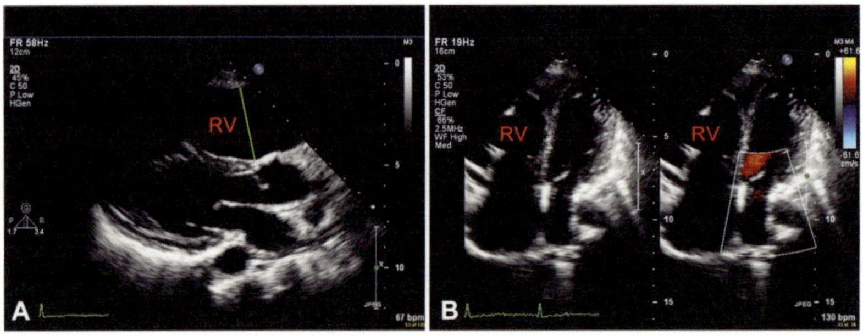


**Figure 4.** Parasternal long axis (A) and apical four-chamber (B) echocardiographic views showing RV dilatation.

http://dx.doi.org/10.5772/65316

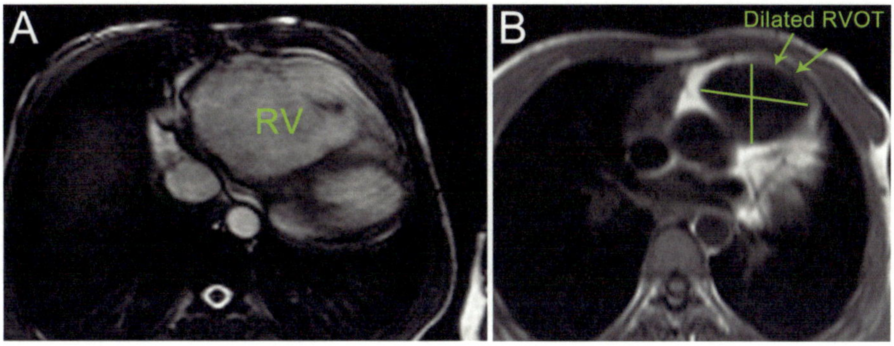


**Figure 5.** (A) Axial cine SSFP (steady-state free precession) MR imaging showing significant RV dilatation and (B) black-blood-prepared HASTE (Half-Fourier Acquired Single-shot Turbo spin Echo) axial slice MRI imaging at the level of RVOT showing RVOT dilatation.

### 6.2. Tissue characterization of wall (endomyocardial biopsy)

Endomyocardial biopsies (EMBs) are infrequently diagnostic, due to the focal nature of the lesions, and the fact that subendocardial layers of the myocardium are usually not affected in an early stage of the disease [131]. Furthermore, EMB sensitivity in ARVC/D is low if samples are taken from the septum, a region uncommonly involved by the disease [132]. Diagnostic values of EMB according to the new Task Force criteria are considered major if histomorphometric analysis of endomyocardial biopsies shows residual myocytes <60% by morphometric analysis (or <50% if estimated), with fibrous replacement of the RV free wall myocardium in ≥1 sample, with or without a fatty replacement of tissue (Task 2010). If the residual myocytes are 60–75% by morphometric analysis (or 50–65% if estimated), it is considered to be a minor criterion [129].

### 6.3. Electrocardiographic changes

The 12-lead ECG has a vital role in ARVC/D for diagnosis. The ECG changes and arrhythmias may precede the histological evidence of myocyte loss and RV changes in radiologic tests. Depolarization and repolarization ECG criteria have to be obtained during sinus rhythm and while off antiarrhythmic drugs.

#### *6.3.1. Depolarization abnormalities*

The hallmark of electrical changes in ARVC/D is the delayed RV activation. This delay may manifest with the presence of an epsilon wave, prolonged terminal activation duration (TAD) in the terminal part and after the QRS complex, and/or by recording late potentials on SAECG. Epsilon waves are defined as low amplitude potentials appearing after, and clearly separated from, the QRS complex in at least one of the precordial leads V1–V3 (**Figure 6**) [133]. Although epsilon waves are highly specific and considered to be one of the major diagnostic criteria, they are observed in only a small minority of patients [134, 135]. TAD has been defined as the longest value measured from the nadir of the S wave to the end of all depolarization deflections in V1–

V3, including the S wave upstroke and both late and fractionated signals and epsilon waves [136]. Prolonged TAD measured in V1–V3 greater than or equal to 55 ms, in the absence of complete RBBB, is considered to be a minor criterion. Prolonged TAD was recorded in 30 of 42 ARVC/D patients and only 1 of 27 patients with idiopathic VT [136]. The detection of late potentials on SAECG or late potentials detected during endocardial mapping in electrophysiologic studies (EPS) are frequently found in ARVC/D patients with documented VT; however, these late potentials can also be observed after myocardial infarction and with other structural heart diseases. Owing to this lack of specificity, SAECG abnormalities are considered a minor criterion. Common to all depolarization criteria is their correlation with disease severity. For instance, a positive correlation has been found between late potentials and the extent of RV fibrosis, reduced RV systolic function and significant morphological abnormalities on imaging [137–139].

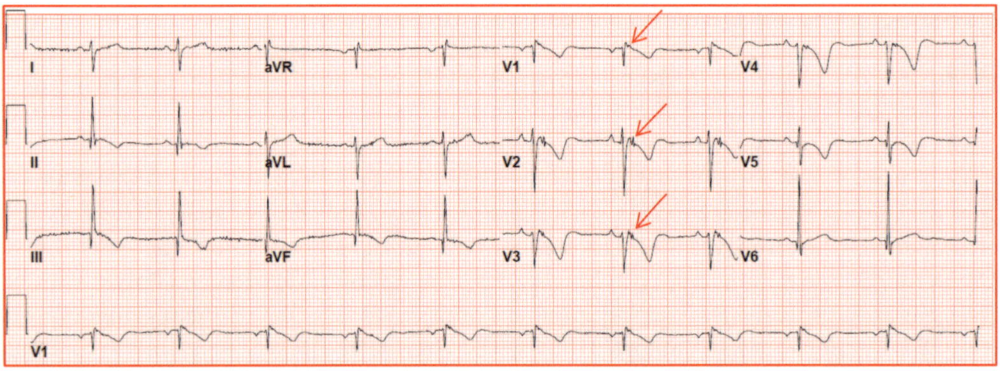


**Figure 6.** ECG of a patient with ARVC/D showing the presence of T-wave inversion in V1-V5 and an epsilon wave (electric potentials after the end of the QRS complex) (arrows).

### *6.3.2. Repolarization abnormalities*

In the new Task Force criteria, negative T-waves in leads V1–V3 form a major ECG criterion in the absence of complete RBBB, but only if the patient is older than 14 years of age (**Figure 6**). T-wave inversion can be a normal feature of the ECG in children and early adolescence. Studies have reported variable prevalence of right precordial T-wave inversion, ranging from 19 to 94% [118–134, 140]. This variation may be due inclusion of family members in some studies and only index cases in others. In a study that considered only at ARVC/D index cases, 67% of them had this criterion but it was not found in patients with idiopathic RV-VT [136]. Other variants of T-wave inversion including T-wave inversion only in leads V1 and V2, T-wave inversion in V4–V6 among individuals older than 14 years of age in the absence of complete RBBB, and inverted T-waves in leads V1–V4 among individuals older than 14 years of age in the presence of RBBB, are considered to be minor repolarization criteria in the new Task Force criteria [119].

### 6.4. Arrhythmia

In ARVC/D, ventricular arrhythmias may range from PVCs to sustained VT or VF, leading to cardiac arrest [136, 141]. Typically, VT originating from RV has a LBBB-like morphology. Furthermore, VT with a superior axis (negative R waves in inferior leads) indicating RV inferior wall or apex origin (**Figure 7**) is considered a major criterion, while VT with inferior axis (positive R waves in inferior leads) indicating RV outflow tract (RVOT) origin is considered a minor criterion (**Figure 8**). VT with LBBB-like morphology and unknown axis is considered a minor criterion. Patients with the extensive disease often show multiple VT morphologies [136]. VT may degenerate into VF and lead to SCD especially in young and athletes individuals with ARVC/D. According to the new Task Force criteria, 500 or more PVCs in a 24-hour Holter recording are considered a minor criterion [119].

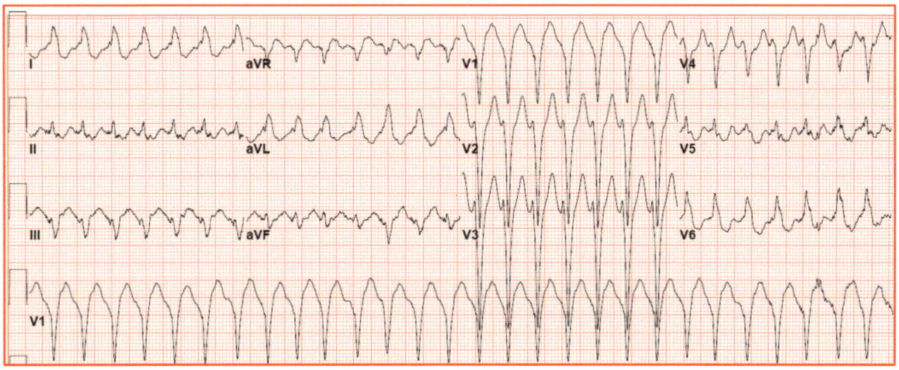


**Figure 7.** ECG showing ventricular tachycardia of RV inferior wall origin (LBBB and superior axis) in a patient with ARVC/D.

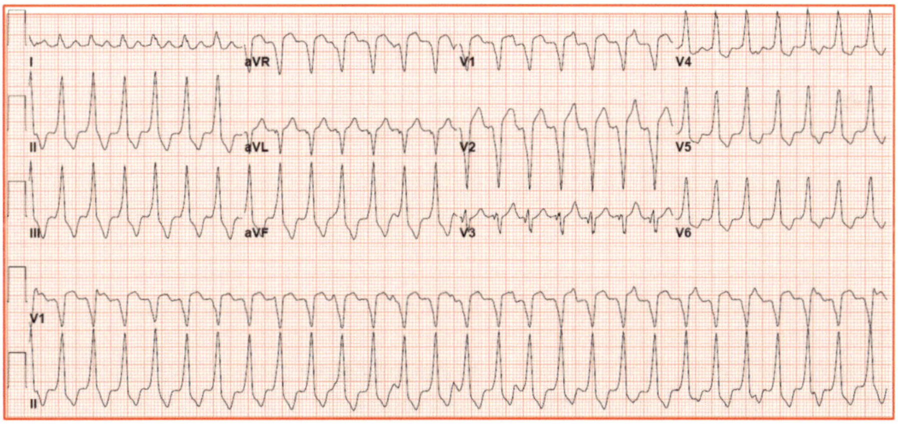


**Figure 8.** ECG showing ventricular tachycardia of RV outflow tract origin (LBBB and inferior axis) in a patient with ARVC/D.

### 6.5. Family history

ARVC/D is a familial disease. Having a first-degree family member with proven ARVC/D is considered an increased risk for other family members to be affected. ARVC/D confirmed in a first-degree relative who meets current Task Force criteria; ARVC/D confirmed pathologically at autopsy or surgery in a first-degree relative, or identification of a pathogenic mutation categorized as associated or probably associated with ARVC/D in the patient under evaluation is each considered as a major diagnostic criteria [119].

If a first-degree relative is diagnosed with ARVC/D but does not fulfill the diagnostic criteria, only a minor criterion is counted. Sudden death of a family member under the age of 35 years, presumably but not proven to be due to ARVC/D related arrhythmias, and ARVC/D confirmed pathologically or by current Task Force criteria in a second-degree relative is a minor criterion [119].

## 7. Differential diagnosis

It is crucial to differentiate ARVC/D from other diseases that primarily involve RV as the prognosis and management are very different. Differential diagnosis of ARVC/D includes:

1. **Right ventricular outflow tract VT (RVOT-VT):** RVOT-VT is a benign disorder that may cause exercise-induced left bundle branch block (LBBB) morphology VT with the inferior axis. In RVOT-VT there is no family history of ARVC/D or SCD, the ECG shows no depolarization or repolarization abnormalities and no RV structural changes can be detected. There is usually no reproducibly inducible VT by premature extrastimuli at programmed stimulation during electrophysiologic studies [142]. Idiopathic RVOT VT may be inducible by regular burst pacing and isoproterenol infusion [143]. The prognosis of RVOT-VT is usually good with very low risk of SCD. Furthermore, catheter ablation is usually curative in idiopathic RVOT-VT.

2. **Dilated cardiomyopathy:** Biventricular dilatation and congestive heart failure may mimic advanced ARVC/D with LV involvement. Characteristic ECG and cardiac MRI (CMRI) abnormalities in ARVC/D help to distinguish the two entities.

3. **Myocarditis:** Myocarditis due to viral infection or other causes may mimic ARVC/D. In general, endomyocardial biopsy is required to distinguish ARVC/D from myocarditis.

4. **Cardiac sarcoidosis:** Sarcoidosis is a disease of unknown etiology, characterized by the presence of noncaseating granulomas. It may affect mainly lungs, but other tissues such as heart, skin, eyes, reticuloendothelial system, kidneys, and central nervous system can be affected. About 5% of sarcoidosis patients may have cardiac involvement, which may manifest as conduction abnormalities, ventricular arrhythmias, valvular dysfunction or congestive heart failure. Although sarcoid patients typically have myocardial sarcoid granulomas and scarring in the LV and interventricular septum, the RV can also be affected. Patients can present with clinical features similar to those of ARVC/D including

http://dx.doi.org/10.5772/65316

arrhythmias, and SCD [144]. Visualization of granuloma in EMB can be a diagnostic value for cardiac sarcoidosis if granulomas are visualized [145]. Gadolinium-enhanced MRI may be beneficial by detecting located abnormalities in the septum, which is typical for sarcoidosis but seldom seen in ARVC/D. Positron emission tomography (PET) scans may show the active foci of sarcoidosis. Therapy with corticosteroids is recommended for patients diagnosed with cardiac sarcoidosis.

5. **Uhl anomaly:** This is a rare disorder characterized by the total lack of RV myocardium and results in a very thin-walled RV (parchment RV) [146]. In ARVC/D, the myocardium is not completely absent and is replaced by a variable degree of fibrosis.

## 8. Management

### 8.1. Risk stratification

The clinical objectives in ARVC/D management are prevention of SCD and death from heart failure; minimizing disease progression to RV, LV, or biventricular heart failure; improvement of quality of life by controlling palpitations, and minimizing appropriate or inappropriate implantable cardioverter defibrillator (ICD) discharges as much as possible; and improving functional capacity by optimization of heart failure management [147].

Therapeutic options consist of lifestyle changes, pharmacological treatment (beta-blockers, heart failure medications, antiarrhythmic medications), electrophysiological study (EPS) and catheter ablation, ICD implantation, and surgical intervention (e.g., RV isolation and heart transplantation).

### 8.2. Therapeutic options

#### *8.2.1. Lifestyle changes*

There is an established relationship between SCD and intense exertion in young individuals with ARVC/D. Competitive sports activity has been shown to increase the risk of SCD by fivefold in adolescent and young adults with ARVC/D [148]. Early identification of affected athletes by preparticipation screening and their disqualification from competitive sports activity may be "life-saving" [149]. Also, physical exercise has been implicated as a factor promoting development and progression of the ARVC/D phenotype [147]. In the animal study, it was demonstrated that in heterozygous plakoglobin-deficient mice, endurance training accelerated the development of RV dilatation, dysfunction, and ventricular ectopy, suggesting that chronically increased ventricular load might contribute to worsening of the ARVC/D phenotype [150].

Studies have shown that repetitive exercise and endurance sports increase age-related penetrance, the risk of VT/VF, and occurrence of heart failure in ARVC/D desmosomal-gene carriers [151, 152]. So, patients with a definite diagnosis of ARVC/D are encouraged not participate in endurance and/or competitive sports.

### 8.2.2. Pharmacological therapy

#### 8.2.2.1. Beta-blockers

VTs and cardiac arrest in ARVC/D are frequently triggered by adrenergic stimulation and occur during or immediately after physical exercise [153–157]. Autonomic dysfunction with increased sympathetic stimulation of ventricular myocardium and subsequent reduction of β-adrenoceptor density were demonstrated with the use of radionuclide imaging and quantitative positron emission tomography [158, 159]. Beta-blockers are useful in the treatment of heart failure, preventing the effort-related VT, and possibly minimizing disease progression by lowering RV wall stress.

Beta-blocker therapy is recommended in ARVC/D patients with recurrent VT, as an adjunct to ICD therapy. It may also be a helpful addition to minimize inappropriate ICD shocks due to sinus tachycardia, supraventricular tachycardia, or atrial fibrillation/flutter with high-ventricular rate [147].

#### 8.2.2.2. Heart failure therapy

For ARVC/D patients who developed right- and/or left-sided heart failure standard pharmacological treatment with angiotensin-converting-enzyme inhibitors, angiotensin II receptor blockers, β-blockers, and diuretics are recommended [147].

ARVC/D patients with severe RV dilatation are at risk of thromboembolism. A 0.5% annual incidence rate of thromboembolic complications is reported during a mean follow-up period of 99±64 months in a cohort of 126 ARVC/D patients [160]. Long-term oral anticoagulation is indicated for secondary prevention in patients with documented intra-cavitary thrombosis or venous/systemic thromboembolism [147].

#### 8.2.2.3. Antiarrhythmic drugs

The aim of antiarrhythmic drug (AAD) therapy in patients with ARVC/D is to improve the quality of life by preventing symptomatic VT and ICD shocks. The data about AAD in ARVC/D are limited due to the lack of randomized control studies, the change in medication regimes over time and the common need for other modalities of treatment like VT ablation or ICD implantation [147, 161–163].

Although initial studies suggest that sotalol, administered at a dosage of 320–640 mg/day, is the most effective therapy with approximately 68% of patients achieving complete or partial arrhythmia suppression [164, 165], more recent available data suggest that amiodarone (loading dose of 400–600 mg daily for 3 weeks and then maintenance dose of 200–400 mg daily), alone or in combination with β-blockers, is the most effective drug for preventing symptomatic VTs and has relatively low proarrhythmic risk even in patients with ventricular dysfunction, although its ability to prevent SCD is unproven [166]. This variation in drugs effect may be partially a result of significant differences in design of the two studies, and the difference in sotalol doses, the difference in the amiodarone loading strategies and the method of medication

http://dx.doi.org/10.5772/65316

selection [161]. There is relatively limited data about the combination of antiarrhythmic therapy. One recent report demonstrated the effective addition of flecainide to patients receiving sotalol with a resultant reduction in recurrent arrhythmias [167]. The addition of flecainide in this study was accomplished without significant adverse events. Several other studies have reported that the combination of amiodarone and beta-blockers may be effective in patients unable to achieve arrhythmia suppression with amiodarone alone [168, 169].

### *8.2.3. Catheter ablation*

Fibrofatty replacement of RV myocardium creates scar regions that form a substrate for re-entry arrhythmias and VT.

Although VT catheter ablation is effective in the short term, the recurrence rate of VT after endocardial ablation procedures is about 50–75% in 3-year follow-up, which is likely secondary to the progressive nature of the disease [148, 170]. The discovery of the epicardial arrhythmogenic substrate in RVC/D patients makes epicardial VT ablation an attractive approach. The combination of endocardial and epicardial ablation approaches resulted in a higher success rate (77–83%) and lower recurrence of VTs over 18 and 36 month follow-up periods [171, 172]. However, this is at the expense of potential complications such as epicardial bleeding and coronary stenosis occurring in approximately 5% of cases [172]. Nevertheless, catheter ablation remains an important therapeutic modality for decreasing patient morbidity in conjunction with ICD implantation and antiarrhythmic medication especially in ARVC/D patients with incessant VT or frequent appropriate ICD interventions on VT despite maximal pharmacological therapy, including amiodarone [147, 161].

### *8.2.4. Implantable cardioverter defibrillator therapy*

High-risk markers for mortality in ARVC/D include the history of syncope, sustained VT, severe RV dysfunction, and LV involvement [173–175]. ICD is the only treatment option that has been shown to reduce mortality. Over a 4-year follow-up period, the survival benefit of ICD implantation was about 25% in one study [176]. In a recent meta-analysis, the estimated annual mortality rate of patients with ARVC/D, who underwent ICD implantation, was 0.9%, significantly lower than those without ICDs [177]. A similar finding was noted in a large cohort of ARVC/D patients and family members where SCD during follow-up occurred more frequently among index-patients without an ICD (16% vs. 0.6%) [178]. The American College of Cardiology, American Heart Association and the European Society of Cardiology recommend ICD implantation for ARCV/D patients with high-risk features [179]. ICD Implantation is recommended in ARVC/D patients who have experienced hemodynamically unstable VT, sustained VT or VF (class I). Also, ICD implantation is recommended in ARVC/D patients with severe RV systolic dysfunction, LV systolic dysfunction or both (Class I). ICD implantation should be considered in ARVC/D patients who have experienced hemodynamically stable, sustained VT or who have "major" risk factors such as unexplained syncope, moderate ventricular dysfunction, or NSVT (Class IIa) [147] (**Figure 9**).

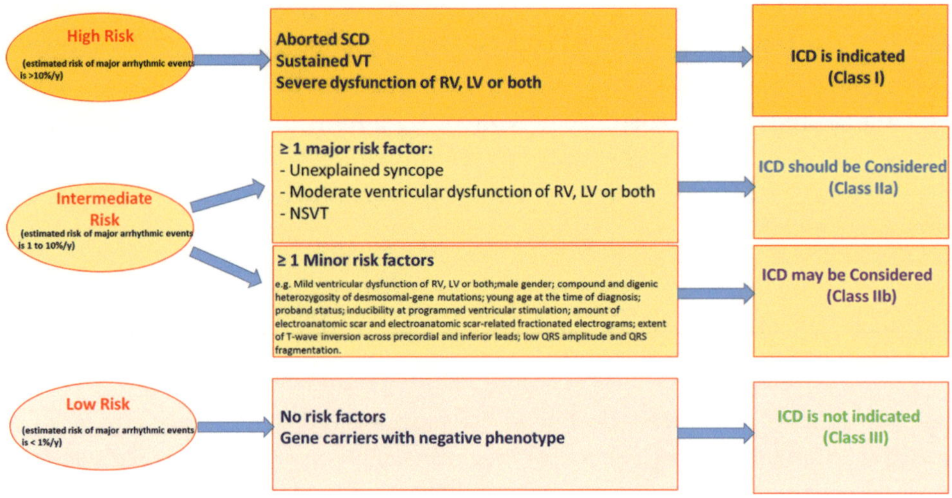


**Figure 9.** Indications for ICD in ARVC/D patients based on risk stratification. Modified with permission from Corrado et al. [147].

### *8.2.5. Surgical interventions*

#### *8.2.5.1. Heart transplantation*

Heart transplantation is recommended as a final therapeutic option in ARVC/D patients with either severe, unresponsive congestive heart failure or recurrent episodes of VT/VF, which are refractory to catheter (and surgical) ablation and/or ICD therapy in experienced centers [147].

The most common indication for heart transplantation in ARVC/D patients is the progression of heart failure followed by intractable VTs [180]. Survival rates after 1-year post-heart transplant after were 94% and at an average follow-up of 6.2 ± 4.8 year it was 88%. In a recent study involving a large cohort of ARVC/D patients, the need for cardiac transplantation was 4% [178].

#### *8.2.5.2. Other surgical therapies*

There is currently no clinical role for surgical therapies such as beating heart cryoablation [181], RV disarticulation [182], RV cardiomyoplasty [183], and left cardiac sympathetic denervation [184] in the treatment of patients with ARVC/D.

## 9. Family screening

ARVC/D is a familial disease and screening the family of affected individuals is important. All first-degree family members of the affected individual should be screened for ARVC/D. Screening should begin during the teenage years unless otherwise indicated. Screening tests

http://dx.doi.org/10.5772/65316

include ECG, signal-averaged ECG, Holter monitoring, echocardiogram, exercise stress test, and cardiac MRI. If a pathogenic mutation is identified in an ARVC/D patient, parents, siblings, and children of this patient can be tested for the mutation via the cascade method. In a recent study that looked at this matter it was found that one-third of family members fulfill conventional diagnostic Task Force criteria. Siblings are at the highest risk of disease even after correcting for age and sex, and an accurate prediction of ARVC/D diagnosis among relatives can be obtained using a model including symptoms, being a sibling, the presence of a pathogenic mutation, and female gender [185]. Meeting Task Force criteria independent of family history had a higher prognostic value for arrhythmic events than conventional Task Force criteria, which include family history. It was also noted that arrhythmic risk prediction is improved by applying modified Task Force criteria that exclude family history. This provides the physician with a reliable risk stratification tool, which does not require a difficult management scheme or additional testing [185].

## 10. Conclusions

ARVC/D is a rare cardiac disease characterized by fibrofatty replacement of myocardial tissue. It affects the RV primarily, but an extension to the LV in more advanced stages of the disease may occur. At the molecular level, both ventricles are affected, presumably in all stages of the disease. Its prevalence has been estimated to vary from 1:2000 to 1:5000. Patients typically present between the second and the fourth decade of life with VT episodes originating from the RV. It is also a major cause of SCD in the young patients and athletes.

The ARVC/D is an inherited cardiomyopathy and the causative genes encode proteins of mechanical cell junctions (e.g., plakoglobin, plakophilin-2, desmoglein-2, desmocollin-2, and desmoplakin) accounting for intercalated disk remodeling. The mode of inherence is mostly an autosomal dominant trait with variable penetrance. The rare recessively inherited variants are often associated with palmoplantar keratoderma and wooly hair. The diagnosis is made according to the modified Task Force criteria, based on functional and structural alterations of the RV, depolarization and repolarization abnormalities, fibrofatty replacement in the endomyocardial biopsy, VT with LBBB morphology, and family history. The use of the Task Force criteria helps to avoid under an overdiagnosis of the disease. Echocardiography and cardiac magnetic resonance imaging (MRI) are the main imaging tools to visualize structural and functional abnormalities. The ARVC/D should be differentiated from other cardiac diseases such as idiopathic RVOT-VT and myocarditis. ARVC/D therapy consists of lifestyle changes, antiarrhythmic drugs, and catheter ablation. Young age at diagnosis, family history of juvenile SCD, LV involvement, VT, syncope, and previous cardiac arrest are the major risk factors for adverse prognosis. Implantable cardioverter defibrillator (ICD) therapy has been demonstrated to affect positively patients' mortality, and it should be considered in all high-risk patients. Heart transplantation may be required in about 4% of the ARVC/D patients. Ongoing research is focused on the understanding of disease pathophysiology and providing a curative therapy that may be able to stop disease progression.

## Acknowledgements

The author would like to express his appreciation to Ms. Sandra Keating and Mrs. Suzanne Tobias for editing the manuscript of this book chapter.


## Author details


Bandar Al-Ghamdi

Address all correspondence to: balghamdi@kfshrc.edu.sa

Heart Centre, King Faisal Specialist Hospital and Research Centre, Alfaisal University, Riyadh, Saudi Arabia


## References


[1] Frank R, Fontaine G, Vedel J, Mialet G, Sol C, Guiraudon G, Grosgogeat Y. Electrocardiologie de quatre cas de dysplasie ventriculaire droite arythmogène (Electrocardiology of 4 cases of right ventricular dysplasia inducing arrhythmia) [Article in French]. Arch Mal Coeur Vaiss. 1978 Sep;71(9):963–972.

[2] Marcus FI, Fontaine GH, Guiraudon G, Frank R, Laurenceau JL, Malergue C, Grosgogeat Y. Right ventricular dysplasia: a report of 24 adult cases. Circulation. 1982 Feb; 65(2):384-398. DOI:10.1161/01.CIR.65.2.384.

[3] Corrado D, Basso C, Thiene G, McKenna WJ, Davies MJ, Fontaliran F, Nava A, Silvestri F, Blomstrom-Lundqvist C, Wlodarska EK, Fontaine G, Camerini F. Spectrum of clinicopathologic manifestations of arrhythmogenic right ventricular cardiomyopathy/dysplasia: a multicenter study. J Am Coll Cardiol. 1997 Nov 15;30(6):1512–1520. DOI:10.1016/S0735-1097(97)00332-X.

[4] Basso C, Thiene G, Corrado D, Angelini A, Nava A, Valente M. Arrhythmogenic right ventricular cardiomyopathy: dysplasia, dystrophy, or myocarditis? Circulation. 1996 Sep 1;94(5):983–991. DOI:10.1161/01.CIR.94.5.983.

[5] Thiene G, Nava A, Corrado D, Rossi L, Pennelli N. Right ventricular cardiomyopathy and sudden death in young people. N Engl J Med. 1988 Jan 21;318(3):129–133. DOI: 10.1056/NEJM198801213180301.

[6] Richardson P, McKenna W, Bristow M, Maisch B, Mautner B, O'Connell J, Olsen E, Thiene G, Goodwin J, Gyarfas I, Martin I, Nordet P. Report of the 1995 World Health Organization/International Society and Federation of Cardiology

Task Force on the Definition and Classification of cardiomyopathies. Circulation. 1996 Mar 1;93(5):841–842. DOI:10.1161/01.CIR.93.5.841.

[7] Lazzarini E, Jongbloed JD, Pilichou K, Thiene G, Basso C, Bikker H, Charbon B, Swertz M, van Tintelen JP, van der Zwaag PA. The ARVD/C genetic variants database: 2014 update.Hum Mutat. 2015 Apr;36(4):403–410. DOI:10.1002/humu.22765.

[8] McKoy G, Protonotarios N, Crosby A, Tsatsopoulou A, Anastasakis A, Coonar A, Norman M, Baboonian C, Jeffery S, McKenna WJ. Identification of a deletion in plakoglobin in arrhythmogenic right ventricular cardiomyopathy with palmoplantar keratoderma and woolly hair (Naxos disease). Lancet. 2000 Jun 17;355(9221):2119–2124. DOI:10.1016/S0140-6736(00)02379-5.

[9] Norgett EE, Hatsell SJ, Carvajal-Huerta L, Cabezas JC, Common J, Purkis PE, Whittock N, Leigh IM, Stevens HP, Kelsell DP. Recessive mutation in desmoplakin disrupts desmoplakin-intermediate filament interactions and causes dilated cardiomyopathy, woolly hair and keratoderma. Hum Mol Genet. 2000 Nov 1;9(18):2761–2766. DOI: 10.1093/hmg/9.18.2761.

[10] Gemayel C, Pelliccia A, Thompson PD. Arrhythmogenic right ventricular cardiomyopathy. J Am Coll Cardiol. 2001;38(7):1773–1781. DOI:10.1016/S0735-1097(01)01654-0.

[11] Corrado D, Thiene G. Arrhythmogenic right ventricular cardiomyopathy/dysplasia: clinical impact of molecular genetic studies. Circulation. 2006;113(13):1634–1637. DOI: 10.1161/CIRCULATIONAHA.105.616490.

[12] Al-Ghamdi B, Shafquat A, Mallawi Y.Arrhythmogenic right ventricular cardiomyopathy/dysplasia in Saudi Arabia: a single-center experience with long-term follow-up. Ann Saudi Med. 2014 Sep-Oct;34(5):415–426. DOI:10.5144/0256-4947.2014.415.

[13] Dalal D, Nasir K, Bomma C, Prakasa K, Tandri H, Piccini J, Roguin A, Tichnell C, James C, Russell SD, Judge DP, Abraham T, Spevak PJ, Bluemke DA, Calkins H. Arrhythmogenic right ventricular dysplasia: a United States experience. Circulation. 2005;112:3823–3832. DOI:10.1161/CIRCULATIONAHA.105.542266.

[14] Corrado D, Fontaine G, Marcus FI, McKenna WJ, Nava A, Thiene G, Wichter T. Arrhythmogenic right ventricular dysplasia/cardiomyopathy: need for an international registry. Study Group on Arrhythmogenic Right Ventricular Dysplasia/Cardiomyopathy of the Working Groups on Myocardial and Pericardial Disease and Arrhythmias of the European Society of Cardiology and of the Scientific Council on Cardiomyopathies of the World Heart Federation. Circulation. 2000 Mar 21;101(11):E101-6. DOI: 10.1161/01.CIR.101.11.e101.

[15] Corrado D, Basso C, Schiavon M, Thiene G. Screening for hypertrophic cardiomyopathy in young athletes. N Engl J Med. 1998;339(6):364–369. DOI:10.1056/NEJM199808063390602.

[16] Shen WK, Edwards WD, Hammill SC, Gersh BJ. Right ventricular dysplasia: a need for precise pathological definition for interpretation of sudden death (abstr). J Am Coll Cardiol. 1994; 23(Suppl):34A.

[17] Romero J, Mejia-Lopez E, Manrique C, Lucariello R. Arrhythmogenic right ventricular cardiomyopathy (ARVC/D): a systematic literature review. Clin Med Insights Cardiol. 2013 May 21;7:97–114. DOI:10.4137/CMC.S10940.

[18] Cheng TO. Ethnic differences in arrhythmogenic right ventricular dysplasia/cardiomyopathy. Int J Cardiol. 2002;83(3):293.Author reply 291. DOI:10.1016/S0167-5273(02)00068-2.

[19] Basso C, Corrado D, Marcus FI, Nava A, Thiene G. Arrhythmogenic right ventricular cardiomyopathy. Lancet. 2009;373:1289–300. DOI:10.1016/S0140-6736(09)60256-7.

[20] Mertens C, Kuhn C, Franke WW. Plakophilins 2a and 2b: constitutive proteins of dual location in the karyoplasm and the desmosomal plaque. J Cell Biol. 1996;135:1009–1025. DOI:10.1083/jcb.135.4.1009.

[21] Gerull B, Heuser A, Wichter T, Paul M, Basson CT, McDermott DA, Lerman BB, Markowitz SM, Ellinor PT, MacRae CA, Peters S, Grossmann KS, Drenckhahn J, Michely B, Sasse-Klaassen S, Birchmeier W, Dietz R, Breithardt G, Schulze-Bahr E, Thierfelder L. Mutations in the desmosomal protein plakophilin-2 are common in arrhythmogenic right ventricular cardiomyopathy. Nat Genet. 2004 Nov;36(11):1162–1164. Erratum in: Nat Genet. 2005 Jan;37(1):106. DOI:10.1038/ng1461.

[22] Syrris P, Ward D, Asimaki A, Sen-Chowdhry S, Ebrahim HY, Evans A, Hitomi N, Norman M, Pantazis A, Shaw AL, Elliott PM, McKenna WJ. Clinical expression of plakophilin-2 mutations in familial arrhythmogenic right ventricular cardiomyopathy. Circulation. 2006 Jan 24;113(3):356–364. DOI:10.1161/CIRCULATIONAHA.105.561654.

[23] Kannankeril PJ, Bhuiyan ZA, Darbar D, Mannens MM, Wilde AA, Roden DM. Arrhythmogenic right ventricular cardiomyopathy due to a novel plakophilin 2 mutation: wide spectrum of disease in mutation carriers within a family. Heart Rhythm. 2006;3:939–944. DOI:10.1016/j.hrthm.2006.04.028.

[24] van der Zwaag PA, Cox MG, van der Werf C, Wiesfeld AC, Jongbloed JD, Dooijes D, Bikker H, Jongbloed R, Suurmeijer AJ, van den Berg MP, Hofstra RM, Hauer RN, Wilde AA, van Tintelen JP. Recurrent and founder mutations in the Netherlands: plakophilin-2 p.Arg79X mutation causing arrhythmogenic right ventricular cardiomyopathy/dysplasia. Neth Heart J. 2010 Dec;18(12):583–591. DOI:10.1007/s12471-010-0839-5.

[25] Li Mura IE, Bauce B, Nava A, Fanciulli M, Vazza G, Mazzotti E, Rigato I, De Bortoli M, Beffagna G, Lorenzon A, Calore M, Dazzo E, Nobile C, Mostacciuolo ML, Corrado D, Basso C, Daliento L, Thiene G, Rampazzo A. Identification of a PKP2 gene deletion in a family with arrhythmogenic right ventricular cardiomyopathy. Eur J Hum Genet. 2013 Nov;21(11):1226–1231. DOI:10.1038/ejhg.2013.39.

[26] Zhou X, Chen M, Song H, Wang B, Chen H, Wang J, Wang W, Feng S, Zhang F, Ju W, Li M, Gu K, Cao K, Wang DW, Yang B. Comprehensive analysis of desmosomal gene mutations in Han Chinese patients with arrhythmogenic right ventricular cardiomyopathy. Eur J Med Genet. 2015 Apr;58(4):258–265. DOI:10.1016/j.ejmg.2015.02.009.

[27] van Tintelen JP, Entius MM, Bhuiyan ZA, Jongbloed R, Wiesfeld AC, Wilde AA, van der Smagt J, Boven LG, Mannens MM, van Langen IM, Hofstra RM, Otterspoor LC, Doevendans PA, Rodriguez LM, van Gelder IC, Hauer RN. Plakophilin-2 mutations are the major determinant of familial arrhythmogenic right ventricular dysplasia/cardiomyopathy. Circulation. 2006 Apr 4;113(13):1650–1658. DOI:10.1161/CIRCULATIONAHA.105.609719.

[28] Groeneweg JA, van der Zwaag PA, Olde Nordkamp LR, Bikker H, Jongbloed JD, Jongbloed R, Wiesfeld AC, Cox MG, van der Heijden JF, Atsma DE, de Boer K, Doevendans PA, Vink A, van Veen TA, Dooijes D, van den Berg MP, Wilde AA, van Tintelen JP, Hauer RN. Arrhythmogenic right ventricular dysplasia/cardiomyopathy according to revised 2010 task force criteria with inclusion of non-desmosomal phospholamban mutation carriers. Am J Cardiol. 2013 Oct 15;112(8):1197–206. DOI:10.1016/j.amjcard.2013.06.017.

[29] Al-Ghamdi B, Alhassnan Z, Al-Fayyadh M, Shafquat A, Manea W, Alhadeq F, Rababh M, Mallawi Y. Clinical and genetic characteristics of arrhythmogenic right ventricular cardiomyopathy/dysplasia patients in Saudi Arabia: a single centre experience. In: Cardiostim-EHRA Europace; 8–11 June 2016; Nice, France: Europace. June 2016;16:Supp 1.

[30] Antoniades L, Tsatsopoulou A, Anastasakis A, Syrris P, Asimaki A, Panagiotakos D, Zambartas C, Stefanadis C, McKenna WJ, Protonotarios N. Arrhythmogenic right ventricular cardiomyopathy caused by deletions in plakophilin-2 and plakoglobin (Naxos disease) in families from Greece and Cyprus: genotype-phenotype relations, diagnostic features and prognosis. Eur Heart J. 2006 Sep;27(18):2208–2216. DOI:10.1093/eurheartj/ehl184.

[31] Cox MG, van der Zwaag PA, van der Werf C, van der Smagt JJ, Noorman M, Bhuiyan ZA, Wiesfeld AC, Volders PG, van Langen IM, Atsma DE, Dooijes D, van den Wijngaard A, Houweling AC, Jongbloed JD, Jordaens L, Cramer MJ, Doevendans PA, de Bakker JM, Wilde AA, van Tintelen JP, Hauer RN.Arrhythmogenic right ventricular dysplasia/cardiomyopathy: pathogenic desmosome mutations in index-patients predict outcome of family screening: Dutch arrhythmogenic right ventricular dysplasia/cardiomyopathy genotype-phenotype follow-up study. Circulation. 2011 Jun 14;123(23):2690–2700. DOI:10.1161/CIRCULATIONAHA.110.988287.

[32] Lahtinen AM, Lehtonen E, Marjamaa A, Kaartinen M, Heliö T, Porthan K, Oikarinen L, Toivonen L, Swan H, Jula A, Peltonen L, Palotie A, Salomaa V, Kontula K. Population-prevalent desmosomal mutations predisposing to arrhythmogenic right ventricular

cardiomyopathy. Heart Rhythm. 2011 Aug;8(8):1214–1221. DOI:10.1016/j.hrthm.2011.03.015.

[33] Sen-Chowdhry S, Syrris P, Ward D, Asimaki A, Sevdalis E, McKenna WJ. Clinical and genetic characterization of families with arrhythmogenic right ventricular dysplasia/cardiomyopathy provides novel insights into patterns of disease expression. Circulation. 2007 Apr 3;115(13):1710–1720. DOI:10.1161/CIRCULATIONAHA.106.660241.

[34] van Tintelen JP, Hofstra RM, Wiesfeld AC, van den Berg MP, Hauer RN, Jongbloed JD. Molecular genetics of arrhythmogenic right ventricular cardiomyopathy: emerging horizon? Curr Opin Cardiol. 2007 May;22(3):185–192. DOI:10.1097/HCO.0b013e3280d942c4.

[35] Awad MM, Calkins H, Judge DP. Mechanisms of disease: molecular genetics of arrhythmogenic right ventricular dysplasia/cardiomyopathy. Nat Clin Pract Cardiovasc Med. 2008 May;5(5):258–267. DOI:10.1038/ncpcardio1182.

[36] den Haan AD, Tan BY, Zikusoka MN, Lladó LI, Jain R, Daly A, Tichnell C, James C, Amat-Alarcon N, Abraham T, Russell SD, Bluemke DA, Calkins H, Dalal D, Judge DP. Comprehensive desmosome mutation analysis in North Americans with arrhythmogenic right ventricular dysplasia/cardiomyopathy. Circ Cardiovasc Genet. 2009 Oct;2(5):428–435. DOI:10.1161/CIRCGENETICS.109.858217.

[37] Bauce B, Nava A, Beffagna G, Basso C, Lorenzon A, Smaniotto G, De Bortoli M, Rigato I, Mazzotti E, Steriotis A, Marra MP, Towbin JA, Thiene G, Danieli GA, Rampazzo A. Multiple mutations in desmosomal proteins encoding genes in arrhythmogenic right ventricular cardiomyopathy/dysplasia. Heart Rhythm. 2010 Jan;7(1):22–29. DOI:10.1016/j.hrthm.2009.09.070.

[38] Fressart V, Duthoit G, Donal E, Probst V, Deharo JC, Chevalier P, Klug D, Dubourg O, Delacretaz E, Cosnay P, Scanu P, Extramiana F, Keller D, Hidden-Lucet F, Simon F, Bessirard V, Roux-Buisson N, Hebert JL, Azarine A, Casset-Senon D, Rouzet F, Lecarpentier Y, Fontaine G, Coirault C, Frank R, Hainque B, Charron P. Desmosomal gene analysis in arrhythmogenic right ventricular dysplasia/cardiomyopathy: spectrum of mutations and clinical impact in practice. Europace. 2010 Jun;12(6):861–868. DOI:10.1093/europace/euq104.

[39] Gerull B. Skin-heart connection: what can the epidermis tell us about the myocardium in arrhythmogenic cardiomyopathy? Circ Cardiovasc Genet. 2014 Jun;7(3):225–227. DOI:10.1161/CIRCGENETICS.114.000647.

[40] Brun F, Barnes CV, Sinagra G, Slavov D, Barbati G, Zhu X, Graw SL, Spezzacatene A, Pinamonti B, Merlo M, Salcedo EE, Sauer WH, Taylor MR, Mestroni L. Titin and desmosomal genes in the natural history of arrhythmogenic right ventricular cardiomyopathy. J Med Genet. 2014 Oct;51(10):669–676. DOI: 10.1136/jmedgenet-2014-102591.

[41] Cerrone M, Lin X, Zhang M, Agullo-Pascual E, Pfenniger A, Chkourko Gusky H, Novelli V, Kim C, Tirasawadichai T, Judge DP, Rothenberg E, Chen HS, Napolitano C,

Priori SG, Delmar M. Missense mutations in plakophilin-2 cause sodium current deficit and associate with a Brugada syndrome phenotype. Circulation. 2014 Mar 11;129(10): 1092–103. DOI:10.1161/CIRCULATIONAHA.113.003077.

[42] Cerrone M, Delmar M. Desmosomes and the sodium channel complex: implications for arrhythmogenic cardiomyopathy and Brugada syndrome. Trends Cardiovasc Med. 2014 Jul;24(5):184–190. DOI:10.1016/j.tcm.2014.02.001

[43] Arnemann J, Spurr NK, Wheeler GN, Parker AE, Buxton RS. Chromosomal assignment of the human genes coding for the major proteins of the desmosome junction, desmoglein DGI (DSG), desmocollins DGII/III (DSC), desmoplakins DPI/II (DSP), and plakoglobin DPIII (JUP). Genomics. 1991 Oct;10(3):640–645. DOI:10.1016/0888-7543(91)90446-L.

[44] Bornslaeger EA, Corcoran CM, Stappenbeck TS, Green KJ. Breaking the connection: displacement of the desmosomal plaque protein desmoplakin from cell-cell interfaces disrupts anchorage of intermediate filament bundles and alters intercellular junction assembly. J Cell Biol. 1996 Aug;134(4):985–1001. DOI:10.1083/jcb.134.4.985.

[45] Carvajal-Huerta L. Epidermolytic palmoplantar keratoderma with woolly hair and dilated cardiomyopathy. J Am Acad Dermatol. 1998 Sep;39(3):418–421. DOI:10.1016/s0190-9622(98)70317-2.

[46] Rampazzo A, Nava A, Malacrida S, Beffagna G, Bauce B, Rossi V, Zimbello R, Simionati B, Basso C, Thiene G, Towbin JA, Danieli GA. Mutation in human desmoplakin domain binding to plakoglobin causes a dominant form of arrhythmogenic right ventricular cardiomyopathy. Am J Hum Genet. 2002 Nov;71(5):1200–1206. DOI:10.1086/344208.

[47] Alcalai R, Metzger S, Rosenheck S, Meiner V, Chajek-Shaul T. A recessive mutation in desmoplakin causes arrhythmogenic right ventricular dysplasia, skin disorder, and woolly hair. J Am Coll Cardiol. 2003 Jul 16;42(2):319–327. DOI:10.1016/s0735-1097(03)00628-4.

[48] Uzumcu A, Norgett EE, Dindar A, Uyguner O, Nisli K, Kayserili H, Sahin SE, Dupont E, Severs NJ, Leigh IM, Yuksel-Apak M, Kelsell DP, Wollnik B. Loss of desmoplakin isoform I causes early onset cardiomyopathy and heart failure in a Naxos-like syndrome. J Med Genet. 2006 Feb;43(2):e5. DOI:10.1136/jmg.2005.032904.

[49] van der Zwaag PA, Jongbloed JD, van den Berg MP, van der Smagt JJ, Jongbloed R, Bikker H, Hofstra RM, van Tintelen JP. A genetic variants database for arrhythmogenic right ventricular dysplasia/cardiomyopathy. Hum Mutat. 2009 Sep;30(9):1278–1283. DOI:10.1002/humu.21064.

[50] Al-Jassar C, Knowles T, Jeeves M, Kami K, Behr E, Bikker H, Overduin M, Chidgey M. The nonlinear structure of the desmoplakin plakin domain and the effects of cardiomyopathy-linked mutations. J Mol Biol. 2011 Sep 2;411(5):1049–1061. DOI:10.1016/j.jmb.2011.06.047.

[51] Whittock NV, Ashton GH, Dopping-Hepenstal PJ, Gratian MJ, Keane FM, Eady RA, McGrath JA. Striate palmoplantar keratoderma resulting from desmoplakin haploinsufficiency. J Invest Dermatol. 1999 Dec;113(6):940–946. DOI:10.1046/j.1523-1747.1999.00783.x.

[52] Arnemann J, Spurr NK, Magee AI, Buxton RS. The human gene (DSG2) coding for HDGC, a second member of the desmoglein subfamily of the desmosomal cadherins, is, like DSG1 coding for desmoglein DGI, assigned to chromosome 18. Genomics. 1992 Jun;13(2):484–446. DOI:10.1016/0888-7543(92)90280-6.

[53] Pilichou K, Nava A, Basso C, Beffagna G, Bauce B, Lorenzon A, Frigo G, Vettori A, Valente M, Towbin J, Thiene G, Danieli GA, Rampazzo A. Mutations in desmoglein-2 gene are associated with arrhythmogenic right ventricular cardiomyopathy. Circulation. 2006 Mar;113(9):1171–1179. DOI:10.1161/CIRCULATIONAHA.105.583674.

[54] Posch MG, Posch MJ, Geier C, Erdmann B, Mueller W, Richter A, Ruppert V, Pankuweit S, Maisch B, Perrot A, Buttgereit J, Dietz R, Haverkamp W, Ozcelik C. A missense variant in desmoglein-2 predisposes to dilated cardiomyopathy. Mol Genet Metab. 2008 Sep-Oct;95(1-2):74–80. DOI:10.1016/j.ymgme.2008.06.005.

[55] Amagai M, Wang Y, Minoshima S, Kawamura K, Green KJ, Nishikawa T, Shimizu N. Assignment of the human genes for desmocollin 3 (DSC3) and desmocollin 4 (DSC4) to chromosome 18q12. Genomics. 1995 Jan;25(1):330–332. DOI:10.1016/0888-7543(95)80154-E.

[56] Syrris P, Ward D, Evans A, Asimaki A, Gandjbakhch E, Sen-Chowdhry S, McKenna WJ. Arrhythmogenic right ventricular dysplasia/cardiomyopathy associated with mutations in the desmosomal gene desmocollin-2. Am J Hum Genet. 2006 Nov;79(5):978–984. DOI:10.1086/509122.

[57] Heuser A, Plovie ER, Ellinor PT, Grossmann KS, Shin JT, Wichter T, Basson CT, Lerman BB, Sasse-Klaassen S, Thierfelder L, MacRae CA, Gerull B. Mutant desmocollin-2 causes arrhythmogenic right ventricular cardiomyopathy. Am J Hum Genet. 2006 Dec;79(6):1081–1088. DOI:10.1086/509044.

[58] Groeneweg JA, van der Zwaag PA, Jongbloed JD, Cox MG, Vreeker A, de Boer RA, van der Heijden JF, van Veen TA, McKenna WJ, van Tintelen JP, Dooijes D, Hauer RN. Left-dominant arrhythmogenic cardiomyopathy in a large family: associated desmosomal or nondesmosomal genotype? Heart Rhythm. 2013 Apr;10(4):548–559. DOI:10.1016/j.hrthm.2012.12.020.

[59] Asimaki A, Syrris P, Wichter T, Matthias P, Saffitz JE, McKenna WJ.A novel dominant mutation in plakoglobin causes arrhythmogenic right ventricular cardiomyopathy. Am J Hum Genet. 2007 Nov;81(5):964–973. DOI:10.1086/521633.

[60] Protonotarios N, Tsatsopoulou A, Patsourakos P. Cardiac abnormalities in familial palmoplantar keratosis. Br Heart J. 1986 Oct;56(4):321–326.

[61] Protonotarios N, Tsatsopoulou A, Fontaine G. Naxos disease: keratoderma, scalp modifications, and cardiomyopathy. J Am Acad Dermatol. 2001 Feb;44(2):309–311. DOI: 10.1067/mjd.2001.110648.

[62] Marian AJ. On the diagnostic utility of junction plakoglobin in arrhythmogenic right ventricular cardiomyopathy. Cardiovasc Pathol. 2013 Sep-Oct;22(5):309–311. DOI: 10.1016/j.carpath.2013.05.002.

[63] McNally E, MacLeod H, Dellefave-Castillo L. Arrhythmogenic right ventricular dysplasia/cardiomyopathy. In: Pagon RA, Adam MP, Ardinger HH, Wallace SE, Amemiya A, Bean LJH, Bird TD, Fong CT, Mefford HC, Smith RJH, Stephens K, editors. GeneReviews® [Internet]. Seattle, WA: University of Washington, Seattle; 1993–2016. 2005 Apr 18 [Updated 2014 Jan 9]. Available from: http://www.ncbi.nlm.nih.gov/books/NBK1131/ [Accessed: 2016-07-20]

[64] Sen-Chowdhry S, Syrris P, McKenna WJ. Role of genetic analysis in the management of patients with arrhythmogenic right ventricular dysplasia/cardiomyopathy. J Am Coll Cardiol. 2007 Nov 6;50(19):1813–1821.DOI:10.1016/j.jacc.2007.08.008.

[65] Tiso N, Stephan DA, Nava A, Bagattin A, Devaney JM, Stanchi F, Larderet G, Brahmbhatt B, Brown K, Bauce B, Muriago M, Basso C, Thiene G, Danieli GA, Rampazzo A. Identification of mutations in the cardiac ryanodine receptor gene in families affected with arrhythmogenic right ventricular cardiomyopathy type 2 (ARVD2). Hum Mol Genet. 2001 Feb 1;10(3):189–194. DOI:10.1093/hmg/10.3.189.

[66] Bauce B, Rampazzo A, Basso C, Bagattin A, Daliento L, Tiso N, Turrini P, Thiene G, Danieli GA, Nava A. Screening for ryanodine receptor type 2 mutations in families with effort-induced polymorphic ventricular arrhythmias and sudden death: early diagnosis of asymptomatic carriers. J Am Coll Cardiol. 2002 Jul 17;40(2):341–349. DOI:10.1016/S0735-1097(02)01946-0.

[67] Priori SG, Napolitano C, Tiso N, Memmi M, Vignati G, Bloise R, Sorrentino V, Danieli GA. Mutations in the cardiac ryanodine receptor gene (hRyR2) underlie catecholaminergic polymorphic ventricular tachycardia. Circulation. 2001 Jan 16;103(2):196–200. DOI:10.1161/01.CIR.103.2.196.

[68] Priori SG, Napolitano C, Memmi M, Colombi B, Drago F, Gasparini M, DeSimone L, Coltorti F, Bloise R, Keegan R, Cruz Filho FE, Vignati G, Benatar A, DeLogu A. Clinical and molecular characterization of patients with catecholaminergic polymorphic ventricular tachycardia. Circulation. 2002 Jul 2;106(1):69–74. DOI:10.1161/01.CIR.0000020013.73106.D8.

[69] Laitinen PJ, Brown KM, Piippo K, Swan H, Devaney JM, Brahmbhatt B, Donarum EA, Marino M, Tiso N, Viitasalo M, Toivonen L, Stephan DA, Kontula K. Mutations of the cardiac ryanodine receptor (RyR2) gene in familial polymorphic ventricular tachycardia. Circulation. 2001 Jan 30;103(4):485–490. DOI:10.1161/01.CIR.103.4.485.

[70] Laitinen PJ, Swan H, Kontula K. Molecular genetics of exercise-induced polymorphic ventricular tachycardia: identification of three novel cardiac ryanodine receptor

mutations and two common calsequestrin 2 amino-acid polymorphisms. Eur J Hum Genet. 2003 Nov;11(11):888–891. DOI:10.1038/sj.ejhg.5201061.

[71] Leask A, Abraham DJ. TGF-beta signaling and the fibrotic response. FASEB J. 2004 May; 18(7):816–827. DOI:10.1096/fj.03-1273rev.

[72] Beffagna G, Occhi G, Nava A, Vitiello L, Ditadi A, Basso C, Bauce B, Carraro G, Thiene G, Towbin JA, Danieli GA, Rampazzo A. Regulatory mutations in transforming growth factor-beta3 gene cause arrhythmogenic right ventricular cardiomyopathy type 1. Cardiovasc Res. 2005 Feb 1;65(2):366–373. DOI:10.1016/j.cardiores.2004.10.005.

[73] Rampazzo A. Genetic bases of arrhythmogenic right ventricular cardiomyopathy. Heart Int. 2006;2(1):17. DOI:10.4081/hi.2006.17.

[74] Wiemann S, Weil B, Wellenreuther R, Gassenhuber J, Glassl S, Ansorge W, Böcher M, Blöcker H, Bauersachs S, Blum H, Lauber J, Düsterhöft A, Beyer A, Köhrer K, Strack N, Mewes HW, Ottenwälder B, Obermaier B, Tampe J, Heubner D, Wambutt R, Korn B, Klein M, Poustka A. Toward a catalog of human genes and proteins: sequencing and analysis of 500 novel complete protein coding human cDNAs. Genome Res. 2001 Mar; 11(3):422–435. DOI:10.1101/gr.154701.

[75] Merner ND, Hodgkinson KA, Haywood AF, Connors S, French VM, Drenckhahn JD, Kupprion C, Ramadanova K, Thierfelder L, McKenna W, Gallagher B, Morris-Larkin L, Bassett AS, Parfrey PS, Young TL. Arrhythmogenic right ventricular cardiomyopathy type 5 is a fully penetrant, lethal arrhythmic disorder caused by a missense mutation in the TMEM43 gene. Am J Hum Genet. 2008 Apr;82(4):809–821. DOI:10.1016/j.ajhg. 2008.01.010.

[76] Christensen AH, Andersen CB, Tybjaerg-Hansen A, Haunso S, Svendsen JH. Mutation analysis and evaluation of the cardiac localization of TMEM43 in arrhythmogenic right ventricular cardiomyopathy. Clin Genet. 2011 Sep;80(3):256–264. DOI:10.1111/j.1399-0004.2011.01623.x.

[77] Haywood AF, Merner ND, Hodgkinson KA, Houston J, Syrris P, Booth V, Connors S, Pantazis A, Quarta G, Elliott P, McKenna W, Young TL. Recurrent missense mutations in TMEM43 (ARVD5) due to founder effects cause arrhythmogenic cardiomyopathies in the UK and Canada. Eur Heart J. 2013 Apr;34(13):1002–1011. DOI:10.1093/eurheartj/ehs383.

[78] Baskin B, Skinner JR, Sanatani S, Terespolsky D, Krahn AD, Ray PN, Scherer SW, Hamilton RM. TMEM43 mutations associated with arrhythmogenic right ventricular cardiomyopathy in non-Newfoundland populations. Hum Genet. 2013 Nov;132(11): 1245–1252. DOI:10.1007/s00439-013-1323-2.

[79] Pilichou K, Thiene G, Bauce B, Rigato I, Lazzarini E, Migliore F, Perazzolo Marra M, Rizzo S, Zorzi A, Daliento L, Corrado D, Basso C. Arrhythmogenic cardiomyopathy. Orphanet J Rare Dis. 2016;11:33. DOI:10.1186/s13023-016-0407-1.

[80] Mallat Z, Tedgui A, Fontaliran F, Frank R, Durigon M, Fontaine G. Evidence of apoptosis in arrhythmogenic right ventricular dysplasia. N Engl J Med. 1996 Oct 17;335(16):1190–1196. DOI:10.1056/NEJM199610173351604.

[81] Fontaine G, Fontaliran F, Lascault G, Frank R, Tonet J, Chomette G, Grosgogeat Y. Congenital and acquired right ventricular dysplasia [Article in French]. Arch Mal Coeur Vaiss. 1990 Jun;83(7):915–920.

[82] Chimenti C, Pieroni M, Maseri A, Frustaci A. Histologic findings in patients with clinical and instrumental diagnosis of sporadic arrhythmogenic right ventricular dysplasia. J Am Coll Cardiol. 2004 Jun 16;43(12):2305–2313. DOI:10.1016/j.jacc. 2003.12.056.

[83] d'Amati G, di Gioia CR, Giordano C, Gallo P. Myocyte transdifferentiation: a possible pathogenetic mechanism for arrhythmogenic right ventricular cardiomyopathy. Arch Pathol Lab Med. 2000 Feb;124(2):287–290. DOI:10.1043/0003-9985(2000)124<0287:MT> 2.0.CO;2.

[84] Huber O. Structure and function of desmosomal proteins and their role in development and disease. Cell Mol Life Sci. 2003 Sep;60(9):1872–1890. DOI:10.1007/s00018-003-3050-7.

[85] Garrod D, Chidgey M. Desmosome structure, composition and function. Biochim Biophys Acta. 2008 Mar;1778(3):572–587. DOI:10.1016/j.bbamem.2007.07.014.

[86] Green KJ, Gaudry CA. Are desmosomes more than tethers for intermediate filaments? Nat Rev Mol Cell Biol. 2000 Dec;1(3):208-16. DOI:10.1038/35043032.

[87] Guiraudon CM. Histological diagnosis of right ventricular dysplasia: a role for electron microscopy? Eur Heart J. 1989 Sep;10(Suppl D):95–96. DOI:10.1093/eurheartj/ 10.suppl_D.95.

[88] Basso C, Czarnowska E, Della Barbera M, Bauce B, Beffagna G, Wlodarska EK, Pilichou K, Ramondo A, Lorenzon A, Wozniek O, Corrado D, Daliento L, Danieli GA, Valente M, Nava A, Thiene G, Rampazzo A. Ultrastructural evidence of intercalated disc remodelling in arrhythmogenic right ventricular cardiomyopathy: an electron microscopy investigation on endomyocardial biopsies. Eur Heart J. 2006 Aug;27(15):1847–1854. DOI:10.1093/eurheartj/ehl095.

[89] Sato PY, Coombs W, Lin X, Nekrasova O, Green KJ, Isom LL, Taffet SM, Delmar M. Interactions between ankyrin-G, Plakophilin-2, and Connexin43 at the cardiac intercalated disc. Circ Res. 2011 Jul 8;109(2):193–201. DOI:10.1161/CIRCRESAHA.111.247023.

[90] Hariharan V, Asimaki A, Michaelson JE, Plovie E, MacRae CA, Saffitz JE, Huang H. Arrhythmogenic right ventricular cardiomyopathy mutations alter shear response without changes in cell-cell adhesion. Cardiovasc Res. 2014 Nov 1;104(2):280–289. DOI: 10.1093/cvr/cvu212.

[91] Asimaki A, Tandri H, Huang H, Halushka MK, Gautam S, Basso C, Thiene G, Tsatsopoulou A, Protonotarios N, McKenna WJ, Calkins H, Saffitz JE. A new diagnostic test

for arrhythmogenic right ventricular cardiomyopathy. N Engl J Med. 2009 Mar 12;360(11):1075–1084. DOI:10.1056/NEJMoa0808138.

[92] Garcia-Gras E, Lombardi R, Giocondo MJ, Willerson JT, Schneider MD, Khoury DS, Marian AJ. Suppression of canonical Wnt/beta-catenin signaling by nuclear plakoglobin recapitulates phenotype of arrhythmogenic right ventricular cardiomyopathy. J Clin Invest. 2006 Jul;116(7):2012–2021. DOI:10.1172/JCI27751.

[93] Swope D, Li J, Muller EJ, Radice GL. Analysis of a Jup hypomorphic allele reveals a critical threshold for postnatal viability. Genesis. 2012 Oct;50(10):717–727. DOI:10.1002/dvg.22034.

[94] Simcha I, Shtutman M, Salomon D, Zhurinsky J, Sadot E, Geiger B, Ben-Ze'ev A. Differential nuclear translocation and transactivation potential of beta-catenin and plakoglobin. J Cell Biol. 1998 Jun 15;141(6):1433–1448. DOI:10.1083/jcb.141.6.1433.

[95] Ross SE, Hemati N, Longo KA, Bennett CN, Lucas PC, Erickson RL, MacDougald OA. Inhibition of adipogenesis by Wnt signaling. Science. 2000 Aug 11;289(5481):950–953. DOI:10.1126/science.289.5481.950.

[96] Chen SN, Gurha P, Lombardi R, Ruggiero A, Willerson JT, Marian AJ. The hippo pathway is activated and is a causal mechanism for adipogenesis in arrhythmogenic cardiomyopathy. Circ Res. 2014 Jan 31;114(3):454–468. DOI:10.1161/CIRCRESAHA.114.302810.

[97] Basso C, Bauce B, Corrado D, Thiene G. Pathophysiology of arrhythmogenic cardiomyopathy. Nat Rev Cardiol. 2011 Nov 29;9(4):223–233. DOI:10.1038/nrcardio.2011.173.

[98] Kaplan SR, Gard JJ, Protonotarios N, Tsatsopoulou A, Spiliopoulou C, Anastasakis A, Squarcioni CP, McKenna WJ, Thiene G, Basso C, Brousse N, Fontaine G, Saffitz JE. Remodeling of myocyte gap junctions in arrhythmogenic right ventricular cardiomyopathy due to a deletion in plakoglobin (Naxos disease). Heart Rhythm. 2004 May;1(1):3–11. DOI:10.1016/j.hrthm.2004.01.001.

[99] Fidler LM, Wilson GJ, Liu F, Cui X, Scherer SW, Taylor GP, Hamilton RM. Abnormal connexin43 in arrhythmogenic right ventricular cardiomyopathy caused by plakophilin-2 mutations. J Cell Mol Med. 2009 Oct;13(10):4219–4228. DOI:10.1111/j.1582-4934.2008.00438.x.

[100] Rizzo S, Lodder EM, Verkerk AO, Wolswinkel R, Beekman L, Pilichou K, Basso C, Remme CA, Thiene G, Bezzina CR. Intercalated disc abnormalities, reduced Na(+) current density, and conduction slowing in desmoglein-2 mutant mice prior to cardiomyopathic changes. Cardiovasc Res. 2012 Sep 1;95(4):409–418. DOI:10.1093/cvr/cvs219.

[101] Cerrone M, Noorman M, Lin X, Chkourko H, Liang FX, van der Nagel R, Hund T, Birchmeier W, Mohler P, van Veen TA, van Rijen HV, Delmar M. Sodium current deficit

and arrhythmogenesis in a murine model of plakophilin-2 haploinsufficiency. Cardiovasc Res. 2012 Sep 1;95(4):460–468. DOI:10.1093/cvr/cvs218.

[102] Zhang Q, Deng C, Rao F, Modi RM, Zhu J, Liu X, Mai L, Tan H, Yu X, Lin Q, Xiao D, Kuang S, Wu S. Silencing of desmoplakin decreases connexin43/Nav1.5 expression and sodium current in HL-1 cardiomyocytes. Mol Med Rep. 2013 Sep;8(3):780–786. DOI: 10.3892/mmr.2013.1594.

[103] Noorman M, Hakim S, Kessler E, Groeneweg JA, Cox MG, Asimaki A, van Rijen HV, van Stuijvenberg L, Chkourko H, van der Heyden MA, Vos MA, de Jonge N, van der Smagt JJ, Dooijes D, Vink A, de Weger RA, Varro A, de Bakker JM, Saffitz JE, Hund TJ, Mohler PJ, Delmar M, Hauer RN, van Veen TA. Remodeling of the cardiac sodium channel, connexin43, and plakoglobin at the intercalated disk in patients with arrhythmogenic cardiomyopathy. Heart Rhythm. 2013 Mar;10(3):412–419. DOI:10.1016/j.hrthm.2012.11.018.

[104] Asimaki A, Kapoor S, Plovie E, Karin Arndt A, Adams E, Liu Z, James CA, Judge DP, Calkins H, Churko J, Wu JC, MacRae CA, Kléber AG, Saffitz JE. Identification of a new modulator of the intercalated disc in a zebrafish model of arrhythmogenic cardiomyopathy. Sci Transl Med. 2014 Jun 11;6(240):240ra74. DOI:10.1126/scitranslmed.3008008.

[105] Protonotarios N, Tsatsopoulou A. Arrhythmogenic right ventricular cardiomyopathy: clinical forms of the disease. Hellenic J Cardiol. 1998;39(Suppl A):78–80.

[106] Protonotarios N, Tsatsopoulou A. Naxos disease and Carvajal syndrome: cardiocutaneous disorders that highlight the pathogenesis and broaden the spectrum of arrhythmogenic right ventricular cardiomyopathy. Cardiovasc Pathol. 2004 Jul-Aug;13(4):185-94. DOI:10.1016/j.carpath.2004.03.609

[107] Bukhari I, Juma'a N. Naxos disease in Saudi Arabia. J Eur Acad Dermatol Venereol. 2004 Sep;18(5):614-6. DOI:10.1111/j.1468-3083.2004.01010.x.

[108] Protonotarios N, Tsatsopoulou A. Naxos disease: cardiocutaneous syndrome due to cell adhesion defect. Orphanet J Rare Dis. 2006 Mar 13;1:4. DOI:10.1186/1750-1172-1-4

[109] Coonar AS, Protonotarios N, Tsatsopoulou A, Needham EW, Houlston RS, Cliff S, Otter MI, Murday VA, Mattu RK, McKenna WJ. Gene for arrhythmogenic right ventricular cardiomyopathy with diffuse nonepidermolytic palmoplantar keratoderma and woolly hair (Naxos disease) maps to 17q21. Circulation. 1998 May 26;97(20):2049-58.

[110] Protonotarios N, Tsatsopoulou A, Anastasakis A, Sevdalis E, McKoy G, Stratos K, Gatzoulis K, Tentolouris K, Spiliopoulou C, Panagiotakos D, McKenna W, Toutouzas P. Genotype-phenotype assessment in autosomal recessive arrhythmogenic right ventricular cardiomyopathy (Naxos disease) caused by a deletion in plakoglobin. J Am Coll Cardiol. 2001 Nov 1;38(5):1477-84. DOI:10.1016/S0735-1097(01)01568-6

[111] Rao BH, Reddy IS, Chandra KS. Familial occurrence of a rare combination of dilated cardiomyopathy with palmoplantar keratoderma and curly hair. Indian Heart J. 1996 Mar-Apr;48(2):161-2.

[112] Kaplan SR, Gard JJ, Carvajal-Huerta L, Ruiz-Cabezas JC, Thiene G, Saffitz JE. Structural and molecular pathology of the heart in Carvajal syndrome. Cardiovasc Pathol. 2004 Jan-Feb;13(1):26-32. DOI:10.1016/S1054-8807(03)00107-8.

[113] De Pasquale CG, Heddle WF. Left sided arrhythmogenic ventricular dysplasia in siblings. Heart 2001;86:128-130 DOI:10.1136/heart.86.2.128

[114] Collett BA, Davis GJ, Rohr WB. Extensive fibrofatty infiltration of the left ventricle in two cases of sudden cardiac death. J Forensic Sci. 1994 Sep;39(5):1182-7. DOI:10.1520/JFS13703J.

[115] Michalodimitrakis M, Papadomanolakis A, Stiakakis J, Kanaki K. Left side right ventricular cardiomyopathy. Med Sci Law. 2002 Oct;42(4):313-7. DOI:10.1177/002580240204200406

[116] Gallo P, d'Amati G, Pelliccia F. Pathologic evidence of extensive left ventricular involvement in arrhythmogenic right ventricular cardiomyopathy. Hum Pathol. 1992 Aug;23(8):948-52.

[117] Sen-Chowdhry S, Syrris P, Prasad SK, Hughes SE, Merrifield R, Ward D, Pennell DJ, McKenna WJ. Left-dominant arrhythmogenic cardiomyopathy: an under-recognized clinical entity. J Am Coll Cardiol. 2008 Dec 16;52(25):2175-87. DOI:10.1016/j.jacc.2008.09.019.

[118] McKenna WJ, Thiene G, Nava A, Fontaliran F, Blomstrom-Lundqvist C, Fontaine G, and Camerini F. Diagnosis of arrhythmogenic right ventricular dysplasia/cardiomyopathy. Task Force of the Working Group Myocardial and Pericardial Disease of the European Society of Cardiology and of the Scientific Council on Cardiomyopathies of the International Society and Federation of Cardiology. Br Heart J. 1994 Mar;71(3):215–218.

[119] Marcus FI, McKenna WJ, Sherrill D, Basso C, Bauce B, Bluemke DA, Calkins H, Corrado D, Cox MG, Daubert JP, Fontaine G, Gear K, Hauer R, Nava A, Picard MH, Protonotarios N, Saffitz JE, Sanborn DM, Steinberg JS, Tandri H, Thiene G, Towbin JA, Tsatsopoulou A, Wichter T, Zareba W. Diagnosis of arrhythmogenic right ventricular cardiomyopathy/dysplasia: proposed modification of the task force criteria. Circulation. 2010;121(13):1533-41. DOI:10.1161/CIRCULATIONAHA.108.840827. Eur Heart J. 2010 Apr;31(7):806-14. DOI:10.1093/eurheartj/ehq025.

[120] White JB, Razmi R, Nath H, Kay GN, Plumb VJ, Epstein AE. Relative utility of magnetic resonance imaging and right ventricular angiography to diagnose arrhythmogenic right ventricular cardiomyopathy. J Interv Card Electrophysiol. 2004 Feb;10(1):19-26. DOI:10.1023/B:JICE.0000011480.66948.c3

[121] Lindstrom L, Wilkenshoff U, Larsson H, Wranne B. Echocardiographic assessment of arrhythmogenic right ventricular cardiomyopathy. Heart 2001;86:31-38 DOI:10.1136/heart.86.1.31

[122] Marcus FI, Fontaine G. Arrhythmogenic right ventricular dysplasia/cardiomyopathy: a review. Pacing Clin Electrophysiol. 1995 Jun;18(6):1298-314. DOI:10.1111/j.1540-8159.1995.tb06971.x.

[123] Yoerger DM, Marcus F, Sherrill D, Calkins H, Towbin JA, Zareba W, Picard MH. Multidisciplinary Study of Right Ventricular Dysplasia Investigators. Echocardiographic findings in patients meeting task force criteria for arrhythmogenic right ventricular dysplasia: new insights from the multidisciplinary study of right ventricular dysplasia. J Am Coll Cardiol. 2005 Mar 15;45(6):860-5. DOI:10.1016/j.jacc.2004.10.070

[124] Mast TP, Teske AJ, Doevendans PA, Cramer MJ. Current and future role of echocardiography in arrhythmogenic right ventricular dysplasia/cardiomyopathy. Cardiol J. 2015;22(4):362-74. DOI:10.5603/CJ.a2015.0018.

[125] Tandri H, Calkins H, Nasir K, Bomma C, Castillo E, Rutberg J, Tichnell C, Lima JA, Bluemke DA. Magnetic resonance imaging findings in patients meeting task force criteria for arrhythmogenic right ventricular dysplasia. J Cardiovasc Electrophysiol. 2003 May;14(5):476-82. DOI:10.1046/j.1540-8167.2003.02560.x.

[126] American College of Cardiology Foundation Task Force on Expert Consensus Documents, Hundley WG, Bluemke DA, Finn JP, Flamm SD, Fogel MA, Friedrich MG, Ho VB, Jerosch-Herold M, Kramer CM, Manning WJ, Patel M, Pohost GM, Stillman AE, White RD, Woodard PK. ACCF/ACR/AHA/NASCI/SCMR 2010 Expert Consensus Document on Cardiovascular Magnetic Resonance: A Report of the American College of Cardiology Foundation Task Force on Expert Consensus Documents. J Am Coll Cardiol. 2010 Jun 8;55(23):2614-62. DOI:10.1016/j.jacc.2009.11.011.

[127] Tandri H, Friedrich MG, Calkins H, Bluemke DA. MRI of arrhythmogenic right ventricular cardiomyopathy/dysplasia. J Cardiovasc Magn Reson. 2004;6(2):557-63. DOI:10.1081/JCMR-120030583

[128] Van der Wall EE, Kayser HW, Bootsma MM, de Roos A, Schalij MJ. Arrhythmogenic right ventricular dysplasia: MRI findings. Herz. 2000 Jun;25(4):356-64.

[129] Jain A, Tandri H, Calkins H, Bluemke DA. Role of cardiovascular magnetic resonance imaging in arrhythmogenic right ventricular dysplasia. J Cardiovasc Magn Reson. 2008;10(1):32. DOI:10.1186/1532-429X-10-32

[130] Tandri H, Castillo E, Ferrari VA, Nasir K, Dalal D, Bomma C, Calkins H, Bluemke DA. Magnetic resonance imaging of arrhythmogenic right ventricular dysplasia: sensitivity, specificity, and observer variability of fat detection versus functional analysis of the

right ventricle. J Am Coll Cardiol. 2006 Dec 5;48(11):2277-84. DOI:10.1016/j.jacc.2006.07.051

[131] Corrado D, Basso C, Thiene G. Arrhythmogenic right ventricular cardiomyopathy: diagnosis, prognosis, and treatment. Heart. 2000 May;83(5):588–595. DOI: 10.1136/heart.83.5.588

[132] Basso C, Ronco F, Marcus F, Abudureheman A, Rizzo S, Frigo AC, Bauce B, Maddalena F, Nava A, Corrado D, Grigoletto F, Thiene G. Quantitative assessment of endomyocardial biopsy in arrhythmogenic right ventricular cardiomyopathy/dysplasia: an in vitro validation of diagnostic criteria. Eur Heart J. 2008 Nov;29(22):2760-71. DOI: 10.1093/eurheartj/ehn415.

[133] Fontaine G, Umemura J, Di Donna P, Tsezana R, Cannat JJ, Frank R. Duration of QRS complexes in arrhythmogenic right ventricular dysplasia. A new noninvasive diagnostic marker [Article in French]. Ann Cardiol Angeiol (Paris). 1993 Oct;42(8):399-405.

[134] Peters S, Trümmel M. Diagnosis of arrhythmogenic right ventricular dysplasia-cardiomyopathy: value of standard ECG revisited. Ann Noninvasive Electrocardiol. 2003 Jul;8(3):238-45. DOI:10.1046/j.1542-474X.2003.08312.x.

[135] Pinamonti B, Sinagra G, Salvi A, Di Lenarda A, Morgera T, Silvestri F, Bussani R, Camerini F. Left ventricular involvement in right ventricular dysplasia. Am Heart J. 1992 Mar;123(3):711-24. DOI:10.1016/0002-8703(92)90511-S.

[136] Cox MG, Nelen MR, Wilde AA, Wiesfeld AC, van der Smagt JJ, Loh P, Cramer MJ, Doevendans PA, van Tintelen JP, de Bakker JM, Hauer RN. Activation delay and VT parameters in arrhythmogenic right ventricular dysplasia/cardiomyopathy: toward improvement of diagnostic ECG criteria. J Cardiovasc Electrophysiol. 2008 Aug;19(8): 775-81. DOI:10.1111/j.1540-8167.2008.01140.x.

[137] Nasir K, Rutberg J, Tandri H, Berger R, Tomaselli G, Calkins H. Utility of SAECG in arrhythmogenic right ventricle dysplasia. Ann Noninvasive Electrocardiol. 2003 Apr; 8(2):112-20. DOI:10.1046/j.1542-474X.2003.08204.x.

[138] Oselladore L, Nava A, Buja G, Turini P, Daliento L, Livolsi B, Thiene G. Signal-averaged electrocardiography in familial form of arrhythmogenic right ventricular cardiomyopathy. Am J Cardiol. 1995 May 15;75(15):1038-41. DOI:10.1016/S0002-9149(99)80720-6

[139] Turrini P, Angelini A, Thiene G, Buja G, Daliento L, Rizzoli G, Nava A. Late potentials and ventricular arrhythmias in arrhythmogenic right ventricular cardiomyopathy. Am J Cardiol. 1999 Apr 15;83(8):1214-9. DOI:10.1016/S0002-9149(99)00062-4

[140] Nava A, Bauce B, Basso C, Muriago M, Rampazzo A, Villanova C, Daliento L, Buja G, Corrado D, Danieli GA, Thiene G. Clinical profile and long-term follow-up of 37 families with arrhythmogenic right ventricular cardiomyopathy. J Am Coll Cardiol. 2000 Dec;36(7):2226-33. DOI:10.1016/S0735-1097(00)00997-9

[141] Zareba W, Piotrowicz K, Turrini P. Electrocardiographic manifestations. In: Marcus FI, Nava A, Thiene G, editors. Arrhythmogenic Right Ventricular Dysplasia/Cardiomyopathy, Recent Advances. Milano: Springer Verlag; 2007. p. 121-8.

[142] Lerman BB, Stein KM, Markowitz SM. Idiopathic right ventricular outflow tract tachycardia: a clinical approach. Pacing Clin Electrophysiol. 1996 Dec;19(12 Pt 1):2120-37. DOI:10.1111/j.1540-8159.1996.tb03287.x.

[143] Markowitz SM, Litvak BL, Ramirez de Arellano EA, Markisz JA, Stein KM, Lerman BB. Adenosine-sensitive ventricular tachycardia, right ventricular abnormalities delineated by magnetic resonance imaging. Circulation. 1997 Aug 19;96(4):1192-200. DOI: 10.1161/01.CIR.96.4.1192

[144] Chapelon C, Piette JC, Uzzan B, Coche E, Herson S, Ziza JM, Godeau P. The advantages of histological samples in sarcoidosis. Retrospective multicenter analysis of 618 biopsies performed on 416 patients. Rev Med Interne. 1987 Mar-Apr;8(2):181-5.

[145] Ladyjanskaia GA, Basso C, Hobbelink MG, Kirkels JH, Lahpor JR, Cramer MJ, Thiene G, Hauer RN, Oosterhout MF V. Sarcoid myocarditis with ventricular tachycardia mimicking ARVD/C. J Cardiovasc Electrophysiol. 2010 Jan;21(1):94-8. DOI:10.1111/j.1540-8167.2009.01479.x.

[146] Gerlis LM, Schmidt-Ott SC, Ho SY, Anderson RH. Dysplastic conditions of the right ventricular myocardium: Uhl's anomaly vs. arrhythmogenic right ventricular dysplasia. Br Heart J. 1993 Feb;69(2):142–150.

[147] Corrado D, Wichter T, Link MS, Hauer RN, Marchlinski FE, Anastasakis A, Bauce B, Basso C, Brunckhorst C, Tsatsopoulou A, Tandri H, Paul M, Schmied C, Pelliccia A, Duru F, Protonotarios N, Estes NM 3rd, McKenna WJ, Thiene G, Marcus FI, Calkins H. Treatment of arrhythmogenic right ventricular cardiomyopathy/dysplasia. Circulation. 2015 Aug 4;132(5):441-53. DOI:10.1161/CIRCULATIONAHA.115.017944.

[148] Dalal D, Jain R, Tandri H, Dong J, Eid SM, Prakasa K, Tichnell C, James C, Abraham T, Russell SD, Sinha S, Judge DP, Bluemke DA, Marine JE, Calkins H. Long-term efficacy of catheter ablation of ventricular tachycardia in patients with arrhythmogenic right ventricular dysplasia/cardiomyopathy. J Am Coll Cardiol. 2007 Jul 31;50(5):432-40. DOI: 10.1016/j.jacc.2007.03.049

[149] Satomi K, Kurita T, Suyama K, Noda T, Okamura H, Otomo K, Shimizu W, Aihara N, Kamakura S. Catheter ablation of stable and unstable ventricular tachycardias in patients with arrhythmogenic right ventricular dysplasia. J Cardiovasc Electrophysiol. 2006 May;17(5):469-76. DOI:10.1111/j.1540-8167.2006.00434.x.

[150] Verma A, Kilicaslan F, Schweikert RA, Tomassoni G, Rossillo A, Marrouche NF, Ozduran V, Wazni OM, Elayi SC, Saenz LC, Minor S, Cummings JE, Burkhardt JD, Hao S, Beheiry S, Tchou PJ, Natale A. Short- and long-term success of substrate-based mapping and ablation of ventricular tachycardia in arrhythmogenic right ventricular

dysplasia. Circulation. 2005 Jun 21;111(24):3209-16. DOI:10.1161/CIRCULATIONAHA.104.510503

[151] Reithmann C, Hahnefeld A, Remp T, Dorwarth U, Dugas M, Steinbeck G, Hoffmann E. Electroanatomic mapping of endocardial right ventricular activation as a guide for catheter ablation in patients with arrhythmogenic right ventricular dysplasia. Pacing Clin Electrophysiol. 2003 Jun;26(6):1308-16. DOI:10.1046/j.1460-9592.2003.t01-1-00188.x.

[152] Ellison KE, Friedman PL, Ganz LI, Stevenson WG. Entrainment mapping and radiofrequency catheter ablation of ventricular tachycardia in right ventricular dysplasia. J Am Coll Cardiol. 1998 Sep;32(3):724-8. DOI:10.1016/S0735-1097(98)00292-7

[153] Corrado D, Basso C, Pavei A, Michieli P, Schiavon M, Thiene G. Trends in sudden cardiovascular death in young competitive athletes after implementation of a preparticipation screening program. JAMA. 2006 Oct 4;296(13):1593-601. DOI:10.1001/jama.296.13.1593

[154] Corrado D, Thiene G, Nava A, Rossi L, Pennelli N. Sudden death in young competitive athletes: clinicopathologic correlations in 22 cases. Am J Med. 1990 Nov;89(5):588-96. DOI:10.1016/0002-9343(90)90176-E.

[155] Corrado D, Basso C, Rizzoli G, Schiavon M, Thiene G. Does sports activity enhance the risk of sudden death in adolescents and young adults? J Am Coll Cardiol. 2003 Dec 3;42(11):1959-63. DOI:10.1016/j.jacc.2003.03.002

[156] James CA, Bhonsale A, Tichnell C, Murray B, Russell SD, Tandri H, Tedford RJ, Judge DP, Calkins H. Exercise increases age-related penetrance and arrhythmic risk in arrhythmogenic right ventricular dysplasia/cardiomyopathy-associated desmosomal mutation carriers. J Am Coll Cardiol. 2013 Oct 1;62(14):1290-7. DOI:10.1016/j.jacc.2013.06.033.

[157] Saberniak J, Hasselberg NE, Borgquist R, Platonov PG, Sarvari SI, Smith HJ, Ribe M, Holst AG, Edvardsen T, Haugaa KH. Vigorous physical activity impairs myocardial function in patients with arrhythmogenic right ventricular cardiomyopathy and in mutation positive family members. Eur J Heart Fail. 2014 Dec;16(12):1337-44. DOI:10.1002/ejhf.181.

[158] Wichter T, Hindricks G, Lerch H, Bartenstein P, Borggrefe M, Schober O, Breithardt G. Regional myocardial sympathetic dysinnervation in arrhythmogenic right ventricular cardiomyopathy. An analysis using $^{123}$I-metaiodobenzylguanidine scintigraphy. Circulation. 1994 Feb;89(2):667–683. DOI:10.1161/01.CIR.89.2.667

[159] Wichter T, Schäfers M, Rhodes CG, Borggrefe M, Lerch H, Lammertsma AA, Hermansen F, Schober O, Breithardt G, Camici PG. Abnormalities of cardiac sympathetic innervation in arrhythmogenic right ventricular cardiomyopathy: quantitative assessment of presynaptic norepinephrine reuptake and postsynaptic beta-adrenergic

receptor density with positron emission tomography. Circulation. 2000 Apr 4;101(13): 1552-8. DOI:10.1161/01.CIR.101.13.1552

[160] Wlodarska EK, Wozniak O, Konka M, Rydlewska-Sadowska W, Biederman A, Hoffman P. Thromboembolic complications in patients with arrhythmogenic right ventricular dysplasia/cardiomyopathy. Europace. 2006 Aug;8(8):596-600. DOI:10.1093/europace/eul053

[161] Ermakov S, Scheinman M. Arrhythmogenic right ventricular cardiomyopathy – antiarrhythmic therapy. Arrhythm Electrophysiol Rev. 2015 Aug;4(2):86-9. DOI: 10.15420/aer.2015.04.02.86.

[162] Nogami A, Sugiyasu A, Tada H, Kurosaki K, Sakamaki M, Kowase S, Oginosawa Y, Kubota S, Usui T, Naito S. Changes in the isolated delayed component as an endpoint of catheter ablation in arrhythmogenic right ventricular cardiomyopathy: predictor for long-term success. J Cardiovasc Electrophysiol. 2008 Jul;19(7):681-8. DOI:10.1111/j. 1540-8167.2008.01104.x.

[163] Breithardt G, Wichter T, Haverkamp W, Borggrefe M, Block M, Hammel D, Scheld HH. Implantable cardioverter defibrillator therapy in patients with arrhythmogenic right ventricular cardiomyopathy, long QT syndrome, or no structural heart disease. Am Heart J. 1994 Apr;127(4 Pt 2):1151-8.DOI:10.1016/0002-8703(94)90103-1

[164] Wichter T, Borggrefe M, Haverkamp W, Chen X, Breithardt G. Efficacy of antiarrhythmic drugs in patients with arrhythmogenic right ventricular disease. Results in patients with inducible and noninducible ventricular tachycardia. Circulation. 1992 Jul;86(1): 29-37. DOI:10.1161/01.CIR.86.1.29

[165] Wichter T, Borggrefe M, Bocker D. Prevention of sudden cardiac death in arrhythmogenic right ventricular cardiomyopathy. In: Aliot E, Clementy J, Prystowsky EN, editors. Fighting Sudden Cardiac Death: A Worldwide Challenge. New York: Futura Publishing Company. 2000. p. 275–95.

[166] Marcus GM, Glidden DV, Polonsky B, Zareba W, Smith LM, Cannom DS, Estes NA 3rd, Marcus F, Scheinman MM; Multidisciplinary Study of Right Ventricular Dysplasia Investigators. Efficacy of antiarrhythmic drugs in arrhythmogenic right ventricular cardiomyopathy: a report from the North American ARVC Registry. J Am Coll Cardiol. 2009 Aug 11;54(7):609-15. DOI:10.1016/j.jacc.2009.04.052.

[167] Ermakov S, Hoffmayer KS, Gerstenfeld EP, Scheinman MM. Combination drug therapy for patients with intractable ventricular tachycardia associated with right ventricular cardiomyopathy. Pacing Clin Electrophysiol. 2014 Jan;37(1):90-4. DOI:10.1111/pace. 12250.

[168] Leclercq JF, Coumel P. Characteristics, prognosis and treatment of the ventricular arrhythmias of right ventricular dysplasia. Eur Heart J. 1989 Sep;10 Suppl D:61-7. DOI: 10.1093/eurheartj/10.suppl_D.61

[169] Tonet J, Frank R, Fontaine G, Grosgogeat Y. Efficacy of the combination of low doses of beta-blockers and amiodarone in the treatment of refractory ventricular tachycardia [Article in French]. Arch Mal Coeur Vaiss. 1989 Sep;82(9):1511–1517.

[170] Bai R, Di Biase L, Shivkumar K, Mohanty P, Tung R, Santangeli P, Saenz LC, Vacca M, Verma A, Khaykin Y, Mohanty S, Burkhardt JD, Hongo R, Beheiry S, Dello Russo A, Casella M, Pelargonio G, Santarelli P, Sanchez J, Tondo C, Natale A. Ablation of ventricular arrhythmias in arrhythmogenic right ventricular dysplasia/cardiomyopathy: arrhythmia-free survival after endoepicardial substrate based mapping and ablation. Circ Arrhythm Electrophysiol 2011 Aug;4(4):478–485. DOI:10.1161/CIRCEP.111.963066.

[171] Garcia FC, Bazan V, Zado ES, Ren JF, Marchlinski FE. Epicardial substrate and outcome with epicardial ablation of ventricular tachycardia in arrhythmogenic right ventricular cardiomyopathy/dysplasia. Circulation. 2009 Aug 4;120(5):366–375. DOI:10.1161/CIRCULATIONAHA.108.834903.

[172] Sacher F, Roberts-Thomson K, Maury P, Tedrow U, Nault I, Steven D, Hocini M, Koplan B, Leroux L, Derval N, Seiler J, Wright MJ, Epstein L, Haissaguerre M, Jais P, Stevenson WG. Epicardial ventricular tachycardia ablation a multicenter safety study. J Am Coll Cardiol. 2010 May 25;55(21):2366–2372. DOI:10.1016/j.jacc.2009.10.084.

[173] Wichter T, Paul TM, Eckardt L, Gerdes P, Kirchhof P, Böcker D, Breithardt G. Arrhythmogenic right ventricular cardiomyopathy: antiarrhythmic drugs, catheter ablation, or ICD. Herz. 2005 Mar;30(2):91–101. DOI:10.1007/s00059-005-2677-6.

[174] Peters S, Peters H, Thierfelder L. Risk stratification of sudden cardiac death and malignant ventricular arrhythmias in right ventricular dysplasia-cardiomyopathy. Int J Cardiol. 1999 Dec 1;71(3):243–250. DOI:10.1016/S0167-5273(99)00142-4.

[175] Lemola K, Brunckhorst C, Helfenstein U, Oechslin E, Jenni R, Duru F. Predictors of adverse outcome in patients with arrhythmogenic right ventricular dysplasia/cardiomyopathy: long-term experience of a tertiary care centre. Heart. 2005 Sep;91(9):1167–1172. DOI:10.1136/hrt.2004.038620.

[176] Corrado D, Leoni L, Link MS, Della Bella P, Gaita F, Curnis A, Salerno JU, Igidbashian D, Raviele A, Disertori M, Zanotto G, Verlato R, Vergara G, Delise P, Turrini P, Basso C, Naccarella F, Maddalena F, Estes NA 3rd, Buja G, Thiene G. Implantable cardioverter defibrillator therapy for prevention of sudden death in patients with arrhythmogenic right ventricular cardiomyopathy/dysplasia. Circulation. 2003 Dec 23;108(25):3084–3091. DOI:10.1161/01.CIR.0000103130.33451.D2.

[177] Schinkel AF. Implantable cardioverter defibrillators in arrhythmogenic right ventricular dysplasia/cardiomyopathy: patient outcomes, incidence of appropriate and inappropriate interventions, and complications. Circ Arrhythm Electrophysiol. 2013 Jun;6(3):562–568. DOI:10.1161/CIRCEP.113.000392.

[178] Groeneweg JA, Bhonsale A, James CA, te Riele AS, Dooijes D, Tichnell C, Murray B, Wiesfeld AC, Sawant AC, Kassamali B, Atsma DE, Volders PG, de

Groot NM, de Boer K, Zimmerman SL, Kamel IR, van der Heijden JF, Russell SD, Jan Cramer M, Tedford RJ, Doevendans PA, van Veen TA, Tandri H, Wilde AA, Judge DP, van Tintelen JP, Hauer RN. Calkins H. Clinical presentation, long-term follow-up, and outcomes of 1001 arrhythmogenic right ventricular dysplasia/cardiomyopathy patients and family members. Circ Cardiovasc Genet. 2015 Jun;8(3):437–446. DOI:10.1161/CIRCGENETICS.114.001003.

[179] European Heart Rhythm Association; Heart Rhythm Society, Zipes DP, Camm AJ, Borggrefe M, Buxton AE, Chaitman B, Fromer M, Gregoratos G, Klein G, Moss AJ, Myerburg RJ, Priori SG, Quinones MA, Roden DM, Silka MJ, Tracy C, Smith SC Jr, Jacobs AK, Adams CD, Antman EM, Anderson JL, Hunt SA, Halperin JL, Nishimura R, Ornato JP, Page RL, Riegel B, Priori SG, Blanc JJ, Budaj A, Camm AJ, Dean V, Deckers JW, Despres C, Dickstein K, Lekakis J, McGregor K, Metra M, Morais J, Osterspey A, Tamargo JL, Zamorano JL; American College of Cardiology; American Heart Association Task Force; European Society of Cardiology Committee for Practice Guidelines. ACC/AHA/ESC 2006 guidelines for management of patients with ventricular arrhythmias and the prevention of sudden cardiac death: a report of the American College of Cardiology/American Heart Association Task Force and the European Society of Cardiology Committee for Practice Guidelines (Writing Committee to Develop Guidelines for Management of Patients With Ventricular Arrhythmias and the Prevention of Sudden Cardiac Death). J Am Coll Cardiol. 2006 Sep 5;48(5):e247–346. DOI: 10.1016/j.jacc.2006.07.010.

[180] Tedford RJ, James C, Judge DP, Tichnell C, Murray B, Bhonsale A, Philips B, Abraham T, Dalal D, Halushka MK, Tandri H, Calkins H, Russell SD. Cardiac transplantation in arrhythmogenic right ventricular dysplasia/cardiomyopathy. J Am Coll Cardiol. 2012 Jan 17;59(3):289–290. DOI:10.1016/j.jacc.2011.09.051.

[181] Bakir I, Brugada P, Sarkozy A, Vandepitte C, Wellens F. A novel treatment strategy for therapy refractory ventricular arrhythmias in the setting of arrhythmogenic right ventricular dysplasia. Europace. 2007 May;9(5):267–269. DOI:10.1093/europace/eum029.

[182] Zacharias J, Forty J, DOIg JC, Bourke JP, Hilton CJ. Right ventricular disarticulation. An 18-year single centre experience. Eur J Cardiothorac Surg. 2005 Jun;27(6):1000–1004. DOI:10.1016/j.ejcts.2005.02.020.

[183] Chachques JC, Argyriadis PG, Fontaine G, Hebert JL, Frank RA, D'Attellis N, Fabiani JN, Carpentier AF. Right ventricular cardiomyoplasty: 10-year follow-up. Ann Thorac Surg. 2003 May;75(5):1464–1468. DOI:10.1016/S0003-4975(02)04823-3.

[184] Coleman MA, Bos JM, Johnson JN, Owen HJ, Deschamps C, Moir C, Ackerman MJ. Videoscopic left cardiac sympathetic denervation for patients with recurrent ventricular fibrillation/malignant ventricular arrhythmia syndromes besides congenital long-QT syndrome. Circ Arrhythm Electrophysiol. 2012 Aug 1;5(4):782–788. DOI:10.1161/CIRCEP.112.971754.

[185] Te Riele AS, James CA, Groeneweg JA, Sawant AC, Kammers K, Murray B, Tichnell C, van der Heijden JF, Judge DP, Dooijes D, van Tintelen JP, Hauer RN, Calkins H, Tandri H. Approach to family screening in arrhythmogenic right ventricular dysplasia/cardiomyopathy. Eur Heart J. 2016 Mar 1;37(9):755–763. DOI:10.1093/eurheartj/ehv387.

[186] Que D, Yang P, Song X, Liu L. Traditional vs. genetic pathogenesis of arrhythmogenic right ventricular cardiomyopathy. Europace Apr 2015.

[187] Thiene G, Corrado and D, Basso C. Arrhythmogenic right ventricular cardiomyopathy/dysplasia. Orphanet J Rare Dis. 2007. 2:45 DOI:10.1186/1750-1172-2-45.

Chapter 9

# Complexity of Sarcomere Protein Gene Mutations in Restrictive Cardiomyopathy

Shuai Wang and Daoquan Peng

Additional information is available at the end of the chapter

http://dx.doi.org/10.5772/66378

**Abstract**

Restrictive cardiomyopathy (RCM) is characterized by impaired filling of the ventricles in the presence of normal wall thickness and systolic function. Although idiopathic RCM is rare compared to other types of cardiomyopathy, the effects are severe. Until recently, many sarcomere genes previously described to be causative mutations in hypertrophic cardiomyopathy and dilated cardiomyopathy have been reported in RCM. Nowadays, it is accepted that primary RCM is also within the spectrum of sarcomere disease. However, the relationship between the identified mutations in sarcomere genes and clinical manifestation are complex, and the possible pathogenic mechanisms are not fully understood. Besides, many RCM-related sarcomere mutations were reported to cause variable clinical phenotype. Occasionally, "phenotype transition" may also be seen in an individual who was previously diagnosed with RCM.

**Keywords:** restrictive cardiomyopathy, sarcomere, gene mutation

## 1. Introduction

Restrictive cardiomyopathy (RCM) is characterized by impaired filling of the ventricles in the presence of normal wall thickness and systolic function. While RCM is rare compared to other primary cardiomyopathies, most affected individuals have severe signs and symptoms of heart failure and majority die shortly after diagnosis unless they receive a cardiac transplant [1]. According to the etiology, RCM has been classified as primary or secondary. Secondary RCM refers to the conditions in association with local inflammation (Loeffler cardiomyopathy, endomyocardial fibrosis, and eosinophilic endomyocardial disease) or infiltrative (amyloidosis and sarcoidosis) or storage disease (hemochromatosis, glycogen storage disease, and Fabry disease, etc.) [2]. Primary RCM includes RCM ascribed to inherited or sporadically acquired mutations or in many cases due to unknown etiology. So far, through mutation screening of different individuals and families presenting the RCM phenotype, mutations in multiple sarcomere genes have been identified to be linked with RCM, which has greatly expanded our understanding about "idiopathic RCM." However, the relationship between the identified sarcomeric mutations and clinical manifestation are complex and many puzzles still exist. The mechanism behind the genotype-phenotype correlation is not clearly understood. Most of these RCM-associated sarcomeric mutations, when mutated at specific sites, are also known to induce HCM or DCM. Even people carrying the same mutation of the same sarcomeric gene may exhibit heterogenetic manifestations. "Phenotype transition" may even been seen at a late stage of RCM resulting in atypical RCM.

## 2. Multiple sarcomeric gene mutations in human RCM

The sarcomere contains different protein involved in muscle contraction. Two major components are actin, which constitutes the backbone of the thin filament, and myosin, which makes up the thick filament. The interaction of myosin and actin causing the sliding of the thin filaments along the thick filaments results in muscle contraction and force development. Association and disassociation of myosin and actin are regulated in a $Ca^{2+}$-dependent manner by the troponin-alphatropomysin (Tm) complex. The actin-myosin contractile apparatus, which consists of five thin filament proteins (actin, tropomyosin, and troponin T, I, and C) and three thick filament proteins (myosin heavy chain, essential light chain, and regulatory light chain), plays a key role in regulating the sarcomere function. So far, except for troponin C, mutations in the other thin filament and thick filament proteins have all been identified in RCM. Besides, a series of mutations in other regulatory sarcomere proteins such as myosin-binding protein C, titin, and Z-disc proteins also have been recognized to induce diastolic dysfunction resulting in a restrictive phenotype.

### 2.1. Cardiac troponin mutation

Cardiac troponin is located at regular intervals along the thin filament and consists of three subunits: cardiac troponin C (cTnC), troponin I (cTnI), and troponin T (cTnT). cTnC acts as a $Ca^{2+}$ sensor, which confers $Ca^{2+}$ sensitivity to muscle contraction [3]. Cardiac TnI is the inhibitory subunit, primarily functioning to prevent actin and myosin from interacting in the absence of $Ca^{2+}$. The cTnT subunit binds to tropomyosin (Tm) and is responsible for transmitting the $Ca^{2+}$-binding signal from cTn to Tm [4]. Electrical depolarization of the cell membrane opens the L-type calcium channels and allows $Ca^{2+}$ influx, which incites release of $Ca^{2+}$ from sarcoplasmic reticulum due to opening of the ryanodine receptors. The released $Ca^{2+}$ binds to cardiac troponin C and induces conformational changes in the troponin T-tropomyosin complex, resulting in displacement of cTnI from actin and subsequent association of actin with myosin. Currently, nine mutations in genes encoding cTnI and three dominant mutations in genes encoding cTnT have been reported in human RCM and no mutations have been identified in cTnC yet.

#### *2.1.1. Troponin I mutation*

The gene of cardiac TnI (*TNNI3*) is situated on the 19th chromosome (19q13.4) and consists of eight exons and seven introns. The mature molecule of cTnI is 209 a.a long and consists of five domains: (1) N-terminal domains, (2) IT-arm, (3) inhibitory domain, (4) regulatory domain, and (5) C-terminal mobile domains [5]. Until now, RCM-related cTnI mutations are found located in the inhibitory domain and the C-terminal domain.

*2.1.1.1. Missense mutations located at the inhibitory domain*

The inhibitory domain of hcTnI spans residues 137–148 [6, 7], some also reported a different border of this region (residues 129–148) [6, 8]. In the absence of $Ca^{2+}$, residues 138–148 of the inhibitory domain interact with actin [9] and shift the tropomyosin molecule, impeding the antomyosin-complex formation [10]. Two of the RCM mutations are localized within this important region. The first one is 797T→A nucleotide substitution of exon 7, which led to a Leu144Gln (L144Q) amino acid substitution [11]. The second mutation is 799C→T nucleotide substitution of exon 7 that leads to an Arg145Trp (R145W) amino acid substitution [11].

Data from *in vitro* experiment showed that both L144Q and R145W alter myofilament sensitivity to $Ca^{2+}$. Skinned cardiac fiber experiment, which measures the $Ca^{2+}$-buffering capacity of the myofilament while measuring the development of tension and maximal force, revealed that these two mutations resulted in increase of $Ca^{2+}$ sensitivity of force development in skinned fibers from transgenic mice. In addition, a significant increase in the basal force was shown compared to WT cardiac fiber [12]. Measurement of myofilament ATPase activity revealed that L144Q and R145W mutant showed an increase in the basal ATPase at low $Ca^{2+}$ concentrations. Besides, fibers from these two mutants exhibited markedly increased $Ca^{2+}$ sensitivity of ATPase activity [13].

*2.1.1.2. Missense mutations located at the mobile C-terminal domain*

The mobile C-terminal domain of hcTnI is further divided into the H4 $\alpha$-helix (residues 164–188) and the C-terminal part (residues 199–210) [5]. 865G→A nucleotide substitution of exon 7 that led to an Ala171Thr amino acid substitution and an 886A→G nucleotide substitution of exon 7, which resulted in a Lys178Glu (K178E) amino acid substitution both occurred within the H4 $\alpha$-helix region and have been identified in RCM patients. Since these two mutations are known to be located within the actin-binding sites (residues 173–181) [14, 15], K178E and Ala171Thr mutations may influence the inhibitory function through actin binding.

Although the structure of the C-terminal part of hcTnI which consists of residues 190–210 is not fully understood, it is critical for a full inhibitory activity and $Ca^{2+}$ sensitivity of force development because it binds to actin and helps to maintain the thin filament in a blocked state [16]. Mutations occurred at the C-terminal domain may destabilize or decrease its interactions with actin in the absence of $Ca^{2+}$, consequently relieving cTnI inhibition [17]. Up to now, RCM-related mutant Asp190His (D190H), Arg192His (R192H), and Arg204His (R204H) have been localized within the conserved C-terminal region of the protein [11, 18]. *In vitro* experiments revealed that two of these mutants D190H and R192H markedly increased the filament sensitivity to $Ca^{2+}$, while another mutation R204H has been reported to result in a disruption of the normal interaction between cTnI-cTnC and cTnI-cTnT. It remains to be further determined what conformational changes happened in these mutant that lead to disrupted interaction between cTnI-actin and cTnI-cTnC.

*2.1.1.3. Two deletion mutations*

Deletion of nucleotides usually causes frame shift and the introduction of a premature stop codon. Two deletion mutations of *TNNI3* which impaired relaxation of myocardium and resulted in a restrictive filling pattern were reported to be located in exon 7 and cause truncation of C-terminal portion of cTnI. The truncated cTnI which lost its C-terminal portion is susceptible to degradation and has reduced inhibitory capacity on the thin filament since C-terminal contains the second binding domain for actin and cTnC [19, 20].

*2.1.2. Troponin T mutation*

cTnT anchors the troponin complex to Tm and plays a critical role in modulating ATPase activation when $Ca^{2+}$ concentrations achieve threshold levels. Until now, three different mutations in the cTnT gene (*TNNT2*) linked to RCM have been identified. However, the molecular pathogenesis of these cTnT mutations is not clear [20–22].

## 3. α-Cardiac actin (*ACTC*)

Actin is a major constituent of the thin filament and spans the length of thin filament. Together with myosin, actin generates force and transmits this force from the sarcomere to the surrounding syncytium via the thin filament [23]. RCM mutations in the ACTC gene are extremely rare and only one ACTC mutation has been reported in RCM (nucleotide substitution in exon 5 g. 4642G→C which lead to an Asp313His amino acid substitution). However, the significance of this variant is uncertain.

## 4. α-Tropomyosin (*TPM1*)

In cardiac muscles, tropomyosin together with troponin forms the principal mechanism by which contractility is regulated in response to the $Ca^{2+}$ concentration. In the absence of $Ca^{2+}$, tropomyosin prevents productive myosin head binding. In systole, tropomyosin moves in response to $Ca^{2+}$ binding to allow partial myosin attachment, which resulted in further shift of tropomyosin to expose fully the interaction site on actin [24]. Recently, a novel missense mutation in α-tropomyosin, c.835A>C p.Asn279His has been identified in a patient with primary RCM [25]. However, the significance of this variant is not clear since family evaluation did not show cosegregation.

## 5. β-Myosin heavy chain (*MYH7*)

Myosin is a dimeric protein consisting of two heavy chains and two associated pairs of light chains. The ~23-kb long human *MYH7* gene, located on chromosome 14, contains 40 exons that direct the synthesis of the 1935 amino acid β-myosin heavy chain [26]. Although over

500 disease-causing point mutations have been found in human *MYH7* gene, most of them are reported in HCM, only four of these variants are identified in patients with primary RCM [27–32]. The understanding about the genotype-phenotype correlation between the reported MYH7 mutation and RCM are very limited. MYH7 contains different functional domains, including the globular head domain (S1), the neck or hinge region (S2), and the tail (light meromyosin) [33, 34]. Although many mutations have been identified to cluster in functional hotspots due to the development of high throughput sequencing, all the above mentioned RCM-related *MYH7* mutations located at regions where no definite function has been assigned to so far [28]. Besides, whether haploinsufficiency may contribute to the consequence of the variants is not clear.

## 6. Ventricular myosin essential light chain (*MYL3*) and ventricular myosin regulatory light chain (*MYL2*)

Myosin assembles into hexamers comprising two heavy chains and two pairs of each light chain isoform. The light chain forms a stabilizing collar around the α-helical neck of the heavy chain, a region of the myosin multimer thought to function as the level arm. Mutation in the gene encoding the essential light chain of myosin (*MYL3* Met149Val) and the regulatory light chain of myosin (MYL2 Glu22Lys) was previously reported to correlate with marked diastolic dysfunction and restrictive physiology both in human and transgenic mice [35]. Interestingly, carriers with simultaneous mutation in both *MYL3* and MYL2 showed different phenotypes. While patients with heterozygous mutation in MYL2 (p.Gly57Glu) and homozygous mutation in *MYL3* (p.Glu143Lys) had severe, early onset RCM, double heterozygote for these variants have no evidence of cardiomyopathy [25, 36]. It is speculated that Glu143Lys substitution may be responsible for this heterogeneity through a loss of function mechanism. This speculation is based on (1) carriers with one mutant allele were clinically silent [36], while homozygotes for the mutation have severe, early-onset cardiomyopathy [25]. If the cardiomyopathy was caused by a dominant-negative mechanism, an intermediate phenotype in heterozygotes would be expected. (2) The substitution occurs in a surface-exposed loop of the essential light chain [37], which makes it less likely to disrupt protein conformation or stability. The site-directed mutagenesis of the corresponding loop domain was confirmed to have no effect on binding between light and heavy chains [38]. Further study using transgenic animal models may help to answer this question.

## 7. Myosin-binding protein C (*MYBPC3*)

Cardiac myosin-binding protein C is a modular polypeptide located at the C-zone in the striated muscles and binds myosin heavy chain in thick filament and titin in elastic filaments [39]. More than 150 mutations identified in MYBPC3 have been reported, which is the most common genetic cause of HCM [40, 41]. Recently, variants of MYBPC3 have also been reported to be RCM-causing mutation [42, 43].

## 8. Titin (*TTN*)

The giant protein titin acts as the third filament system of the sarcomere, in addition to the actin and myosin filament. It physically connects myosin fibers to actin polymers and is attached to the Z-line. Titin consists of four structurally and functionally distinct regions. (1) The N-terminal titin binds to various Z-disk proteins and acts as an anchor, which is composed of Z-repeats and multiple immunoglobulin (Ig) domains. (2) Elastic I-band region contains the important PEVK portion (proline, glutamate, valine, and lysine) and acts as the molecular spring. (3) Stabilizing A-band region binds to the thick muscle filaments and contains Ig-like, fibronectin type III (fibronection3) domain. (4) M-band region contains the unique serine-threonine kinase domain modulating titin expression and turnover, with C-terminus of titin embedding in the M-line [44–46]. When the sarcomere is stretched during diastole, the I-band segments gradually lengthen and develop passive tension and therefore, titin is a major determinant of the stiffness of myocardium [47].

Currently, two mechanisms are known to modulate titin's passive stiffness. (1) Titin-based passive tension is critically defined by the ratio of the two major adult cardiac isoforms (N2BA and N2B). As a general rule, longer titin isoforms with longer PEVK repeats in the I-band have more elasticity, whereas shorter isoforms provide more passive stiffness [48]. In adult cardiac muscle, two major isoforms are present: the long compliant N2BA and the shorter stiff N2B. In healthy adult, the ratio of N2BA to N2B in human left ventricle is 40:60 [49]. Moreover, the right ventricle expresses more N2BA than does the left ventricle [50]. In conditions with concentric remodeling such as hypertension or aortic stenosis with diastolic function, a decreased N2BA:N2B ratio was shown [51, 52]. (2) Another more short-term mechanism modulating titin's passive stiffness is caused by post-translational modification influencing phosphorylation states. Titin could be phosphorylated at the PEVK domain and the cardiac-specific N2B domain, and phosphorylated titin exhibited decreased titin-based passive tension [53].

Titin, known to be the major disease-causing gene for DCM, is encoded by a single gene *TTN* on chromosome 2q31 [54]. Interestingly, recent clinical and genetic studies have established the role of titin defects in the pathophysiology of diastolic dysfunction and RCM. A de novo missense mutation of Titin c.22862A > G replacing adenine by guanine at position 109 of exon 226, resulting in the substitution of an evolutionally conserved tyrosine by cysteine (p.Y7621C) has been reported to result in early-onset family RCM with severe heart failure [55]. Structural analysis revealed that p.Y7621C mutation is likely to disrupt the hydrophobic core within fibronectin3 domain, which locates in the A/I junction region [55]. However, how this *TTN* mutation might affect cardiac function and lead to the consecutive development of RCM is unknown.

## 9. Myopalladin (*MYPN*)

Myopalladin (MYPN) is an Ig-domain family member protein that has been reported to be a key intermediate molecule at the Z-disc involved in sarcomere/Z-disc assembly and regulation of gene expression in cardiac cells [56]. Through genetic screening for *MYPN* mutations in large cohorts of patients with cardiomyopathy, 15 *MYPN* variants were identified, of which a nonsense mutation (p.Q529X) was identified in an RCM family with variable penetrance [57]. Q529X was found to disturb different functional domains of MYNP. MYNP contains five Ig domains (two N-terminal and three C-terminal). Central and C-terminal domains of MYPN bind at the Z-disc to $\alpha$-actinin and nebulette (NEBL), respectively. This actinin-MYPN-NEBL complex tethers actin and titin to the Z-disc and may play roles in the signaling and regulation of gene expression in response to muscle stress. The N-terminal domain of MYNP binds cardiac ankyrin repeat protein (CARP), which is involved in the control of muscle gene expression [58]. Q529X mutation truncates the C-terminus of MYNP, including the NEBL- and $\alpha$-actinin-binding domains. Comparative immunohistochemistry of human heart tissue was performed on specimens from the siblings with RCM and from normal control subjects without *MYPN* mutation as well as in neonatal rat cardiomyocytes (NRCs) expressing green fluorescent protein (GFP) chimeras of WT- and Q529X-MYPN. Disrupted sarcomeric Z-discs with abnormally diffuse MYPN codistributed focally with abnormal sarcomeric $\alpha$-actin, localization were seen in the specimen from siblings with RCM and NRCs expressing Q529X-MYPN [57]. Therefore, losing the NEBL and $\alpha$-actinin-binding domain results in severe disturbance of sarcomere/Z-disc assembly, which may have impact on early myofibrillogenesis and resulted in RCM. Besides, since MYPN localizes both at sarcoplasm and nucleus, mutant MPPN-Q529X protein in the nucleus was reported to result in downregulation of CARP expression and upregulation of MLP and desmin, augmenting fibrotic restrictive remodeling [59]. In addition, truncated proteins are usually unstable due to decay of mRNA and/or protein degradation through the lysosome or ubiquitin-proteasome system. Although *MYPN* mRNA was not affected by the Q529X-MYPN mutation in the myocardium, mutant MYPN was relatively unstable compared with WT protein [57]. Therefore, insufficient quantities of the protein (haploinsufficiency) may be partly involved in dysfunction of the protein.

## 10. Mutations cause variable phenotypes

The molecular mechanisms by which gene mutation cause cardiomyopathy can usually be explained by two alternative ways. One is mutation may cause structural and functional change in the protein, which should be analyzed in four different levels: (1) change in the deoxyribonucleic acid sequence, (2) the actual amino acid change, (3) the changes in $Ca^{2+}$ sensitivity of force development and ATPase activity, and (4) the change in protein-protein interaction. The other mechanism may involve insufficient quantities of the protein due to instability of the mutant protein leading to haploinsufficiency [23].

However, it is now evident that different mutations in one gene could cause multiple phenotypes. It is also intriguing that even for a given single mutation and even within a single family disparate phenotypes can be seen. For example, the cTnT lle79Asn mutation has been shown to be associated with HCM, DCM, and RCM within a single pedigree [60]. This implies that factors just beyond the pathogenic sarcomere mutation influence the phenotype. Therefore, the model of sarcomeric cardiomyopathy as monogenic disease following simple Mendelian pattern of inheritance is an oversimplification. Theoretically, a discrete number of reasons can account for phenotypic diversity. (1) First of all, patients may carry more than one disease-associated mutations, which is underestimated in most cases. Recent genotyping suggests that multiple cardiomyopathy patients have more than one mutation in the same gene or mutations in different genes. For example, in a study carried out in 292 HCM patients, 13 were found to carry at least 2 mutations [61, 62]. However, the number of patients carrying at least two mutations is likely to be significantly underestimated since many genetic studies typically investigate less than 15 genes for mutations associated with cardiomyopathy [63]. (2) Secondly, different expression and the incorporation rate of the mutant sarcomeric proteins in the heart may also contribute to the heterogeneity of the disease. A few examples in HCM have been published. Heterozygous individuals carrying the βMHC Lys207Gln mutation developed an HCM phenotype, but a homozygous individual developed a DCM-like phenotype [61]. In another case, homozygous carriers of cTnT Ser179Phe mutation exhibited profound left and right ventricular hypertrophy [64] while heterozygous carriers had little or no hypertrophy [65]. (3) Third, mutant proteins are usually unstable due to decay of mRNA and/or degradation through the lysosome or ubiquitin-proteasome system, especially in the case of nonsense mutation [66]. Because of genetic polymorphisms, individuals with RCM are likely to have substantial difference in their genome sequence including disease-modifier genes which are involved in post-translational or translational regulation, resulting in different amounts of mutant protein. This mechanism may interfere with the development of the phenotype and explain different penetrance of a specific mutation. (4) Lastly, sarcomere gene mutation induces serials of maladaptive features, ranging from the prolongation of cardiomyocyte action potential to microvascular dysfunction, from intracellular calcium abnormality to dysregulation of collagen turn-over, and from energetic derangement to abnormal sympathetic activation [67]. The extent and the rate at which each of these features occur and evolve are quite variable within individual patients. Therefore, the clinical heterogeneity of a specific sarcomere gene mutation may partly be ascribed to different stages of disease progression [68]. Although epigenetics and environmental factors are likely to be relevant in sarcomeric cardiomyopathies, there have been no studies yet describing how epigenetic modification and environmental factors may affect phenotype in sarcomeric RCM.

## 11. Phenotype transition

Occasionally, with the progression of disease, "phenotype transition" may be seen in a given individual who was initially diagnosed with a specific type of cardiomyopathy. This situation could often be seen in patients who was initially diagnosed with HCM and gradually developed into end-stage of the disease. The morpho-functional manifestation in this advanced stage usually exhibits two extremes: hypokinetic-dilated from or hypokinetic-restrictive form which could be hard to distinguish from primary DCM and RCM [68]. The "HCM to RCM" transition has been discussed above. There is another situation that patients initially diagnosed with primary RCM could undergo persistent cardiac remodeling resulting atypical phenotype at a later stage of the disease. Although the main impairment of RCM is diastolic dysfunction, deterioration of systolic function has been observed in some patients. In a retrospective study, it was reported that 16% of 94 primary RCM patients was observed to have systolic dysfunction [69]. Another study carried out in pediatric RCM reveals that although all the 18 children had preserved ventricular systolic function at diagnosis, 6 of them later presented a deteriorated ventricular systolic function and eventually required inotropic support [70]. In the RCM model using transgenic mice noticeable impaired systolic was observed over a time of 10 months. By the time, those RCM mice presented with signs of severely aggravated congestive heart failure and some of them died [71]. This disease progression is consistent with some of the clinical observation, suggesting that systolic dysfunction may be responsible for the end-stage lethal heart failure. As for the mechanism, some proposed that ischemia may be a bridge between the progression of diastolic dysfunction and the development of systolic function, based on evidence of ischemia observed in hearts for autopsy from RCM patients and transgenic RCM mice [71–73]. Besides, it is presumed that reduced capillary density due to interstitial fibrosis and increased extravascular compressive force in the restrictive heart may also induce ischemia [74]. Of note, although an RCM patient may appear to have systolic dysfunction and low cardiac output, enlargement of ventricle is seldom seen, probably because the molecular mechanism and sarcomeric mechanics of RCM and DCM are opposite [75].

## 12. Summary

In the past decades, clinical and genetic studies suggest that primary RCM is part of a spectrum of sarcomeric disease. Since RCM is associated with severe prognosis, ongoing and future basic science will continue to dissect the precise pathways driving how these mutations remodel the heart, and identify rational therapies targeting pathophysiological aspects to interrupt the emergency of pathology. On the other hand, it is also important to realize that genes contain information that is essential for the development of the phenotype but not necessarily complete. The final phenotype is determined not only by the causal mutation but also by the modifier genes, each exerting a modest effect, epigenetic factors, which link the gene to the phenotype, and the environmental factors, as in the case of complex phenotypes observed in single-gene disorders with Mendelian pattern of inheritance. Thus, while advances in molecular genetics of cardiovascular diseases are gradually changing our classical understanding of the disease and the phenotype-based approach to the practice of medicine, currently they are unlikely to be sufficient to trigger a full switch from a phenotype-based to genotyped-based medicines. A comprehensive understanding of molecular mechanism of the pathogenesis integrating the genetic, epigenetic, transcriptomic, and proteomic profiles is necessary.

## Author details

Shuai Wang and Daoquan Peng*

*Address all correspondence to: pengdq@hotmail.com

1 Department of Cardiovascular Medicine, The Second Xiangya Hospital of Central South University, Changsha, Hunan, China

## References


[1] Mogensen J, Arbustini E. Restrictive cardiomyopathy. *Curr Opin Cardiol*. 2009;24:214–220.

[2] Kushwaha SS, Fallon JT, Fuster V. Restrictive cardiomyopathy. *N Engl J Med*. 1997;336:267–276.

[3] Gordon AM, Homsher E, Regnier M. Regulation of contraction in striated muscle. *Physiol Rev*. 2000;80:853–924.

[4] Gordon AM, Regnier M, Homsher E. Skeletal and cardiac muscle contractile activation: tropomyosin "rocks and rolls". *News Physiol Sci*. 2001;16:49–55.

[5] Katrukha IA. Human cardiac troponin complex. Structure and functions. *Biochemistry (Mosc)*. 2013;78:1447–1465.

[6] Takeda S, Yamashita A, Maeda K, Maeda Y. Structure of the core domain of human cardiac troponin in the $Ca^{2+}$-saturated form. *Nature*. 2003;424:35–41.

[7] Kobayashi T, Patrick SE, Kobayashi M. Ala scanning of the inhibitory region of cardiac troponin i. *J Biol Chem*. 2009;284:20052–20060.

[8] Brown LJ, Sale KL, Hills R, Rouviere C, Song L, Zhang X, Fajer PG. Structure of the inhibitory region of troponin by site directed spin labeling electron paramagnetic resonance. *Proc Natl Acad Sci U S A*. 2002;99:12765–12770.

[9] Lindhout DA, Sykes BD. Structure and dynamics of the c-domain of human cardiac troponin c in complex with the inhibitory region of human cardiac troponin i. *J Biol Chem*. 2003;278:27024–27034.

[10] Farah CS, Miyamoto CA, Ramos CH, da Silva AC, Quaggio RB, Fujimori K, Smillie LB, Reinach FC. Structural and regulatory functions of the $NH_2$- and COOH-terminal regions of skeletal muscle troponin i. *J Biol Chem*. 1994;269:5230–5240.

[11] Mogensen J, Kubo T, Duque M, Uribe W, Shaw A, Murphy R, Gimeno JR, Elliott P, McKenna WJ. Idiopathic restrictive cardiomyopathy is part of the clinical expression of cardiac troponin i mutations. *J Clin Invest*. 2003;111:209–216.

[12] Gomes AV, Liang J, Potter JD. Mutations in human cardiac troponin i that are associated with restrictive cardiomyopathy affect basal atpase activity and the calcium sensitivity of force development. *J Biol Chem*. 2005;280:30909–30915.

[13] Kobayashi T, Solaro RJ. Increased $Ca^{2+}$ affinity of cardiac thin filaments reconstituted with cardiomyopathy-related mutant cardiac troponin i. *J Biol Chem*. 2006;281:13471–13477.

[14] Gomes AV, Potter JD. Cellular and molecular aspects of familial hypertrophic cardiomyopathy caused by mutations in the cardiac troponin i gene. *Mol Cell Biochem*. 2004;263:99–114.

[15] Tripet B, Van Eyk JE, Hodges RS. Mapping of a second actin-tropomyosin and a second troponin c binding site within the c terminus of troponin i, and their importance in the $Ca^{2+}$-dependent regulation of muscle contraction. *J Mol Biol*. 1997;271:728–750.

[16] Galinska A, Hatch V, Craig R, Murphy AM, Van Eyk JE, Wang CL, Lehman W, Foster DB. The c terminus of cardiac troponin i stabilizes the $Ca^{2+}$-activated state of tropomyosin on actin filaments. *Circ Res*. 2010;106:705–711.

[17] Rarick HM, Tu XH, Solaro RJ, Martin AF. The c terminus of cardiac troponin i is essential for full inhibitory activity and $Ca^{2+}$ sensitivity of rat myofibrils. *J Biol Chem*. 1997;272:26887–26892.

[18] Gambarin FI, Tagliani M, Arbustini E. Pure restrictive cardiomyopathy associated with cardiac troponin i gene mutation: mismatch between the lack of hypertrophy and the presence of disarray. *Heart*. 2008;94:1257.

[19] Kostareva A, Gudkova A, Sjoberg G, Morner S, Semernin E, Krutikov A, Shlyakhto E, Sejersen T. Deletion in tnni3 gene is associated with restrictive cardiomyopathy. *Int J Cardiol*. 2009;131:410–412.

[20] Kaski JP, Syrris P, Burch M, Tome-Esteban MT, Fenton M, Christiansen M, Andersen PS, Sebire N, Ashworth M, Deanfield JE, McKenna WJ, Elliott PM. Idiopathic restrictive cardiomyopathy in children is caused by mutations in cardiac sarcomere protein genes. *Heart*. 2008;94:1478–1484.

[21] Peddy SB, Vricella LA, Crosson JE, Oswald GL, Cohn RD, Cameron DE, Valle D, Loeys BL. Infantile restrictive cardiomyopathy resulting from a mutation in the cardiac troponin t gene. *Pediatrics*. 2006;117:1830–1833.

[22] Miller T, Szczesna D, Housmans PR, Zhao J, de Freitas F, Gomes AV, Culbreath L, McCue J, Wang Y, Xu Y, Kerrick WG, Potter JD. Abnormal contractile function in transgenic mice expressing a familial hypertrophic cardiomyopathy-linked troponin t (i79n) mutation. *J Biol Chem*. 2001;276:3743–3755.

[23] Xu Q, Dewey S, Nguyen S, Gomes AV. Malignant and benign mutations in familial cardiomyopathies: insights into mutations linked to complex cardiovascular phenotypes. *J Mol Cell Cardiol*. 2010;48:899–909.

[24] McKillop DF, Geeves MA. Regulation of the interaction between actin and myosin subfragment 1: evidence for three states of the thin filament. *Biophys J*. 1993;65:693–701.

[25] Caleshu C, Sakhuja R, Nussbaum RL, Schiller NB, Ursell PC, Eng C, De Marco T, McGlothlin D, Burchard EG, Rame JE. Furthering the link between the sarcomere and primary cardiomyopathies: restrictive cardiomyopathy associated with multiple mutations in genes previously associated with hypertrophic or dilated cardiomyopathy. *Am J Med Genet A*. 2011;155A:2229–2235.

[26] Buvoli M, Hamady M, Leinwand LA, Knight R. Bioinformatics assessment of beta-myosin mutations reveals myosin's high sensitivity to mutations. *Trends Cardiovasc Med*. 2008;18:141–149.

[27] Greenway SC, Wilson GJ, Wilson J, George K, Kantor PF. Sudden death in an infant with angina, restrictive cardiomyopathy, and coronary artery bridging: an unusual

phenotype for a beta-myosin heavy chain (myh7) sarcomeric protein mutation. *Circ Heart Fail*. 2012;5:e92–e93.

[28] Colegrave M, Peckham M. Structural implications of beta-cardiac myosin heavy chain mutations in human disease. *Anat Rec (Hoboken)*. 2014;297:1670–1680.

[29] Karam S, Raboisson MJ, Ducreux C, Chalabreysse L, Millat G, Bozio A, Bouvagnet P. A de novo mutation of the beta cardiac myosin heavy chain gene in an infantile restrictive cardiomyopathy. *Congenit Heart Dis*. 2008;3:138–143.

[30] Rai TS, Ahmad S, Ahluwalia TS, Ahuja M, Bahl A, Saikia UN, Singh B, Talwar KK, Khullar M. Genetic and clinical profile of Indian patients of idiopathic restrictive cardiomyopathy with and without hypertrophy. *Mol Cell Biochem*. 2009;331:187–192.

[31] Koppole S, Smith JC, Fischer S. Simulations of the myosin ii motor reveal a nucleotide-state sensing element that controls the recovery stroke. *J Mol Biol*. 2006;361:604–616.

[32] Yu BL, Xiang R, Hu D, Peng DQ. A novel myh7 mutation in a family with cardiomyopathy presenting with restrictive physiology and varying degrees of left ventricle hypertrophy. *Eur Heart J*. 2015;36:178.

[33] Miroshnichenko NS, Balanuk IV, Nozdrenko DN. Packing of myosin molecules in muscle thick filaments. *Cell Biol Int*. 2000;24:327–333.

[34] Walsh R, Rutland C, Thomas R, Loughna S. Cardiomyopathy: a systematic review of disease-causing mutations in myosin heavy chain 7 and their phenotypic manifestations. *Cardiology*. 2010;115:49–60.

[35] Sanbe A, Nelson D, Gulick J, Setser E, Osinska H, Wang X, Hewett TE, Klevitsky R, Hayes E, Warshaw DM, Robbins J. In vivo analysis of an essential myosin light chain mutation linked to familial hypertrophic cardiomyopathy. *Circ Res*. 2000;87:296–302.

[36] Olson TM, Karst ML, Whitby FG, Driscoll DJ. Myosin light chain mutation causes autosomal recessive cardiomyopathy with mid-cavitary hypertrophy and restrictive physiology. *Circulation*. 2002;105:2337–2340.

[37] Rayment I, Holden HM, Whittaker M, Yohn CB, Lorenz M, Holmes KC, Milligan RA. Structure of the actin-myosin complex and its implications for muscle contraction. *Science*. 1993;261:58–65.

[38] Ho G, Chisholm RL. Substitution mutations in the myosin essential light chain lead to reduced actin-activated atpase activity despite stoichiometric binding to the heavy chain. *J Biol Chem*. 1997;272:4522–4527.

[39] Oakley CE, Hambly BD, Curmi PM, Brown LJ. Myosin binding protein c: structural abnormalities in familial hypertrophic cardiomyopathy. *Cell Res*. 2004;14:95–110.

[40] Bahrudin U, Morisaki H, Morisaki T, Ninomiya H, Higaki K, Nanba E, Igawa O, Takashima S, Mizuta E, Miake J, Yamamoto Y, Shirayoshi Y, Kitakaze M, Carrier L, Hisatome I. Ubiquitin-proteasome system impairment caused by a missense cardiac myosin-binding protein c mutation and associated with cardiac dysfunction in hypertrophic cardiomyopathy. *J Mol Biol*. 2008;384:896–907.

[41] Olivotto I, d'Amati G, Basso C, Van Rossum A, Patten M, Emdin M, Pinto Y, Tomberli B, Camici PG, Michels M. Defining phenotypes and disease progression in sarcomeric cardiomyopathies: contemporary role of clinical investigations. *Cardiovasc Res*. 2015;105:409–423.

[42] Wu W, Lu CX, Wang YN, Liu F, Chen W, Liu YT, Han YC, Cao J, Zhang SY, Zhang X. Novel phenotype-genotype correlations of restrictive cardiomyopathy with myosin-binding protein c (mybpc3) gene mutations tested by next-generation sequencing. *J Am Heart Assoc*. 2015; Jul 10;4(7)

[43] Zou Y, Wang J, Liu X, Wang Y, Chen Y, Sun K, Gao S, Zhang C, Wang Z, Zhang Y, Feng X, Song Y, Wu Y, Zhang H, Jia L, Wang H, Wang D, Yan C, Lu M, Zhou X, Song L, Hui R. Multiple gene mutations, not the type of mutation, are the modifier of left ventricle hypertrophy in patients with hypertrophic cardiomyopathy. *Mol Biol Rep*. 2013;40:3969–3976.

[44] Bang ML, Centner T, Fornoff F, Geach AJ, Gotthardt M, McNabb M, Witt CC, Labeit D, Gregorio CC, Granzier H, Labeit S. The complete gene sequence of titin, expression of an unusual approximately 700-kDa titin isoform, and its interaction with obscurin identify a novel z-line to i-band linking system. *Circ Res*. 2001;89:1065–1072.

[45] Lange S, Xiang F, Yakovenko A, Vihola A, Hackman P, Rostkova E, Kristensen J, Brandmeier B, Franzen G, Hedberg B, Gunnarsson LG, Hughes SM, Marchand S, Sejersen T, Richard I, Edstrom L, Ehler E, Udd B, Gautel M. The kinase domain of titin controls muscle gene expression and protein turnover. *Science*. 2005;308:1599–1603.

[46] Labeit S, Kolmerer B. Titins: giant proteins in charge of muscle ultrastructure and elasticity. *Science*. 1995;270:293–296.

[47] Gerull B. The rapidly evolving role of titin in cardiac physiology and cardiomyopathy. *Can J Cardiol*. 2015;31:1351–1359.

[48] Freiburg A, Trombitas K, Hell W, Cazorla O, Fougerousse F, Centner T, Kolmerer B, Witt C, Beckmann JS, Gregorio CC, Granzier H, Labeit S. Series of exon-skipping events in the elastic spring region of titin as the structural basis for myofibrillar elastic diversity. *Circ Res*. 2000;86:1114–1121.

[49] Cazorla O, Freiburg A, Helmes M, Centner T, McNabb M, Wu Y, Trombitas K, Labeit S, Granzier H. Differential expression of cardiac titin isoforms and modulation of cellular stiffness. *Circ Res*. 2000;86:59–67.

[50] Neagoe C, Opitz CA, Makarenko I, Linke WA. Gigantic variety: expression patterns of titin isoforms in striated muscles and consequences for myofibrillar passive stiffness. *J Muscle Res Cell Motil*. 2003;24:175–189.

[51] Williams L, Howell N, Pagano D, Andreka P, Vertesaljai M, Pecor T, Frenneaux M, Granzier H. Titin isoform expression in aortic stenosis. *Clin Sci (Lond)*. 2009;117:237–242.

[52] Warren CM, Jordan MC, Roos KP, Krzesinski PR, Greaser ML. Titin isoform expression in normal and hypertensive myocardium. *Cardiovasc Res*. 2003;59:86–94.

[53] Hidalgo C, Granzier H. Tuning the molecular giant titin through phosphorylation: role in health and disease. *Trends Cardiovasc Med*. 2013;23:165–171.

[54] Hinson JT, Chopra A, Nafissi N, Polacheck WJ, Benson CC, Swist S, Gorham J, Yang L, Schafer S, Sheng CC, Haghighi A, Homsy J, Hubner N, Church G, Cook SA, Linke WA, Chen CS, Seidman JG, Seidman CE. Heart disease. Titin mutations in ips cells define sarcomere insufficiency as a cause of dilated cardiomyopathy. *Science*. 2015;349:982–986.

[55] Peled Y, Gramlich M, Yoskovitz G, Feinberg MS, Afek A, Polak-Charcon S, Pras E, Sela BA, Konen E, Weissbrod O, Geiger D, Gordon PM, Thierfelder L, Freimark D, Gerull B, Arad M. Titin mutation in familial restrictive cardiomyopathy. *Int J Cardiol*. 2014;171:24–30.

[56] Bang ML, Mudry RE, McElhinny AS, Trombitas K, Geach AJ, Yamasaki R, Sorimachi H, Granzier H, Gregorio CC, Labeit S. Myopalladin, a novel 145-kilodalton sarcomeric protein with multiple roles in z-disc and i-band protein assemblies. *J Cell Biol*. 2001;153:413–427.

[57] Purevjav E, Arimura T, Augustin S, Huby AC, Takagi K, Nunoda S, Kearney DL, Taylor MD, Terasaki F, Bos JM, Ommen SR, Shibata H, Takahashi M, Itoh-Satoh M, McKenna WJ, Murphy RT, Labeit S, Yamanaka Y, Machida N, Park JE, Alexander PM, Weintraub RG, Kitaura Y, Ackerman MJ, Kimura A, Towbin JA. Molecular basis for clinical heterogeneity in inherited cardiomyopathies due to myopalladin mutations. *Hum Mol Genet*. 2012;21:2039–2053.

[58] Otey CA, Dixon R, Stack C, Goicoechea SM. Cytoplasmic ig-domain proteins: cytoskeletal regulators with a role in human disease. *Cell Motil Cytoskeleton*. 2009;66:618–634.

[59] Huby AC, Mendsaikhan U, Takagi K, Martherus R, Wansapura J, Gong N, Osinska H, James JF, Kramer K, Saito K, Robbins J, Khuchua Z, Towbin JA, Purevjav E. Disturbance in z-disk mechanosensitive proteins induced by a persistent mutant myopalladin causes familial restrictive cardiomyopathy. *J Am Coll Cardiol*. 2014;64:2765–2776.

[60] Menon SC, Michels VV, Pellikka PA, Ballew JD, Karst ML, Herron KJ, Nelson SM, Rodeheffer RJ, Olson TM. Cardiac troponin t mutation in familial cardiomyopathy with variable remodeling and restrictive physiology. *Clin Genet*. 2008;74:445–454.

[61] Alpert NR, Mohiddin SA, Tripodi D, Jacobson-Hatzell J, Vaughn-Whitley K, Brosseau C, Warshaw DM, Fananapazir L. Molecular and phenotypic effects of heterozygous, homozygous, and compound heterozygote myosin heavy-chain mutations. *Am J Physiol Heart Circ Physiol*. 2005;288:H1097–H1102.

[62] Friedrich FW, Bausero P, Sun Y, Treszl A, Kramer E, Juhr D, Richard P, Wegscheider K, Schwartz K, Brito D, Arbustini E, Waldenstrom A, Isnard R, Komajda M, Eschenhagen T, Carrier L, Project EHF. A new polymorphism in human calmodulin iii gene promoter is a potential modifier gene for familial hypertrophic cardiomyopathy. *Eur Heart J*. 2009;30:1648–1655.

[63] Frisso G, Limongelli G, Pacileo G, Del Giudice A, Forgione L, Calabro P, Iacomino M, Detta N, Di Fonzo LM, Maddaloni V, Calabro R, Salvatore F. A child cohort study from

southern Italy enlarges the genetic spectrum of hypertrophic cardiomyopathy. *Clin Genet*. 2009;76:91–101.

[64] Maron BJ, Thompson PD, Puffer JC, McGrew CA, Strong WB, Douglas PS, Clark LT, Mitten MJ, Crawford MH, Atkins DL, Driscoll DJ, Epstein AE. Cardiovascular preparticipation screening of competitive athletes. A statement for health professionals from the sudden death committee (clinical cardiology) and congenital cardiac defects committee (cardiovascular disease in the young), American Heart Association. *Circulation*. 1996;94:850–856.

[65] Ho CY, Lever HM, DeSanctis R, Farver CF, Seidman JG, Seidman CE. Homozygous mutation in cardiac troponin t: implications for hypertrophic cardiomyopathy. *Circulation*. 2000;102:1950–1955.

[66] Vosberg HP. The ubiquitin-proteasome system may be involved in the pathogenesis of hypertrophic cardiomyopathy. *Cardiovasc Res*. 2005;66:1–3.

[67] Ferrantini C, Belus A, Piroddi N, Scellini B, Tesi C, Poggesi C. Mechanical and energetic consequences of hcm-causing mutations. *J Cardiovasc Transl Res*. 2009;2:441–451.

[68] Olivotto I, Cecchi F, Poggesi C, Yacoub MH. Patterns of disease progression in hypertrophic cardiomyopathy: an individualized approach to clinical staging. *Circ Heart Fail*. 2012;5:535–546.

[69] Ammash NM, Seward JB, Bailey KR, Edwards WD, Tajik AJ. Clinical profile and outcome of idiopathic restrictive cardiomyopathy. *Circulation*. 2000;101:2490–2496.

[70] Weller RJ, Weintraub R, Addonizio LJ, Chrisant MR, Gersony WM, Hsu DT. Outcome of idiopathic restrictive cardiomyopathy in children. *Am J Cardiol*. 2002;90:501–506.

[71] Du J, Liu J, Feng HZ, Hossain MM, Gobara N, Zhang C, Li Y, Jean-Charles PY, Jin JP, Huang XP. Impaired relaxation is the main manifestation in transgenic mice expressing a restrictive cardiomyopathy mutation, r193h, in cardiac tni. *Am J Physiol Heart Circ Physiol*. 2008;294:H2604–H2613.

[72] Jean-Charles PY, Li YJ, Nan CL, Huang XP. Insights into restrictive cardiomyopathy from clinical and animal studies. *J Geriatr Cardiol*. 2011;8:168–183.

[73] Palka P, Lange A, Ward C. A fatal case of idiopathic restrictive cardiomyopathy. *Cardiol Young*. 2003;13:469–471.

[74] Maron MS, Olivotto I, Maron BJ, Prasad SK, Cecchi F, Udelson JE, Camici PG. The case for myocardial ischemia in hypertrophic cardiomyopathy. *J Am Coll Cardiol*. 2009;54:866–875.

[75] Robinson P, Mirza M, Knott A, Abdulrazzak H, Willott R, Marston S, Watkins H, Redwood C. Alterations in thin filament regulation induced by a human cardiac troponin t mutant that causes dilated cardiomyopathy are distinct from those induced by troponin t mutants that cause hypertrophic cardiomyopathy. *J Biol Chem*. 2002;277:40710–40716.

Section 4

# Specific Cardiomyopathies

Chapter 10

# Infective Cardiomyopathy

Agnieszka Pawlak and Robert Julian Gil

Additional information is available at the end of the chapter

http://dx.doi.org/10.5772/66095

## Abstract

Both the infectious agent and development of inflammatory response to infection can lead to irreversible myocardial injury, which affects the outcome of short- and long-term prognosis. In the case of the rapid elimination of the infectious agent and rapid withholding of inflammatory process, changes in myocardium are small. If the immune response does not lead to complete elimination of infectious agent or inflammation progresses after removing the virus, chronic myocardial damage may develop. Persistence of the virus in myocardium, postinfectious immune reaction, autoimmunity, and primary cardiac damage may result in the development of progressive ventricular dysfunction, development of cardiac arrhythmias, and exacerbation of symptom. Because of the long-term consequences, it is important to diagnose infective cardiomyopathy (IC) quickly and start appropriate treatment. However, IC is still a diagnostic challenge. Infective cardiomyopathy is often underdiagnosed because of a wide spectrum of factors causing IC—infectious, toxic, immunologic, and various clinical manifestation. The processes responsible for the development of IC take place at the cellular level, which is why it is important to make the diagnosis not only based on clinical symptoms and imaging but also to confirm it with the use of histological, immunohistochemical, and molecular studies. Progress in the diagnosis and understanding of the pathomechanisms responsible for the development of IC contributed to the use of new therapeutic options. Immunosuppresive and immunomodulative treatment is still of limited use. However, in some cases of viral IC, targeted antiviral treatment can be added to the standard heart failure therapy resulting in improvement of the prognosis.

**Keywords:** myocarditis, infective heart disease, cardiomyoapthy

## 1. Introduction

Infective cardiomyopathy (IC) is a disease in which structural or/and functional heart disorders are observed as a result of present or past infection caused by various infectious agents. In the course of infective cardiomyopathy heart chambers' dilatation, heart walls' hypertrophy or restriction may occur. A relation between infection and chronic heart disease was suggested as early as 1806, when Corvisart described a cardiac inflammatory disorder that could result in progressive abnormalities of cardiac function after all the evidence of the infective agent had disappeared [1]. Because of a variety of symptoms, diagnosis of IC can be difficult [2]. Usually, the suspicion of IC is based on clinical presentation and results of noninvasive diagnostic imaging, e.g., cardiac magnetic resonance (CMR) [3]. Although endomyocardial biopsy (EMB), which can confirm myocarditis, is the gold standard in making a diagnosis, it is not often performed because of its still low availability and invasiveness. However, the interest in this method is increasing lately [2]. Although more is known about the pathophysiology of the disease, many questions remain unanswered. There are many controversions about the treatment of patients with IC, especially the most common form—viral myocarditis [3].

## 2. Etiology

Infective cardiomyopathy may be caused by many etiological factors including viruses, bacteria, rickettsiae, fungi, protozoa, and parasites. However, the spectrum of pathogens has changed over the decades and also varies geographically as, for example, *Trypanosoma cruzi* [4]. Moreover, it can result from noninfectious agents, such as allergic agents, autoimmunity, toxins, and drugs [5]. Etiological factors that could cause IC are presented in **Table 1**.

| **The most popular infective agents** | |
|---|---|
| **Viruses** | RNA viruses:<br>Coxsackieviruses A and B, Echoviruses, Polioviruses, Influenza A and B viruses, Respiratory Syncytial virus, Mumps virus, Measles virus, Rubella virus, Hepatitis C virus, Dengue virus, Yellow fever virus, Chikungunya virus, Junin virus, Lassa fever virus, Rabies virus, Human immunodeficiency virus-1<br>DNA viruses:<br>Adenoviruses, Parvovirus B19, Cytomegalovirus, Human herpesvirus-6, Epstein-Barrvirus, Varicella-zoster virus, Herpes Simplex virus, Variola virus, Vaccinia virus |
| **Bacteria** | Staphylococcus, Streptococcus, Pneumococcus, Meningococcus, Gonococcus, Salmonella, Corynebacterium diphtheria, Haemophilus influenzae, Mycobacterium tuberculosis, Mycoplasma pneumoniae, Brucella |
| **Spirochete** | Borrelia, Leptospira |
| **Fungi** | Aspergillus, Actinomyces, Blastomyces, Candida, Coccidioides, Cryptococcus, Histoplasma, Mucormyces, Nocardia, Sporothrix |
| **Protozoa** | *Trypanosoma cruzi, Toxoplasma gondii,* Entamoeba, Leishmania |
| **Parasites** | *Trichella spiralis, Echinococcus granulosus, Taenia solium* |
| **Rickettsiae** | *Coxiella burnetti, R. rickettsii, R. tsutsugamuschi* |

Source: Modified based on Ref. [2].

**Table 1.** Etiological factors of IC.

## 3. Diagnostic criteria for myocarditis

The common feature of the diseases that are called "infective heart disease" is myocarditis. Changes in myocarditis affect cardiomyocytes, interstitial tissue, vessels, and sometimes also the pericardium. Recent prospective postmortem data have implicated myocarditis in sudden cardiac death of young adults at rates of 8.6–12% [6, 7]. Furthermore, it has been identified as a cause of dilated cardiomyopathy in 9% of the cases in a large prospective series [8]. The diagnosis of myocarditis is based on histological, immunohistochemical, and immunological criteria [4].

### 3.1. Histological criteria—Dallas criteria

The Dallas criteria were proposed in 1986 and provided a histopathological categorization by which the diagnosis of myocarditis could be established (**Figure 1A** and **B**). Dallas criteria (acute) myocarditis requires an inflammatory infiltrate and necrosis or damage of adjacent muscle cells not characteristic of an ischemic event. Borderline myocarditis requires a less intense inflammatory infiltrate and no light microscopic evidence of myocyte destruction [8]. The histological diagnosis of myocarditis includes different forms, classified according to the type of inflammatory cell infiltrate: lymphocytic, eosinophilic, polymorphic, giant cell myocarditis, and cardiac sarcoidosis. The distribution and diffusion of the cellular infiltrate can be focal, confluent or diffuse, and mild, moderate or severe.

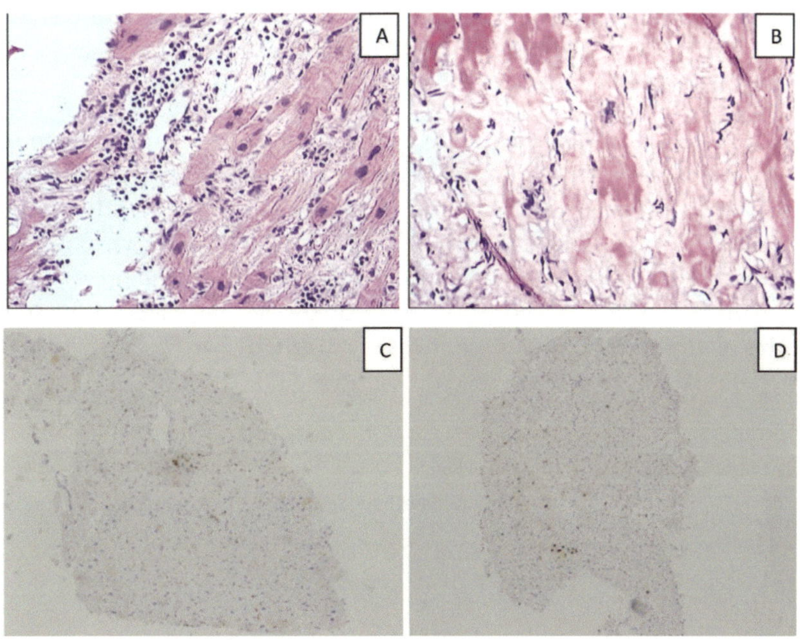


**Figure 1.** H&E staining, presenting numerous leucocytes (A) and myocyte damage (B). Immunohistochemical staining of leucocytes (C) and CD 3 lymphocytes (D).

### 3.2. Immunohistochemical criteria

The Dallas criteria are limited by the high interobserver variability in interpreting biopsy specimens (in particular with regard to borderline myocarditis) and because noncellular inflammatory processes cannot be detected (**Figure 1C** and **D**). Thus, immunohistochemistry is gaining further acceptance in the diagnosis of myocarditis. Monoclonal antibodies allow the characterization and localization of the mononuclear cell infiltrates: for example, CD3 for T cells, CD68 for activated macrophages, and human leukocyte antigen to assess HLA class II cells. With the use of these immunohistological methods, the number of EMB revealing myocarditis markedly increased. According to the World Health Organization/International Society and Federation of Cardiology Task Force on the Definition and Classification of Cardiomyopathies, EMB is considered to be inflamed by immunohistochemical detection of the inflammatory infiltration defined as: ≥14 leukocytes/mm$^2$ (including ≥7 cells/mm$^2$ CD3 + and <4 monocytes/mm$^2$) [2].

Histological assessment and immunohistochemical analysis of biopsy allow the determination of the presence of inflammation in the heart. In order to determine the etiology, many frequent further studies, including polymerase chain reaction (PCR), should be performed.

## 4. Viral infection

Viral infections are considered to be the main cause of myocarditis in Europe and in USA [9]. It is characterized by myocardial infiltrate with lymphocytes as the predominant inflammatory cell (Lymphocytic (viral) myocarditis).

With the use of molecular techniques, EMB detection of viruses is possible in up to 67% of idiopathic left ventricular dysfunction [10]. In the past, enteroviruses (especially Coxsackie B3 and B4 viruses) were assigned to be the most common cause of IC; currently, the most common viral etiologic agents are parvovirus B19 (PVB19), human herpes virus 6 (HHV 6), and cytomegalovirus (CMV) [5, 11]. It is still not known to what extent the presence of PVB19 and HHV 6 genome detected in the myocardium affects the development of inflammation. The following forms of viral heart diseases are currently distinguished based on histopathological, genetic examinations, and results of echocardiography [12] (**Table 2**):

| The form of heart disease caused by viruses | Dallas and immunohistochemical criteria | The presence of viral genome | Dilatation of left ventricle |
|---|---|---|---|
| Viral myocarditis with normal ejection fraction | + | + | – |
| Viral inflammatory cardiomyopathy | + | + | + |
| Viral heart disease | – | + | +/– |

**Table 2.** The forms of heart diseases caused by viruses based on histopathology, genetics, and echocardiography.

http://dx.doi.org/10.5772/66095

### 4.1. Parvovirus B19 (PVB19)

Parvovirus B19 is the most common cause of viral cardiomyopathy, both in the presence or without inflammation. The presence of PVB19 has been observed significantly more often in patients with an ejection fraction (EF) <45% as compared to those of EF >45% [13]. The incidence of PVB19 DNA in patients with IC ranges from 11 to 56% according to various sources [14, 15]. The presence of PVB19 is associated with a gradual deterioration of EF, and the elimination of PVB19 from the myocardium resulted in significant improvement of ventricular function [16].

### 4.2. Human hepresvirus 6 (HHV 6)

The genome of HHV 6, beside PVB19, is now one of the most frequently detected pathogens during EMB [11]. Its presence has been found in 11–18% of the EMB samples [10, 15]. What is important, HHV6 can activate infections caused by other viruses such Epstein-Barr virus (EBV) and PVB19 [17]. Both HHV 6, as well as PVB19, may remain in the infected cells for a lifetime. Therefore, such a high proportion of the genome of the virus among patients with IC can be associated with the previous infection [16, 18].

### 4.3. Enterovirus

Presently, in patients with IC, enteroviral etiology is less frequently observed. According to various sources, enteroviral RNA is found in from 3 to 53% of the patients with IC. The majority of data is related to Coxsackievirus B3 [16]. It is important that, in contrast to PVB19 and HHV 6, up to 50% of the patients with IC, spontaneous elimination of the enteroviral genome was observed, with improvement of EF [11].

### 4.4. Adenovirus

Currently, adenovirus genome is less often detected during EMB, and it is present in <2% of the biopsies [19]. Patients with adenovirusal IC often present only mild clinical symptoms, and the results of biopsies analyzed according to the Dallas criteria show mild myocarditis or borderline fulfill these criteria. Therefore, adenoviral IC may have been underestimated for many years [20].

### 4.5. Cytomegalovirus (CMV)

Currently, CMV DNA is rarely detected during EMB performed in patients with myocardial dysfunction, and the incidence is <3%; according to some sources, it is even <1% [10, 19]. However, there are reports that the presence of CMV in immunocompetent patients is associated with the occurrence of severe IC [21].

### 4.6. Influenza virus

The influenza virus may also be responsible for the development of IC [20, 22, 23], and its genome is detected in <1% of the patients with IC [16]. Infectious cardiomyopathy caused by influenza A virus may result in the development of heart failure, leading to patient's death or myocardial fibrosis with conduction defects [24]. The relationship between pandemic influenza virus H1N1 and IC is studied carefully. There are cases of acute IC observed mainly among young patients, which are associated with this pandemia [25].

### 4.7. The human immunodeficiency virus (HIV)

HIV infection may also cause myocarditis [26]. In a postmortem study of HIV-infected patients, myocarditis was established by histopathological criteria in more than 60% of the cases. However, most of these patients have discrete and unspecific abnormalities on the echocardiogram. In general, patients with advanced forms of HIV infection are subject to a high risk of developing overt myocarditis. HIV-related myocarditis is associated with a poor prognosis, especially in patients with low CD4+ counts (<400 cells/mm$^3$). These high-risk patients may develop severe left ventricular dysfunction, which could progress to advanced forms of dilated cardiomyopathy [27]. Nevertheless, it is still discussed, whether the virus, the medical treatment, or the coinfections are responsible for the development of IC in patients infected with HIV [27]. It is known that the IC related to HIV infection is characterized by a significantly worse prognosis than other lymphocytic IC [28].

### 4.8. Hepatitis C virus (HCV)

Hepatitis C virus is also considered to be the cause of IC [29]. HCV-associated cardiomyopathy can develop in genetically susceptible patients infected with HCV in whom viral, immunologic, and apoptotic mechanisms may lead to myocardial damage [30]. Hepatitis C virus not only causes myocarditis but also involved in the development of dilated cardiomyopathy, hypertrophic cardiomyopathy, and arrhythmogenic right ventricular cardiomyopathy. Frequency of HCV genomes in cardiomyopathies varies in different regions or in different populations. Major histocompatibility complex class II (MHC class II) genes may be important in the susceptibility to HCV infection and may play a role in the development of different types of cardiomyopathies. It has been suggested that interferon (IFN) treatment can be useful among these patients [31].

### 4.9. Clinical presentation

Infectious cardiomyopathy can be completely asymptomatic [32]. The most common symptoms in patients with IC are shortness of breath, chest pain, and palpitations [33]. Often cardiac manifestation of IC is preceded by flu-like symptoms, infection of upper respiratory tract, or gastrointestinal tract. Fatigue, shortness of breath, palpitations, and atypical chest pain may occur a few days or weeks later [34]. Infectious cardiomyopathy can result in development of fulminant heart failure [27]. Since some of the symptoms may resemble acute coronary syndrome (ACS), it is important to exclude coronary artery disease (CAD) and other diseases of the cardiovascular system [2]. In some cases, the only abnormality may be nonspecific ECG changes [27]. In some cases, laboratory examinations can reveal increased troponin I, troponin T, and CK-MB, suggesting myocardial injury [35]. There are four main clinical presentations of IC (**Table 3**):

http://dx.doi.org/10.5772/66095

1. Acute coronary syndrome-like
2. New onset or worsening heart failure in the absence of CAD and known causes of heart failure
3. Chronic heart failure in the absence of CAD and known causes of heart failure
4. "Life-threatening condition," in the absence of CAD and known causes of heart failure comprising

| **Clinical presentation of patients with inflammatory heart disease** | |
|---|---|
| 1. | **Acute coronary syndrome-like:** |
| | a. Acute chest pain frequently presents after respiratory or gastrointestinal infection, associated with severe or recurrent symptoms in the absence of angiographic evidence of coronary artery disease (CAD) |
| | b. ST/T wave changes: ST-segment elevation or depression or T-wave inversion |
| | c. With or without normal global or regional LV and/or RV dysfunction on echocardiography or CMR |
| | d. With or without increased TnT/TnI that may have a time course similar to acute myocardial infarction or a prolonged and sustained release over several weeks or months |
| 2. | **New onset or worsening heart failure in the absence of CAD and known causes of heart failure** |
| | a. New onset or progressive heart failure over 2 weeks to 3 months |
| | b. Impaired systolic LV and/or RV function, with or without dilated LV and/or RV on echocardiography or CMR |
| | c. Symptoms possibly started after a respiratory or a gastrointestinal infection, or in the peripartum period |
| | d. Nonspecific ECG signs, sometimes bundle branch block and/or ventricular arrhythmias and/or AV-block |
| 3. | **Chronic heart failure in the absence of CAD and known causes of heart failure (see Point 2 above)** |
| | a. Heart failure symptoms (with recurrent exacerbations) of >3 months duration |
| | b. Fatigue, palpitation, dyspnoea, atypical chest pain, and arrhythmia in ambulant patient |
| | c. Impaired systolic LV and/or RV function on echocardiography or CMR suggestive of dilated cardiomyopathy or nonischemic cardiomyopathy |
| | d. Nonspecific ECG signs, sometimes bundle branch block and/or ventricular arrhythmias and/or AV-block |
| 4. | **Life-threatening condition', in the absence of CAD and known causes of heart failure comprising:** |
| | a. Life-threatening arrhythmias and aborted sudden death |
| | b. Cardiogenic shock |
| | c. Severely impaired LV function |

Source: Based on Ref. [2].

**Table 3.** Clinical presentation of patients with IC.

### 4.10. Clinicopathological classification

Myocarditis is classified based on clinical presentation, function of left ventricle, Dallas, and immunohistochemical criteria on the following:

1. Fulminant myocarditis: a presentation with acute illness following a distinct viral syndrome. Histological study reveals multiple foci of active myocarditis. Clinical presentation consists of severe cardiovascular compromise and ventricular dysfunction. This subgroup typically either resolves spontaneously or results in death. Fulminant myocarditis in most of the cases is associated with giant cell or eosinophilic myocarditis.

2. Acute myocarditis: a presentation with insidious onset of illness and evidence of established ventricular dysfunction. This subgroup may progress to dilated cardiomyopathy.

3. Chronic active myocarditis: a presentation with insidious onset of illness with clinical and histological relapses with development of left ventricular dysfunction and associated chronic recurrent inflammatory changes.

4. Chronic persistent myocarditis: a presentation with insidious onset of illness characterized by a persistent histological infiltrate frequently with foci of myocyte necrosis. Clinically, no ventricular dysfunction is present despite other cardiovascular symptoms (such as palpitations or chest pain).

### 4.11. Diagnostics

#### *4.11.1. Electrocardiography*

Infectious cardiomyopathy is often accompanied by nonspecific ECG abnormalities (**Table 4**). The spectrum changes to include ST-segment elevation in multiple leads, generally concave, rarely of another shape. The occurrence of atrioventricular block with a mild enlargement of the left ventricle may suggest, e.g., IC in the course of Lyme disease, sarcoidosis, or multicellular myocarditis [2]. Infectious cardiomyopathy may also result in "idiopathic" atrial or ventricular arrhythmias and reduction of PQ-segment [36, 37]. The sensitivity of the ECG is determined at 47%, but the specificity remains unknown [38]. It is recommended to perform standard 12-lead ECG in patients with suspected IC [2].

#### *4.11.2. Echocardiography*

Abnormalities revealed by echocardiography are not specific for IC. However, the use of this method allows assessing both size of heart chambers and systolic and diastolic function of the heart in patients with IC. This modality can be also useful to exclude other causes of heart failure, such as valvular heart disease or other forms of cardiomyopathy (hypertrophic cardiomyopathy and restrictive cardiomyopathy). Performing echocardiography plays especially important role in the assessment of the heart before EMB—to exclude pericardial effusion and blood clots in the cavities of the heart, which are present in 25% of the patients [39]. Moreover, evaluation of echocardiographic parameters has a prognostic significance. Patients with fulminant IC often have normal heart chamber dimensions but increased intraventricular septum thickness due to myocardial edema, while in patients with acute IC dilatation of left ventricle and normal wall thickness can be observed [3, 40].

| Diagnostic criteria | |
|---|---|
| 1. | **ECG/Holter/stress test features**<br>Newly abnormal 12 lead ECG and/or Holter and/or stress testing, any of the following: I to III degree atrioventricular block, or bundle branch block, ST/T wave change (ST or non-ST elevation, T-wave inversion), sinus arrest, ventricular tachycardia or fibrillation ora systole, atriafl fibrillation, reduced R-wave height, intraventricular conduction delay (widened QRS complex), abnormal Q-waves, low voltage, frequent premature beats, supraventricular tachycardia |
| 2. | **Myocardiocytolysis markers**<br>Elevated TnT/TnI |
| 3. | **Functional and structural abnormalities on cardiac imaging (echo/angio/CMR)** new, otherwise unexplained LV and/or RV structure and function abnormality (including incidental finding in apparently asymptomatic subjects): regional wall motion nor global systolic or diastolic function abnormality, with or without ventricular dilatation, with or without increased wall thickness, with or without pericardial effusion, with or without endocavitary thrombi |
| 4. | **Tissue characterization by CMR**<br>Edema and/or LGE of classical myocarditic pattern |

Source: Based on Ref. [2].

**Table 4.** Diagnostic criteria for clinically suspected IC.

#### *4.11.3. Cardiac magnetic resonance*

The use of CMR, with the assessment of early gadolinium enhancement (EGE) and late gadolinium enhancement (LGE), is helpful in making the diagnosis of IC. In T1-weighted imaging with the assessment of the EGE, hyperintense areas show myocardium with a good blood supply, whereas the assessment of the LGE in T1-weighted imaging allows to visualize the irreversible myocardial injury resulting from the replacement of myocardial cells by fibrous tissue. Scarring and fibrosis delineated with the use of LGE-imaging are hyperechoic in contrast to normal myocardial cells. Scarring that is present in IC is located intramuscularly (typically in chronic IC) or subepicardially (typically in acute IC) [41, 42]. Location of changes in CMR enables to distinguish postinfarction scars that occur subendocardially or include the entire myocardial wall from the scars arising in the course of IC. Moreover, T2-weighted imaging reveals swelling of the myocardium, which is visible as a hyperechogenic area. Swelling in IC can be both global and regional. It reflects the reversible myocardial damage and can be present even in the absence of LGE hyperintense regions [43–45]. Cardiac magnetic resonance should be performed before EMB in hemodynamically stable patients, however, in life-threatening conditions, in which urgent EMB is necessary, it is not recommended to perform CMR [2, 46, 47].

### *4.11.4. Endomyocardial biopsy*

Endomyocardial biopsy plays an important role in the diagnosis of IC. Nevertheless, in many clinics, it is performed only in the minority of cases with a suspicion of IC or it is not performed at all because of the lack of technical possibilities and experience. However, it is important to perform EMB in every patient with suspected IC, as it is considered to be a gold standard in making the diagnosis of IC [2, 3]. In the absence of feasibility of performing EMB, patients should be transferred to a reference center [48]. According to Schultheiss, EMB should be performed in every case of suspected IC [18, 49]. This method indicates the etiology and shows type of inflammatory infiltration, which may have therapeutic implications. According to Dallas criteria, making the diagnosis of acute IC is possible based on the presence of both lymphocyte infiltration and necrosis of cardiomyocytes, while borderline IC is defined as the presence of lympocyte infiltration and lack of cardiomyocytes necrosis [48]. Together with molecular, histological, and immunohistochemical examinations, EMB allows to start antiviral treatment or immunosuppression safely. Performing EMB has the highest level of recommendation in life-threatening IC [46]. Endomyocardial biopsy should be performed early in the course of a disease and at least 8–10 specimens should be taken, each 1–2 mm in size. Samples should be examined histologically, by immunohistochemistry and for the presence of viral genome with the use of PCR (to exclude systemic infection, it is recommended to perform viral PCR in peripheral blood at the same time). If it is necessary, EMB should be repeated to monitor the effectiveness of therapy or when sampling error is suspected [2].

When ≥1 clinical presentation and ≥1 diagnostic criteria are fulfilled, coronary angiography and EMB are recommended [2].

Infectious cardiomyopathy is clinically suspected if ≥1 clinical presentation and ≥1 diagnostic criteria from different categories are fulfilled, in the absence of:

1. angiographically detectable coronary artery disease (coronary stenosis ≥50%);
2. known pre-existing cardiovascular disease or extra-cardiac causes that could explain the syndrome (e.g., valve disease, congenital heart disease, and hyperthyroidism). Suspicion is higher with higher number of fulfilled criteria. If the patient is asymptomatic, ≥2 diagnostic criteria should be met [2].

## 4.12. Treatment

In the course of IC, cardiomyocytes can be damaged by direct action of the virus, antiviral immune response, or autoimmune response. As the cardiomyocytes are not able to regenerate, improvement of myocardial function mainly depends on the tissue not affected by inflammation. Response to treatment depends on the cause of IC, and the severity of irreversible changes presents at the moment of initiation of treatment [50].

Regardless of the cause, IC therapy is based on optimal treatment of heart failure, consisting of the use of angiotensin-converting enzyme inhibitors (ACE-I)/angiotensin receptor blockers and/or β-adrenergic receptors' blockers [50–52]. There are well-known studies that confirm the efficacy of captopril and candesartan in the treatment of IC [53, 54]. Moreover, it is recommended to reduce physical activity during the acute phase of IC and for at least 6 months after the onset of the disease [2].

### 4.12.1. Antiviral treatment

Elimination of viruses from cardiomyocytes results in decrease in the symptoms reported by patients. It also affects the heart chambers' size, improvement of left ventricle EF, and reduction of long-term mortality [55]. Targeted antiviral therapy can result in total elimination of the virus genome or, even if the total elimination is not possible, it can reduce the patient's complaints. Nevertheless, starting antiviral therapy is useful only early in the course of a disease, when irreversible changes in the myocardium are not present yet [18]. In IC caused by HHV6, valacyclovir, and ganciclovir can be used [2, 17]. The use of interferon β (IFN-β) enables to eliminate adenoviruses and enteroviruses from cardiomyocytes, improving also heart efficiency. After treatment with IFN-β, increase in EF, decrease in left ventricle, reduction in heart failure symptoms, and smaller inflammatory infiltration were observed [55]. Interferon β can also be used in IC caused by PVB19—it can reduce the symptoms and endothelium dysfunction, but it has only little effect on the elimination of the virus [18]. Mechanism of beneficial clinical effects of IFN-β is not known, but IFN-β inhibits reactivation of PVB19 and improves the viability of endothelial cells [56]. Similarly, in IC caused by HHV6, treatment with IFN-β or ganciclovir does not eliminate virus from the myocardial tissue, probably because of viral genome integration with host genome. However, in patients with HHV6, IC ganciclovir reduces clinical symptoms [57].

### 4.12.2. Immunosuppression

Immunosuppression with the use of steroids, combination of steroids and azathioprine or azathioprine, cyclosporine A, and steroids is safe and efficient in IC. So far there is no data about the use of other Immunosuppresive drugs in IC treatment [2]. It is important to perform EMB before initiation of immunosuppression to exclude viral etiology of IC [50] because only patients with autoimmune IC benefit from immunosuppression [58–60]. Therefore, immunosuppression should be considered in patients with autoimmune IC, including giant-cell IC, sarcoidosis, IC in the course of "noncardiac" autoimmune diseases, who do not have contraindications for immunosuppressive therapy. The use of steroids is indicated in sarcoidosis with ventricle dysfunction and/or arrhythmia and in some cases of noninfectious eozynophilic IC or toxic IC with concomitant heart failure and/or arrhythmia. When there are no contraindications, immunosuppression can be also considered in noninfectious lymphocytic IC resistant to standard therapy [2].

### 4.12.3. High-dose intravenous immunoglobulin

No consensus exists on the benefits of high-dose intravenous immunoglobulin (IVIG) in the treatment of IC. Although there are reports confirming the improvement of left ventricular function and increase in one-year survival after application of IVIG [61], finally, it appears that this therapy has no positive effect on progression of IC [62, 63].

#### *4.12.4. Immunoabsorption*

The aim of immunoabsorption (IA) is elimination of antibodies against cardiac proteins [64]. There are some studies that confirm the efficacy of IA in dilated cardiomyopathy [65, 66]. However, multicenter, randomized studies are needed to recommend the use of IA in a standard IC therapy.

## 5. Other heart infections

### 5.1. Bacterial infections

Bacterial myocarditis with no coexisting endocarditis occurs extremely rarely. Usually, it results from massive bacteremia. *Staphylococcus aureus* is a main etiological factor of bacterial myocarditis. Nevertheless, cardiac involvement in the course of streptococcal (*Streptococcus pyogenes, Streptococcus viridans,* and *Streptococcus pneumoniae*) infection has also been reported [67]. Moreover, myocarditis can be the result of meningococcal disease or can be associated with *Salmonella, Listeria monocytogens,* or *Corynebacterium diphtheria* infection [68–71]. Bacteremia, neutropenia, myocardial infarction, osteomyelitis, and recent surgical procedures are considered to be main risk factors of bacterial myocarditis. Clinical manifestation is dominated by sepsis and heart failure symptoms. To confirm the diagnosis, EMB should be performed, revealing active myocarditis with evidence of bacterial invasion or positive tissue cultures [71]. Standard treatment consists of aggressive targeted antibiotic or antitoxin therapy and appropriate hemodynamic support, in conjunction with the treatment of arrhythmias or mechanical complications [67, 71].

#### *5.1.1. Mycobacterium tuberculosis*

Myocarditis is a very rare manifestation of Mycobacterium tuberculosis infection. There are three types of myocardial tuberculosis: nodular tubercles of the myocardium, miliary tubercles of the myocardium, and diffuse infiltrative type associated with tuberculous pericarditis. Cardiac tissue can be infected by hematogenous spread, by retrograde lymphatic spread from mediastinal lymph nodes, or directly from the pericardium. In patients with strong suspicion of cardiac tuberculosis, EMB should be performed to confirm the diagnosis. Clinical presentation is nonspecific and varies from ventricular fibrillation, long QT syndrome, congestive heart failure, and DCM to sudden cardiac arrest. However, a large number of patients are completely asymptomatic. Anti-tuberculosis therapy is usually effective; nevertheless, it does not reduce the risk of sudden cardiac death [72].

#### *5.1.2. Tropheryma whipplei*

Whipple's disease is a rare bacterial infection, which usually affects the intestinal tract, but it can also involve other organs. Cardiac manifestation of Whipple's disease occurs in 35–60% of affected patients. Infectious endocarditis with negative blood cultures develops most commonly. Whipple's disease may also present as adhesive pericarditis and myocardial fibrosis.

Lymphocytic myocarditis is unusual [73]. Cardiac involvement can clinically present as congestive heart failure, conduction disturbances, arrhythmias, or even sudden cardiac death. It is suggested that chronic damage of heart tissue is the cause of death in most patients with end-stage disease [74]. It is difficult to confirm the diagnosis due to lack of culture and serodiagnostic methods. Currently, detection of *T. whipplei* by PCR is a method of choice to establish the diagnosis. Treatment of Whipple's disease remains empirical; it is suggested to use trimethoprim-sulfamethoxazole for at least 1 year, or, alternatively, an initial parenteral therapy with penicillin and streptomycin for 2 weeks followed by trimethoprim-sulfamethoxazole [73].

### 5.2. Spirochetes infection

#### 5.2.1. *Borrelia burgdorferi*

Lyme disease (LD) that is caused by *B. burgdorferi* mostly affects skin, heart, nervous system, and joints [75]. The most common cardiac manifestation of LD is conduction and rhythm disturbances, most frequent of which is atrioventricular (AV) block [76]. However, LD can also result in myocarditis and new-onset of DCM, especially in the highly endemic area for LD [75, 77]. Serological diagnosis in patients with cardiac LD may be difficult, as IgM and IgG antibodies against *B. burgdorferi* are frequently negative at first; a measurable level of antibodies develops in the course of illness [75, 78]. Therefore, EMB can be extremely useful in making the diagnosis of DCM caused by *B. burgdorferi* [79]. Early treatment with antibiotic therapy (intravenous infusion of ceftriaxone) is effective and leads to significant improvement of left ventricle ejection fraction and reduction of heart failure symptoms [75, 79].

### 5.3. Fungal infection

Fungal myocarditis mostly develops in immunodeficient patients. Therefore, it can be often clinically latent or masked by neurological or respiratory symptoms [80].

#### 5.3.1. *Aspergillus*

Cardiac aspergillosis occurs mostly in patients with immunodeficiency or immunosuppression such as cancer, hematological conditions, or organ transplantation. Cardiac involvement occurs as a result of disseminated *Aspergillus* infection. It is associated with high mortality rate because of late diagnosis and lack of effective therapy [81].

#### 5.3.2. *Blastomycosis*

Cardiac blastomycosis can develop by an extension from pericardial blastomycosis, by a direct involvement of heart tissue, or by a lymphatic spread from mediastinal lymph nodes. It often leads to congestive heart failure, with heart chambers dilatation and little hypertrophy. The course of cardiac blastomycosis has many common features with cardiac tuberculosis [82].

#### 5.3.3. *Candida*

*Candida* is not pathogenic among immunocompetent hosts, but it can cause severe mucosal or systemic infections in immunocompromised patients [83]. *Candida* invasion of the heart significantly complicates the clinical course of candidiasis and aggravates the patients' condition and should be suspected when arrhythmia, conduction disturbance, or other QRS changes occur in patients with systemic candidiasis [84].

### 5.4. Protozoan infections

#### 5.4.1. *Trypanosoma cruzi*

Chagas disease is caused by infection with *Trypanosoma cruzi* (*T. cruzi*), which is transmitted by blood-sucking insects and small mammals. The disease is common in the southwestern part of United States, Mexico, Central, and South America [85]. Contact of skin lesions, mucosal surfaces, or the conjunctiva with parasites present in the feces of the insect leads to infection with *T. cruzi*. In nonendemic countries, transmission is also possible with blood transfusion, organ transplantation, and vertical way [86].

In the course of Chagas disease, two phases are described: an acute and a chronic phase [86]. Patients with acute Chagas disease may present nonspecific symptoms or may be completely asymptomatic. Moreover, acute myocarditis, pericardial effusion, and/or meningoencephalitis can develop in the course of acute infection [85]. In a majority of patients, the acute phase subsides spontaneously after 6–8 weeks [86]. In some of the infected patients, chronic Chagas disease develops with the symptoms from various organs [86]. Patients with chronic Chagas cardiomyopathy can present symptoms of heart failure, arrhythmias, thromboembolism (systemic or pulmonary), and chest pain [85]. Echocardiography may be useful in making the diagnosis of Chagas cardiomyopathy. It can reveal a specific pattern of segmental myocardial contractility disturbance, mainly localized in left ventricular apex and inferior-posterior wall [86]. Moreover, in chronic Chagas cardiomyopathy, echocardiography can show severe dilation of the heart chambers characteristic aneurysm localized in left ventricle's apex [85]. Because of high risk of thromboembolism, transesophageal echocardiography can be helpful to identify cardiac sources of emboli and make decision about anticoagulant treatment [85]. Histopathologically myocytolysis, reparative fibrosis, and lymphocytic infiltrates are seen in Chagas heart disease. Treatment of Chagas cardiac disease consists of targeted antiparasitic therapy and treatment of heart failure, arrhythmias, and thromboembolism [86]. Benznidazole is used to eliminate *T.cruzi*, and it is effective in acute phase [87]. Its efficacy in chronic Chagas cardiomyopathy is still discussed [86]. Angiotensin-converting enzyme (ACE) inhibitors and $\beta$-blockers can be useful in heart failure therapy. Because of high risk of thromboembolism in Chagas disease, oral anticoagulation should be considered with cardioembolic risk score for Chagas disease patients [86]. Moreover, pacemaker or ICD implantation may contribute to a better survival in some patients with Chagas disease [87].

http://dx.doi.org/10.5772/66095

### 5.5. Parasitic infection

#### *5.5.1. Echinococcus*

Echinococcal infection develops after consumption of *Echinococcus* eggs from the feces of infected dogs or other canids. In the majority of cases, the disease involves liver or lungs. Heart is a very rare localization of parasites' cysts. Cardiac echinococcosis can manifest as arrhythmias, myocardial infarction, cardiac tamponade, pulmonary hypertension syncope, purulent pericarditis, and sudden cardiac death. The basis of making the diagnosis is serology and echocardiography, which can visualize myocardial or pericardial hydatid cysts. Moreover, with the use of CMR or computed tomography calcification of the cysts' walls can be shown. Albendazole or mebendazole should be used in the treatment of cardiac echonococcosis [88].

## 6. Autoimmune heart inflammation

### 6.1. Sarcoidosis

Sarcoidosis is a systemic granulomatous disease of unknown etiology. Clinical presentation varies among patients. Sarcoidosis mostly affects skin, lymph nodes, lungs, eyes, and the central nervous system. Cardiac involvement will occur in approximately 5% of the patients with sarcoidosis [89] and varies in the different geographical regions, but it is considered to be very important prognostic factor in this disease [90]. Cardiac sarcoidosis may present as acute heart failure, ventricular arrhythmia, conduction disturbances, and even sudden death. Diagnosing cardiac sarcoidosis may be difficult due to nonspecific ECG and echocardiographic findings; therefore, it is often misdiagnosed. To make the right diagnosis, the use of endomyocardial biopsy (EMB), cardiac magnetic resonance (CMR), and $^{18}$F-fluorodeoxyglucose positron emission tomography may be helpful. Patients should be treated with corticosteroids, which help to control inflammatory process, prevent fibrosis, and protect from aggravation of the cardiac function [90].

### 6.2. Churg-Strauss syndrome (CSS)

Churg-Strauss syndrome is a rare systemic vasculitis, which affects small- and medium-sized blood vessels, characterized by eosinophil infiltration of various tissues [91]. It occurs in patients with an atopic condition, typically with a previous history of asthma or allergy disease. According to different sources, cardiac involvement is reported in 16–92% of patients with CCS [92, 93]. Cardiac changes are associated with a poor prognosis and high mortality, if not treated [94]. There are two types of cardiac involvement in CSS: vasculitis-related ischemia and eosinophilic infiltration of the myocardium. It can present as myocarditis with cardiomyopathy, pericarditis, pericardial effusion, heart failure, ventricular and supraventricular arrhythmias, and sudden cardiac death. Heart involvement is characterized by both fibrosis and an active inflammatory process. Changes visualized by CMR with LGE are mostly localized in the subendocardium [95, 96], but they can be also observed in the intramural and subepicardial myocardium [97]. Patients with cardiac involvement are mainly antineutrophil cytoplasmic antibody (ANCA)-negative. The management of myocarditis in the course of CCS includes standard therapy for heart failure and immunosuppressive treatment with steroids [98]. Initiation of treatment allows recovery of cardiac function and reduces symptoms of heart failure.

### 6.3. Systemic lupus erythematosus (SLE)

Systemic lupus erythematosus is an autoimmune disease, which usually occurs in young females. Cardiac involvement is one of the most frequent manifestations. All anatomical heart structures can be affected: pericardium, myocardium, valves, coronary arteries, and the conduction system [99]. Several autoantibodies, such as anti-phospholipid antibodies (aPL), anti-SSA/Ro antibodies, and anti-endothelial cells antibodies, can contribute to heart damage in SLE. Antibodies-SSA/Ro and anti-SSB/La antigens are responsible for the development of heart conduction disorders in the neonatal lupus syndrome.

Myocarditis is uncommon, but a serious presentation of SLE can lead to cardiac dysfunction or even sudden cardiac death [100]. Early diagnosis of lupus myocarditis is important because of the likely progression to arrhythmias, conduction disturbances, dilated cardiomyopathy, and heart failure [101]. Echocardiography is a sensitive and specific technique, and it can not only reveal global hypokinesis in patients with SLE myocarditis but also visualize other cardiac manifestations of SLE, such as pericarditis or valvular lesions [102]. In patients with lupus myocarditis, CMR shows LGE; however, it cannot differentiate these changes from myocarditis of other etiology [99]. Therefore, endomyocardial biopsy is the gold standard technique in making the diagnosis [103]. Histopathological examination shows immune complexes with mononuclear cell infiltrates, perivascular inflammation or arteriopathy, and necrosis of the cardiomyocytes [99]. Early treatment with high-dose steroids is the basis of lupus myocarditis therapy. In severe cases, intravenous pulse corticosteroid should be administered. Azathioprine, cyclophosphamide, or intravenous immunoglobulines (IVIG) may be useful [103].

## 7. Summary

Both the infectious agent and development of inflammatory response to infection can lead to irreversible myocardial injury, which affects the outcome of short- and long-term prognosis. In the case of the rapid elimination of the infectious agent and rapid withholding of inflammatory process, changes in myocardium are small. If the immune response does not lead to complete elimination of infectious agent or inflammation progresses after removing the virus, chronic myocardial damage may develop. Persistence of the virus in myocardium, postinfectious immune reaction, autoimmunity, and primary cardiac damage may result in the development of progressive ventricular dysfunction, development of cardiac arrhythmias, and exacerbation of symptoms [18]. Because of long-term consequences, it is important to diagnose IC quickly and start appropriate treatment. However, IC is still diagnostic challenge.

http://dx.doi.org/10.5772/66095

Infective cardiomyopathy is often underdiagnosed because of a wide spectrum of factors causing IC—infectious, toxic, immunologic, and various clinical manifestations [3]. The processes responsible for the development of IC take place at the cellular level, which is why it is important to make the diagnosis not only based on clinical symptoms and imaging but also to confirm it with the use of histological, immunohistochemical, and molecular studies [18]. Progress in the diagnosis and understanding of the pathomechanisms responsible for the development of IC contributed to the use of new therapeutic options. Immunosuppresive and immunomodulative treatment is still of limited use [2]. However, in some cases of viral IC, targeted antiviral treatment can be added to standard heart failure therapy resulting in improvement of the prognosis [18].

## Acknowledgements

Funding provided by The National Science Center (Poland) grant No. 2014/13/B/NZ4/03832.

## Author details

Agnieszka Pawlak[1,2*] and Robert Julian Gil[1,2]

*Address all correspondence to: a.pawlak1@wp.pl

1 Mossakowski Medical Research Centre, Polish Academy of Sciences, Warsaw, Poland

2 Central Clinical Hospital of the Ministry of Interior, Department of Invasive Cardiology, Warsaw, Poland

## References

[1] Kearney, M.T., et al., Viral myocarditis and dilated cardiomyopathy: mechanisms, manifestations, and management. Postgrad Med J, 2001. 77(903): pp. 4–10.

[2] Caforio, A.L., et al., Current state of knowledge on aetiology, diagnosis, management, and therapy of myocarditis: a position statement of the European Society of Cardiology Working Group on Myocardial and Pericardial Diseases. Eur Heart J, 2013. 34(33): pp. 2636–48, 48a–d.

[3] Kindermann, I., et al., Update on myocarditis. J Am Coll Cardiol, 2012. 59(9): pp. 779–92.

[4] Richardson, P., et al., Report of the 1995 World Health Organization/International Society and Federation of Cardiology Task Force on the Definition and Classification of cardiomyopathies. Circulation, 1996. 93(5): pp. 841–2.

[5] Maisch, B. and S. Pankuweit, Standard and etiology-directed evidence-based therapies in myocarditis: state of the art and future perspectives. Heart Fail Rev, 2013. 18(6): pp. 761–95.

[6] Fabre, A. and M.N. Sheppard, Sudden adult death syndrome and other non-ischaemic causes of sudden cardiac death. Heart, 2006. 92(3): pp. 316–20.

[7] Doolan, A., N. Langlois, and C. Semsarian, Causes of sudden cardiac death in young Australians. Med J Aust, 2004. 180(3): pp. 110–2.

[8] Felker, G.M., et al., The spectrum of dilated cardiomyopathy. The Johns Hopkins experience with 1,278 patients. Medicine (Baltimore), 1999. 78(4): pp. 270–83.

[9] Andreoletti, L., et al., Viral causes of human myocarditis. Arch Cardiovasc Dis, 2009. 102(6–7): pp. 559–68.

[10] Kuhl, U., et al., High prevalence of viral genomes and multiple viral infections in the myocardium of adults with "idiopathic" left ventricular dysfunction. Circulation, 2005. 111(7): pp. 887–93.

[11] Kuhl, U., et al., Viral persistence in the myocardium is associated with progressive cardiac dysfunction. Circulation, 2005. 112(13): pp. 1965–70.

[12] Maisch, B., V. Ruppert, and S. Pankuweit, Management of fulminant myocarditis: a diagnosis in search of its etiology but with therapeutic options. Curr Heart Fail Rep, 2014. 11(2): pp. 166–77.

[13] Maisch, B. and S. Pankuweit, Current treatment options in (peri)myocarditis and inflammatory cardiomyopathy. Herz, 2012. 37(6): pp. 644–56.

[14] Klein, R.M., et al., Frequency and quantity of the parvovirus B19 genome in endomyocardial biopsies from patients with suspected myocarditis or idiopathic left ventricular dysfunction. Z Kardiol, 2004. 93(4): pp. 300–9.

[15] Mahrholdt, H., et al., Presentation, patterns of myocardial damage, and clinical course of viral myocarditis. Circulation, 2006. 114(15): pp. 1581–90.

[16] Pankuweit, S. and K. Klingel, Viral myocarditis: from experimental models to molecular diagnosis in patients. Heart Fail Rev, 2013. 18(6): pp. 683–702.

[17] Krueger, G.R. and D.V. Ablashi, Human herpesvirus-6: a short review of its biological behavior. Intervirology, 2003. 46(5): pp. 257–69.

[18] Kuhl, U. and H.P. Schultheiss, Viral myocarditis. Swiss Med Wkly, 2014. 144: p. w14010.

[19] Kandolf, R., et al., Molecular mechanisms and consequences of cardiac viral infections. Pathologe, 2008. 29(Suppl. 2): pp. 112–7.

[20] Bowles, N.E., et al., Detection of viruses in myocardial tissues by polymerase chain reaction. Evidence of adenovirus as a common cause of myocarditis in children and adults. J Am Coll Cardiol, 2003. 42(3): pp. 466–72.

[21] Kyto, V., et al., Cytomegalovirus infection of the heart is common in patients with fatal myocarditis. Clin Infect Dis, 2005. 40(5): pp. 683–8.

[22] Calabrese, F., et al., Overexpression of tumor necrosis factor (TNF)alpha and TNFalpha receptor I in human viral myocarditis: clinicopathologic correlations. Mod Pathol, 2004. 17(9): pp. 1108–18.

[23] Mamas, M.A., D. Fraser, and L. Neyses, Cardiovascular manifestations associated with influenza virus infection. Int J Cardiol, 2008. 130(3): pp. 304–9.

[24] Kuiken, T. and J.K. Taubenberger, Pathology of human influenza revisited. Vaccine, 2008. 26(Suppl. 4): pp. D59–66.

[25] Gdynia, G., et al., Sudden death of an immunocompetent young adult caused by novel (swine origin) influenza A/H1N1-associated myocarditis. Virchows Arch, 2011. 458(3): pp. 371–6.

[26] Sudano, I., et al., Cardiovascular disease in HIV infection. Am Heart J, 2006. 151(6): pp. 1147–55.

[27] Magnani, J.W. and G.W. Dec, Myocarditis: current trends in diagnosis and treatment. Circulation, 2006. 113(6): pp. 876–90.

[28] Barbaro, G., et al., Incidence of dilated cardiomyopathy and detection of HIV in myocardial cells of HIV-positive patients. Italian Group for the Study of Cardiology Patients Suffering from AIDS. N Engl J Med, 1998. 339(16): pp. 1093–9.

[29] Matsumori, A., et al., Myocarditis and heart failure associated with hepatitis C virus infection. J Card Fail, 2006. 12(4): pp. 293–8.

[30] Sanchez, M.J. and N.V. Bergasa, Hepatitis C associated cardiomyopathy: potential pathogenic mechanisms and clinical implications. Med Sci Monit, 2008. 14(5): pp. RA55–63.

[31] Matsumori, A., Role of hepatitis C virus in cardiomyopathies. Ernst Schering Res Found Workshop, 2006. 55: pp. 99–120.

[32] Maze, S.S. and R.J. Adolph, Myocarditis: unresolved issues in diagnosis and treatment. Clin Cardiol, 1990. 13(2): pp. 69–79.

[33] Hufnagel, G., et al., The European Study of Epidemiology and Treatment of Cardiac Inflammatory Diseases (ESETCID). First epidemiological results. Herz, 2000. 25(3): pp. 279–85.

[34] Dec, G.W., Jr., et al., Active myocarditis in the spectrum of acute dilated cardiomyopathies. Clinical features, histologic correlates, and clinical outcome. N Engl J Med, 1985. 312(14): pp. 885–90.

[35] Schultz, J.C., et al., Diagnosis and treatment of viral myocarditis. Mayo Clin Proc, 2009. 84(11): pp. 1001–9.

[36] Wang, K., R.W. Asinger, and H.J. Marriott, ST-segment elevation in conditions other than acute myocardial infarction. N Engl J Med, 2003. 349(22): pp. 2128–35.

[37] Dennert, R., H.J. Crijns, and S. Heymans, Acute viral myocarditis. Eur Heart J, 2008. 29(17): pp. 2073–82.

[38] Liu, P.P. and A.T. Yan, Cardiovascular magnetic resonance for the diagnosis of acute myocarditis: prospects for detecting myocardial inflammation. J Am Coll Cardiol, 2005. 45(11): pp. 1823–5.

[39] Blauwet, L.A. and L.T. Cooper, Myocarditis. Prog Cardiovasc Dis, 2010. 52(4): pp. 274–88.

[40] Felker, G.M., et al., Echocardiographic findings in fulminant and acute myocarditis. J Am Coll Cardiol, 2000. 36(1): pp. 227–32.

[41] Petryka, J., et al., Cardiovascular magnetic resonance in the diagnosis of myocarditis. Kardiol Pol, 2010. 68(7): pp. 824–9.

[42] Hunold, P., et al., Myocardial late enhancement in contrast-enhanced cardiac MRI: distinction between infarction scar and non-infarction-related disease. Am J Roentgenol, 2005. 184(5): pp. 1420–6.

[43] Friedrich, M.G., et al., Cardiovascular magnetic resonance in myocarditis: A JACC White Paper. J Am Coll Cardiol, 2009. 53(17): pp. 1475–87.

[44] Abdel-Aty, H., et al., Delayed enhancement and T2-weighted cardiovascular magnetic resonance imaging differentiate acute from chronic myocardial infarction. Circulation, 2004. 109(20): pp. 2411–6.

[45] Aletras, A.H., et al., Retrospective determination of the area at risk for reperfused acute myocardial infarction with T2-weighted cardiac magnetic resonance imaging: histopathological and displacement encoding with stimulated echoes (DENSE) functional validations. Circulation, 2006. 113(15): pp. 1865–70.

[46] Cooper, L.T., et al., The role of endomyocardial biopsy in the management of cardiovascular disease: a scientific statement from the American Heart Association, the American College of Cardiology, and the European Society of Cardiology. Endorsed by the Heart Failure Society of America and the Heart Failure Association of the European Society of Cardiology. J Am Coll Cardiol, 2007. 50(19): pp. 1914–31.

[47] Yilmaz, A., et al., Comparative evaluation of left and right ventricular endomyocardial biopsy: differences in complication rate and diagnostic performance. Circulation, 2010. 122(9): pp. 900–9.

[48] Aretz, H.T., Myocarditis: the Dallas criteria. Hum Pathol, 1987. 18(6): pp. 619–24.

[49] Kuhl, U., et al., Interferon-Beta improves survival in enterovirus-associated cardiomyopathy. J Am Coll Cardiol, 2012. 60(14): pp. 1295–6.

[50] Schultheiss, H.P., U. Kuhl, and L.T. Cooper, The management of myocarditis. Eur Heart J, 2011. 32(21): pp. 2616–25.

[51] Dickstein, K., et al., ESC Guidelines for the diagnosis and treatment of acute and chronic heart failure 2008: the Task Force for the Diagnosis and Treatment of Acute and Chronic Heart Failure 2008 of the European Society of Cardiology. Developed in collaboration with the Heart Failure Association of the ESC (HFA) and endorsed by the European Society of Intensive Care Medicine (ESICM). Eur Heart J, 2008. 29(19): pp. 2388–442.

[52] Hunt, S.A., et al., 2009 Focused update incorporated into the ACC/AHA 2005 Guidelines for the Diagnosis and Management of Heart Failure in Adults. A Report of the American College of Cardiology Foundation/American Heart Association Task Force on Practice Guidelines Developed in Collaboration With the International Society for Heart and Lung Transplantation. J Am Coll Cardiol, 2009. 53(15): pp. e1–e90.

[53] Rezkalla, S.H., S. Raikar, and R.A. Kloner, Treatment of viral myocarditis with focus on captopril. Am J Cardiol, 1996. 77(8): pp. 634–7.

[54] Saegusa, S., et al., Oral administration of candesartan improves the survival of mice with viral myocarditis through modification of cardiac adiponectin expression. Cardiovasc Drugs Ther, 2007. 21(3): pp. 155–60.

[55] Kuhl, U., et al., Interferon-beta treatment eliminates cardiotropic viruses and improves left ventricular function in patients with myocardial persistence of viral genomes and left ventricular dysfunction. Circulation, 2003. 107(22): pp. 2793–8.

[56] Schmidt-Lucke, C., et al., Interferon beta modulates endothelial damage in patients with cardiac persistence of human parvovirus b19 infection. J Infect Dis, 2010. 201(6): pp. 936–45.

[57] Kuhl, U., et al., Chromosomally integrated human herpesvirus 6 in heart failure: prevalence and treatment. Eur J Heart Fail, 2015. 17(1): pp. 9–19.

[58] Juhl, U., B.E. Strauer, and H.P. Schultheiss, Methylprednisolone in chronic myocarditis. Postgrad Med J, 1994. 70(Suppl. 1): pp. S35–42.

[59] Frustaci, A., et al., Immunosuppressive therapy for active lymphocytic myocarditis: virological and immunologic profile of responders versus nonresponders. Circulation, 2003. 107(6): pp. 857–63.

[60] Frustaci, A., M.A. Russo, and C. Chimenti, Randomized study on the efficacy of immunosuppressive therapy in patients with virus-negative inflammatory cardiomyopathy: the TIMIC study. Eur Heart J, 2009. 30(16): pp. 1995–2002.

[61] Drucker, N.A., et al., Gamma-globulin treatment of acute myocarditis in the pediatric population. Circulation, 1994. 89(1): pp. 252–7.

[62] McNamara, D.M., et al., Controlled trial of intravenous immune globulin in recent-onset dilated cardiomyopathy. Circulation, 2001. 103(18): pp. 2254–9.

[63] Klugman, D., et al., Pediatric patients hospitalized with myocarditis: a multi-institutional analysis. Pediatr Cardiol, 2010. 31(2): pp. 222–8.

[64] Felix, S.B., et al., Removal of cardiodepressant antibodies in dilated cardiomyopathy by immunoadsorption. J Am Coll Cardiol, 2002. 39(4): pp. 646–52.

[65] Felix, S.B., et al., Hemodynamic effects of immunoadsorption and subsequent immunoglobulin substitution in dilated cardiomyopathy: three-month results from a randomized study. J Am Coll Cardiol, 2000. 35(6): pp. 1590–8.

[66] Doesch, A.O., et al., Effects of protein A immunoadsorption in patients with advanced chronic dilated cardiomyopathy. J Clin Apher, 2009. 24(4): pp. 141–9.

[67] Wasi, F. and J. Shuter, Primary bacterial infection of the myocardium. Front Biosci, 2003. 8: pp. s228–31.

[68] Taldir, G., et al., Acute right-sided heart failure caused by *Neisseria meningitidis*. J Clin Microbiol, 2013. 51(1): pp. 363–5.

[69] Childs, L. and S. Gupta, *Salmonella enteritidis* induced myocarditis in a 16-year-old girl. BMJ Case Rep, 2012. Nov 27. doi: 10.1136/bcr-2012-007628.

[70] Sagar, S., P.P. Liu, and L.T. Cooper, Jr., Myocarditis. Lancet, 2012. 379(9817): pp. 738–47.

[71] Haddad, F., et al., Active bacterial myocarditis: a case report and review of the literature. J Heart Lung Transplant, 2007. 26(7): pp. 745–9.

[72] Michira, B.N., F.O. Alkizim, and D.M. Matheka, Patterns and clinical manifestations of tuberculous myocarditis: a systematic review of cases. Pan Afr Med J, 2015. 21: p. 118.

[73] Dutly, F. and M. Altwegg, Whipple's disease and *Tropheryma whippelii*. Clin Microbiol Rev, 2001. 14(3): pp. 561–83.

[74] de Takats, P.G., et al., Symptomatic cardiomyopathy as a presentation in Whipple's disease. Postgrad Med J, 1995. 71(834): pp. 236–9.

[75] Palecek, T., et al., Presence of *Borrelia burgdorferi* in endomyocardial biopsies in patients with new-onset unexplained dilated cardiomyopathy. Med Microbiol Immunol, 2010. 199(2): pp. 139–43.

http://dx.doi.org/10.5772/66095

[76] Lelovas, P., et al., Cardiac implications of Lyme disease, diagnosis and therapeutic approach. Int J Cardiol, 2008. 129(1): pp. 15–21.

[77] Cox, J. and M. Krajden, Cardiovascular manifestations of Lyme disease. Am Heart J, 1991. 122(5): pp. 1449–55.

[78] Bateman, H. and L. Sigal, Update on Lyme Carditis. Curr Infect Dis Rep, 2000. 2(4): pp. 299–301.

[79] Kuchynka, P., et al., Recent-onset dilated cardiomyopathy associated with *Borrelia burgdorferi* infection. Herz, 2015. 40(6): pp. 892–7.

[80] Hofman, P., et al., Fungal myocarditis in acquired immunodeficiency syndrome. Arch Mal Coeur Vaiss, 1992. 85(2): pp. 203–8.

[81] Xie, L., et al., Cardiac aspergillosis in patients with acquired immunodeficiency syndrome: a case report and review of the literature. Arch Pathol Lab Med, 2005. 129(4): pp. 511–5.

[82] Baker, R.D. and E.W. Brian, Blastomycosis of the heart: Report of two cases. Am J Pathol, 1937. 13(1): pp. 139–147.

[83] Smeekens, S.P., et al., Genetic susceptibility to Candida infections. EMBO Mol Med, 2013. 5(6): pp. 805–13.

[84] Franklin, W.G., A.B. Simon, and T.M. Sodeman, *Candida* myocarditis without valvulitis. Am J Cardiol, 1976. 38(7): pp. 924–8.

[85] Aiello, V.D. and F.P. de Campos, Chronic Chagas cardiomyopathy. Autops Case Rep, 2015. 5(3): pp. 7–9.

[86] Biolo, A., A.L. Ribeiro, and N. Clausell, Chagas cardiomyopathy—where do we stand after a hundred years? Prog Cardiovasc Dis, 2010. 52(4): pp. 300–16.

[87] Rassi, A., Jr., A. Rassi, and W.C. Little, Chagas heart disease. Clin Cardiol, 2000. 23(12): pp. 883–9.

[88] Hidron, A., et al., Cardiac involvement with parasitic infections. Clin Microbiol Rev, 2010. 23(2): pp. 324–49.

[89] Birnie, D.H., et al., Cardiac manifestations of sarcoidosis: diagnosis and management. Eur Heart J, 2016 Jul 28. pii: ehw328.

[90] Kusano, K.F. and K. Satomi, Diagnosis and treatment of cardiac sarcoidosis. Heart, 2016. 102(3): pp. 184–90.

[91] Correia, A.S., et al., Churg-Strauss syndrome presenting with eosinophilic myocarditis: a diagnostic challenge. Rev Port Cardiol, 2013. 32(9): pp. 707–11.

[92] Sinico, R.A., et al., Prevalence and clinical significance of antineutrophil cytoplasmic antibodies in Churg-Strauss syndrome. Arthritis Rheum, 2005. 52(9): pp. 2926–35.

[93] Guillevin, L., et al., Churg-Strauss syndrome. Clinical study and long-term follow-up of 96 patients. Medicine (Baltimore), 1999. 78(1): pp. 26–37.

[94] Knockaert, D.C., Cardiac involvement in systemic inflammatory diseases. Eur Heart J, 2007. 28(15): p. 1797–804.

[95] Wassmuth, R., et al., Cardiovascular magnetic resonance imaging detects cardiac involvement in Churg-Strauss syndrome. J Card Fail, 2008. 14(10): pp. 856–60.

[96] Neumann, T., et al., Cardiac involvement in Churg-Strauss syndrome: impact of endomyocarditis. Medicine (Baltimore), 2009. 88(4): pp. 236–43.

[97] Szczeklik, W., et al., Multimodality assessment of cardiac involvement in Churg-Strauss syndrome patients in clinical remission. Circ J, 2011. 75(3): pp. 649–55.

[98] Chen, M.X., et al., Eosinophilic myocarditis due to Churg-Strauss syndrome mimicking reversible dilated cardiomyopathy. Heart Lung, 2014. 43(1): pp. 45–7.

[99] Miner, J.J. and A.H. Kim, Cardiac manifestations of systemic lupus erythematosus. Rheum Dis Clin North Am, 2014. 40(1): pp. 51–60.

[100] Zhang, L., et al., Lupus Myocarditis: a case-control study from China. Chin Med J (Engl), 2015. 128(19): pp. 2588–94.

[101] Wijetunga, M. and S. Rockson, Myocarditis in systemic lupus erythematosus. Am J Med, 2002. 113(5): pp. 419–23.

[102] Doria, A., et al., Cardiac involvement in systemic lupus erythematosus. Lupus, 2005. 14(9): pp. 683–6.

[103] Tincani, A., et al., Heart involvement in systemic lupus erythematosus, anti-phospholipid syndrome and neonatal lupus. Rheumatology (Oxford), 2006. 45(Suppl. 4): pp. iv8–13.

Chapter 11

# Novel Insights into the Pathophysiology of Chagas' Cardiomyopathy

Philipp Stahl and Thomas Meyer

Additional information is available at the end of the chapter

http://dx.doi.org/10.5772/65945

**Abstract**

The protozoan hemoflagellate *Trypanosoma cruzi* (*T. cruzi*) is the etiologic agent of the zoonotic Chagas' disease that affects approximately six to seven million people in Central and South America, causing dilated cardiomyopathy and megavisceral disease. Although Chagas' disease is the leading cause of heart failure in Latin America among people living in poverty and places an immense socioeconomic burden on society, it is still currently classified as a neglected tropical disease (NTD). The disease is typically transmitted by *reduviid* bugs or orally by contaminated food, while the transmission of parasitic organisms by other routes such as blood transfusion, organ transplantation, and transplacental infection is relatively rare. Given the wide cellular tropism infecting virtually all nucleated cells, the protozoan is able to persist asymptomatically for decades until ultimately causing organ-specific symptoms of chronic Chagas' disease such as chronic heart failure. The acute phase of the disease triggers an immune response that often does not restrict the dissemination of the parasite and may cause skin lesions, fever, enlarged lymph nodes, pallor, swelling, and abdominal and chest pain. Despite recent advances in our knowledge about the pathogenesis of this disease, the complex host-parasite interactions are not completely understood and, in particular, the persistence of parasites in host cells for such a long time remains largely undefined. In this book chapter, we focus on the pathophysiology of American trypanosomiasis and emphasize the role of host-specific transcription factors executing antiparasitic immune reactions.

**Keywords:** *Trypanosoma cruzi*, Chagas' disease, dilated cardiomyopathy, immune response, STAT transcription factors, apoptosis

## 1. Introduction

The pathogenic protozoan *Trypanosoma cruzi* (*T. cruzi*) is the causative agent of Chagas' disease, and more than 150 species of mammals are affected by this unicellular parasite, including humans. The parasite was discovered in 1909 by the Brazilian physician Carlos Chagas, while dissecting assassin bugs (*Reduviidae*) from the subfamily *Triatominae* that act as vectors and hosts for the parasite, and was later named after Chagas' scientific mentor Oswaldo Cruz [1].

Chagas' disease, also termed American trypanosomiasis, causes the third largest disease burden of the tropics after malaria and schistosomiasis [2] and is responsible for higher morbidity and mortality than any other parasitic infection in America [3]. According to surveys of the World Health Organization (WHO) from 2014, six to seven million people worldwide are estimated to be infected with *T. cruzi*, while around 14,000 patients die annually as a result of the parasitosis. An overview of the geographic distribution of Chagas' disease is presented in **Figure 1**.

The link between poverty and dissemination of Chagas' disease is striking, as it particularly affects people living in simple huts made of mud and wood with roofs of straw or palm leaves in rural areas of Latin America, where the predatory bugs have easy access. In the most important endemic areas, vectors include *Panstrongylus megistus, Triatoma infestans, T. dimidiata, T. pallidipennis,* and *Rhodnius prolixus* [4] (**Figure 2**). Non-vectorial transmission, such as the ingestion of *T. cruzi*-contaminated food and congenital transmission from the mother to the fetus [5] as well as blood transfusion and organ transplantation, increase the number of people at risk, estimated at 100 million worldwide. Owing to international migration, isolated cases of Chagas' disease in nonendemic countries are increasingly being recognized.

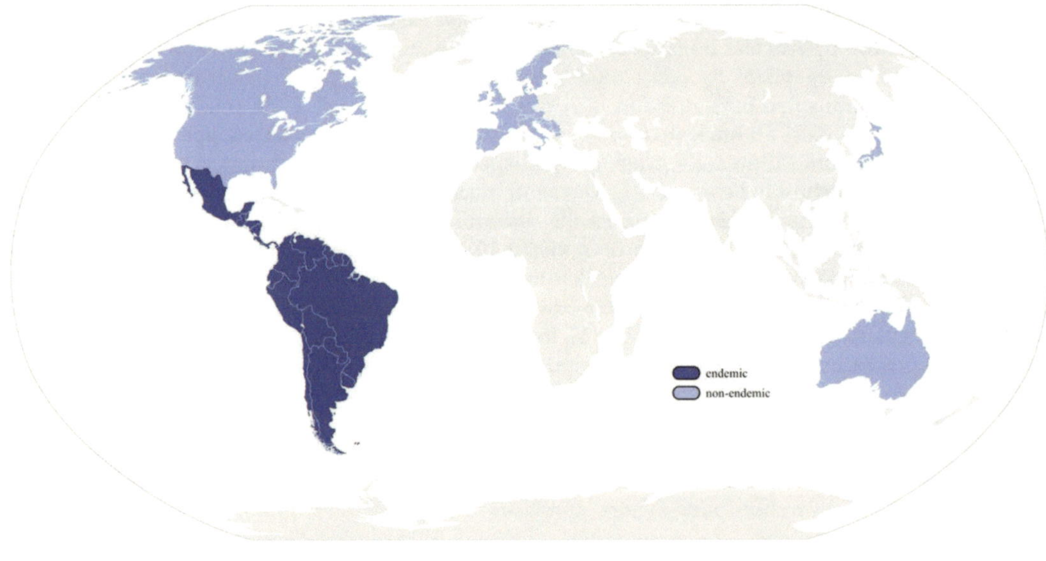


**Figure 1.** Geographical distribution of Chagas' disease. Dark blue indicates endemic countries and light blue nonendemic countries.

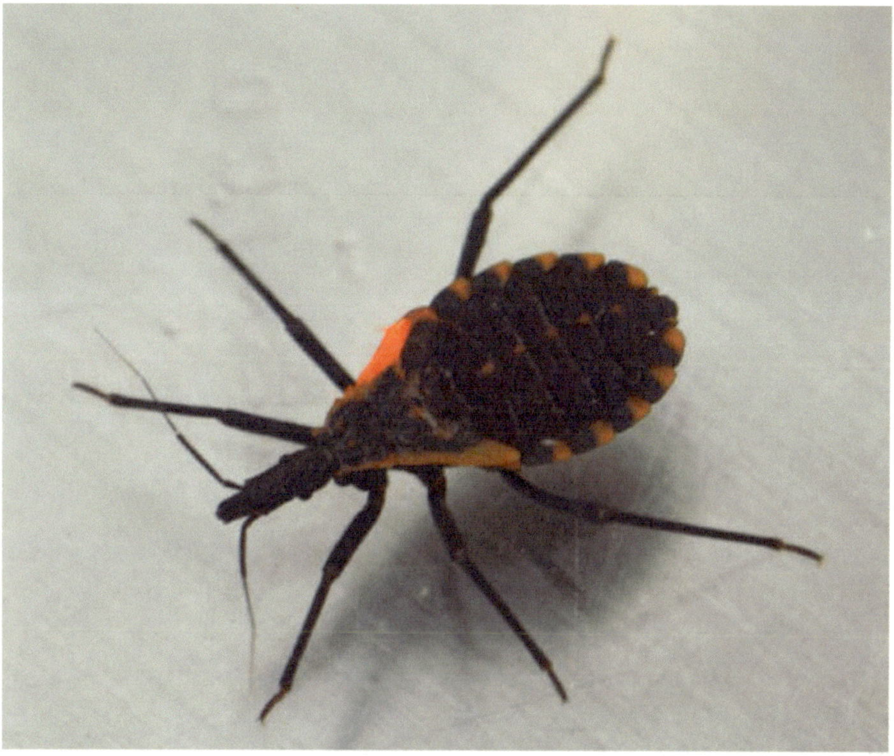

**Figure 2.** *Meccus pallidipennis* (syn. *Triatoma pallidipennis*, Hemiptera: *Reduviidae*) from the subfamily *Triatominae* as a vector for *T. cruzi*.

## 2. Biology and life cycle of *T. cruzi*

Assassin bugs infected with *T. cruzi* preferably sting sleeping victims and usually suck their blood unnoticed. After the blood meal, the pressure in the bug's gastrointestinal tract increases and the insect defecates on the skin near the wound. This behavior of *Triatominae* is crucial for their ability to act as a vector for *T. cruzi*, since infective stages of *T. cruzi* reach the stab wound only when the bugs defecate during food intake. The assassin bug transmits the parasites to the definitive host, by spreading excrement on the wound while escaping. When the pathogen-containing feces are rubbed into the fresh puncture wound by the victim or when the pathogen penetrates into uninjured mucosa, especially those of the eye, highly infectious and very motile metacyclic trypomastigotes of *T. cruzi* are transmitted into the blood flow of the host [6, 7] (**Figure 3**). The trypomastigotes are then disseminated successively into the organism of the host, and preferably infect cells of the reticuloendothelial and mononuclear phagocytic system [8]. A parasitophorous vacuole is formed only briefly during the life cycle of *T. cruzi*, while the intracellular parasites multiply in the cytoplasm of the host cell by binary division [9, 10].

*T. cruzi* can infect any nucleated cell but predominantly replicates in cardiac muscle cells as well as in cells of the nervous system, gonads, intestinal mucosa, and placenta [11]. After penetration into the cytoplasm of the host cell, the morphology of the metacyclic trypomastigotes

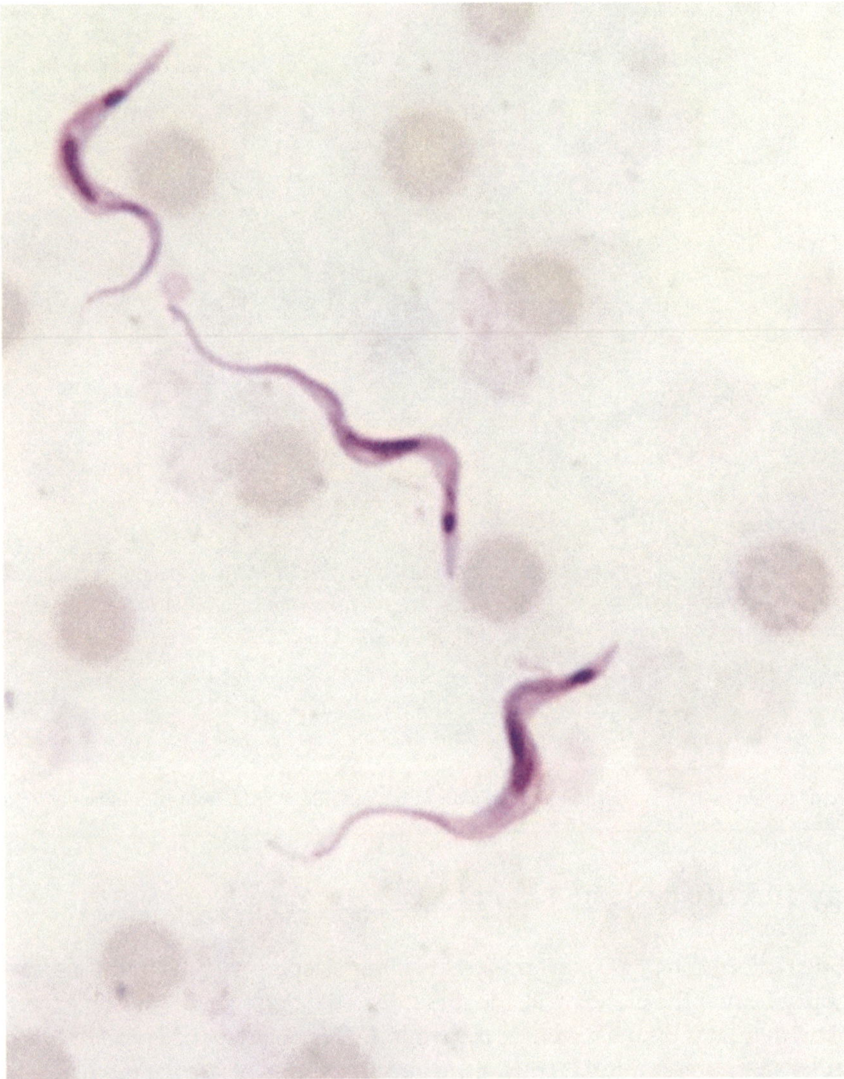

**Figure 3.** *Trypanosoma cruzi* metacyclic trypomastigotes on a peripheral blood smear shown by Giemsa staining.

changes to intracellular amastigotes with diameters of 3–5 μm, when they lose their undulating membrane which is a characteristic feature of mobile trypomastigotes [9, 12] (**Figure 4**). Intracellular amastigotes undergo several rounds of division and are then transformed into trypomastigotes, approximately 20-μm long, which leave the host cell and spread further into the organism to infect new host cells [13]. Unlike the African sleeping sickness caused by *T. brucei*, intracellular replication of *T. cruzi* in host cells is mandatory, since the pathogenic agent of American trypanosomiasis is not able to divide in the blood. For this reason, the intracellular amastigote form of *T. cruzi* is always present and can be histopathologically detected in tissue samples from spleen, liver, brain, and heart muscle. The life cycle of *T. cruzi* continues when the bug takes a blood meal from an infected host, and the parasites transform in the

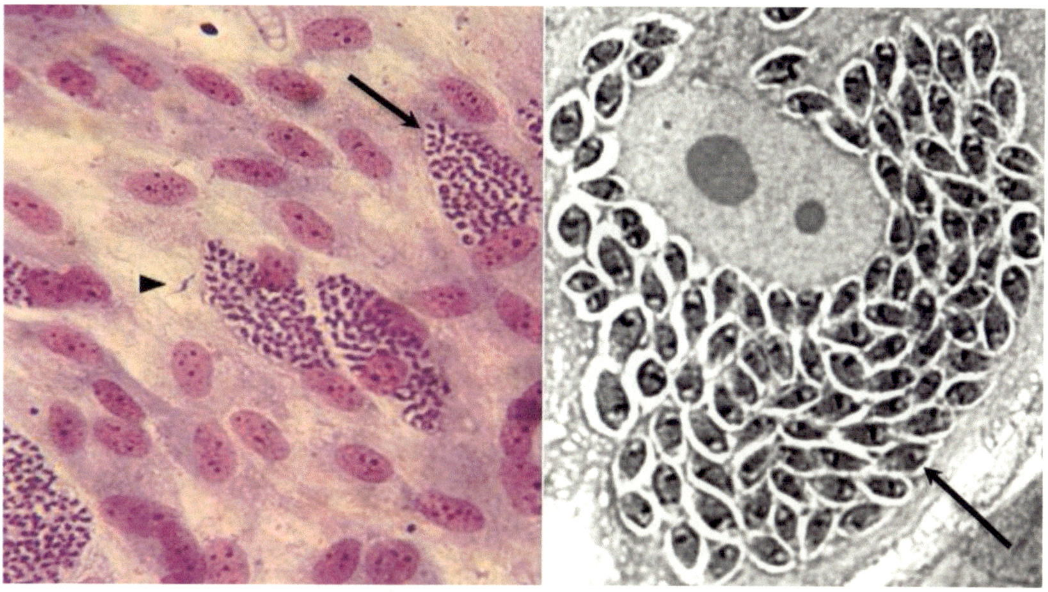

**Figure 4.** Intracytoplasmic localization of *T. cruzi* amastigotes in cultured fibroblasts stained with Giemsa at low (left) and high (right) magnification. Arrows mark intracellular amastigotes, and the arrow head (left) indicates an extracellular trypomastigote.

bug´s midgut to epimastigote forms and multiply by binary fission. Finally, the highly infectious metacyclic trypomastigotes develop in the rectum of the bug, and will be passed again with the feces during a subsequent second blood meal [14].

## 3. Epidemiology

Following a decline in incidence in endemic countries of Latin America, recorded in the mid-1990s up to the beginning of this millennium due to vector-eradication campaigns, Chagas' disease is currently worldwide on the rise again even in Europe [15–21]. Alternative transmission modes of Chagas' disease, such as congenital infection and infection through contaminated blood and organ donations, now play a major role both in classical endemic areas and in countries outside Latin America due to an increase in worldwide migration. The disease is, therefore, increasingly being detected in Europe, since more than 14 million people have left the endemic areas of South America, four to five million for Europe [22]. In a statement from the WHO for Chagas' disease in Europe in 2010, the number of *T. cruzi*-infected individuals in Europe is estimated at 80,000–100,000. Switzerland is home to a group of people at risk, and it is estimated that of the approximately 40,000 legal immigrants from Latin America, 2000–4000 people may have become infected with this pathogen [23]. In Spain, the estimated number of people infected with *T. cruzi*, most of these being legal immigrants from South America, is 25,000–48,000 [17, 18].

Chagas' disease can also pose a threat to Germany. The data collection among the approximately 85,000 immigrants coming from endemic areas is, however, incomplete. It is estimated that the prevalence of seropositive immigrants is 1.3–1.7% (1100–1450-infected individuals); however, it is assumed that the number of patients is significantly underdiagnosed with Chagas' disease [18, 24]. Epidemiological data from the United States of America estimated up to a million people infected with *T. cruzi*, and for the entire American continent including Mexico up to seven million [25]. In South America, Bolivia is the country with by far the highest infection rate, and serological screening in maternity hospitals detected up to 23.6% pregnant women infected with the parasite [26]. Recent data also underline the spread with increasing prevalence of Chagas' disease in Australia and New Zealand [27].

## 4. Symptomatology of Chagas' disease

Infection with *T. cruzi* can be divided into three distinct phases: the acute, indeterminate (latent), and chronic phase. The acute phase is characterized by the detection of circulating trypomastigotes in the blood. The majority of patients infected in adulthood are asymptomatic or show only mild and nonspecific symptoms. Children, however, are much more susceptible to a recognizable acute infection with *T. cruzi* and often have a higher parasitemia than adults. After an incubation period of 1–3 weeks, local inflammatory reactions develop at the entry point. In about half of all cases, the eye is the primary portal of entry. Parasites penetrate transconjunctivally into mesenchymal cells or are phagocytosed by macrophages and cause a local inflammatory reaction. Characteristic for acute Chagas' disease is a periorbital edema accompanied by conjunctivitis, which is termed Româna's sign.

Inflammatory lesions or nodules on the puncture wound in the face are less frequently observed manifestations of the acute stage (Chagoma), indicating a local inflammatory response with tissue destruction. Invasion of neutrophils and activation of tissue macrophages result in the secretion of pro-inflammatory cytokines such as tumor necrosis factor-$\alpha$ (TNF-$\alpha$) and interferon-$\gamma$ (IFN-$\gamma$). After a further 1–2 weeks, the stage of hematogenous and lymphatic spread is achieved, and further clinical symptoms of the acute phase may develop such as fever, anemia, muscle and bone pain, fatigue, diarrhea, lymphadenopathy, and hepatosplenomegaly. Whereas these symptoms typically disappear after 3–4 months, a small number of individuals, especially children, die from complications such as myocarditis or meningoencephalitis. The fatal course is highly dependent on the immune system and nutritional status of the host as well as the parasite load during transmission. The subsequent indeterminate phase is characterized by a very low parasitemia in the blood and can last for decades. Cellular immunity is at this stage an important endogenous strategy of the host to keep the parasites under control. Usually, 20–30% of seropositive patients develop the chronic phase of Chagas' disease [28]. In 40–50% of the affected patients, a progressive cardiomyopathy and less frequently neuronal dysfunction of the autonomic nerves of the gastrointestinal tract can develop [29]. These symptoms are often found clinically only at a later stage, as many patients are initially asymptomatic. During routine analysis, radiological signs of left heart failure and cardiomegaly can be found. Damage to the heart may result in atrioventricular (AV), His-bundle or intraventricular blocks with Adam-Stokes seizures and syncopes [30]. Cellular hypertrophy and subsequent chamber enlargement lead to systolic heart failure and may result in arrhythmias. Patients often die of sudden cardiac death induced by ventricular tachycardia and congestive heart failure [31]. Histopathologic examination of endomyocardial biopsies shows myocardial fibrosis, resulting from cell lysis by trypanosomes and/or immune-pathological mechanisms. Development of gastrointestinal mega-syndrome, particularly the esophagus and colon, are additional clinical manifestations of chronic Chagas' disease. The formation of mega-organs results from the destruction of the parasympathetic ganglia of the Meissner and Auerbach plexus in the gastrointestinal tract, which critically impairs peristalsis and leads to the ballooning of the organs. Clinically, these patients show symptoms of dysphagia, regurgitation, constipation, and secondary achalasia resulting from the dysfunction of the lower esophageal sphincter.

## 5. Diagnosis and treatment

Based on the aforementioned clinical signs of *T. cruzi* infection, chronic Chagas' disease is diagnosed using conventional methods in clinical cardiology. The electrocardiogram (ECG) is the diagnostic tool of choice in the question of Chagas' cardiomyopathy. Magnetic resonance imaging (MRI) allows noninvasive and accurate assessment of inflammatory infiltrates of the heart muscle and the identification of an apical ventricular aneurysm. To confirm the diagnosis, a series of laboratory tests should be employed. The classic laboratory diagnostic measure to confirm an acute infection is a blood smear, which is stained after fixation with Giemsa and typically shows motile trypanomastigotes. The serological diagnosis comprises detection of both immunoglobulin (Ig) M and IgG antibodies against *T. cruzi* using enzyme-linked immunosorbent assay (ELISA), indirect hemagglutination assay (IHA) or indirect immunofluorescence assay (IFA). For suspected Chagas' disease, the WHO recommends two mutually independent tests [32]. The polymerase chain reaction (PCR) for the detection of nucleic acid sequences of parasites can be used to detect parasites in organ transplants, as well as to test the parasite load during and after chemotherapy. Finally, in unclear serological cases and when the blood smear is repeatedly negative, the xenodiagnosis developed by the French parasitologist Alexander Joseph Émile Brumpt may be applied using confirmed *T. cruzi*-negative assassin bugs, which take a blood meal on the patient´s skin. After 10–30 days, in the case of an infection of the patient with *T. cruzi*, even at low parasitemia, metacyclic trypomastigotes of *T. cruzi* can be demonstrated in the intestine of the bug and confirm the diagnosis [33].

In principle, two drugs for the treatment of acute Chagas' disease are available, nifurtimox and benznidazole, which require prolonged treatment and may cause significant side effects [34]. Nifurtimox, a nitrofuran with antiparasitic activity against both life cycle stages in the host, causes the accumulation of free radicals and superoxides and is generally genotoxic [35]. The nitroimidazole derivate benznidazole is an antiparasitic medication equally effective against the two life-cycle stages. This drug inhibits the synthesis of RNA and generates the accumulation of superoxides [35]. Although the parasite burden can be reduced below the detection limit in about 70% of all pharmacologically treated cases in acute Chagas' disease, there is still no evidence that antiparasitic treatment can cure the patient completely from *T. cruzi* [36–38]. Data for the treatment of patients with chronic Chagas' heart disease are not sufficiently validated to recommend a basic chemotherapy for these patients due to the unfavorable side-effect profile. In nonrandomized clinical or animal studies, some authors conclude that treatment with benznidazole may also be of benefit during the chronic phase, since thus severe courses of Chagas' cardiomyopathy can be avoided [39, 40]. However, results from the multicenter, randomized Benznidazole Evaluation for Interrupting Trypanosomiasis (BENEFIT) trial to assess the efficacy and safety of benznidazole treatment in patients with chronic Chagas' cardiomyopathy demonstrated that anti-trypanocidal therapy does not significantly reduce clinical deterioration through 5 years of follow-up as compared to placebo, despite reductions in the parasite load in serum samples [41]. These findings emphasize the urgent need for the development of new pharmacological agents against chronic Chagas' disease.

## 6. Prevention

Hitherto, the only sure prevention of the disease is the exposure prophylaxis by aerial spraying of insecticides and by modernization of traditional huts in rural areas. *T. cruzi*-infected pets, especially dogs and cats, provide a large reservoir of pathogens. Some countries perform an obligatory blood bank screening for the pathogen of Chagas' disease. These include, for example, Brazil, Uruguay, Argentina, Colombia, and the United States, but also Spain and Portugal. A vaccination against *T. cruzi* does not yet exist. Surface components of the parasite, particularly glycolipids such as glycosylphosphatidylinositol (GPI) anchors, have been well studied for their role in infectivity [42]. Trypanosomal trans-sialidase, belonging to the family of GPI-anchored proteins which transfer sialic acids from the cell membrane of the host to glycoproteins on the parasite surface, is involved in the infection of the host cell, and trans-sialidase inhibitors have been successfully tested *in vitro* [43].

## 7. Innate immune response to infections with *T. cruzi*

The innate immune system is essential in order to control the spread of *T. cruzi* parasites in the body and to ensure the survival of the host [44]. Pattern recognition receptors (PRRs), particularly the transmembrane toll-like receptors (TLRs), recognize the so-called pathogen-associated molecular patterns (PAMPs) in microorganisms [45]. Binding of glycoinositol-phospholipids (GIPL), GPI anchors, DNA, and RNA fragments of *T. cruzi* to TLR2, TLR4, TLR7, and TLR9 initiates a signaling cascade that finally activates important pro-inflammatory processes [46–52]. In myocarditis, genes for the endogenous TLR-7 and TLR-9 receptors are upregulated and their gene products serve as potential biomarkers for inflammatory heart disease [53]. Through the adapter molecule myeloid differentiation factor 88 (MyD88), a signal pathway is activated that finally leads to the upregulation of pro-inflammatory genes, such as interleukin-(IL)-1$\beta$ [54], IL-6 [55], IL-12 [56–60], TNF-$\alpha$ [57, 58, 61], IFN-$\beta$ [62–64], and IFN-$\gamma$ [54, 59–61, 65–67].

Activation of these pathways is critical for resistance to infection with *T. cruzi*. Mice functionally deficient in MyD88 expression are more susceptible to infection by this protozoan, which is probably due to a defect in the production of pro-inflammatory cytokines [68]. In *T. cruzi*-infected macrophages, the expression of pro-inflammatory cytokines is mediated by two transcription factors: nuclear factor-κB (NF-κB) [69–71] and interferon-regulatory factor 3 (IRF3) [64]. NF-kB also activates inducible NO synthase (iNOS) which catalyzes the production of microbicidal nitric oxide (NO). Mice with a deficiency of iNOS or IFN-γ receptor are sensitive to infection with *T. cruzi*, showing a high rate of parasitemia, and, furthermore, macrophages from these mice have impaired trypanocidal activity due to lower amounts of NO [72].

## 8. Apoptosis of cardiac myocytes in Chagas' disease

The chronic stage of Chagas' disease usually leads to symptoms of dilated cardiomyopathy, which is characterized by an enlargement of the heart muscle with a steadily progressive loss of systolic function. The decrease in the biventricular ejection volume is presumably reflecting altered heart muscle remodeling and may include apoptotic cell death. Apoptosis is a form of programmed cell death which differs from necrosis by actively carrying out a cell-death program [73]. Apoptosis-regulating genes such as Bax and Apaf-1 are involved in the execution of apoptosis, whereas Bcl-2 is an antiapoptotic protein.

Proteolytic enzymes termed caspases play a central role in the execution of apoptotic cell death. The activation of the caspase cascade can be initiated by both intra- and extracellular stimuli. Extracellular stimuli induce the activation of caspases 8 and 10 through the Fas ligand and TNF receptors, whereas the intracellular pathway consists of the cytochrome C-regulated apoptosome which activates caspase 9. The JAK-STAT-signaling pathway regulates apoptosis via STAT3 (signal transducer and activator of transcription 3) by promoting the expression of antiapoptotic genes coding for the Bcl-2 protein family [74]. Cytotoxic T lymphocytes (CTLs, $CD8^+$ T-cells) activate caspases 3 and 7. These are key caspases in which caspases 8 and 9 converge and henceforth result in a common final pathway of the signaling cascade. Apoptosis of cardiomyocytes in the context of *T. cruzi* infection is a potential mechanism of the host to limit the spread of parasites.

In autopsy samples from Chagas' cardiomyopathy patients, signs of apoptotic cell death were detected post mortem in cardiac myocytes [75], confirming earlier results that *T. cruzi*-infected cardiomyocytes undergo fibrosis and apoptotic cell death [76, 77]. Zhang and colleagues detected apoptosis in a canine model of acute chagasic myocarditis characterized by the presence of amastigotes and trypomastigotes of *T. cruzi* within the cytoplasm of cardiac muscle cells [76]. In a gene expression study, Manque and colleagues showed that the infection of murine cardiomyocytes with *T. cruzi* resulted in the upregulation of the two classical pro-apoptotic genes *bid*, encoding BH3-interacting domain death agonist, and *fas* which encodes a member of the TNF receptor gene. In addition, the *gadd45b* gene engaged in cell cycle control, DNA repair, and apoptosis was upregulated upon infection [78].

However, there are conflicting results on the role of apoptosis in murine cardiomyocytes during infection with *T. cruzi* trypomastigotes. De Souza et al. reported that cardiomyocytes became apoptotic after infection with different strains of *T. cruzi* [79], whereas Aoki et al.

showed that the cysteine protease cruzipain on the surface of *T. cruzi* appears to have a protective effect on the host cell and serves as a survival factor supporting the propagation of the parasites [80]. Our group demonstrated apoptotic rat cardiomyocytes upon infection with either trypomastigote or amastigote stages of *T. cruzi* [81]. Petersen et al. showed that both *T. cruzi* infection and activation of NF-κB prevented apoptotic cell death in isolated neonatal rat cardiomyocytes [82]. Another study reported that amastigotes presented higher rates of apoptosis-like cell death as compared to trypomastigotes [83].

The JAK-STAT-signaling pathway has an important role in cardiomyopathy, myocarditis, and myocardial infarction [84]. Cardiomyocytes express various receptors for cytokines and growth factors (among others, TNF$\alpha$ and EGF) on their surface. Secreted cytokines or growth factors may be involved in the apoptotic cell death of cardiomyocytes and chronic cardiomyopathy. Specifically, the balance in the activation state of the two related transcription factors STAT1 and STAT3 may determine the outcome between cell death and survival of cardiac muscle cells during infection with *T. cruzi* [85].

In the context of chronic Chagas' disease, which can develop up to 25 years after parasitic infection, the question arises as to how the parasite can persist and replicate for such a long period of time in the host without causing an exacerbating immune response. The most obvious explanation is that the parasite has developed effective mechanisms to circumvent the immune response which affects the steady balance between parasite load and apoptosis-induced destruction of host cells. Various parasitological studies highlight the dogma that the replication of parasites in the cardiac myocytes is required to initiate the complete picture of Chagas' heart disease ranging from acute myocarditis to chronic cardiomyopathy [86].

## 9. The role of STAT proteins in Chagas' cardiomyopathy

There is growing evidence that not only NF-kB but also STAT transcription factors are engaged in *T. cruzi* infection. Recently, we have demonstrated that serine phosphorylation of STAT1 at position 727 is targeted by *T. cruzi*, suggesting that the parasite inhibits the antiparasitic effects of STAT1 [87] (**Figure 5**). Ponce and coworkers reported that the secretion of endogenous IL-6 or the addition of recombinant IL-6 protects cardiomyocytes from cell death by apoptosis during an infection with *T. cruzi* [88]. Furthermore, the authors showed the phosphorylation of STAT3 at tyrosine 705 by IL-6 in response to infection with *T. cruzi*. In cardiac tissues, the expression of the STAT3-regulated antiapoptotic factor Bcl-2 was increased, suggesting that, during the acute phase of infection with *T. cruzi*, tyrosine-phosphorylated STAT3 acts as a mediator of cell survival. In summary, the results of this important study suggest that STAT3 executes pro-survival effects in cardiac muscle cells evoked by the parasite.

In addition, Ponce et al. demonstrated that, in *T. cruzi*-infected cells, the release of IL-6 via a TLR2-dependent pathway is required to induce survival of cardiomyocytes [88]. The enzymatic activity of cruzipain, the main cysteine protease secreted by this parasite, critically interferes with IL-6-mediated STAT3 phosphorylation by means of cleavage of the ectodomain of glycoprotein gp130, which is the shared receptor of several IL-6-type cytokines [89]. The parasite cysteine protease inhibitor chagasin inhibits cruzipain-induced gp130 cleavage,

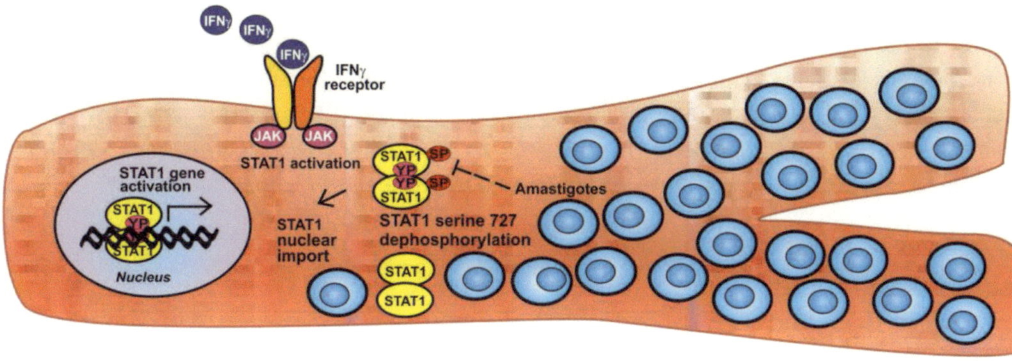


**Figure 5.** Illustration of a cardiac myocyte showing replicating intracellular *T. cruzi* parasites that evade the protective role of IFN-γ signaling by targeting essential components of the JAK-STAT pathway such as the dephosphorylation of STAT1 at serine 727. While phosphorylation of STAT1 serine 727 is required for full transcriptional activity, its dephosphorylation inhibits antiparasitic effects of STAT1.

suggesting that the pro-inflammatory IL-6 response in *T. cruzi*-infected cells is modified by cysteine protease activity. In addition, it has been well established that STAT transcription factors activate genes whose products have been identified as suppressors of cytokine signaling (SOCS) which act as inhibitors of the JAK-STAT pathway in a negative feedback loop [90].

Previous studies have described how STAT3 is activated by the two cytokines IL-6 or IL-10 [91, 92] and how the expression of SOCS3 is upregulated by the anti-inflammatory IL-10 in *T. cruzi*-infected cardiomyocytes [71]. During chronic infection with *T. cruzi*, the expression of SOCS2 is upregulated and most probably plays a significant role in the etiopathogenesis of Chagas' heart disease by influencing heart muscle damage [93].

Another member of the STAT family, the transcription factor STAT4, is activated in response to the cytokine IL-12, which acts as a pro-inflammatory cytokine and drives Th cells along a Th1 lineage. STAT6 is activated by receptor binding of two cytokines with anti-inflammatory properties, IL-4 and IL-13, which provide an alternative signal for the development along a Th2 lineage. Tarleton and coworkers demonstrated that STAT4-deficient mice were highly susceptible to infection with *T. cruzi*, whereas STAT6-deficient mice showed enhanced resistance with lower parasitemia and little or no evidence of inflammatory processes in the heart muscle as compared to their wild-type littermates [94]. The apparent absence of disease in chronically infected STAT6-deficient mice is remarkable despite their inability to achieve entire parasite clearance. The findings in this investigation suggest that the severity of inflammation critically depends on STAT4- and STAT6-mediated cytokine-driven immune reactions which modulate tissue parasite load [94]. Finally, the authors infer that the clearance of intracellular parasites may not be required to prevent the progression of the disease to cardiomyopathy.

## 10. Concluding remarks

In summary, the pathogenic protozoan *T. cruzi* has evolved complex and still undefined mechanisms to circumvent an effective immune response in the human myocardium. The bypassing of protective signaling pathways by the parasite such as the JAK-STAT pathway may account for the intracellular multiplication and long-lasting persistence of *T. cruzi* in the host. Amastigotes of *T. cruzi* proliferating in the cytoplasm of infected cardiomyocytes have developed effective strategies to counteract the attack executed by STAT proteins, which are crucial for an effective immune defense against the protozoan. Further research efforts are required to elucidate the role of cytokine-driven gene expression in the fight against the parasite.

## Acknowledgement

The research on this subject was funded by grants from Deutsche Forschungsgemeinschaft (DFG), Deutsche Gesellschaft für Kardiologie (DGK), and Deutsches Zentrum für Herz- und Kreislaufforschung (DZHK).

## Author details

Philipp Stahl[1, 2] and Thomas Meyer[3, 4*]

*Address all correspondence to: thomas.meyer@med.uni-goettingen.de

1 Institute of Virology, Parasitology Unit, University of Marburg, Marburg, Germany

2 Department of Internal Medicine, Section of Gastroenterology and Infectious Diseases, University Hospital Gießen and Marburg, Marburg, Germany

3 Department of Psychosomatic Medicine and Psychotherapy, University of Göttingen, Göttingen, Germany

4 German Center for Cardiovascular Research, partner site Göttingen, Göttingen, Germany

## References

[1] Chagas C. Nova tripanozomiase humana. Estudos sobre a morfologia e o ciclo evolutivo do Schizotrypanum cruzi n. gen., n. sp., agente etiológico de nova entidade mórbida do homem. Mem. Inst. Oswaldo Cruz 1909;**1**:159–218.

[2] Moncayo A. Progress towards the elimination of transmission of Chagas disease in Latin America. World Health Stat. Q. 1997;**50**:195–198.

[3] Rassi A Jr, Rassi A, Marin-Neto JA. Chagas disease. Lancet 2010;**375**:1388–1402.

[4] Schaub GA. Pathogenicity of trypanosomatids on insects. Parasitol. Today 1994; **10**:463–468.

[5] Sánchez LV, Ramírez JD. Congenital and oral transmission of American trypanosomiasis: an overview of physiopathogenic aspects. Parasitology 2013;**140**:147–159.

[6] Brener Z. Biology of *Trypanosoma cruzi*. Annu. Rev. Microbiol. 1973;**27**:347–382.

[7] Vickerman K. Developmental cycles and biology of pathogenic trypanosomes. Br. Med. Bull. 1985:**41**:105–114.

[8] De Souza W. Basic cell biology of *Trypanosoma cruzi*. Curr. Pharm. Des. 2002;**8**:269–285.

[9] Andrews NW. Living dangerously: how *Trypanosoma cruzi* uses lysosomes to get inside host cells, and then escapes into the cytoplasm. Biol. Res. 1993:**26**:65–67.

[10] Tan H, Andrews NW. Don't bother to knock—the cell invasion strategy of *Trypanosoma cruzi*. Trends Parasitol. 2002;**18**:427–428.

[11] Burleigh BA, Andrews NW. The mechanisms of *Trypanosoma cruzi* invasion of mammalian cells. Annu. Rev. Microbiol. 1995;**49**:175–200.

[12] Tyler KM, Engman DM. The life cycle of *Trypanosoma cruzi* revisited. Int. J. Parasitol. 2001;**31**:472–481.

[13] Ferreira ER, Bonfim-Melo A, Mortara RA, Bahia D. *Trypanosoma cruzi* extracellular amastigotes and host cell signaling: more pieces to the puzzle. Front. Immunol. 2012;**3**:363.

[14] De Souza W. Cell biology of *Trypanosoma cruzi*. Int. Rev. Cytol. 1984;**86**:197–283.

[15] Schofield CJ, Dias JC. The Southern Cone Initiative against Chagas disease. Adv. Parasitol. 1999;**42**:1–27.

[16] Moncayo A, Silveira AC. Current epidemiological trends for Chagas disease in Latin America and future challenges in epidemiology, surveillance and health policy. Mem. Inst. Oswaldo Cruz 104 Suppl 2009;**1**:17–30.

[17] Gascon J, Bern C, Pinazo MJ. Chagas disease in Spain, the United States and other non-endemic countries. Acta Trop. 2010;**115**:22–27.

[18] Basile L, Jansá JM, Carlier Y, Salamanca DD, Angheben A, Bartoloni A, Seixas J, Van Gool T, Canavate C, Flores-Chávez M, Jackson Y, Chiodini PL, Albajar-Vinas P, and Working Group on Chagas Disease. Chagas disease in European countries: the challenge of a surveillance system. Euro. Surveill. 2011;**16**.

[19] Angheben A, Anselmi M, Gobbi F, Marocco S, Monteiro G, Buonfrate D, Tais S, Talamo M, Zavarise G, Strohmeyer M, Bartalesi F, Mantella A, Di Tommaso M, Aiello KH, Veneruso G, Graziani G, Ferrari M, Spreafico I, Bonifacio E, Gaiera G, Lanzafame M, Mascarello M, Cancrini G, Albajar-Vinas P, Bisoffi Z, Bartoloni A. Chagas disease in Italy: breaking an epidemiological silence. Euro. Surveill. 2011:**16**.

[20] Perez-Molina JA, Perez-Ayala A, Parola P, Jackson Y, Odolini S, Lopez-Velez R, and EuroTravNet Network. EuroTravNet: imported Chagas disease in nine European countries, 2008 to 2009. Euro Surveill. Bull. 2011;**16**.

[21] Albajar-Vinas P, Jannin J. The hidden Chagas disease burden in Europe. Euro Surveill. 2011;**16***.

[22] Schmunis GA, Yadon ZE. Chagas disease: a Latin American health problem becoming a world health problem. Acta Trop. 2010;**115**:14–21.

[23] Jackson Y, Chappuis F. Chagas disease in Switzerland: history and challenges. Euro. Surveill. 2011;**16**.

[24] Strasen J, Williams T, Ertl G, Zoller T, Stich A, Ritter O. Epidemiology of Chagas disease in Europe: many calculations, little knowledge. Clin. Res. Cardiol. 2014;**103**:1–10.

[25] Hotez PJ, Dumonteil E, Betancourt Cravioto M, Bottazzi ME, Tapia-Conyer R, Meymandi S, Karunakara U, Ribeiro I, Cohen RM, Pecoul B. An unfolding tragedy of Chagas disease in North America. PLoS Negl. Trop. Dis. 2013;**7**:e2300.

[26] Salas Clavijo NA, Postigo JR, Schneider D, Santalla JA, Brutus L, Chippaux JP. Prevalence of Chagas disease in pregnant women and incidence of congenital transmission in Santa Cruz de la Sierra, Bolivia. Acta Trop. 2012;**124**:87–91.

[27] Jackson Y, Pinto A, Pett S. Chagas disease in Australia and New Zealand: risks and needs for public health interventions. Trop. Med. Int. Health 2014,**19**:212–218.

[28] Rossi MA, Bestetti RB. The challenge of chagasic cardiomyopathy. The pathologic roles of autonomic abnormalities, autoimmune mechanisms and microvascular changes, and therapeutic implications. Cardiology 1995;**86**:1–7.

[29] Rassi A Jr, Rassi A, Marcondes de Rezende J. American Trypanosomiasis (Chagas Disease). Infect. Dis. Clin. North Am. 2012;**26**:275–291.

[30] Marin-Neto JA, Cunha-Neto E, Maciel BC, Simões MV. Pathogenesis of chronic Chagas heart disease. Circulation 2007;**115**:1109–1123.

[31] de Lourdes Higuchi M, Benvenuti LA, Martins Reis M, Metzger M. Pathophysiology of the heart in Chagas' disease: current status and new developments. Cardiovasc. Res. 2003;**60**:96–107.

[32] Otani MM, Vinelli E, Kirchhoff LV, del Pozo A, Sands A, Vercauteren G, Sabino EC. WHO comparative evaluation of serologic assays for Chagas disease. Transfusion (Paris) 2009;**49**:1076–1082.

[33] Brumpt E. Le xenodiagnostic. Application au diagnostic de quelques infections parasitaires et en particulier à la trypanosome de Chagas. Bull. Soc. Path. Exot. 1914;**77**:706–710.

[34] Lattes R, Lasala MB. Chagas disease in the immunosuppressed patient. Clin. Microbiol. Infect. 2014;**20**:300–309.

[35] Le Loup G, Pialoux G, Lescure FX. Update in treatment of Chagas disease. Curr. Opin. Infect. Dis. 2011;**24**:428–434.

[36] Marin-Neto JA, Rassi A, Avezum A, Mattos AC, Rassi A, Morillo CA, Sosa-Estani S, Yusuf S, and BENEFIT Investigators. The BENEFIT trial: testing the hypothesis that trypanocidal therapy is beneficial for patients with chronic Chagas heart disease. Mem. Inst. Oswaldo Cruz 104 Suppl 2009;**1**:319–324.

[37] Apt W. Current and developing therapeutic agents in the treatment of Chagas disease. Drug Des. Devel. Ther. 2010;**4**:243–253.

[38] Bern C. Chagas' Disease. N. Engl. J. Med. 2015;**373**:456–466.

[39] Garcia S, Ramos CO, Senra JFV, Vilas-Boas F, Rodrigues MM, Campos-de-Carvalho AC, Ribeiro-dos-Santos R, Soares MBP. Treatment with benznidazole during the chronic phase of experimental Chagas' disease decreases cardiac alterations. Antimicrob. Agents Chemother. 2005;**49**:1521–1528.

[40] Viotti R, Vigliano C, Lococo B, Bertocchi G, Petti M, Alvarez MG, Postan M, Armenti A. Long-term cardiac outcomes of treating chronic Chagas disease with benznidazole versus no treatment: a nonrandomized trial. Ann. Intern. Med. 2006:**144**:724–734.

[41] Morillo CA, Marin-Neto JA, Avezum A, Sosa-Estani S, Rassi A Jr, Rosas F, Villena E, Quiroz R, Bonilla R, Britto C, Guhl F, Velazquez E, Bonilla L, Meeks B, Rao-Melacini P, Pogue J, Mattos A, Lazdins J, Rassi A, Connolly SJ, Yusuf S, and BENEFIT Investigators. Randomized trial of benznidazole for chronic Chagas' cardiomyopathy. N. Engl. J. Med. 2015;**373**:1295–1306.

[42] Debierre-Grockiego F. Glycolipids are potential targets for protozoan parasite diseases. Trends Parasitol. 2010;**26**:404–411.

[43] Schauer R, Kamerling JP. The chemistry and biology of trypanosomal trans-sialidases: virulence factors in Chagas disease and sleeping sickness. ChemBioChem 2011;**12**:2246–2264.

[44] Machado FS, Dutra WO, Esper L, Gollob KJ, Teixeira MM, Factor SM, Weiss LM, Nagajyothi F, Tanowitz HB, Garg NJ. Current understanding of immunity to *Trypanosoma cruzi* infection and pathogenesis of Chagas disease. Semin. Immunopathol. 2012;**34**:753–770.

[45] Takeda K, Akira S. Toll-like receptors in innate immunity. Int. Immunol. 2005;**17**:1–14.

[46] Campos MA, Almeida IC, Takeuchi O, Akira S, Valente EP, Procópio DO, Travassos LR, Smith JA, Golenbock DT, Gazzinelli RT. Activation of Toll-like receptor-2 by glycosylphosphatidylinositol anchors from a protozoan parasite. J. Immunol. 2001;**167**:416–423.

[47] Ropert C, Gazzinelli RT. Regulatory role of Toll-like receptor 2 during infection with *Trypanosoma cruzi*. J. Endotoxin Res. 2004;**10**:425–430.

[48] Oliveira AC, Peixoto JR, de Arruda LB, Campos MA, Gazzinelli RT, Golenbock DT, Akira S, Previato JO, Mendonça-Previato L, Nobrega A, Bellio M. Expression of functional TLR4 confers proinflammatory responsiveness to *Trypanosoma cruzi* glycoinositolphospholipids and higher resistance to infection with *T. cruzi*. J. Immunol. 2004;**173**:5688–5696.

[49] Bafica A, Santiago HC, Goldszmid R, Ropert C, Gazzinelli RT, Sher A. Cutting edge: TLR9 and TLR2 signaling together account for MyD88-dependent control of parasitemia in *Trypanosoma cruzi* infection. J. Immunol. 2006;**177**:3515–3519.

[50] Medeiros MM, Peixoto JR, Oliveira AC, Cardilo-Reis L, Koatz VLG, Van Kaer L, Previato JO, Mendonça-Previato L, Nobrega A, Bellio M. Toll-like receptor 4 (TLR4)-dependent proinflammatory and immunomodulatory properties of the glycoinositolphospholipid (GIPL) from *Trypanosoma cruzi*. J. Leukoc. Biol. 2007;**82**:488–496.

[51] Caetano BC, Carmo BB, Melo MB, Cerny A, dos Santos SL, Bartholomeu DC, Golenbock DT, Gazzinelli RT. Requirement of UNC93B1 reveals a critical role for TLR7 in host resistance to primary infection with *Trypanosoma cruzi*. J. Immunol. 2011;**187**:1903–1911.

[52] Gravina HD, Antonelli L, Gazzinelli RT, Ropert C. Differential use of TLR2 and TLR9 in the regulation of immune responses during the infection with *Trypanosoma cruzi*. PloS One 2013;**8**:e63100.

[53] Heidecker B, Kittleson MM, Kasper EK, Wittstein IS, Champion HC, Russell SD, Hruban RH, Rodriguez ER, Baughman KL, Hare JM. Transcriptomic biomarkers for the accurate diagnosis of myocarditis. Circulation 2011;**123**:1174–1184.

[54] Gonçalves VM, Matteucci KC, Buzzo CL, Miollo BH, Ferrante D, Torrecilhas AC, Rodrigues MM, Alvarez JM, Bortoluci KR. NLRP3 controls *Trypanosoma cruzi* infection through a caspase-1-dependent IL-1R-independent NO production. PLoS Negl. Trop. Dis. 2013;**7**:e2469.

[55] Truyens C, Angelo-Barrios A, Torrico F, Van Damme J, Heremans H, Carlier Y. Interleukin-6 (IL-6) production in mice infected with *Trypanosoma cruzi*: effect of its paradoxical increase by anti-IL-6 monoclonal antibody treatment on infection and acute-phase and humoral immune responses. Infect. Immun. 1994:**62**:692–696.

[56] Aliberti JC, Cardoso MA, Martins GA, Gazzinelli RT, Vieira LQ, Silva, JS. Interleukin-12 mediates resistance to *Trypanosoma cruzi* in mice and is produced by murine macrophages in response to live trypomastigotes. Infect. Immun. 1996;**64**:1961–1967.

[57] Camargo MM, Almeida IC, Pereira ME, Ferguson MA, Travassos LR, Gazzinelli RT. Glycosylphosphatidylinositol-anchored mucin-like glycoproteins isolated from *Trypanosoma cruzi* trypomastigotes initiate the synthesis of proinflammatory cytokines by macrophages. J. Immunol. 1997;**158**:5890–5901.

[58] Almeida IC, Camargo MM, Procópio DO, Silva LS, Mehlert A, Travassos LR, Gazzinelli RT, Ferguson MA. Highly purified glycosylphosphatidylinositols from *Trypanosoma cruzi* are potent proinflammatory agents. EMBO J. 2000;**19**:1476–1485.

[59] Antúnez MI, Cardoni RL. IL-12 and IFN-$\gamma$ production, and NK cell activity, in acute and chronic experimental *Trypanosoma cruzi* infections. Immunol. Lett. 2000;**71**:103–109.

[60] Michailowsky V, Silva NM, Rocha CD, Vieira LQ, Lannes-Vieira J, Gazzinelli RT. Pivotal role of interleukin-12 and interferon-gamma axis in controlling tissue parasitism and inflammation in the heart and central nervous system during *Trypanosoma cruzi* infection. Am. J. Pathol. 2001;**159**:1723–1733.

[61] Bastos KRB, Barboza R, Sardinha L, Russo M, Alvarez JM, Lima MRD. Role of endogenous IFN-$\gamma$ in macrophage programming induced by IL-12 and IL-18. J. Interferon Cytokine Res. 2007;**27**:399–410.

[62] Kierszenbaum F, Sonnenfeld G. Beta-interferon inhibits cell infection by *Trypanosoma cruzi*. J. Immunol. 1984;**132**:905–908.

[63] Koga R, Hamano S, Kuwata H, Atarashi K, Ogawa M, Hisaeda H, Yamamoto M, Akira S, Himeno K, Matsumoto M, Takeda K. TLR-dependent induction of IFN-β mediates host defense against *Trypanosoma cruzi*. J. Immunol. 2006;**177**:7059–7066.

[64] Chessler ADC, Ferreira LRP, Chang TH, Fitzgerald KA, Burleigh BA. A novel IFN regulatory factor 3-dependent pathway activated by trypanosomes triggers IFN-β in macrophages and fibroblasts. J. Immunol. 2008;**181**:7917–7924.

[65] Wirth JJ, Kierszenbaum F, Sonnenfeld G, Zlotnik A. Enhancing effects of gamma interferon on phagocytic cell association with and killing of *Trypanosoma cruzi*. Infect. Immun. 1985:**49**:61–66.

[66] Müller U, Köhler G, Mossmann H, Schaub GA, Alber G, Di Santo JP, Brombacher F, Hölscher C. IL-12-independent IFN-γ production by T cells in experimental Chagas' disease is mediated by IL-18. J. Immunol. 2001;**167**:3346–3353.

[67] Rodrigues AA, Saosa JSS, da Silva GK, Martins FA, da Silva AA, da Silva Souza Neto CP, Horta CV, Zamboni DS, da Silva JS, Ferro EAV, da Silva CV. IFN-γ plays a unique role in protection against low virulent *Trypanosoma cruzi* strain. PLoS Negl. Trop. Dis. 2012;**6**:e1598.

[68] Campos MA, Closel M, Valente EP, Cardoso JE, Akira S, Alvarez-Leite JI, Ropert C, Gazzinelli RT. Impaired production of proinflammatory cytokines and host resistance to acute infection with *Trypanosoma cruzi* in mice lacking functional myeloid differentiation factor 88. J. Immunol. 2004;**172**:1711–1718.

[69] Huang H, Calderon TM, Berman JW, Braunstein VL, Weiss LM, Wittner M, Tanowitz HB. Infection of endothelial cells with *Trypanosoma cruzi* activates NF-kappaB and induces vascular adhesion molecule expression. Infect. Immun. 1999;**67**:5434–5440.

[70] Hall BS, Tam W, Sen R, Pereira ME. Cell-specific activation of nuclear factor-kappaB by the parasite *Trypanosoma cruzi* promotes resistance to intracellular infection. Mol. Biol. Cell 2000;**11**:153–160.

[71] Hovsepian E, Penas F, Siffo S, Mirkin GA, Goren NB. IL-10 inhibits the NF-κB and ERK/MAPK-mediated production of pro-inflammatory mediators by up-regulation of SOCS-3 in *Trypanosoma cruzi*-infected cardiomyocytes. PloS One 2013;**8**:e79445.

[72] Hölscher C, Köhler G, Müller U, Mossmann H, Schaub GA, Brombacher F. Defective nitric oxide effector functions lead to extreme susceptibility of *Trypanosoma cruzi*-infected mice deficient in gamma-interferon receptor or inducible nitric oxide synthase. Infect. Immun. 1998;**66**:1208–1215.

[73] Böhm I, Schild H. Apoptosis: the complex scenario for a silent cell death. Mol. Imaging Biol. 2003;**5**:2–14.

[74] Fukada T, Hibi M, Yamanaka Y, Takahashi-Tezuka M, Fujitani Y, Yamaguchi T, Nakajima K, Hirano T. Two signals are necessary for cell proliferation induced by a cytokine receptor gp130: involvement of STAT3 in anti-apoptosis. Immunity. 1996;**5**:449–460.

[75] Tostes S Jr, Bertulucci Rocha-Rodrigues D, de Araujo Pereira G, Rodrigues V Jr. Myocardiocyte apoptosis in heart failure in chronic Chagas' disease. Int. J. Cardiol. 2005:**99**:233–237.

[76] Zhang J, Andrade ZA, Yu ZX, Andrade SG, Takeda K, Sadirgursky M, Ferrans VJ. Apoptosis in a canine model of acute Chagasic myocarditis. J. Mol. Cell. Cardiol. 1999;**31**:581–596.

[77] Henriques-Pons A, Oliveira GM, Paiva MM, Correa AFS, Batista MM, Bisaggio RC, Liu CC, Cotta-de-Almeida V, Coutinho CMLM, Persechini PM, Araújo-Jorge. Evidence for a perforin-mediated mechanism controlling cardiac inflammation in *Trypanosoma cruzi* infection. Int. J. Exp. Pathol. 2002;**83**:67–79.

[78] Manque PA, Probst CM, Probst CM, Pereira MCS, Rampazzo RCP, Ozaki LS, Ozaki LS, Pavoni DP, Silva Neto DT, Carvalho MR, Xu P, Serrano MG, Alves JMP, de Nazareth SL Meirelles M, Goldenberg S, Krieger MA, Buck GA. *Trypanosoma cruzi* infection induces a global host cell response in cardiomyocytes. Infect. Immun. 2011;**79**:1855–1862.

[79] De Souza EM, Araújo-Jorge TC, Bailly C, Lansiaux A, Batista MM, Oliveira GM, Soeiro MN. Host and parasite apoptosis following *Trypanosoma cruzi* infection in in vitro and in vivo models. Cell Tissue Res. 2003:**314**:223–235.

[80] Aoki MP, Guiñazú NL, Pellegrini AV, Gotoh T, Masih DT, Gea S. Cruzipain, a major *Trypanosoma cruzi* antigen, promotes arginase-2 expression and survival of neonatal mouse cardiomyocytes. Am. J. Physiol. Cell Physiol. 2004;**286**:C206–212.

[81] Stahl P, Ruppert V, Meyer T, Schmidt J, Campos MA, Gazzinelli RT, Maisch B, Schwarz RT, Debierre-Grockiego F. Trypomastigotes and amastigotes of *Trypanosoma cruzi* induce apoptosis and STAT3 activation in cardiomyocytes in vitro. Apoptosis 2013;**18**:653–663.

[82] Petersen CA, Krumholz KA, Carmen J, Sinai AP, Burleigh BA. *Trypanosoma cruzi* infection and nuclear factor kappa B activation prevent apoptosis in cardiac cells. Infect. Immun. 2006;**74**:1580–1587.

[83] De Souza EM, Nefertiti ASG, Bailly C, Lansiaux A, Soeiro MN. Differential apoptosis-like cell death in amastigote and trypomastigote forms from *Trypanosoma cruzi*-infected heart cells in vitro. Cell Tissue Res. 2010;**341**:173–180.

[84] Barry SP, Townsend PA, Latchman DS, Stephanou A. Role of the JAK-STAT pathway in myocardial injury. Trends Mol. Med. 2007;**13**:82–89.

[85] Stahl P, Schwarz RT, Debierre-Grockiego F, Meyer T. *Trypanosoma cruzi* parasites fight for control of the JAK-STAT pathway by disarming their host. JAK-STAT 2015;**3**:e1012964.

[86] Tarleton RL, Zhang L. Chagas disease etiology: autoimmunity or parasite persistence? Parasitol. Today 1999;**15**:94–99.

[87] Stahl P, Ruppert V, Schwarz RT, Meyer T. *Trypanosoma cruzi* evades the protective role of interferon-gamma-signaling in parasite-infected cells. PLoS One 2014;**9**:e110512.

[88] Ponce NE, Cano RC, Carrera-Silva EA, Lima AP, Gea S, Aoki MP. Toll-like receptor-2 and interleukin-6 mediate cardiomyocyte protection from apoptosis during *Trypanosoma cruzi* murine infection. Med. Microbiol. Immunol. 2012;**201**:145–155.

[89] Ponce NE, Carrera-Silva EA, Pellegrini AV, Cazorla SI, Malchiodi EL, Lima AP, Gea S, Aoki MP. *Trypanosoma cruzi,* the causative agent of Chagas disease, modulates interleukin-6-induced STAT3 phosphorylation via gp130 cleavage in different host cells. Biochim. Biophys. Acta 2013;**1832**:485–494.

[90] Starr R, Willson TA, Viney EM, Murray LJ, Rayner JR, Jenkins BJ, Gonda TJ, Alexander WS, Metcalf D, Nicola NA, Hilton DJ. A family of cytokine-inducible inhibitors of signalling. Nature 1997;**387**:917–921.

[91] Zhong Z, Wen Z, Darnell JE Jr. Stat3: a STAT family member activated by tyrosine phosphorylation in response to epidermal growth factor and interleukin-6. Science 1994;**264**:95–98.

[92] Riley JK, Takeda K, Akira S, Schreiber RD. Interleukin-10 receptor signaling through the JAK-STAT pathway. Requirement for two distinct receptor-derived signals for anti-inflammatory action. J. Biol. Chem. 1999;**274**:16513–16521.

[93] Esper L, Roman-Campos D, Lara A, Brant F, Castro LL, Barroso A, Araujo RRS, Vieira LQ, Mukherjee S, Gomes ERM, Rocha NN, Ramos IPR, Lisanti MP, Campos CF, Arantes RME Guatimosim S, Weiss LM, Cruz JS, Tanowitz HB, Teixeira MM, Machado FS. Role of SOCS2 in modulating heart damage and function in a murine model of acute Chagas disease. Am. J. Pathol. 2012;**181**:130–140.

[94] Tarleton RL, Grusby MJ, Zhang L. Increased susceptibility of Stat4-deficient and enhanced resistance in Stat6-deficient mice to infection with *Trypanosoma cruzi*. J. Immunol. 2000;**165**:1520-1525.

Chapter 12

# Diabetic Cardiomyopathy: Focus on Oxidative Stress, Mitochondrial Dysfunction and Inflammation

Sara Nunes, Anabela Pinto Rolo,
Carlos Manuel Palmeira and Flávio Reis

Additional information is available at the end of the chapter

http://dx.doi.org/10.5772/65915

**Abstract**

Diabetic cardiomyopathy (DCM) is an independent clinical entity defined as structural and functional changes in the myocardium because of metabolic and cellular abnormalities induced by diabetes, resulting in cardiac failure. Hyperglycemia has been seen as a major cause of DCM due to activation of different mechanisms leading to oxidative stress. Several body of evidence show that distinct pathways of oxygen and nitrogen reactive species formation contribute to myocardial impairment. Abnormal mitochondrial morphology and energetics, evoked by abnormal $Ca^{2+}$ handling, metabolic changes and oxidative stress, are observed in DCM, suggesting a pivotal role of mitochondrial dynamics in disease pathogenesis. In addition, insulin resistance compromises myocardial glucose uptake due to cellular depletion of glucose transporter proteins, together with increased myocardial uptake of free fatty acids and augmented triglyceride levels, which cause cardiomyocyte lipotoxicity. Finally, the state of chronic low-grade inflammation, a feature of obese type 2 diabetes, seems to also play a major role in DCM progression, whose mechanisms have been progressively disclosed. In this book chapter, we review the cellular mechanism contributing to DCM development, focusing on oxidative stress, mitochondrial dysfunction and inflammation of cardiomyocytes, as well as on possible therapeutic strategies.

**Keywords:** diabetic cardiomyopathy, oxidative stress, mitochondrial dysfunction, inflammation, therapeutic strategies

## 1. Introduction

Type 2 diabetes mellitus (T2DM) is one of the most common endocrine deregulation worldwide, reaching pandemic proportions on a global scale [1]. In 2015, there were 415 million people with diabetes globally and an increase to 642 million by 2040 is estimated by the International Diabetes Federation [2]. In addition, T2DM is one of the leading causes of illness and premature death, with 5 million deaths in 2015, mainly affecting developed regions ("Occidental World"), as well as many countries in development, particularly due to unhealthy lifestyle habits, such as physical inactivity and high fat and sugar diets [1].

T2DM is a major risk factor for the development of cardiovascular diseases (CVD), which are responsible for up to 65% of all deaths in diabetic patients, as well as for substantial morbidity and loss of quality of life. As T2DM progresses, the heart and blood vessels undergo changes, leading to a number of different cardiovascular complications, including coronary artery disease (CAD), stroke, peripheral arterial disease, as well as diabetic cardiomyopathy (DCM) [2].

The original finding of Rubler et al. [3] of the existence of heart failure (HF) in postmortem diabetic patients free of detectable CAD was the basis of the first use of DCM terminology. Subsequent clinical and epidemiological studies have confirmed these observations [4, 5], suggesting that diabetes can damage the cardiac tissue independently of other cardiovascular risk factors. Such associations have provided a credible existence of DCM as a unique clinical entity, independent of hypertension, CAD, left ventricular hypertrophy (LVH), atrial fibrillation, or any other known cardiac diseases, leading to HF, caused by complex relationships between metabolic abnormalities that accompany diabetes and its cellular consequences [6].

Despite the development of asymptomatic DCM for a long period of time, the metabolic anomalies at the cardiac myocyte level progresses, leading to structural and functional abnormalities. Although hyperglycemia has been classically indicated as the primary responsible, other factors seem to be involved in the evolution of the disease and several substrates have been suggested [7]. During the last years, the structural, functional, pathological and molecular aspects of the disease have been increasingly investigated, but the issue is far to be elucidated and no specific markers and therapeutics have been found so far. Unravelling the molecular mechanisms underlying DCM development and progression is crucial to identify relevant therapeutic targets and generate novel therapies tailored to reduce the risk of HF in diabetic patients.

In this book chapter, we revisit some of the main features of DCM, focusing on pathophysiological mechanisms associated with cardiomyocyte oxidative stress, mitochondrial dysfunction and inflammation. We also indicate possible therapeutic strategies targeting those important cellular events that seem to play a major role in DCM development and progression.

## 2. Structural and functional cardiac changes

Increasing evidences from experimental, pathologic, epidemiologic and clinical studies have been shown that diabetes results in structural and functional cardiac changes. Anatomic changes in DCM, mainly assessed by echocardiography or magnetic resonance imaging, are essentially characterized by myocardial hypertrophy and fibrosis. In addition, although many studies have shown that diabetic patients have abnormal diastolic function but preserved systolic function, which might be due to the lower sensitivity to detect systolic dysfunction by

http://dx.doi.org/10.5772/65915

some of the techniques used, the current knowledge points to the existence of a continuum of diastolic and systolic dysfunction in DCM.

### 2.1. Cardiac hypertrophy

One of the most important structural hallmarks of DCM is cardiac hypertrophy, which is a powerful predictor of cardiovascular events. Apoptotic and necrotic loss of cardiomyocytes causes compensatory hypertrophy of the remaining viable cardiomyocyte. Although the right ventricle can also become hypertrophic, LVH is more common and generally represents a more advanced stage of the disease. Even though the causes and mechanisms underlying LVH development in diabetic patients remain poorly understood, experimental and clinical studies have been suggesting that hyperinsulinemia, insulin resistance, hyperglycemia, and increased nonesterified fatty acids (NEFAs) may collectively play a major role. Insulin, in particular, is viewed as a growth factor in the myocardium, which is sustained by experimental findings that sustained hyperinsulinemia causes increased myocardial mass and decreased cardiac output in rats [8]. In addition, clinical and experimental data have been shown increased markers of cardiomyocyte hypertrophy, including augmented width and myofiber disarray of cardiomyocyte, as well overexpression of hypertrophic genes, namely β-myosin heavy chain, atrial natriuretic peptide (ANP) and brain natriuretic peptide (BNP) [9, 10].

### 2.2. Myocardial fibrosis, apoptosis and necrosis

Myocardial fibrosis has been indicated as another major mechanism contributing to cardiac alterations in DCM. This pathological feature of DCM that have been observed in diabetic patients without significant CAD and in animal models, results from the accumulation of interstitial glycoproteins and increased extracellular collagen matrix, which potentiates stiffening and inhibits ventricles relaxation [11, 12]. The echocardiographic features of increased left ventricular fibrosis appear in the form of impaired relaxation and diastolic dysfunction; consequently, alterations in collagen phenotype may play an important role in the impaired left ventricular diastolic filling that is typical of DCM [11]. It has been suggested that collagen is a major determinant of ventricular stiffness. In a study with rats, a correlation between increased extracellular collagen content and decrease in early mitral peak flow (decreased E/A ratio) was reported [12]. The cause for the accumulation of cardiac fibrosis in diabetes is believed to result from decreased degradation of glycosylated collagen by matrix metalloproteinases and, conversely, from excessive production of collagen by fibroblasts due to increased renin–angiotensin–aldosterone system (RAAS) activation [11]. Furthermore, increased formation in myocardial advanced glycation end-products (AGEs) has also been reported in diabetic patients, which has been attributed to hyperglycemia [13]. In fact, collagen cross-linked with AGEs causes myocardial stiffness and inhibits collagen degradation, which promotes additional collagen accumulation and fibrosis [11, 13]. This mechanism seems to be also a major contributor for the impaired left ventricular diastolic function observed in diabetic patients [13].

Finally, DCM is associated with increased myocyte cell death and apoptosis. Accelerated necrosis and apoptosis is caused by hyperglycemia, increased formation of ROS, overactivation of local RAAS system and of insulin-like growth factor-1 and transforming growth factor beta 1

(TGF-β1) [14]. While apoptosis does not cause scar formation or accumulation of interstitial collagen, because nuclear fragmentation and cell shrinkage is replaced by the surrounding cells, necrosis is able to promote the widening of extracellular compartments among myocytes and increased deposition of collagen, which causes replacement fibrosis and connective cell proliferation [15].

### 2.3. Diastolic dysfunction

In many cases, it has been found that abnormalities of diastolic function may advertise the subsequent progressive deterioration of cardiac function. Diastolic dysfunction is the basic hemodynamic feature and the earliest findings of DCM that can be detected using imaging techniques. The noninvasive assessment of diastolic dysfunction mainly relies on Doppler studies of diastolic transmitral inflow, flow velocities, flow patterns, isovolumic relaxation time and deceleration time, which are the most common criteria used in its evaluation. The criteria of the consensus statement on the diagnosis of heart failure with normal left ventricular ejection fraction by the Heart Failure and Echocardiography Associations of the European Society of Cardiology have been used to assess left ventricular diastolic dysfunction [16].

Diastolic dysfunction is characterized by an abnormal myocardial relaxation and filling. This condition is typically manifested by reduced early diastolic filling and increased atrial filling, by augmented isovolumetric relaxation and increased number of supraventricular premature beats, as well as by amplified left ventricular end-diastolic pressure and diminished left ventricular end-diastolic volume [17–19].

Diastolic dysfunction is found in several other cardiovascular diseases, such as hypertension, hypertrophic cardiomyopathy and CAD, even with intact systolic function. However, experimental and clinical studies have shown impaired diastolic function in the absence of manifestations of congestive HF, even in prediabetes or in early stages of diabetes [19], thus suggesting that could be a useful early marker for disease prognosis. Furthermore, left ventricular diastolic dysfunction may progress to a systolic dysfunction, causing reduced left ventricular ejection fraction (LVEF) in years. Therefore, it is very important to detect left ventricular diastolic dysfunction in diabetic patients, both for early diagnosis and treatment of DCM, as well as for prevention of further systolic dysfunction.

### 2.4. Systolic dysfunction

Systolic dysfunction, defined as impaired ability of the heart to pump arterial blood in the periphery, is typically associated with a reduced LVEF and cardiac output. In DCM, systolic dysfunction occurs late, often when patients have already developed significant diastolic dysfunction. The presence of systolic dysfunction in the early years of diabetes has been a controversial issue, while diastolic dysfunction is more easily detected by Doppler echocardiography. The controversy relies on the fact that current techniques used to assess systolic function are less sensitive than those used for diastolic dysfunction evaluation. For this reason, more sensitive and accurately techniques for systolic assessment have been developed, such as tissue Doppler imaging (TDI) and strain rate imaging techniques, which are able to estimate left ventricular function in longitudinal, radial and circumferential ways, thus allowing the detection of preclinical systolic abnormalities in diabetic patients. Currently, shortened left ventricular ejection time, decreased peak systolic velocity (S′), and smaller left ventricular fractional shortening can be the detectable parameters for identification of systolic dysfunction [20]. The prognosis in patients with depressed systolic dysfunction is poor with an annual mortality of 15–20%.

## 3. Overview of the molecular mechanisms involved in DCM development

The pathophysiological molecular mechanisms underlying the development and progression of DCM are multifactorial and complex and have been progressively disclosed. Some of the main features of DM are also pivotal elements in the pathogenesis of DCM, including hyperglycemia, hyperinsulinemia and insulin resistance, as well as hyperlipidemia (**Figure 1**).

Hyperglycemia has been seen as a major cause of DCM development due to activation of the classical oxidative stress pathways (polyol, hexosamine, AGEs and protein kinase C—PKC). These mechanisms cause increased production of mitochondrial reactive oxygen species (ROS), nonenzymatic glycation of proteins and glucose auto-oxidation, thus leading to cellular (cardiac) injury—glucotoxicity. Glucose and collagen interact to form Schiff bases and the fibrous network is reorganized with the so-called Amadori products, which can be transformed in AGEs. As above mentioned, the increased formation of AGEs is highly associated

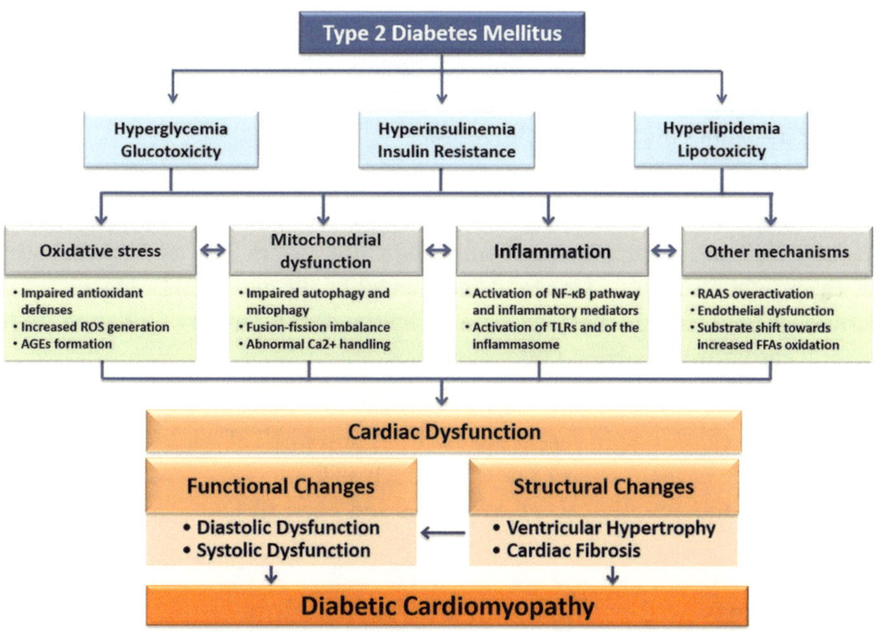


**Figure 1.** Metabolic abnormalities underlying T2DM that are considered the main triggers for the cellular and molecular pathways associated with structural and functional changes in DCM. Adapted with permission from Ref. [24]. *Abbreviations:* AGEs, advanced glycation end products; FFAs, free fatty acids, NF-κB, nuclear factor-κB; RAAS, renin–angiotensin–aldosterone system; ROS, reactive oxygen species; TLRs, Toll-like receptors.

with myocardial fibrosis in diabetic hearts by affecting the structural components of the extracellular matrix, such as collagen. This stable cross-linked collagen accumulate in vessel walls and in myocardial tissue, increasing diastolic stiffness of the heart and contributing to endothelial dysfunction, thus suggesting a key role of AGEs in DCM development.

Insulin resistance originates cellular depletion of glucose transporter proteins (GLUT-1 and GLUT-4) leading to reduced glucose uptake in the diabetic heart, which facilitates a substrate shift towards increased fatty acids (FAs) oxidation, resulting in reduced cardiac efficiency [21]. In brief, once inside the cardiomyocytes, the free fatty acids (FFAs) are converted into acetyl coenzyme A derivatives that will activate PKC isoforms responsible for blocking insulin cascade elevated levels of FFAs compete with glucose as energy substrate, with a shift in energy production from β-oxidation of FFAs. As a result, there is a reduced glucose utilization and oxidation, increased glucose and insulin levels, promoting insulin resistance.

Additionally, the increase concentration of FFAs and of its metabolism causes intracellular accumulation of toxic FA intermediates (such as ceramide and diacylglycerol) and formation of ROS. These mechanisms originates cardiac lipotoxicity by means of oxidative stress, cardiomyocyte apoptosis and increased myocardial consumption of oxygen, resulting in impaired contractility, mitochondrial uncoupling and decreased adenosine triphosphate (ATP) availability [22]. Intracellular deposition of FFAs is also responsible for the saturation of the mitochondrial capacity of oxidation, thus activating transcription factors, including the peroxisome proliferator-activated receptors (PPARs), which has been indicated as an inductor of cardiac lipotoxicity and dysfunction [23]. Several body of evidences show that distinct pathways of oxygen and nitrogen reactive species formation contribute to myocardial injury. Impaired mitochondrial morphology and energetics, evoked by abnormal $Ca^{2+}$ handling, metabolic changes and oxidative stress, are observed in DCM, suggesting a pivotal role of mitochondrial dynamics in disease pathogenesis.

In addition, the state of chronic low-grade inflammation, a feature of obese T2DM, seems to also play a major role in DCM progression, whose mechanisms have been progressively disclosed [24]. The epicardial adipose tissue (EAT) that covers 80% of the heart surface and constitutes approximately 20% of the total heart weight have endocrine and paracrine properties that interfere with cardiac function, namely by the development of inflammation, insulin resistance and cardiac dysfunction [25].

As above mentioned, activation of the RAAS, locally and systemically, has been associated with the development of insulin resistance and the onset of T2DM. In addition, it has been associated with some of the hallmarks of DCM, such as increased fibrosis, oxidative damage, and cardiomyocyte and endothelial cell apoptosis and necrosis [26].

## 4. Oxidative stress and mitochondrial dysfunction

Mitochondria are dynamic organelles with a key role in energy transduction, signaling and cell death pathways. Consequently, mitochondrial dysfunction and oxidative stress are broadly relevant in the development of cardiovascular diseases, in both acquired and inherited disease [27]. Tissues with high aerobic metabolism demands, such as the heart muscle, are severely affected by a decline in mitochondrial efficiency such as in the context of diabetes, ischemia-reperfusion and aging [28, 29], associated with loss of calcium homeostasis and impaired contractile function. In fact, mitochondria comprise one-third of the volume of the heart and support the vast majority of ATP production derived from oxidation of fatty acids (FAs) and glucose, being FAs the preferred substrate in the normal adult myocardium, while failing human hearts shift to oxidizing glucose for energy production.

In the inner mitochondrial membrane, electrons deriving from the oxidation of NADH and FADH2 are funneled through the electron transport chain. This flow is coupled with the translocation of protons across the inner mitochondrial membrane to the intermembrane space, generating an electrochemical gradient. Under normal conditions, much of the energy of this gradient is used to generate ATP, as the collapse of the proton gradient through ATP synthase drives the ATP synthetic machinery. However, when the electrochemical potential difference generated by the electrochemical gradient is high (such as in high-fat or high-glucose states), or under conditions of inhibition of the ETC complexes, the life of superoxide-generating electron transport intermediates, such as ubisemiquinone radical, is prolonged [30], resulting in increased ROS generation. Although ROS are produced in multiple cell compartments, the majority of cellular ROS (approximately 90%) are mitochondrial, mainly at the level of complexes I and III of the ETC [31]. The activity of detoxifying enzymes and uncoupling proteins limits ROS generation. In the healthy myocardium, ROS concentration is tightly controlled to low steady-state level by superoxide dismutase (SOD) [32]. Superoxide anion is dismutated by mitochondrial manganese SOD into hydrogen peroxide, which is detoxified into water by the mitochondrial glutathione peroxidase (GPx), an action dependent on mitochondrial reduced glutathione (GSH) content. Mitochondrial catalase has a detoxifying effect against overproduction of hydrogen peroxide. An imbalance of antioxidant defenses that favors the accumulation of oxidants, expose mitochondria to oxidative stress, with ROS reacting with DNA, proteins and lipids, inactivating the ETC complexes and mitochondrial proteins, thus impairing both oxidative phosphorylation (OXPHOS) and inducing ROS accumulation. In the diabetic heart, increased FAs accumulation and metabolism is linked to oxidative stress [33]. Also, in the context of myocardial ischemia/reperfusion, oxidative stress is implicated in ATP depletion and cardiomyocyte death. At the onset of reperfusion, increased ROS and mitochondrial calcium influx favor induction of the mitochondrial permeability transition (MPT) and loss of mitochondrial inner membrane impermeability [34]. Recently, it has been shown that offspring of diabetic pregnancies are at risk of cardiovascular disease at birth and throughout life, with high-fat diet-exposed offspring exhibiting mitochondrial dysfunction and lipid peroxidation [35]. Each cell has normally several copies of mitochondrial DNA (mtDNA) which encodes ribosomal and transfer RNAs necessary for the synthesis of the mtDNA-encoded 13 OXPHOS polypeptides in the mitochondrial matrix [36]. The proximity to the inner membrane, the absence of protective histones, and incomplete repair mechanisms in mitochondria, renders mtDNA extremely sensitive to oxidative damage. The accumulation of mtDNA mutations due to oxidative damage results in further unbalanced ETC and increased ROS generation, perpetuating oxidative damage and enhancing inflammatory, hypertrophic, fibrotic, and cell death events in the myocardium [37]. Therefore, mechanisms able to eliminate dysfunctional mitochondria are essential to prevent the cytotoxic impact of ROS and thus maintain cellular homeostasis.

Autophagy is a tightly regulated cellular process which promotes the turnover of dysfunctional mitochondria along with the elimination of long-lived proteins and other damaged organelles, being essential for maintaining normal cardiac function [38]. Autophagy also maintains cell viability under stress conditions by supplying amino acids for de novo protein synthesis and providing substrates for the tricarboxylic acid cycle [39], as shown by myocardial survival promoted by activation of autophagy upon starvation or ischemia [40, 41]. Autophagy is redox-dependent due to redox regulation of metabolic alterations as well as ROS-mediated modification of autophagy-regulatory proteins. Disruption of ATG5, an autophagy-related gene, results in heart failure under basal and stress conditions [42]. In turn, autophagy regulates intracellular ROS by selective elimination of dysfunctional mitochondria (mitophagy) [43] and degradation of KEAP1 and activation of the nuclear factor erythroid 2-related factor 2 (NRF2), activating the expression of antioxidant genes such as glutathione peroxidase, superoxide dismutase and thioredoxin [44]. A decline in autophagy with aging, leading to increased levels of oxidative damage and the accumulation of dysfunctional mitochondria has been proposed as an underlying cause for the pathogenesis of cardiovascular diseases prevalent in late life [45].

Besides mitophagy, mitochondrial quality control is dependent on balanced fusion and fission events that continually alter mitochondrial morphology by undergoing fission to generate discrete fragmented mitochondria or fusion to form an interconnected elongated network. This dynamic behavior shapes mitochondria to adapt metabolism to the energetic needs of the cell, allows mixing of mtDNA, lipids, proteins and metabolites, enhances communication with the endoplasmic reticulum or segregates dysfunctional or depolarized mitochondria away from the healthy network, facilitating its clearance [46]. These two processes are under the control of mitochondrial fission and fusion proteins: mitofusins (MFN1 and MFN2) and optic atrophy 1 (OPA1) mediate mitochondrial fusion while dynamin-related protein 1 (DRP1) mediates mitochondrial fission by interaction with other fission mediators such as fission protein (FIS1) [47]. Changes on mitochondrial morphology, linked to altered expression of DRP1 and MFN2, are evident during stem cell differentiation into cardiomyocytes, transitioning from fragmented rounded mitochondria into an elongated network with well-developed cristae and an efficient OXPHOS system [48]. The essential role of MFN proteins is also shown by mitochondrial fragmentation, impaired mitochondrial function and development of heart failure in models of conditional cardiac ablation of MFN 1 and 2 [49]. In post-mitotic tissues with high metabolic demands, such as the heart, abnormal mitochondrial dynamics results in the development of cardiovascular disease, due to impaired mitochondrial turnover and accumulation of fragmented and depolarized mitochondria, sources of increased ROS generation [50]. Recently, it has also been shown that DRP1 ablation results in cardiomyocyte necrosis and dilated cardiomyopathy in mice, mitophagic mitochondrial depletion and favors MPT induction, probably linked to spatiotemporal alterations in calcium signaling [51]. When exposed to calcium overload, both neonatal and adult rat cardiomyocytes exhibited increased ROS generation and mitochondrial fragmentation, which suggested that activation of the fission machinery may be an event preceding ROS generation regulated by calcium signaling [52]. Giant or mega-mitochondria have been described in a variety of

http://dx.doi.org/10.5772/65915

cardiomyopathies, including those associated with mtDNA mutations [53]. The observation of increased mtDNA content, induction of genes involved in mitochondrial biogenesis, fatty acid metabolism, and glucose transport, as well as uncoupling proteins and antioxidant enzymes in mitochondrial cardiomyopathies hearts, may indicate a compensatory response, although unable to prevent energy depletion and increased ROS generation [54].

Balanced fusion–fission events are essential for normal mitochondrial biogenesis, the process by which cells increase mitochondrial mass and copy number. Among the transcription factors involved in this process, peroxisome proliferator-activated receptor-$\gamma$ coactivator-1, PGC-1$\alpha$, is the master regulator. This inducible coactivator acts as a coactivator of the transcription factors involved in the expression of nuclear/mitochondrial genes and bioenergetic capacity, as well as regulates cardiac fuel selection and mitochondrial ATP-producing capacity [55]. An interplay between PGC-1$\alpha$ and MFN-2 has been shown as follows: MFN2 is critical for the stimulatory effect of PGC-1$\alpha$ on mitochondrial membrane potential while PGC-1$\alpha$ may regulate mitochondrial fusion/fission events [56]. Besides stimulating mitochondrial biogenesis and OXPHOS, PGC-1$\alpha$ prevents oxidative stress by inducing ROS-detoxifying enzymes [57]. Sirtuin 3 (SIRT3) has been shown essential for the stimulatory effect of PGC-1$\alpha$ on both mitochondrial biogenesis and ROS-detoxifying enzymes [58]. Sirtuins (1–7) are a conserved family of NAD+-dependent lysine-modifying acylases that regulate a variety of cellular functions such as metabolic responses to diet and exercise [59]. The decline in NAD+ during aging decreases sirtuin activity thus impairing the transcription of mitochondrial OXPHOS genes which leads to cardiovascular disease, an event precipitated by SIRT1 deletion [60]. Cardiac SIRT1 is upregulated during nutrient starvation, exercise and ischemic preconditioning while downregulated during I/R [61]. SIRT3, which exhibits mitochondrial deacetylase activity, deacetylates and increases the activity of mitochondrial metabolic and antioxidant enzymes [62] as well as regulates mitochondrial fusion–fission dynamics [63]. By deacetylating and suppressing the activity of cyclophilin D, SIRT3 increases resistance to MPT induction, preventing cell death and cardiac hypertrophy [64].

## 5. Inflammation

Chronic low-grade inflammation is commonly associated with obesity and T2DM, and clear evidence has emerged to suggest that inflammatory process also contributes to the pathogenesis of DCM. The inflammatory signaling in cardiomyocytes usually occurs as an early response to myocardial injury and involves an increased formation of cytosolic and mainly mitochondrial ROS. Several molecular pathways have been classically associated with the inflammatory response in the cardiac tissue: increased activation of the proinflammatory nuclear transcription factor-$\kappa$B (NF-$\kappa$B), overexpression of cytokines [namely the tumor necrosis factor-$\alpha$ (TNF$\alpha$), some interleukins (such as IL-1$\beta$ and IL-6), chemokines (i.e., monocyte chemotactic protein-1: MCP-1), adhesion molecules (i.e., selectins and adhesion molecules (ICAM-1, VCAM-1)] and migration of leukocytes into the myocardium [24]. There is evidence that chronic progression of hypertrophy, fibrosis and ventricular dysfunction is correlated with a local increase in cytokines and activation of NF-$\kappa$B [65]. Activation of NF-$\kappa$B is associated with the increased release of cytokines, such as TNF-α and IL-6, which are often involved in cardiac damage (hypertrophy and fibrosis) and left ventricular dysfunction [65, 66]. Accumulating data have been demonstrated that increased IL-1β and TNF-α are implicated in DCM, increasing epicardial thickness, promoting myocyte contractile dysfunction, thus depressing myocardial function and contributing to HF [67]. The inflammatory stimuli in the diabetic heart include hyperglycemia, hyperlipidemia, ROS, angiotensin II and the activation of Toll-like receptors (TLRs). Hyperglycemia-induced oxidative stress and inflammation seem to be deeply correlated with development of DCM. In fact, hyperglycemia activates several oxidative stress-responsive/proinflammatory transcription factors, including NF-κB, which is able to induce collagen and fibronectin synthesis, as well as to stimulate the production of inflammatory cytokines. Hyperglycemia-evoked diastolic dysfunction may be mediated partly by the macrophage migration inhibitory factor, suggesting that the NF-κB pathways may be involved in this process [68].

RAAS overactivation seems to also play an important role in the modulation of inflammation associated with DCM. In fact, Ang II not only induces vasoconstriction, cell growth and oxidative stress but also stimulates inflammation, namely by inducting cytokines release, by stimulating the production of PAI-1 and pro-inflammatory transcription factors, such as NF-κB, which in turn regulate adhesion molecules (VCAM-1 and ICAM-1) and the expression of several cytokines [69].

Activation of TLRs and the inflammasome complex has been recently proposed to play a pivotal role in cardiac inflammation and likely in the pathogenesis of DCM [70]. Accumulating evidences support the hypothesis that hyperglycemia and FFA are able to stimulate TLRs, thus inducing proinflammatory pathways in DCM. In fact, TLR-dependent NF-κB and ROS seem to be able to regulate both the priming and the posttranslational pathways required for the assembly and activation of the inflammasome, thus opening new therapeutic opportunities to DCM treatment, as further discussed.

## 6. Therapeutic strategies

Despite a specific therapy for the treatment or prevention of DCM is still lacking, some therapeutic strategies could present potential benefits. The advances on the knowledge of DCM pathogenesis provides us with improved management options, including lifestyle measures, strategies to improve diabetic control, lipid lowering therapy, as well as agents directed to target some of the main molecular events and mechanisms underlying DCM development and progression, including fibrosis, hypertrophy, oxidative stress and inflammation.

### 6.1. Physical exercise

Regular physical activity (training) has been associated with improved glycemic control and insulin sensitivity, as well as with amelioration of the metabolism of glucose and fatty acids in heart muscle, thus improving left ventricular function and attenuating diabetes induced-cardiac alterations. Physical exercise has also greater anti-inflammatory effects by decreasing the release of inflammatory cytokines from the skeletal muscles endothelial cells and immune system, together with increasing the anti-inflammatory cytokines, such as adiponectin [71]. In an animal model of T2DM, the Zucker Diabetic Fatty (ZDF) rat regular aerobic exercise (training) was able to not only improve the glycemic control and attenuate dyslipidaemia, but also to promote an anti-inflammatory effect, viewed by the reduction in pro-inflammatory cytokines, such as TNF-$\alpha$ and CRP, and by the increment of adiponectin levels [72–74]. This effect occurred independently of weight loss and was not observed when an acute extenuating exercise was used [75].

### 6.2. Antidiabetic agents

Improvement of glycemic control has been shown to be associated with better outcomes in diabetic microvascular complications in many clinical trials. Even though the impact of strict glycemic control on macrovascular outcomes remains debatable, the recognized role of microvascular disease in DCM development suggests that a better glycemic control would benefit patients.

#### *6.2.1. Insulin-sensitizing agents*

Insulin resistance is a hallmark of T2DM and plays an important role in the pathogenesis of DCM. Accordingly, agents used to ameliorate insulin resistance might be useful to prevent DCM progression. The beneficial effects of insulin may rely not only on the improved glycemic control in some patients but also on cardioprotective anti-inflammatory properties. Several data show a reduction in adhesion molecules, such as ICAM-1 and E-selection, circulating CRP, IL-6 and PAI-1 due to insulin-sensitizing therapy [76]. Metformin, one of the most commonly prescribed anti-diabetic drugs and a known insulin-sensitizing agent, improves peripheral sensitivity to insulin and promotes intensive glucose control [77]. Besides, cardioprotective actions of metformin have been described, namely inhibition of hypertrophy and pro-authophagic and anti-inflammatory actions [78].

The possible beneficial effects of thiazolidinediones (TZDs) and PPAR agonists on the myocardium have been demonstrated in several studies. Pioglitazone was associated with improved diabetic cardiac function in animal models, by raising myocardial glucose uptake and improving myocardial fatty acid metabolism [79]. In addition, rosiglitazone showed an amelioration of myocardial diastolic function in T2DM patients, which was related to an antioxidant and anti-inflammatory effect [80]. Other factors involved in improved cardiac function with TZDs therapy include decreased collagen accumulation and fibrosis, as well as inhibition of cardiomyocyte hypertrophy [79, 81]. Pioglitazone and rosiglitazone stimulate the PPAR-$\gamma$, which regulates important genes for the metabolism of glucose and fat and enhance insulin sensitivity in skeletal muscle and adipose tissue [82]. Additionally, PPAR activators may have anti-inflammatory effects by inhibition of TNF-$\alpha$ expression at the transcriptional level due to attenuation of NF-$\kappa$B activity in cardiomyocytes [83]. However, the effects of this therapy on cardiac function in patients with T2DM have not yet been fully elucidated. On the other hand, experimental studies using PPAR$\alpha$ agonists suggested cardiac benefits related to apoptosis and hypertrophy [84]. However, further research is still required in order to fully understand the role of PPAR$\alpha$ agonists, as well as TZDs, in DCM.

#### *6.2.2. Incretin-based therapies*

Glucagon-like peptide-1 (GLP-1), an incretin hormone rapidly released by the L-cells of the small intestine after a meal intake, presents several actions that contribute to glucose homeostasis, including stimulation of postprandial insulin secretion by pancreatic beta cells, thus improving insulin sensitivity. GLP-1 is metabolized by the enzyme dipeptidyl peptidase 4 (DPP-4), thus inactivating their insulinotropic activities. In diabetic patients, the incretin effect is partially blunted, which contributes to a poor glycemic control. The incretin-based therapies, a new class of antidiabetic drugs currently available for the treatment of diabetic patients, include DPP-4 inhibitors (such as sitagliptin) and GLP-1 receptor (GLP-1R) agonists (namely exenatide). GLP-1R and DPP-4 are expressed in several extra-pancreatic tissues, including the heart, which has encouraged studies concerning its role in cardiac physiology, as well putative cardiac and cardiovascular benefits of incretin-based therapies.

Several body of experimental and clinical data have suggested a considerable cardioprotective role of GLP-1 agonists in the myocardium. Myocardial ischemia-reperfusion injury was attenuated by GLP-1 in vitro rat hearts, showing cardioprotective and inotropic effects [85]. Furthermore, it has been shown that mice with genetic deletion of GLP-1 receptor display reduced heart rate, elevated left ventricular end-diastolic pressure and impaired left ventricular contractility and diastolic function after insulin administration. Furthermore, infusion of GLP-1 resulted in improved left ventricular function, hemodynamic status and efficiency, indicating a direct role of GLP-1 on the cardiac physiology [86]. Apart the clinical pharmacological effects on body weight reduction, amelioration of blood pressure and improvement of glycemic control and lipid profile, GLP-1R agonists have been experimentally shown to exert antioxidant, vasoprotective and anti-inflammatory properties. One of these studies showed that liraglutide exerts anti-inflammatory effect on vascular endothelial cells through increased NO production and suppressed NF-κB activation, which is at least partly mediated via AMPK activation [87]. In another study, liraglutide was able to ameliorate cardiac hypertrophy in mice [88]. However, further research is advisory to better understand the complete benefits of GLP-1R agonists in the treatment of DCM.

DPP-4 inhibitors are able to increase the endogenous contents of incretins, such as GLP-1. Besides their effect on glycemic control, beneficial actions on other tissues, including on the heart tissue, have been shown, which might be due to anti-inflammatory, antioxidant and anti-apoptotic properties [89–94]. DPP-IV inhibitors have the advantage of being available for oral administration and do not raise supra-physiological concentration of GLP-1. However, further research is needed to elucidate the effective relevance of DPP-IV inhibitors in DCM.

### 6.3. Other non-antidiabetic agents

#### *6.3.1. Statins*

Statins are primarily inhibitors of cholesterol biosynthesis and the control of hyperlipidemia will benefit T2DM patients. However, although the key benefits of statins were initially attributed to their lipid lowering effects, it is now known that they directly act through other cellular mechanisms, known as pleiotropic effects [95]. Statins increase the expression and

http://dx.doi.org/10.5772/65915

activation of eNOS thus causing an increase in the bioavailability of nitric oxide (NO), which contribute to the reduction in blood thrombogenicity, of oxidative stress and of cell proliferation. In addition, statins may also exert anti-inflammatory effects by several pathways, including reduced activity of VCAM-1 and ICAM-1, decreased function and levels of MCP-1 and decreased CRP [96]. Atorvastatin have been associated with improved left ventricular function, reduced fibrosis and hypertrophy; the protective effects on cardiac remodeling have been attributed to its anti-inflammatory actions [97]. However, further studies should be conducted to better evaluate the possible beneficial effects in DCM.

### *6.3.2. RAAS inhibitors*

Angiotensin converting enzyme inhibitors (ACEIs) and angiotensin receptor blockers (ARBs) are the most used drugs to block the RAAS, and there are numerous evidences suggesting that these antihypertensive agents reduce cardiovascular mortality in diabetic patients due to improvement of cardiac dysfunction [98]. ACEI and ARBs have been associated with several beneficial properties at cardiac level, including improved cardiac fibrosis, reduced collagen synthesis and deposition, amelioration of cardiomyocyte apoptosis and cardiac hypertrophy [98–100]. Experimental and clinical studies also suggest a beneficial effect on T2DM by ameliorating insulin sensitivity, enhancing glucose uptake, improving pancreatic and skeletal muscle blood flow and stimulating proliferation and differentiation of adipocytes, beyond the reduction in blood pressure [99]. Additionally, inhibition of Ang II production and/or action with ACEI and ARBs attenuate its pro-inflammatory actions. In fact, although further clinical evidences are still needed, several studies have showed beneficial effect on markers of inflammation (such as TNF-$\alpha$, IL-6 and IFN-$\gamma$) in heart failure patients [100].

### *6.3.3. Modulators of mitochondrial function*

Numerous studies have highlighted the pivotal importance of impaired mitochondrial metabolism and increased formation of ROS in the pathogenesis of cardiac dysfunction, as discussed previously. Therefore, strategies aiming at modulation of different aspects of mitochondria such as biogenesis, fusion and fission, mitophagy, MPT and ROS generation may lead to effective treatments for cardiomyopathies [101]. Modulation of sirtuins activity, exercise-induced PGC-1 activation, fission and fusion as well as autophagy/mitophagy [102–105] are examples. Interestingly, although increased ROS generation and consequent oxidative damage is associated with pathological processes, mild levels of mitochondrial-derived ROS have been proposed to induce a hormetic response. The concept of mitohormesis proposes that a mild increase in mitochondrial ROS may act as a sublethal trigger of cytoprotective long-lasting metabolic and biochemical changes against larger subsequent stresses [106]. This approach was addressed in mice as a pathway to stimulate mitochondrial energy metabolism and to induce antioxidant defenses, thus preventing cardiomyopathy induced by the cardiotoxic doxorubicin [107], an effect that was also triggered by exercise [108]. Moreover, it has been shown that the development of cardiomyopathy due to impaired mitophagy and consequent accumulation of damaged ROS-forming mitochondria can be surprisingly improved by ROS-dependent activation of compensatory autophagic pathways of mitochondrial quality control, preventing a vicious cycle of ROS formation and mitochondrial dysfunction [109].

## 7. Concluding remarks

Over the years, DCM has evolved from a nebulous concept to concrete reality and is now viewed as a specific clinical entity caused by the complex relationships between metabolic abnormalities that accompany diabetes, resulting in functional and structural changes in the myocardium that ultimately leads to HF. DCM involves the damage of the myocardium through several mechanisms, namely hypertrophy, fibrosis, apoptosis and necrosis of cardiomyocytes. Some of the main factors involved in diabetes pathogenesis are also pivotal in DCM development, including hyperglycemia-evoked oxidative stress and mitochondrial dysfunction (by impaired autophagy, mitophagy and fusion–fission balance), hyperlipidemia, accompanied by inflammation and a switch of substrate supply to FFAs, as well as insulin resistance. Increasing body of evidence suggests the existence of relevant links between some of these pathways, including between oxidative energy metabolism dysregulation, impaired mitochondrial morphology and energetics evoked by abnormal $Ca^{2+}$ handling, metabolic changes and oxidative stress, as well as chronic low-grade inflammation. The improved knowledge regarding the molecular mechanisms underlying DCM development has contributed to identify novel putative targets and therapeutic opportunities for the management of DCM. Pharmacological options targeting hyperglycemia, insulin resistance and reduced sensitivity, hyperlipidemia, inflammation, oxidative stress and mitochondrial dysfunction have been increasingly investigated, and it is hoped that could significantly improve the ability to prevent and/or improve management of DCM.

## Acknowledgements

Authors thank the financial support of Fundação para a Ciência e Tecnologia through (FCT) for the Sara Nunes PhD scholarship (SFRH/BD/109017/2015) and UID/NEU/04539/2013 (CNC.IBILI Consortium), as well as FEDER-COMPETE (FCOMP-01-0124-FEDER-028417 and POCI-01-0145-FEDER-007440).

## Author details

Sara Nunes[1†], Anabela Pinto Rolo[2†], Carlos Manuel Palmeira[2*] and Flávio Reis[1*]

*Address all correspondence to: palmeira@uc.pt; freis@fmed.uc.pt

1 Laboratory of Pharmacology and Experimental Therapeutics, Institute for Biomedical Imaging and Life Sciences (IBILI), Faculty of Medicine and CNC.IBILI Consortium, University of Coimbra, Coimbra, Portugal

2 Department of Life Sciences and Center for Neurosciences and Cell Biology, University of Coimbra, Coimbra, Portugal

† These authors contributed equally for this work.

## References

[1] Hossain P, Kawar B, El Nahas M. Obesity and diabetes in the developing world: a growing challenge. N Engl J Med. 2007;**356**:213–5. doi:10.1056/NEJMp068177.

[2] Tuomilehto J, Lindström J. The major diabetes prevention trials. Curr Diab Rep. 2003;**3**:115–22. doi:10.1007/s11892-003-0034-9.

[3] Rubler S,Dlugash J, Yuceoglu YZ, Kumral T, Branwood AW, Grishman A. New type of cardiomyopathy associated with diabetic glomerulosclerosis. Am J Cardiol. 1972;**30**:595–602. doi:10.1016/0002-9149(72)90595-4.

[4] Shrestha NR, Sharma SK, Karki P, Shrestha NK, Acharya P. Echocardiographic evaluation of diastolic function in asymptomatic type 2 diabetes. JNMA J Nepal Med Assoc. 2009;**48**:20–3.

[5] Wilson Tang WH. Glycemic control and treatment patterns in patients with heart failure. Curr Cardiol Rep. 2007;**9**:242–7. doi:10.1007/BF02938357.

[6] Letonja M, Petrovič D. Is diabetic cardiomyopathy a specific entity? World J Cardiol. 2014;**6**:8–13. doi:10.4330/wjc.v6.i1.8.

[7] Boudina S, Abel ED. Diabetic cardiomyopathy, causes and effects. Rev Endocr Metab Disord. 2010;**11**:31–9. doi:10.1007/s11154-010-9131-7.

[8] Karason K, Sjostrom L, Wallentin I, Peltonen M. Impact of blood pressure and insulin on the relationship between body fat and left ventricular structure. Eur Heart J. 2003;**24**:1500–5. [pii]:S0195668X03003129.

[9] Rosenkranz AC, Hood SG, Woods RL, Dusting GJ, Ritchie RH. B-type natriuretic peptide prevents acute hypertrophic responses in the diabetic rat heart: importance of cyclic GMP. Diabetes. 2003;**52**:2389–95. doi:10.2337/diabetes.52.9.2389.

[10] Nunes S, Soares E, Fernandes J, Viana S, Carvalho E, Pereira FC, et al. Early cardiac changes in a rat model of prediabetes: brain natriuretic peptide overexpression seems to be the best marker. Cardiovasc Diabetol. 2013;**12**:44. doi:10.1186/1475-2840-12-44.

[11] van Heerebeek L, Hamdani N, Handoko ML, Falcao-Pires I, Musters RJ, Kupreishvili K, et al. Diastolic stiffness of the failing diabetic heart: importance of fibrosis, advanced glycation end products, and myocyte resting tension. Circulation. 2008;**117**:43–51. doi:10.1161/CIRCULATIONAHA.107.728550.

[12] Mizushige K, Yao L, Noma T, Kiyomoto H, Yu Y, Hosomi N, et al. Alteration in left ventricular diastolic filling and accumulation of myocardial collagen at insulin-resistant prediabetic stage of a type II diabetic rat model. Circulation. 2000;**101**:899–907. doi:10.1161/01.CIR.101.8.899.

[13] Aronson D. Cross-linking of glycated collagen in the pathogenesis of arterial and myocardial stiffening of aging and diabetes. J Hypertens. 2003;**21**:3–12. doi:10.1097/01.hjh.0000042892.24999.92.

[14] D'Souza A, Howarth FC, Yanni J, Dobrzynski H, Boyett MR, Adeghate E, et al. Chronic effects of mild hyperglycaemia on left ventricle transcriptional profile and structural remodelling in the spontaneously type 2 diabetic Goto-Kakizaki rat. Heart Fail Rev. 2014;**19**:65–74. doi:10.1007/s10741-013-9376-9.

[15] Eckhouse SR, Spinale FG. Changes in the myocardial interstitium and contribution to the progression of heart failure. Heart Fail Clin. 2012;**8**:7–20. doi:10.1016/j.hfc.2011.08.012.

[16] Paulus WJ, Tschöpe C, Sanderson JE, Rusconi C, Flachskampf FA, Rademakers FE, et al. How to diagnose diastolic heart failure: a consensus statement on the diagnosis of heart failure with normal left ventricular ejection fraction by the Heart Failure and Echocardiography Associations of the European Society of Cardiology. Eur Heart J. 2007;**28**:2539–50. doi:10.1093/eurheartj/ehm037.

[17] Schannwell CM, Schneppenheim M, Perings S, Plehn G, Strauer BE. Left ventricular diastolic dysfunction as an early manifestation of diabetic cardiomyopathy. Cardiology. 2002;**98**:33–9. doi:64682.

[18] Hamblin M, Friedman DB, Hill S, Caprioli RM, Smith HM, Hill MF. Alterations in the diabetic myocardial proteome coupled with increased myocardial oxidative stress underlies diabetic cardiomyopathy. J Mol Cell Cardiol. 2007;**42**:884–95. doi:10.1016/j.yjmcc.2006.12.018.

[19] Von Bibra H, St John Sutton M. Diastolic dysfunction in diabetes and the metabolic syndrome: promising potential for diagnosis and prognosis. Diabetologia. 2010;**53**:1033–45. doi:10.1007/s00125-010-1682-3.

[20] Yilmaz S, Canpolat U, Aydogdu S, Abboud HE. Diabetic cardiomyopathy; summary of 41 years. Korean Circ J. 2015;**45**:266–72. doi:10.4070/kcj.2015.45.4.266.

[21] Jia G, DeMarco VG, Sowers JR. Insulin resistance and hyperinsulinaemia in diabetic cardiomyopathy. Nat Rev Endocrinol. 2016;**12**:144–53. doi:10.1038/nrendo.2015.216.

[22] Khullar M, Al-Shudiefat AA-RS, Ludke A, Binepal G, Singal PK. Oxidative stress: a key contributor to diabetic cardiomyopathy. Can J Physiol Pharmacol. 2010;**88**:233–40. doi:10.1139/Y10-016.

[23] Son NH, Park TS, Yamashita H, Yokoyama M, Huggins LA, Okajima K, et al. Cardiomyocyte expression of PPARgamma leads to cardiac dysfunction in mice. J Clin Invest. 2007;**117**:2791–801. doi:10.1172/JCI30335.

[24] Nunes S, Soares E, Pereira F, Reis F. The role of inflammation in diabetic cardiomyopathy. Int J Interf Cytokine Mediat Res. 2012;**4**:59. doi:10.2147/IJICMR.S21679.

[25] Iacobellis G, Sharma AM. Epicardial adipose tissue as new cardio-metabolic risk marker and potential therapeutic target in the metabolic syndrome. Curr Pharm Des. 2007;**13**:2180–4.

[26] Singh VP, Le B, Khode R, Baker KM, Kumar R. Intracellular angiotensin II production in diabetic rats is correlated with cardiomyocyte apoptosis, oxidative stress, and cardiac fibrosis. Diabetes. 2008;**57**:3297–306. doi:10.2337/db08-0805.

[27] Dorn GW, Vega RB, Kelly DP. Mitochondrial biogenesis and dynamics in the developing and diseased heart. Genes Dev. 2015;**29**:1981–91. doi:10.1101/gad.269894.115.

[28] Huss JM, Kelly DP. Mitochondrial energy metabolism in heart failure: a question of balance. J Clin Invest. 2005;**115**:547–55. doi:10.1172/JCI200524405.

[29] Lesnefsky EJ, Chen Q, Hoppel CL. Mitochondrial metabolism in aging heart. Circ Res. 2016;**118**:1593–611. doi:10.1161/CIRCRESAHA.116.307505.

[30] Korshunov SS, Skulachev VP, Starkov AA. High protonic potential actuates a mechanism of production of reactive oxygen species in mitochondria. FEBS Lett. 1997;**416**:15–8. doi:10.1016/S0014-5793(97)01159-9.

[31] Turrens JF. Mitochondrial formation of reactive oxygen species. J Physiol. 2003;**552**:335–44. doi:10.1113/jphysiol.2003.049478.

[32] Giordano FJ. Oxygen, oxidative stress, hypoxia, and heart failure. J Clin Invest. 2005;**115**:500–8. doi:10.1172/JCI200524408.

[33] Di Filippo C, Cuzzocrea S, Rossi F, Marfella R, D'Amico M. Oxidative stress as the leading cause of acute myocardial infarction in diabetics. Cardiovasc Drug Rev. 2006;**24**:77–87. doi:10.1111/j.1527-3466.2006.00077.x.

[34] Halestrap AP. Mitochondria and reperfusion injury of the heart—A holey death but not beyond salvation. J Bioenerg Biomembr. 2009;**41**:113–21. doi:10.1007/s10863-009-9206-x.

[35] Mdaki KS, Larsen TD, Wachal AL, Schimelpfenig MD, Weaver LJ, Dooyema SDR, et al. Maternal high-fat diet impairs cardiac function in offspring of diabetic pregnancy through metabolic stress and mitochondrial dysfunction. Am J Physiol Heart Circ Physiol. 2016:ajpheart.00795.2015. doi:10.1152/ajpheart.00795.2015.

[36] Wallace DC, Fan W. Energetics, epigenetics, mitochondrial genetics. Mitochondrion 2010;**10**:12–31. doi:10.1016/j.mito.2009.09.006.

[37] Ricci C, Pastukh V, Leonard J, Turrens J, Wilson G, Schaffer D, et al. Mitochondrial DNA damage triggers mitochondrial-superoxide generation and apoptosis. Am J Physiol Cell Physiol. 2008;**294**:C413–22. doi:10.1152/ajpcell.00362.2007.

[38] Filomeni G, Zio D De, Cecconi F, De Zio D, Cecconi F. Oxidative stress and autophagy: the clash between damage and metabolic needs. Cell Death Differ. 2015;**22**:377–88. doi:10.1038/cdd.2014.150.

[39] Rabinowitz JD, White E. Autophagy and metabolism. Science. 2010;**330**:1344–8. doi:10.1126/science.1193497.

[40] Yan L, Vatner DE, Kim SJ, Ge H, Masurekar M, Massover WH, et al. Autophagy in chronically ischemic myocardium. Proc Natl Acad Sci USA. 2005;**102**:13807–12. doi:10.1073/pnas.0506843102.

[41] Matsui Y, Takagi H, Qu X, Abdellatif M, Sakoda H, Asano T, et al. Distinct roles of autophagy in the heart during ischemia and reperfusion: roles of AMP-activated protein

kinase and beclin 1 in mediating autophagy. Circ Res. 2007;**100**:914–22. doi:10.1161/01.RES.0000261924.76669.36.

[42] Nakai A, Yamaguchi O, Takeda T, Higuchi Y, Hikoso S, Taniike M, et al. The role of autophagy in cardiomyocytes in the basal state and in response to hemodynamic stress. Nat Med. 2007;**13**:619–24. doi: 10.1038/nm1574. pii:nm1574.

[43] Wang K, Klionsky DJ. Mitochondria removal by autophagy. Autophagy. 2011;**7**:297–300. doi:10.4161/auto.7.3.14502.

[44] Komatsu M, Kurokawa H, Waguri S, Taguchi K, Kobayashi A, Ichimura Y, et al. The selective autophagy substrate p62 activates the stress responsive transcription factor Nrf2 through inactivation of Keap1. Nat Cell Biol. 2010;**12**:213–23. doi:10.1038/ncb2021.

[45] Wohlgemuth SE, Calvani R, Marzetti E. The interplay between autophagy and mitochondrial dysfunction in oxidative stress-induced cardiac aging and pathology. J Mol Cell Cardiol. 2014;**71**:62–70. doi:10.1016/j.yjmcc.2014.03.007.

[46] Liesa M, Palacín M, Zorzano A. Mitochondrial dynamics in mammalian health and disease. Physiol Rev. 2009;**89**:799–845. doi:10.1152/physrev.00030.2008.

[47] Lee Y, Jeong S-Y, Karbowski M, Smith CL, Youle RJ. Roles of the mammalian mitochondrial fission and fusion mediators Fis1, Drp1, and Opa1 in apoptosis. Mol Biol Cell. 2004;**15**:5001–11. doi:10.1091/mbc.E04-04-0294.

[48] Papanicolaou KN, Kikuchi R, Ngoh GA, Coughlan KA, Dominguez I, Stanley WC, et al. Mitofusins 1 and 2 are essential for postnatal metabolic remodeling in heart. Circ Res. 2012;**111**:1012–26. doi:10.1161/CIRCRESAHA.112.274142.

[49] Chen Y, Liu Y, Dorn GW. Mitochondrial fusion is essential for organelle function and cardiac homeostasis. Circ Res. 2011;**109**:1327–31. doi:10.1161/CIRCRESAHA.111.258723.

[50] Ong S-B, Hausenloy DJ. Mitochondrial morphology and cardiovascular disease. Cardiovasc Res. 2010;**88**:16–29. doi:10.1093/cvr/cvq237.

[51] Song M, Mihara K, Chen Y, Scorrano L, Dorn GW. Mitochondrial fission and fusion factors reciprocally orchestrate mitophagic culling in mouse hearts and cultured fibroblasts. Cell Metab. 2015;**21**:273–85. doi:10.1016/j.cmet.2014.12.011.

[52] Hom J, Yu T, Yoon Y, Porter G, Sheu S-S. Regulation of mitochondrial fission by intracellular Ca(2+) in rat ventricular myocytes. Biochim Biophys Acta. 2010;**1797**:913–21. doi:10.1016/j.bbabio.2010.03.018.

[53] Tandler B, Dunlap M, Hoppel CL, Hassan M. Giant mitochondria in a cardiomyopathic heart. Ultrastruct Pathol. 2002;**26**:177–83. doi:10.1080/01913120290076847.

[54] Sebastiani M, Giordano C, Nediani C, Travaglini C, Borchi E, Zani M, et al. Induction of mitochondrial biogenesis is a maladaptive mechanism in mitochondrial cardiomyopathies. J Am Coll Cardiol. 2007;**50**:1362–9. doi:10.1016/j.jacc.2007.06.035.

[55] Kelly DP, Scarpulla RC. Transcriptional regulatory circuits controlling mitochondrial biogenesis and function. Genes Dev. 2004;**18**:357–68. doi:10.1101/gad.1177604.

[56] Soriano FX, Liesa M, Bach D, Chan DC, Palacín M, Zorzano A. Evidence for a mitochondrial regulatory pathway defined by peroxisome proliferator-activated receptor-gamma coactivator-1 alpha, estrogen-related receptor-alpha, and mitofusin 2. Diabetes. 2006;**55**:1783–91. doi:10.2337/db05-0509.

[57] St-Pierre J, Drori S, Uldry M, Silvaggi JM, Rhee J, Jäger S, et al. Suppression of reactive oxygen species and neurodegeneration by the PGC-1 transcriptional coactivators. Cell. 2006;**127**:397–408. doi:10.1016/j.cell.2006.09.024.

[58] Kong X, Wang R, Xue Y, Liu X, Zhang H, Chen Y, et al. Sirtuin 3, a new target of PGC-1alpha, plays an important role in the suppression of ROS and mitochondrial biogenesis. PLoS One. 2010;**5**:e11707. doi:10.1371/journal.pone.0011707.

[59] Haigis MC, Sinclair DA. Mammalian sirtuins: biological insights and disease relevance. Annu Rev Pathol. 2010;**5**:253–95. doi:10.1146/annurev.pathol.4.110807.092250.

[60] Gomes AP, Price NL, Ling AJY, Moslehi JJ, Montgomery MK, Rajman L, et al. Declining NAD+ induces a pseudohypoxic state disrupting nuclear-mitochondrial communication during aging. Cell. 2013;**155**:1624–38. doi:10.1016/j.cell.2013.11.037.

[61] Matsushima S, Sadoshima J. The role of sirtuins in cardiac disease. Am J Physiol Hear Circ Physiol. 2015;**1**:ajpheart.00053.2015. doi:10.1152/ajpheart.00053.2015.

[62] Horton JL, Martin OJ, Lai L, Riley NM, Richards AL, Vega RB, et al. Mitochondrial protein hyperacetylation in the failing heart. JCI Insight. 2016;1. doi:10.1172/jci.insight.84897.

[63] Samant S a, Zhang HJ, Hong Z, Pillai VB, Sundaresan NR, Wolfgeher D, et al. SIRT3 deacetylates and activates OPA1 to regulate mitochondrial dynamics during stress. Mol Cell Biol. 2014;**34**:807–19. doi:10.1128/MCB.01483-13.

[64] Hafner A V, Dai J, Gomes AP, Xiao CY, Palmeira CM, Rosenzweig A, et al. Regulation of the mPTP by SIRT3-mediated deacetylation of CypD at lysine 166 suppresses age-related cardiac hypertrophy. Aging (Albany NY). 2010;**2**:914–23. doi:10.18632/aging.100252.

[65] Lorenzo O, Picatoste B, Ares-Carrasco S, Ramírez E, Egido J, Tuñón J. Potential role of nuclear factor-kb in diabetic cardiomyopathy. Mediators Inflamm. 2011;2011. doi:10.1155/2011/652097.

[66] Sun M, Dawood F, Wen WH, Chen M, Dixon I, Kirshenbaum LA, et al. Excessive tumor necrosis factor activation after infarction contributes to susceptibility of myocardial rupture and left ventricular dysfunction. Circulation. 2004;**110**:3221–8. doi:10.1161/01.CIR.0000147233.10318.23.

[67] Westermann D, Rutschow S, Van Linthout S, Linderer A, Bücker-Gärtner C, Sobirey M, et al. Inhibition of p38 mitogen-activated protein kinase attenuates left ventricular dysfunction by mediating pro-inflammatory cardiac cytokine levels in a mouse model of diabetes mellitus. Diabetologia. 2006;**49**:2507–13. doi:10.1007/s00125-006-0385-2.

[68] Yu X-Y, Chen H-M, Liang J-L, Lin Q-X, Tan H-H, Fu Y-H, et al. Hyperglycemic myocardial damage is mediated by proinflammatory cytokine: macrophage migration inhibitory factor. PLoS One. 2011;**6**:e16239. doi:10.1371/journal.pone.0016239.

[69] Schieffer B, Luchtefeld M, Braun S, Hilfiker a, Hilfiker-Kleiner D, Drexler H. Role of NAD(P)H oxidase in angiotensin II-induced JAK/STAT signaling and cytokine induction. Circ Res. 2000;**87**:1195–201. doi:10.1161/01.RES.87.12.1195.

[70] Fuentes-Antrás J, Ioan AM, Tuñón J, Egido J, Lorenzo O. Activation of toll-like receptors and inflammasome complexes in the diabetic cardiomyopathy-associated inflammation. Int J Endocrinol. 2014;2014:847827. doi:10.1155/2014/847827.

[71] Hopps E, Canino B, Caimi G. Effects of exercise on inflammation markers in type 2 diabetic subjects. Acta Diabetol. 2011;**48**:183–9. doi:10.1007/s00592-011-0278-9.

[72] de Lemos ET, Reis F, Baptista S, Pinto R, Sepodes B, Vala H, et al. Exercise training is associated with improved levels of C-reactive protein and adiponectin in ZDF (type 2) diabetic rats. Med Sci Monit. 2007;**13**:BR168–74.

[73] Teixeira de Lemos E, Reis F, Baptista S, Pinto R, Sepodes B, Vala H, et al. Exercise training decreases proinflammatory profile in Zucker diabetic (type 2) fatty rats. Nutrition. 2009;**25**:330–9. doi:10.1016/j.nut.2008.08.014.

[74] Teixeira-Lemos E, Nunes S, Teixeira F, Reis F. Regular physical exercise training assists in preventing type 2 diabetes development: focus on its antioxidant and anti-inflammatory properties. Cardiovasc Diabetol. 2011;**10**:12. doi:10.1186/1475-2840-10-12.

[75] Teixeira De Lemos E, Pinto R, Oliveira J, Garrido P, Sereno J, Mascarenhas-Melo F, et al. Differential effects of acute (extenuating) and chronic (training) exercise on inflammation and oxidative stress status in an animal model of type 2 diabetes mellitus. Mediators Inflamm. 2011;2011. doi:10.1155/2011/253061.

[76] Dandona P, Chaudhuri A, Ghanim H, Mohanty P. Insulin as an anti-inflammatory and antiatherogenic modulator. J Am Coll Cardiol. 2009;53. doi:10.1016/j.jacc.2008.10.038.

[77] Group UP. Effects of Intensive blood glucose control with metformin on complications in overweight patients with type 2 diabetes (UKPDS 34). Lancet. 1998;**352**:854–65.

[78] Gundewar S, Calvert JW, Jha S, Toedt-Pingel I, Ji SY, Nunez D, et al. Activation of AMP-activated protein kinase by metformin improves left ventricular function and survival in heart failure. Circ Res. 2009;**104**:403–11. doi:10.1161/CIRCRESAHA.108.190918.

[79] Tsuji T, Mizushige K, Noma T, Murakami K, Ohmori K, Miyatake A, et al. Pioglitazone improves left ventricular diastolic function and decreases collagen accumulation in prediabetic stage of a type II diabetic rat. J Cardiovasc Pharmacol. 2001;**38**:868–74. doi:10.1097/00005344-200112000-00008.

[80] von Bibra H, Diamant M, Scheffer PG, Siegmund T, Schumm-Draeger P-M. Rosiglitazone, but not glimepiride, improves myocardial diastolic function in association with reduction

in oxidative stress in type 2 diabetic patients without overt heart disease. Diabetes Vasc Dis Res. 2008;**5**:310–8. doi:10.3132/dvdr.2008.045.

[81] Terui G, Goto T, Katsuta M, Aoki I, Ito H. Effect of pioglitazone on left ventricular diastolic function and fibrosis of type III collagen in type 2 diabetic patients. J Cardiol. 2009;**54**:52–8. doi:10.1016/j.jjcc.2009.03.004.

[82] Hayat SA, Patel B, Khattar RS, Malik RA. Diabetic cardiomyopathy: mechanisms, diagnosis and treatment. Clin Sci (Lond). 2004;**107**:539–57. doi:10.1042/CS20040057.

[83] Takano H, Nagai T, Asakawa M, Toyozaki T, Oka T, Komuro I, et al. Peroxisome proliferator-activated receptor activators inhibit lipopolysaccharide-induced tumor necrosis factor-alpha expression in neonatal rat cardiac myocytes. Circ Res. 2000;**87**:596–602.

[84] Ares-Carrasco S, Picatoste B, Camafeita E, Carrasco-Navarro S, Zubiri I, Ortiz A, et al. Proteome changes in the myocardium of experimental chronic diabetes and hypertension. Role of PPAR$\alpha$ in the associated hypertrophy. J Proteomics. 2012;**75**:1816–29. doi:10.1016/j.jprot.2011.12.023.

[85] Ossum A, van Deurs U, Engstrøm T, Jensen JS, Treiman M. The cardioprotective and inotropic components of the postconditioning effects of GLP-1 and GLP-1(9–36)a in an isolated rat heart. Pharmacol Res. 2009;**60**:411–7. doi:10.1016/j.phrs.2009.06.004.

[86] Hansotia T, Drucker DJ. GIP and GLP-1 as incretin hormones: lessons from single and double incretin receptor knockout mice. Regul Pept. 2005;**128**:125–34. doi:10.1016/j.regpep.2004.07.019.

[87] Hattori Y, Jojima T, Tomizawa A, Satoh H, Hattori S, Kasai K, et al. A glucagon-like peptide-1 (GLP-1) analogue, liraglutide, upregulates nitric oxide production and exerts anti-inflammatory action in endothelial cells. Diabetologia. 2010;**53**:2256–63. doi:10.1007/s00125-010-1831-8.

[88] Mells JE, Fu PP, Sharma S, Olson D, Cheng L, Handy J a., et al. Glp-1 analog, liraglutide, ameliorates hepatic steatosis and cardiac hypertrophy in C57BL/6J mice fed a Western diet. AJP Gastrointest Liver Physiol. 2012;**302**:G225–35. doi:10.1152/ajpgi.00274.2011.

[89] Ferreira L, Teixeira-De-Lemos E, Pinto F, Parada B, Mega C, Vala H, et al. Effects of sitagliptin treatment on dysmetabolism, inflammation, and oxidative stress in an animal model of type 2 diabetes (ZDF rat). Mediators Inflamm. 2010;2010. doi:10.1155/2010/592760.

[90] Mega C, Teixeira De Lemos E, Vala H, Fernandes R, Oliveira J, Mascarenhas-Melo F, et al. Diabetic nephropathy amelioration by a low-dose sitagliptin in an animal model of type 2 diabetes (Zucker diabetic fatty rat). Exp Diabetes Res. 2011;2011. doi:10.1155/2011/162092.

[91] Gonçalves A, Leal E, Paiva A, Teixeira Lemos E, Teixeira F, Ribeiro CF, et al. Protective effects of the dipeptidyl peptidase IV inhibitor sitagliptin in the blood-retinal

barrier in a type 2 diabetes animal model. Diabetes Obes Metab. 2012;**14**:454–63. doi:10.1111/j.1463-1326.2011.01548.x.

[92] Gonçalves A, Marques C, Leal E, Ribeiro CF, Reis F, Ambrósio AF, et al. Dipeptidyl peptidase-IV inhibition prevents blood-retinal barrier breakdown, inflammation and neuronal cell death in the retina of type 1 diabetic rats. Biochim Biophys Acta Mol Basis Dis. 2014;**1842**:1454–63. doi:10.1016/j.bbadis.2014.04.013.

[93] Marques C, Mega C, Gonçalves A, Rodrigues-Santos P, Teixeira-Lemos E, Teixeira F, et al. Sitagliptin prevents inflammation and apoptotic cell death in the kidney of type 2 diabetic animals. Mediators Inflamm. 2014;2014. doi:10.1155/2014/538737.

[94] Mega C, Vala H, Rodrigues-Santos P, Oliveira J, Teixeira F, Fernandes R, et al. Sitagliptin prevents aggravation of endocrine and exocrine pancreatic damage in the Zucker Diabetic Fatty rat—focus on amelioration of metabolic profile and tissue cytoprotective properties. Diabetol Metab Syndr. 2014;**6**:42. doi:10.1186/1758-5996-6-42.

[95] Davignon J. Beneficial cardiovascular pleiotropic effects of statins. Circulation. 2004;**109**:III39–43. doi:10.1161/01.CIR.0000131517.20177.5a.

[96] Blanco-Colio LM, Tuñón J, Martín-Ventura JL, Egido J. Anti-inflammatory and immunomodulatory effects of statins. Kidney Int. 2003;**63**:12–23. doi:10.1046/j.1523-1755.2003.00744.x.

[97] Sola S, Mir MQS, Lerakis S, Tandon N, Khan B V. Atorvastatin improves left ventricular systolic function and serum markers of inflammation in nonischemic heart failure. J Am Coll Cardiol. 2006;**47**:332–7. doi:10.1016/j.jacc.2005.06.088.

[98] Shekelle PG, Rich MW, Morton SC, Atkinson SW, Tu W, Maglione M, et al. Efficacy of angiotensin-converting enzyme inhibitors and beta-blockers in the management of left ventricular systolic dysfunction according to race, gender, and diabetic status: a meta-analysis of major clinical trials. J Am Coll Cardiol. 2003;**41**:1529–38. doi:10.1016/S0735-1097(03)00262-6.

[99] Scheen a J. Prevention of type 2 diabetes mellitus through inhibition of the renin-angiotensin system. Drugs. 2004;**64**:2537–65. doi:10.2165/00003495-200464220-00004.

[100] Proudfoot JM, Croft KD, Puddey IB, Beilin LJ. Angiotensin II type 1 receptor antagonists inhibit basal as well as low-density lipoprotein and platelet-activating factor-stimulated human monocyte chemoattractant protein-1. J Pharmacol Exp Ther. 2003;**305**:846–53. doi:10.1124/jpet.102.047795.

[101] Muntean DM, Sturza A, Dănilă MD, Borza C, Duicu OM, Mornoș C. The role of mitochondrial reactive oxygen species in cardiovascular injury and protective strategies. Oxid Med Cell Longev. 2016;**2016**:8254942. doi:10.1155/2016/8254942.

[102] Wu Y-T, Wu S-B, Wei Y-H. Roles of sirtuins in the regulation of antioxidant defense and bioenergetic function of mitochondria under oxidative stress. Free Radic Res. 2014;**48**:1070–84. doi:10.3109/10715762.2014.920956.

[103] Wang H, Bei Y, Lu Y, Sun W, Liu Q, Wang Y, et al. Exercise prevents cardiac injury and improves mitochondrial biogenesis in advanced diabetic cardiomyopathy with PGC-1$\alpha$ and Akt activation. Cell Physiol Biochem. 2015;**35**:2159–68. doi:10.1159/000374021.

[104] Hall AR, Burke N, Dongworth RK, Hausenloy DJ. Mitochondrial fusion and fission proteins: novel therapeutic targets for combating cardiovascular disease. Br J Pharmacol. 2014;**171**:1890–906. doi:10.1111/bph.12516.

[105] Disatnik MH, Hwang S, Ferreira JCB, Mochly-Rosen D. New therapeutics to modulate mitochondrial dynamics and mitophagy in cardiac diseases. J Mol Med. 2015;**93**:279–87. doi:10.1007/s00109-015-1256-4.

[106] Ristow M, Zarse K. How increased oxidative stress promotes longevity and metabolic health: the concept of mitochondrial hormesis (mitohormesis). Exp Gerontol. 2010;**45**:410–8. doi:10.1016/j.exger.2010.03.014.

[107] Schulz TJ, Westermann D, Isken F, Voigt A, Laube B, Thierbach R, et al. Activation of mitochondrial energy metabolism protects against cardiac failure. Aging (Albany NY). 2010;**2**:843–53.

[108] Marques-Aleixo I, Santos-Alves E, Mariani D, Rizo-Roca D, Padrão AI, Rocha-Rodrigues S, et al. Physical exercise prior and during treatment reduces sub-chronic doxorubicin-induced mitochondrial toxicity and oxidative stress. Mitochondrion. 2015;**20**:22–33. doi:10.1016/j.mito.2014.10.008.

[109] Song M, Chen Y, Gong G, Murphy E, Rabinovitch PS, Dorn GW. Super-suppression of mitochondrial reactive oxygen species signaling impairs compensatory autophagy in primary mitophagic cardiomyopathy. Circ Res. 2014;**115**:348–53. doi:10.1161/CIRCRESAHA.115.304384.

Chapter 13

# Cirrhotic Cardiomyopathy

Coskun Celtik, Nelgin Gerenli,

Halil Haldun Emiroglu and Nimet Cındık

Additional information is available at the end of the chapter

http://dx.doi.org/10.5772/65318

**Abstract**

Cirrhotic cardiomyopathy (CCMP) is a functional disorder characterized by electrophysiologic disturbances and diastolic and/or systolic dysfunction in patients with chronic liver disease, especially those with ascites and portal hypertension. This disorder is a well-defined entity in adults, but pediatric data are limited. Clinical and laboratory findings are generally latent. The diagnostic criteria are prolonged QT on electrocardiography due to metabolic and extrahepatic causes, in addition to some abnormal echocardiography findings. If echocardiographic findings are normal and only specific prolonged QT is present, this disorder is named as "latent CCMP"; otherwise, it is "manifest CCMP." This disorder is important because it may lead to problems such as cardiac failure and dysrhythmia before or after liver transplantation. Moreover, it may worsen the prognosis.

**Keywords:** cirrhosis, portal hypertension, cardiomyopathy, prolonged QT, liver

## 1. Introduction

Portal hypertension (PHT) is an important disorder that increases morbidity and mortality rates. Many hemodynamic changes related to PHT occur in the human body. The majority of these changes are associated with hyperdynamic circulation, which is characterized by elevated heart rate and cardiac output accompanied by vasodilatation in the splanchnic area and systemic circulation and decreased systemic vascular resistance [1–9]. Moreover, disturbances of the autonomic nerve system and baroreceptors and the increased arterial compliance in patients with cirrhosis aggravate the condition [10–12]. Hemodynamic changes that occur in portal hypertension are shown in **Table 1**.

Cardiovascular disorders associated with cirrhosis were first defined in alcoholic cirrhotic patients, in 1953 by Kowalski and Abelmann, but for many years, it was thought that these disorders were associated with chronic alcohol intake [10–12]. Similar disturbances were described in patients with cirrhosis who had hemochromatosis in some later research, but this time the changes were associated with hemochromatosis [13]. Consequently, cirrhotic cardiomyopathy was not known in those years.

| | |
|---|---|
| **Systemic circulation** | |
| Plasma volume ↑<br>Total blood volume ↑<br>Noncentral blood volume ↑<br>Central arterial blood volume → ↓ (↑) | Cardiac flow (→) ↑<br>Arterial blood tension → ↓<br>Heart rate ↑<br>Systemic vascular resistance ↓ |
| **Heart** | |
| Left atrial volume ↑<br>Left ventricle volume → (↓)<br>Right atrial volume → ↑ ↓<br>Right ventricle volume → ↑ ↓ | Right atrial tension → ↑<br>Right ventricle end-diastole tension →<br>Pulmonary arterial tension → ↑<br>Pulmonary capillary wedge tension →<br>Left ventricle end-diastole tension → |
| **Pulmonary circulation** | |
| Pulmonary blood flow ↑ | Pulmonary vascular resistance ↓ (↑) |
| **Renal circulation** | |
| Renal blood flow ↓ | Renal vascular resistance ↑ |
| **Cerebral circulation** | |
| Cerebral blood flow ↓ → | |
| **Skin, muscular, and skeletal circulation** | |
| Skin blood flow → ↑ | Muscular and skeletal circulation → ↑ ↓ |
| ↑, increased; ↓, decreased; →, not changed | |

**Table 1.** The hemodynamic changes due to cirrhotic portal hypertension [6].

Caremelo et al. first described cirrhotic cardiomyopathy in 1986. The authors demonstrated cardiac function disturbances due to cirrhosis in an experimental rat model and suggested the cirrhotic cardiomyopathy hypothesis. Their hypothesis was supported by subsequent research, and cardiac disorders due to cirrhosis and portal hypertension were named "cirrhotic cardiomyopathy" in 1989 [1–12, 14]. Although the name "hepatocardiac syndrome" was proposed by some authors instead of "cirrhotic cardiomyopathy," this term was not accepted [14].

## 2. Definition

Cirrhotic cardiomyopathy (CCMP) is defined as a functional disorder characterized by electrophysiologic disturbances and diastolic and/or systolic dysfunction in patients with cirrhotic PHT. Even though similar hemodynamic changes have been defined in long-term non-cirrhotic PHT, the development of CCMP in such patients has not been reported. Therefore, this term is usually used for patients with cirrhosis [10, 15–18].

## 3. Pathogenesis

In general, arterial vasodilatation, central hypovolemia, and hyperdynamic circulation which occur as a result of cirrhosis and portal hypertension lead to the development of CCMP together with hepatorenal syndrome and hepatopulmonary syndrome (**Figure 1**) [11, 19–23]. Effects of vasoactive agents are very important in pathogenesis of CCMP. Experimentally, some changes were defined in CCMP, such as downregulation of the density of β receptors, impaired β-adrenergic signaling, alternations of calcium-ion channels, and alternations in plasma membrane fluidity in cardiomyocytes. In addition, the increased serum bile acids, cytokines, and endotoxins have been shown to create negative effects on cardiomyocytes [9–12, 14, 22].

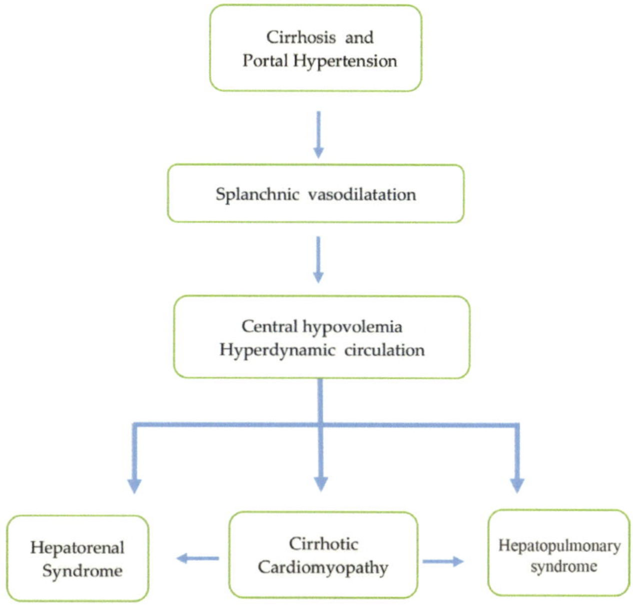


**Figure 1.** Cirrhotic cardiomyopathy pathogenesis.

Vasoconstrictor substances are high in the early stages of PHT, and vasodilator substances gradually increase in advanced stages; the balance tips in favor of vasodilators and a receptor insensitivity develops against vasoconstrictors [10–12, 19, 23–30]. As a result of these events, arterial vasodilatation results and the severity of PHT increases [19, 23–30].

The splanchnic vasodilatation that develops in PHT is combined with a hyperkinetic systemic circulation, low arterial tension, decreased peripheral resistance, and increased cardiac flow.

Although total plasma volume increases, as a result of collection of blood in the splanchnic area, effective blood capacity cannot be achieved, and central hypovolemia develops. After these changes, activation of the sympathetic nervous system and renin-aldosterone system occurs; vasopressin release from the hypothalamus increases, which results in fluid and salt retention [30–33].

The vasoconstrictor and vasodilator substances in the pathogenesis PHT become effective together. The most important vasoconstrictor substances are norepinephrine, angiotensin II, vasopressin, thromboxane (TX), and leukotrienes. The effects of these substances are related with activation of the sympathetic nervous system and renin-angiotensin-aldosterone system. Researches have shown that portal venous tension can be decreased using alpha-adrenergic antagonists (prazosin), beta-adrenergic antagonists (propranolol), angiotensin-II antagonists, cyclooxygenase isoenzyme blockers, and TX antagonists. Results of these researches support the pathogenesis [22, 29–34].

Endothelin (ET) can show vasoconstrictor or vasodilator effects according to the type. Endothelins are classified as ET-1, ET-2, and ET-3 according to their region in the body. ET-1 is mainly found in endothelial cells, the kidney, and the brain and ET-2 in the small intestine and kidney, and ET-3 is found in the blood. ET-1 and ET-2 create a vasoconstrictor effect, whereas ET-3 has a vasodilator effect. These two opposite effects are associated with the induction of nitric oxide and prostacyclin release. The most potent vasoconstrictor substance in the body is ET-1, and it is reported that this substance is very effective in the development of PHT complications [22, 29–34].

Nitric oxide (NO) is another very potent substance in the pathogenesis of PHT. NO is synthesized from arginine by nitric oxide synthetase (NOS) and causes vasodilatation by increasing cyclic guanosine monophosphate. NO initially increases to compensate against the elevated vasoconstrictor agents in the early stage of PHT, but secondary systemic and splanchnic vasodilatation develops because of excessive NO production. This event is a result of stimulation of NOS by cytokines such as TNF-alpha, which increases in cirrhosis [22, 30–36].

The other important vasodilator substances in the pathogenesis of PHT are carbon monoxide (CO), hydrogen sulfide ($H_2S$), prostaglandins, glucagon, and endocannabinoids. CO formed through the heme-oxygenase system is a weaker vasodilator agent than NO, but it is important for regulation of intrahepatic vascular tone. $H_2S$ is formed by intestinal microbiota and increases the effects of other vasodilator substances and PHT severity [22, 30–36].

Prostaglandins are endogen vasodilators produced in the endothelium and are important for hyperdynamic circulation. Prostacyclin is produced from the vascular endothelium. It leads to vasodilatation, which increases the level of intracellular cyclic adenosine monophosphate (c-AMP) through the activation of adenylate cyclase. In recent studies, it was shown that indomethacin, a prostacyclin inhibitor, decreased the hyperdynamic circulation and balanced the vasoconstrictor effect [22, 30–36].

Glucagon is a hormone released from the pancreas. Glucagon levels increase as a result of low hepatic clearance and stimulation of pancreatic alpha cells in patients with cirrhosis. Glucagon also has the effect of reducing endogenous vasoconstrictor activity in addition to having a vasodilator effect. The use of somatostatin and synthetic glucagon analogs for PHT therapy has been proposed in some studies; however, these agents may constitute a risk because they can aggravate the splanchnic vasodilatation in advanced stages [22, 30–36].

Endocannabinoids such as anandamide are vasodilator substances that increase in PHT, worsen hepatic microcirculation, and accelerate apoptosis. These substances act by stimulating CB1 and CB2 receptors in the vascular endothelium. It has been reported that endogen cannabinoids show a negative inotropic effect on myocardial contractions, and therefore these substances are very important for the development of cirrhotic cardiomyopathy [39–41]. These negative effects can be blocked by CB-1 receptor antagonists (AM251) [22, 30–40].

## 4. Clinical finding and diagnosis

Cirrhotic cardiomyopathy (CCMP) represents a condition in which no real cardiac disease is present but a functional cardiac abnormality exists. With time, CCMP progresses to the chronic phase. In a resting state, there is no real disease, but with stress, the cardiac muscle does not contract appropriately and and/or electrophysiologic abnormalities appear [10–12]. There is no exact classification for CCMP and the criteria proposed by Moller et al. are still used (**Table 2**). These data are taken from an adult studies, pediatric data are very limited [41–45]. The most important points from these criteria are (1) at rest, normal, or increased left ventricular contractibility; (2) abnormal systolic contraction or diastolic relaxation with pharmacologic, physiologic, or surgical stress; and (3) cardiac electrical abnormalities [10, 11].

Diagnosis of CCMP in children with cirrhosis is difficult, because invasive methods are life-threatening and noninvasive tests are unreliable for them. In recent years, a new article was published in which CCMP criteria for children were reviewed [45]. According to this literature, a prolonged QT interval on electrocardiography (ECG) is an important finding after all non-liver causes are excluded, and shows latent cardiomyopathy due to cirrhotic changes. If there is the presence of echocardiographic abnormalities, this event is a manifest CCMP [45].

Cirrhotic cardiomyopathy is a latent disease in which there is no abnormality except under stress conditions. In such patients, there is no cardiac disease till end-stage disease. At end stage, infrequent arrhythmias or cardiac insufficiency may be seen. If these findings exist in an early cirrhotic stage, other causes of cardiomyopathy such as infections, metabolic disorders, endocrinopathies, ischemic or toxic causes, and genetic and systemic diseases should be investigated [46].

Cirrhotic cardiomyopathy is more likely dilated cardiomyopathy where some stress factors cause cardiac dysfunction. With stress, the clinical status of the patient deteriorates and decompensation may exist. These stress factors are exercise, infection, positional changes, feeding, paracentesis with high volumes, changes in intravascular volume, the use of vasoconstrictor drugs, transjugular intrahepatic portosystemic shunts (TIPS), or surgical procedures such as minor operations or liver transplantation [10–12]. Exercise tolerance in patients with cirrhosis is abnormal due to cardiac function abnormalities, and this correlates with the patient's Child score [47].

| Systolic dysfunction criteria | Supporting criteria |
| --- | --- |
| • Inadequate cardiac flow to pharmacologic agents, exercise, blood volume changes | • Electrophysiologic abnormalities |
| | • Abnormal chronotropic response |
| • Resting ejection fraction under 55 % | • Electromechanical uncoupling/dyssynchronism |
| **Diastolic dysfunction** | • Prolonged QT intervals |
| • E/A ratio <1,0 (corrected according to age) | • Expended left atrium |
| • Prolonged deceleration time (>200 milliseconds) | • Increased myocardial mass |
| • Prolonged isovolumetric relaxation time (>80 milliseconds) | • Increased BNP and pro-BNP levels |
| | • Increased troponin I levels |

BNP, brain natriuretic peptide; E/A ratio, the ratio between the early (E) and late atrial (A) phases of ventricular velocity

**Table 2.** Diagnostic criteria of cirrhotic cardiomyopathy.

There is a relationship between CCMP and hepatorenal syndrome (HRS), which has been reported in many articles published in recent years, so patients with HRS are at more risk [5, 25, 48].

Cardiac functions in patients with liver cirrhosis are determined by physical examination, ECG, and telecardiography besides of echocardiography. Cardiac functions such as systolic, diastolic, and electromechanical functions should be evaluated in suspected CCMP. ECG is sufficient for determining electrophysiologic function. Systolic and diastolic functions are checked using M-Mod, two- and three-dimensional echocardiocardiography, and spectral and tissue Doppler echocardiocardiography. Cardiac magnetic resonance imaging, radio nuclear angiography, and myocardial perfusion techniques are more advanced methods. Many times, for a diagnosis of CCMP, the findings on ECG and echocardiocardiography are enough.

Firstly, systolic function worsens in the late stage of CCMP. After then, the diastolic functions gradually decay. Diastolic dysfunction is best shown with echocardiographic measurement of the E/A ratio. Deceleration time (DT) and the isovolumetric relaxation time (IVRT) also are used. The E/A ratio results from blood velocity from the left atrium to the left ventricle, the velocity of which during early systole causes the E wave and the same flow causes the A wave during late diastole.

The measurement of E and A waves is expressed as cm/sec and best is done from mitral valve projection. A normal E/A ratio in healthy individuals until the age of 50 years is 1–2 cm/s, but in older people, it decreases below 1 cm/s. An E/A ratio in healthy individuals aged less than 50 years below 1 cm/s shows diastolic dysfunction. However, the restrictive pattern can be observed in advanced stages depending on the severity of the disorder in the patients with CCMP; the E/A ratio may reverse in these cases and may be determined >2 [10, 11, 49] (**Figure 2**).

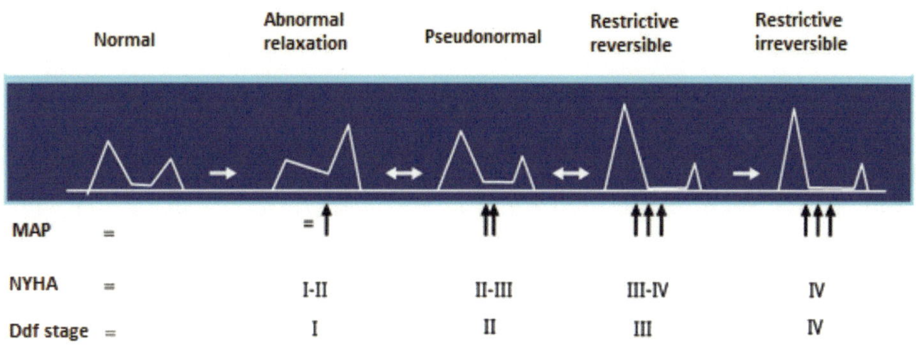


**Figure 2. Diastolic dysfunction stages** [49]. MAP, mean atrial pressure; NYHA, New York Heart Association; Ddf stage, diastolic dysfunction stage.

| Indicator | Normal pattern | Abnormal relaxation (stage I) | Pseudonormal pattern (stage II) | Restrictive pattern (stages III–IV) |
|---|---|---|---|---|
| E/A | >1 | <1 | 1–2 | ≥2 |
| DT (msn) | 160–210 | >220 | 150–200 | <150 |
| IVGT (msn) | 70–90 | >95 | 60–95 | <60 |

DT, deceleration time; E/A, transmitral early diastolic flow (E)/transmitral late diastolic flow (atrial) (A) ratio; IVGT, isovolumetric relaxation time (msn).

**Table 3.** Echocardiographic stages of left ventricular diastolic dysfunction [49].

There are different stages in CCMP. Clinical findings differ according to stage (**Table 3**). The E/A ratio worsens according to the severity of hepatic disease and it is worse in patients with ascites than in patients with non-ascites and normal persons. The E/A ratio improves after paracentesis and this event supports that ascites is the negative effect on cardiac functions [50–53]. There are no publications on these themes in children. There is no definitive normal value for the E/A ratio in children, but in some publications, it is proposed to be between 1.7 and 2.5 cm/s.

Electrical conduction abnormalities and arrhythmias can be seen in the patients according to severity of cirrhosis [8, 9] [54–58]. There are three types of electrophysiologic abnormalities caused by cirrhosis: (1) prolonged QT on ECG, (2) inadequate response to chronotropic stress, and (3) electromagnetic dyssynchronism [10, 11, 14]. The prolonged QT on ECG means a corrected QT interval (QTc) is longer than 0.440 value [41, 54, 55]. Prolonged QT shows abnormal myocardial repolarization as a sign of CCMP [10–12, 56–58]. QT prolongation proportionally increases with cirrhotic stage [56]. Prolonged QT on ECG is frequently seen in patients with CCMP. The rate of determination of prolonged QT is 30–60 % in adults with CCMP and in 18–45 % of pediatric patients [5, 41, 44, 56].

Actually, a prolonged QT interval may cause life-threatening arrhythmias [55], but in many patients with CCMP, despite a prolonged QT interval, no significant clinical problem and arrhythmia are not observed. Cardiac arrhythmias in cirrhotic patients are frequently related to vasopressin use. There is no evidence that a prolonged QT interval in patients with CCMP causes life-threatening arrhythmias. Probably, some compensatory mechanisms in cirrhotic patients prevent the disturbances and the disease occurs latent until end stage.

## 5. Treatment

Treatment consists of preventing stress exposure in patients with CCMP; rest and oxygen supplementation are important [10, 59]. There is no need for pharmacotherapy when there is no cardiac insufficiency. Drugs have adverse effects and pharmacotherapy response is weak in patients with CCMP. In recent years, aldosterone antagonists, cannabinoid receptor antagonists, and spironolactone have been used, but only the effectiveness of beta-blockers has been proved [10, 35, 59]. Beta-blockers can decrease QT wave duration [10, 32, 33]. Diagnosis of CCMP at an early stage is important. Early diagnosis and proper treatment with cardioprotective agents are important for decreasing complications during and after liver transplantation. There are no exact data on prognosis for liver transplantation in patients with CCMP. Data from the past showed that CCMP worsens in the early period after liver transplantation, and later cardiac functions and cardiac electromechanical dysfunctions improve gradually by supplying hemodynamic stabilization of the patient [10, 59–64]. Liver transplantation can be a definitive treatment for CCMP. New pharmacologic agents are needed to help these patients because many patients do not have the chance to receive a transplant.

## Author details

Coskun Celtik[1*], Nelgin Gerenli[1], Halil Haldun Emiroglu[2] and Nimet Cındık[3]

*Address all correspondence to: cceltik2001@yahoo.com

1 Pediatric Gastroenterology, Health Sciences University, Istanbul Umraniye Training and Research Hospital, Istanbul, Turkey

2 Pediatric Gastroenterology, Selcuk University, Faculty of Medicine, Konya, Turkey

3 Pediatric Cardiology, Health Sciences University, Istanbul Umraniye Training and Research Hospital, Istanbul, Turkey

## References

[1] Baik SK, Lee SS. Cirrhotic cardiomyopathy; causes and consequences. *J Gastroenterol Hepatol*, 2004;19(7): 185–190, DOI: 10.1111/j.1440-1746.2004.03639.x.

[2] Mandell MS, Tsou MY. Cardiovascular dysfunction in patient with end-stage liver disease. *J Clin Med Assoc*, 2008;71(7): 331-335, DOI: 10.1016/S1726-4901(08)70134-5.

[3] Liu H., Lee S. Cardiopulmonary dysfunction in cirrhosis. *J Gastroenterol Hepatol*, 1999;14(6): 600-608. DOI: 10.1046/j.1440-1746.1999.01920.x.

[4] Lee, R., Glenn T., Lee S. Cardiac dysfunction in cirrhosis. *Best Pract Res Clin Gastroenterol*, 2007;21(1): 125-140. DOI: 10.1016/j.bpg.2006.06.003.

[5] Baik S, Fouad T, Lee S. Cirrhotic cardiomyopathy. *Orphanet J Rare Dis*, 2007;2(15): 1-8. DOI: 10.1186/1750-1172-2-15.

[6] Møller S., Henriksen J. Cardiovascular dysfunction in cirrhosis. Pathophysiological evidence of a cirrhotic cardiomyopathy. *Scand J Gastroenterol*, 2001;36(8): 785-794. DOI: 10.1080/00365520120972.

[7] Liu H., Song D., Lee S. Cirrhotic cardiomyopathy. *Gastroenterol Clin Biol*, 2002;26(10), 842-847. DOI: GCB-10-2002-26-10-0399-8320-101019-ART4.

[8] Blendis L., Wong F. Is there a cirrhotic cardiomyopathy? *Am J Gastroenterol*, 2000;95, 3026-3028. DOI: 10.1111/j.1572-0241.2000.03306.x.

[9] Hamoudi WA, Lee SS. (2006): Cirrhotic cardiomyopathy. *Ann Hepatol*, 5, 132-139. PMID: 17060868.

[10] Wong, F. Cirrhotic cardiomyopathy. *Hepatol Int*, 2009;3(1), 294-304. DOI: 10.1007/s12072-008-9109-7

[11] Moller S, Henricsen JH. Cardiovascular complications of cirrhosis. *Postgrad Med J*, 2009;85,44-54. DOI: 10.1136/gut.2006.112177.

[12] Swanson KL., Krowka MJ. Pulmonary complications associated with portal hypertension. In: Sanyal AJ, Shah VH, editors. Portal Hypertension; Pathobiology, Evaluation, and Treatment, Humana Press, Totowa, 2005. p. 455-468. ISBN 1-58829-386-6

[13] Niederau C, Fischer R, Sonnenberg A, Stremmel W, Trampisch HJ, Strohmeyer G. Survival and causes of death in cirrhotic and in noncirrhotic patients with primary hemochromatosis. *N Engl J Med*. 1985;313(20),1256-1262. DOI: 10.1056/NEJM198511143132004

[14] Milani, A., Zaccaria R., Bombardieri G., Gasbarrini A., Pola P. (2007): Cirrhotic cardiomyopathy. *Dig Liver Dis*, 39, 507-515. DOI: 10.1016/j.dld.2006.12.014

[15] Sarin SK, Wadhawan M. Noncirrhotic portal hypertension and portal vein thrombosis. In: Sanyal AJ, Shah VH, editors. Portal Hypertension: Pathobiology,

Evaluation, and Treatment, Humana Press Inc, Totowa, NJ. 2005. p. 411-432. ISBN 1-58829-386-6

[16] Molina, E. & K. Reddy. Noncirrhotic portal hypertension. *Clin Liver Dis*, 2001;5(3), 769-87. PMID: 11565140

[17] Sarin SK, Kapoor D. Non-cirrhotic portal fibrosis; current concept and management. *J Gastroenterol Hepatol*, 2002;17(5), 526-534. DOI: 10.1046/j.1440-1746.2002.02764.x

[18] Okudaira M., Ohbu M., Okuda K. Idiopathic portal hypertension and its pathology. *Semin Liver Dis*, 2002;22(1), 59-72. DOI: 10.1055/s-2002-23207.

[19] Gunaratnam NT., Su GL. Pathogenesis and consequences of portal hypertension. In: Rose S, editor. Gastrointestinal and Hepatobiliary Pathophysiology, Fence Creek Publising, Madison, 1998. p.315-326. ISBN: 1-59377-181-9

[20] Møller S, Henriksen JH. Cardiovascular complications of cirrhosis. *Gut*, 2008;57(2), 268-278. DOI: 10.1136/gut.2006.112177

[21] Ma Z., Lee S. Cirrhotic cardiomyopathy; getting to the heart of the matter. *Hepatology*, 1996;24 (2), 451-459. DOI: 10.1002/hep.510240226

[22] Wiese S, Hove JD, Bendtsen F, Moller S. Cirrhotic cardiomyopathy: pathogenesis and clinical relevance. *Nat Rev Gastroenterol Hepatol*,2014; 11(3), 177–186. DOI: 10.1038/nrgastro.2013.210

[23] Treiber G., Csepregi A., Malfertheiner P. The pathophysiology of portal hypertension. *Dig Dis*, 2005;23 (1), 6-10. DOI: 10.1159/000084720

[24] Bosch J., Garcia-Pagàn JC. Complications of cirrhosis. I. Portal hypertension. *J Hepatol*, 2000; 32 (Suppl. 1), 141-156.DOI: 10.1016/S0168-8278(00)80422-5

[25] Liu H., Gaskari S., Lee S. Cardiac and vascular changes in cirrhosis; pathogenic mechanisms. *World J Gastroenterol*, 2006;12(6), 837-42. DOI: 10.3748/WJG.v12.i6.837

[26] Niederberger M., Schrier R. Pathogenesis of sodium and water retention in liver disease. *Prog Liver Dis*, 1992;10, 329-47. PMID:1296235

[27] Møller S., Bendtsen F., Henriksen J. Splanchnic and systemic hemodynamic derangement in decompensated cirrhosis. *Can J Gastroenterol*, 2001;15 (2), 94-106. DOI: 10.1155/2001/603012

[28] Møller S, Bendtsen F, Henriksen JH. Vasoactive substances in the circulatory dysfunction of cirrhosis. *Scand J Clin Lab Invest*, 2001;61, 421-429. DOI: 10.1080/0036551 0152567059

[29] Møller S., Henriksen JH. Cirrhotic cardiomyopathy: a pathophysiological review of circulatory dysfunction in liver disease. *Heart*, 2002;87 (1), 9-15. DOI:10.1136/heart. 87.1.9

[30] Pinzani M, Vizzutti F. Anatomy and vascular biology of the cells in the portal circulation. In: Sanyal AJ., Shah VH, editors. Portal Hypertension; Pathobiology,

Evaluation, and Treatment, Humana Press Inc, Totowa, NJ, 2005, p.15-35. ISBN 1-58829-386-6

[31] Ryckman FC., Alonso MH., Tiao G. Causes and management of portal hypertension in the pediatric population. In: Sanyal AJ, Shah VH, editors. Portal Hypertension; Pathobiology, Evaluation, and Treatment, Humana Press Inc, Totowa, 2005, p.383-410. ISBN 1-58829-386-6

[32] Zambruni A, Trevisani F, Di Micoli A, Savelli F, Berzigotti A, Bracci E, Caraceni P, Domenicali M, Felline P, Zoli M, Bernardi M. Effect of chronic beta-blockade on QT interval in patients with liver cirrhosis. *J Hepatol*, 2008;48(3), 415–421. DOI: 10.1016/j.jhep.2007.11.012

[33] Henriksen JH, Bendtsen F, Hansen EF, Møller S. Acute nonselective beta-adrenergic blockade reduces prolonged frequency adjusted Q-T interval (QTc) in patients with cirrhosis. *J Hepatol*, 2004;40(2), 239–246. DOI: 10.1016/j.jhep.2003.10.026

[34] Pozzi M., Ratti L., Guidi C., Milanese M., Mancia G. Potential therapeutic targets in cirrhotic cardiomyopathy. *Cardiovasc Hematol Disord Drug Targets*, 2007;7(1), 21-26. DOI: 10.2174/187152907780059074

[35] Mallat A., Lotersztajn S. Cannabinoid receptors as therapeutic targets in the management of liver diseases. *Drug News Perspect*, 2008;21(7), 363-8. DOI: 10.1358/dnp.2008.21.7.1255306

[36] Liu H., Ma Z., Lee S. (2000): Contribution of nitric oxide to the pathogenesis of cirrhotic cardiomyopathy in bile duct-ligated rats. *Gastroenterology*, 118(5), 937-944. DOI: 10.1016/S0016-5085(00)70180-6

[37] Pacher P., Bátkai S., Kunos G. Cirrhotic cardiomyopathy: an endocannabinoid connection? *Br J Pharmacol*, 2005;146 (3), 313-314. DOI: 10.1038/sj.bjp.0706332

[38] Caraceni P., Domenicali M, Giannone F, Bernardi M. The role of the endocannabinoid system in liver diseases. *Best Pract Res Clin Endocrinol Metab*, 2009;23 (1), 65-77. DOI: 10.1016/j.beem.2008.10.009

[39] Gaskari, S., Liu H., Moezi L., Li Y., Baik S., Lee S. Role of endocannabinoids in the pathogenesis of cirrhotic cardiomyopathy in bile duct-ligated rats. *Br J Pharmacol*, 2005;146 (3), 315-23. DOI: 10.1038/sj.bjp.0706331

[40] Bátkai S., Pacher P. Endocannabinoids and cardiac contractile function; pathophysiological implications. *Pharmacol Res*, 2009;60 (2), 99-106. DOI: 10.1016/j.phrs.2009.04.003

[41] Fishberger SB., Pittman NS., Rossi AF. Prolongation of the QT interval in children with liver failure. *Clin Cardiol*, 1999; 22(10), 658-60. DOI: 10.1002/clc.4960221013

[42] Ozçay F, Tokel K, Varan B, Saygılı A. Cardiac evaluation of pediatric liver transplantation candidates. *Transplant Proc*, 2002; 34 (6), 2150-2152. DOI: 10.1016/S0041-1345(02)02886-5

[43] Polat, T., Urganci N., Yalcin Y., Akdeniz C., Zeybek C., Erdem A., Celebi A. Evaluation of cardiac function by tissue Doppler imaging in children with chronic hepatitis. *J Pediatr Gastroenterol Nutr*, 2006;43 (2), 222-227. DOI: 10.1097/01.mpg.0000228101.12326.6f

[44] Arikan C., Kilic M., Tumgor G., Levent E., Yuksekkaya HA., Yagci RV., Aydogdu S. (2009): Impact of liver transplantation on rate-corrected QT interval and myocardial function in children with chronic liver disease. *Pediatr Transplant*, 13(3), 300-306. DOI: 10.1111/j.1399-3046.2008.00909.x

[45] Celtik C, Durmaz O, Oner N, Yavuz T, Gökce S, Aydogan A, Nisli K, Emiroglu HH, Ömeroglu RE, Söküсü S. Investigation of cardiomyopathy in children with cirrhotic and noncirrhotic portal hypertension. *J Pediatr Gastroenterol Nutr*. 2015;60(2):177-81. DOI: 10.1097/MPG.0000000000000580.

[46] Towbin JA, Lowe AM, Colan SD, Sleeper LA, Orav EJ, Clunie S, Messere J, Cox GF, Lurie PR, Hsu D, Canter C, Wilkinson JD, Lipshultz SE. Incidence, causes, and outcomes of dilated cardiomyopathy in children. *JAMA*, 2006;296 (15), 1867-1876. DOI: 10.1001/jama.296.15.1867

[47] Terziyski K, Andonov V, Marinov B and Kostianev S. Exercise performance and ventilatory efficiency in patients with mild and moderate liver cirrhosis. *Clin Exp Pharmacol Physiol*, 2007;35 (2),135-140. DOI: 10.1111/j.1440-1681.2007.04751.x

[48] Ruiz-del-Arbol L, Monescillo A, Arocena C, Valer P, Ginès P, Moreira V, Milicua JM, Jiménez W, Arroyo V. Circulatory function and hepatorenal syndrome in cirrhosis. *Hepatology*, 2005;42(2), 439-447. DOI: 10.1002/hep.20766

[49] Tezel T. Evaluation of Diastolic Functions [Diyastolik fonksiyonların değerlendirilmesi]. Nobel Tıp Kitapevleri, Istanbul, Turkey 2007. p. 1-216. ISBN: 97897524205725.

[50] Moller S, Henriksen JH. Cardiopulmonary complications in chronic liver disease. *World J Gastroenterol*, 2006;12(4), 526-538. DOI: 10.3748/WJG.v12.i4.526

[51] Pozzi M, Carugo S, Boari G, Pecci V, de Ceglia S, Maggiolini S, Bolla GB, Roffi L, Failla M, Grassi G, Giannattasio C, Mancia G. Evidence of functional and structural cardiac abnormalities in cirrhotic patients with and without ascites. *Hepatology*, 1997;26(5), 1131-1137. DOI: 10.1002/hep.510260507

[52] Valeriano, V., S. Funaro, R. Lionetti, O. Riggio, G. Pulcinelli, P. Fiore, A. Masini, S. De Castro & M. Merli. Modification of cardiac function in cirrhotic patients with and without ascites. *Am J Gastroenterol*, 2000;95 (11), 3200-3205. DOI: 10.1111/j.1572-0241.2000.03252.x

[53] Finucci G, Desideri A, Sacerdoti D, Bolognesi M, Merkel C, Angeli P, Gatta A. Left ventricular diastolic function in liver cirrhosis. *Scand J Gastroenterol*, 1996;31(3), 279-284. DOI: 10.3109/00365529609004879

[54] Miller MD, Porter CJ, Ackerman MJ. Diagnostic accuracy of screening electrocardiograms in long QT syndrome I. *Pediatrics*, 2001;108 (1), 8–12. DOI: 10.1542/peds.108.1.8

[55] Friedman MJ, Mull CC, Sharieff GQ, Tsarouhas N. Prolonged QT syndrome in children: uncommon but potentially fatal entity. *J Emerg Med*, 2003;24(2), 173–179. DOI: 10.1016/S0736-4679(02)00721-7

[56] Bernardi M, Calandra S, Colantoni A, Trevisani F, Raimondo ML, Sica G, Schepis F, Mandini M, Simoni P, Contin M, Raimondo G. Q-T interval prolongation in cirrhosis: prevalence, relationship with severity, and etiology of the disease and possible pathogenetic factors. *Hepatology*, 1998;27(1), 28-34. DOI: 10.1002/hep.510270106

[57] Bal JS, Thuluvath PJ. Prolongation of QTc interval: relationship with etiology and severity of liver disease, mortality and liver transplantation. *Liver Int*, 2003;23, 243-248. DOI: 10.1034/j.1600-0676.2003.00833.x

[58] Zambruni A, Trevisani F, Caraceni P, Bernardi M. Cardiac electrophysiological abnormalities in patients with cirrhosis. *J Hepatol*, 2006;44(5), 994-1002. DOI: 10.1016/j.jhep.2005.10.034

[59] Gaskari S., Honar H., Lee S. Therapy insight; cirrhotic cardiomyopathy. *Nat Clin Pract Gastroenterol Hepatol*, 2006;3(6), 329-37. DOI: 10.1038/ncpgasthep0498

[60] Acosta F, De La Morena G, Villegas M, Sansano T, Reche M, Beltran R, Roques V, Contreras RF, Robles R, Bueno FS, Ramirez P, Parrilla P. Evaluation of cardiac function before and after liver transplantation. *Transplant Proc*, 1999;31(6), 2369–2370. DOI: 10.1016/S0041-1345(99)00383-8

[61] Myers R., Lee S. Cirrhotic cardiomyopathy and liver transplantation. *Liver Transpl*, 2000;6(4 suppl 1), 44-52. DOI: 10.1002/lt.500060510

[62] Liu H., Lee S. What happens to cirrhotic cardiomyopathy after liver transplantation? *Hepatology*, 2005; 42(5), 1203-5. DOI: 10.1002/hep.20911

[63] Torregrosa M, Aguadé S, Dos L, Segura R, Gónzalez A, Evangelista A, Castell J, Margarit C, Esteban R, Guardia J, Genescà J. Cardiac alterations in cirrhosis; reversibility after liver transplantation, *J Hepatol*, 2005;42(1), 68-74. DOI: 10.1016/j.jhep.2004.09.008

[64] Mandell MS, Lindenfeld J, Tsou MY, Zimmerman M. (2008): Cardiac evaluation of liver transplant candidates. *World J Gastroenterol*, 14(22), 3445-3451. DOI: 10.3748/wjg.14.3445

Chapter 14

# Takotsubo Cardiomyopathy as a Neurocardiogenic Injury after Subarachnoid Hemorrhage: Hemodynamics and Fluid Management

Tatsushi Mutoh, Tomoko Mutoh, Yasuyuki Taki and Tatsuya Ishikawa

Additional information is available at the end of the chapter

http://dx.doi.org/10.5772/65011

**Abstract**

Takotsubo cardiomyopathy (TCM) is a life-threatening systemic disorder that may occur early after aneurysmal subarachnoid hemorrhage (SAH), but precise hemodynamics and fluid management remain unclear. Although TCM is often regarded as a reversible or self-limited phenomenon, it contributes significantly to morbidity and mortality of SAH patients, especially when it is complicated with other neurogenic injuries such as severe left ventricular dysfunction, pulmonary edema, and pneumonia. The purpose of this chapter is to introduce the current practice in intensive hemodynamic monitoring and goal-directed fluid management of post-SAH TCM using advanced hemodynamic devices based on our institutional protocol and the relevant literature and to evaluate their effects on clinical outcomes.

**Keywords:** Takotsubo cardiomyopathy, neurogenic stress cardiomyopathy, fluid therapy, pulmonary edema, subarachnoid hemorrhage

## 1. Introduction

Postoperative management of aneurysmal subarachnoid hemorrhage (SAH) is sometimes complicated by systemic cardiopulmonary complications to affect a significant impact on the morbidity and mortality of the patients [1, 2]. The neuro-cardiac injury of SAH is of particular importance because of their impact on the ability to manage blood pressure and volume status, especially in the setting of cerebral vasospasm or delayed cerebral ischemia (DCI). The pattern of injury produced is commonly referred to as neurogenic stress cardiomyopathy [3]. One distinct morphological variant of stress cardiomyopathy is Takotsubo cardiomyopathy (TCM), which was first described by the Japanese physician in the early 1990s to be a reversible cardiomyopathy, the shape of which named after an octopus trap used by the native fishermen [4]. Although TCM is typically associated with acute emotional stress in postmenopausal women [5], triggers may also include physical stressors such as head trauma, intracranial bleeding, ischemic stroke, medical, and surgical procedures and catecholaminergic drugs [6]. Previous reports suggest the demographics and clinical characteristics of TCM are similar irrespective of their etiologies. However, there are notable differences in post-SAH TCM from other non-neurologic stressors in that the patients tended to be younger and more frequent in females than what is typically reported and had high in-hospital mortality (25%) [7].

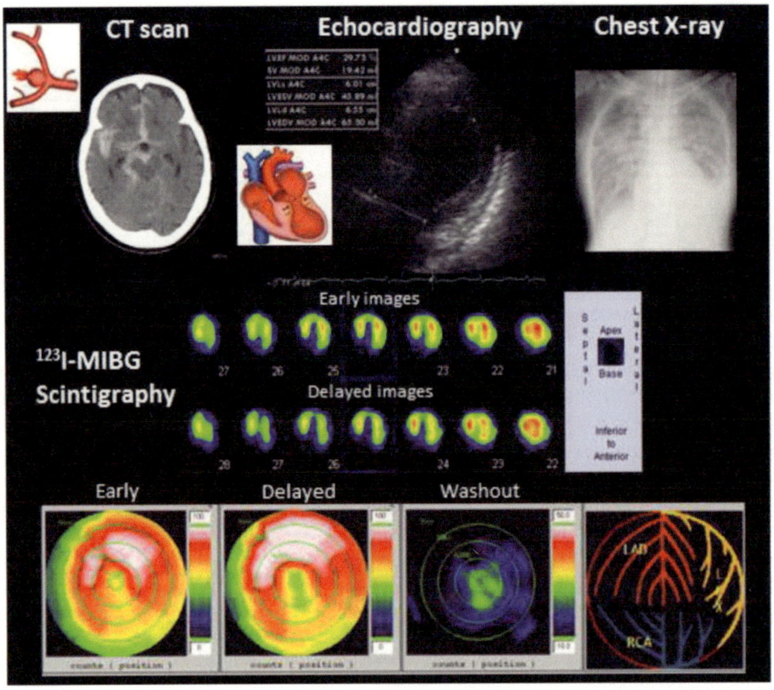


**Figure 1.** Subarachnoid hemorrhage-induced neurogenic injuries. Note that apical ballooning suggestive of Takotsubo cardiomyopathy (TCM) and left ventricular dysfunction detected by apical two-chamber view on initial echocardiogram. Acute pulmonary edema was also observed on chest X-ray. $^{123}$I-metaiodobenzylguanidine (MIBG) SPECT depicting apical defect in the two-chamber view and the analysis of two-dimensional polar maps (bull's eyes) show decreased myocardial perfusion in apex. In 4-h delayed images, washout is increased, suggesting the presynaptic sympathetic dysfunction caused by TCM.

TCM is originally characterized by transient hypokinesis which results from apical wall motion abnormalities with sparing of the base. Although most of the TCM patients (>65%) can present such typical patterns on echocardiography (**Figure 1**), there are several different variants of regional wall motion abnormalities (RWMA) that spares the cardiac apex, as well as one that affects the right ventricle. The right ventricle involvement is noted in 26% of the patients with TCM and bilateral pleural effusions are commonly seen in these patients [8].

The diagnosis of TCM is made based on a modified version of the Mayo Clinic Criteria [9] as described in **Table 1**.

| |
|---|
| 1. Transient hypokinesis, akinesis or dyskinesis of the LV mid-segments with or without apical involvement; the RWMA extend beyond a single epicardial vascular distribution; a stressful trigger is often, but not always, present. |
| 2. Absence of obstructive coronary artery disease or angiographic evidence of acute plaque rupture. |
| 3. New ECG abnormalities (either ST elevation and/or T wave inversion) or modest elevation in cardiac troponin. |
| 4. Absence of other precipitants such as pheochromocytoma and myocarditis. |

LV: left ventricular; RWMA: regional wall motion abnormalities; ECG: electrocardiogram.

**Table 1.** The Mayo Clinic published diagnostic criteria for TCM after SAH.

Patients with akinesis or hypokinesis of left ventricular (LV) apical segments with preserved contractility of the basal segments are considered to have the apical variant of TCM (apical ballooning), while those with akinesis of the basal segments with preserved contractility of the apex and mid-ventricular segments are classified as having reverse TCM (non-apical ballooning).

A massive release of catecholamines into the systemic circulation after aneurysmal rupture has been considered responsible for SAH-induced TCM. In view of the literature reviews (**Table 1**), the incidence of TCM in SAH patients ranges from 0.8 to 17% [1, 2, 7, 10–12], which makes it a relatively common postoperative complication. However, the management of TCM becomes cumbersome in the setting of volumetric and hemodynamic therapy for DCI. In this chapter, we will review the current practice in intensive hemodynamic monitoring and goal-directed fluid management of post-SAH TCM using advanced hemodynamic devices based on our institutional protocol and the relevant literature and to evaluate their effects on clinical outcomes (**Table 2** ).

| | Total number | TCM [*n* (%)] | LVEF <40% [*n* (%)] | Mean age (years) | Female (%) | Poor grade (%) | DCI (%) | Poor outcome (%) |
|---|---|---|---|---|---|---|---|---|
| Mutoh et al. [12] | 575 | 46 (8) | 20 (43) | 64 | 70 | 87 | 33 | 48 |
| Talahma et al. [1] | 800 | 18 (2.2) | N/A | 63 | 78 | 33 | N/A | 44 |
| Kilbourn et al. [2] | 63 | 11 (17) | N/A | 61 | 72 | 82 | N/A | 80 |
| Inamasu et al. [10] | 391 | 30 (7.7) | 8 (27) | 62 | 63 | 83 | 27 | 57 |
| Abd et al. [7] | 2276 | 19 (0.8) | 14 (74) | 45 | 100 | 58 | N/A | N/A |
| Lee et al. [11] | 661 | 8 (1.2) | 4 (50) | 56 | 100 | 88 | 38 | N/A |

**Table 2.** Incidence and characteristics of TCM in patients after subarachnoid hemorrhage.

## 2. Pathophysiology of post-SAH TCM

The underlying mechanism of TCM is not fully understood. Several theories have been proposed to explain its pathophysiology including excessive sympathetic stimulation, microvascular dysfunction, coronary artery vasospasm, and abnormal myocardial tissue metabolism [1]. An excessive release of catecholamines (catecholamine surge or sympathetic storming) immediately after insult associated with aneurysm rupture seems to have a pivotal role in the development of TCM. In fact, patients with TCM are at risk for fatal arrhythmias particularly those with SAH combined with intra-sylvian/intracerebral hematoma that involves the right insular cortex where sympathetic hyperactivation can occur [13, 14].

The deleterious effect of such brain–heart interactions may contribute to explain the observation that the outcome of patients with SAH can be predicted by measuring the levels of circulating catecholamine or myocardial sympathetic function. Using an isotope dilution technique, Naredi et al. [15] suggest that patients with subarachnoid hemorrhage exhibited a threefold increase in plasma norepinephrine within 48 h persisted throughout 7–10 days and normalized thereafter. Indeed, nuclear imaging using $^{123}$I-meta-iodobenzylguanidine (MIBG), a radioactive marker allowing mapping of the autonomic nervous system of the heart also support the existence of sympathetic dysfunction (**Figure 1**) as a result of overactivation in the area of ventricular wall dysfunction with preserved coronary blood flow [16].

Histopathological findings support this theory since patients presented with typical TCM showed extensive area of myocardial thinning and myocyte edema at the cardiac apex in which degenerative myocardium with histiocyte and lymphocyte infiltration, and contracture-like necrotic bands, but a less severe pathology at the base [17, 18]. Oxidative stress can lead to myocardial necrosis, remodelling, and contractility disturbances [8]. Neuropathological evidence of Lewy body-like cytoplasmic inclusions in both dorsal nuclei of the vagus nerve suggests that disorders of the parasympathetic nervous system may also be associated with a consequence of TCM [17].

On the other hand, the predominance of TCM in female subjects implicates possible properties of genetic predisposition and/or estrogen deficiency [8]. Goodloe et al. [19] investigated functional adrenergic polymorphisms in 28 TCM patients to suggest that TCM was enriched for variants within functional domains, although the polymorphism frequencies were similar to population controls as described previously. Kuo et al. [20] presented a case series of 18 TCM patients and concluded that the lack of estrogen replacement in the postmenopausal state may predispose women to Takotsubo cardiomyopathy. Based on the results from TCM in a mother–sister pair, it has been suggested that the segregating rare variants in four genes (ADH5, CACNG1, EPHA4, and PRKCA) [19] may synergistically confer myocardial vulnerability and risk for TCM in the setting of a postmenopausal hormonal environment and a catecholamine trigger.

The available literature provides no clear answer about the safety of general anesthesia in SAH patients complicated with TCM, and whether the treatment of the aneurysms should be surgical or endovascular. However, it appears that TCM may not be a contraindication to surgical obliteration of the aneurysms as long as the patient is hemodynamically stable [10], while multiple other reports showed that endovascular intervention is the preferred modality of treatment in these patients [21]. In fact, 37–61% of patients underwent surgical clipping for their aneurysms which elucidate the safety of anesthesia for microsurgical clipping even in the setting of TCM [1, 10, 12]. Furthermore, neither clipped nor coiled patients developed serious perioperative cardiopulmonary complications, although relatively higher incidence of fatal procedure-related complications was demonstrated in patients underwent coiling [10].

## 3. Hemodynamics of TCM after SAH

The hemodynamic changes of TCM that occur during the course of SAH are not fully understood, presumably because of the complicated underlying acute pathophysiological mechanisms that could merely be an innocent finding reflecting the general population.

Although the RWMA associated with TCM is transient with resolution generally within several days to weeks [22, 23], it contributes significantly to cardiopulmonary hemodynamics following SAH, especially when it is combined with other neurogenic injuries such as pulmonary edema, cardiogenic shock, and life-threatening arrhythmia [24, 25]. The RWMA diagnosed on echocardiography have been reported in up to 20% of patients after SAH [2], which is sometimes extensive enough to reduce left ventricular ejection fraction (LVEF). Therefore, in addition to pulmonary edema and hypoxia, TCM may lead to low cardiac output (CO) and hypotension to reduce cerebral perfusion pressure. The incidence of SAH-induced LV dysfunction has been estimated at around 5–10% [26], the development of which following TCM can increase the risk of DCI [11, 27] and poor outcome [12]. Moreover, TCM is associated with a 25% incidence of left ventricular outflow tract (LVOT) obstruction [28], and thus we have to be carefully monitor the cardiac functions to avoid increased intraventricular pressure gradient particularly when treating the related cardiogenic shock or post-SAH DCI.

## 4. Intensive fluid management for post-SAH TCM

### 4.1. Hemodynamic monitoring

Cardiovascular monitoring is essential for the diagnostic and therapeutic management of critically ill patients. Of particular, early hemodynamic assessment is importance for adequate cerebral circulation in patients with SAH. Echocardiography is currently the most frequently used noninvasive imaging modality for bedside assessment of LV function [29–31], but is not ideal for real-time monitoring of systolic function because of its high intra- and inter-observer variability [32].

Hemodynamic monitoring is essential for the diagnosis and therapeutic management of critically ill patients. Several different methods and techniques are used to monitor patients with cardiopulmonary complications, although none are ideal (i.e., noninvasive, safe, reproducible, assessing both preload and lung edema volumes, as well as cardiac function) [33]. Unfortunately, the use of such monitoring devices has been limited in neurocritical care, presumably due to inexperience and complexity of handling multiple hemodynamic parameters (e.g., pulmonary artery catheter) [34]. Recently, several studies examined acute hemodynamic changes following SAH using an advanced bedside transpulmonary thermodilution (TPTD) device [12, 35–38].

The single-indicator TPTD method incorporated into the PiCCO/PulsioFlex (Pulsion Medical Systems, Munich, Germany) or EV-1000 (Edwards Lifesciences, Irvine, CA, USA) system measures the change in temperature over time at a thermistor-tipped peripheral arterial catheter inserted into the femoral or brachial artery by triplicate injections of 15-mL boluses of ice-cold saline via the central venous line [39]. The TPTD algorithm calculates CO by analysis of the thermodilution curve using the Stewart–Hamilton equations, which are less-invasive but comparable with those by the established PAC technique [40].

The accuracy of continuous CO measurements, superiority of the TPTD-derived volumetric parameters for estimating cardiac preload (based on global end-diastolic volume (GEDV)) compared with measurement using fluid balance, central venous pressure or a pulmonary artery catheter [41], and the utility of EVLW to discriminate pulmonary edema [37, 42] have been validated in clinical studies in SAH. These hemodynamic data can provide to analyze the cardiac function index (CFI, normal value: 4.5–6.5 per minute), which is the ratio of CO to GEDV [39]. Previous data suggest that CFI is closely related to the LV fractional area of change measured by echocardiography [43] and that CFI can be used to accurately assess the effects of positive inotropic therapy with dobutamine in acute circulatory failure [29].

### 4.2. Hemodynamic parameters for monitoring TCM

We have recently demonstrated that CFI measured by TPTD provides reliable real-time estimation of LV systolic function in 46 patients with TCM [12]. This study has an advantage of including the *largest* reported number of patients with post-SAH TCM who were successfully monitored for cardiac performance and volume status for approximately 14 days. CFI behaves like an index of LV systolic function because (1) it is fairly well correlated with the echocardiographic LVEF and reliably tracks treatment-induced changes in LVEF, and (2) it is not affected by fluid loading, but increased after administration of an inotropic agent. The decrease in CFI of <4.0 per minute is valuable for detecting LV dysfunction in TCM defined by LVEF <40% (sensitivity of 82% and specificity of 84%), which is the point at which inotropic support should be considered.

At initial measurement on day 0 during the first 24 h after SAH, depression of LV systolic function (CFI 3.3 per minute) mainly attributable to low CO (2.2 L/min/$m^2$) was observed for patients with TCM. Hypovolemia defined by decreased GEDV (635 mL/$m^2$) was notable in patients with LV dysfunction (LVEF <40%). In our population, we could not detect any significant difference in HR, MAP, CVP, or SVRI between the groups with and without LV dysfunction throughout the acute period of 2 weeks after SAH. It has also been suggested that TCM combined with LV dysfunction has a longer duration of low CFI

(<4.0 per minute, corresponding to predicted LVEF <40% [29]) with a mean difference of 4 days and more frequencies of pulmonary edema defined by EVLW > 14 mL/kg after day 4 (55%) (**Figure 2**).

### 4.3. Choice of drugs for post-SAH TCM patients

Medical treatment of arterial vasospasm following aneurysmal subarachnoid hemorrhage (SAH) generally consists of triple H (hypertensive-hypervolemia-hemodilution) therapy [44, 45] or its modification [46–48], which frequently relies on inotropic agents in order to increase CO. Although the optimal treatment is still a matter of debate, given the relationship between catecholamine hypersecretion and subsequent development of TCM, intensivists are often

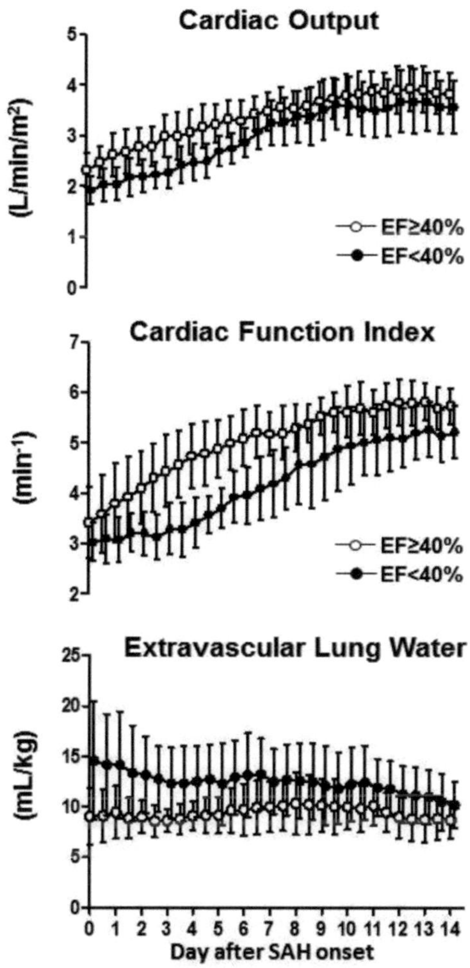


**Figure 2.** Changes in hemodynamic parameters over 2 weeks in 30 patients with Takotsubo cardiomyopathy following subarachnoid hemorrhage. Note that cardiac function index more clearly traces changes in cardiac function than cardiac output particularly in patients with left ventricular dysfunction [ejection fraction (EF) < 40%]. Increased extravascular lung water in this subgroup can also be detected. Modified with permission from Ref. [12].

reluctant to use inotropes and vasopressors even in patients who may benefit from cardiogenic shock or hemodynamic therapy for DCI. Although there is general agreement in the literature about avoiding vasopressors in TCM patients because of the adverse effects on catecholamine hypersensitivity, the recent data suggest that vasopressors may be used safely by careful monitoring of the hemodynamic parameters [1, 49]. In fact, most patients (61%) had already been administered vasopressors prior to the diagnosis of TCM, in which more than 60% remained on the same treatment and most of them (86%) had good outcome [1]. There is only a case of TCM reported as a direct effect of catecholamine stimulation, including an anecdotal case of de novo TCM in a patient treated with dobutamine for symptomatic SAH vasospasm [50]. In select patients, the use of intra-aortic balloon pump (IABP) may be beneficial as an adjunctive therapy of patients with comorbid DCI and TCM who become intolerant to aggressive pharmacologic hemodynamic augmentation [51].

Milrinone could be a good alternative when inotropes are required in TCM and when dobutamine infusion is associated with tachycardia [52]. The use of milrinone has been proposed to augment the cerebral perfusion in TCM giving its combined inotropic and vasodilating properties [53]. Milrinone is a phosphodiesterase-III inhibitor that increases calcium influx in the myocardium which leads to increased cardiac contractility without β-agonist action, resulting in less tachycardia [52] and myocardial oxygen consumption [54]. However, milrinone may induce hypotension as a result of peripheral vasodilatory property, which may require intensive hemodynamic monitoring during the management.

In the case of concurrent LVOT obstruction associated with post-SAH TCM that may have a paradoxical decrease in CO following administration of inotropic pressors, discontinuation of the inotropes and maintenance of hypervolemia may be required in order to optimize cerebral perfusion and prevent ischemia [27]. If a patient with TCM is deteriorating and has a low CO with LVOT, cardiogenic shock, and progressive multiorgan failure, temporary LV assist devices (LVAD) or extracorporeal membrane oxygenation (ECMO) as a bridge-to-recovery may be useful, as there is a possibility that the ventricular function will recover fully [55].

The role of β-blockers in SAH patients with TCM remains unclear. Patients who had been treated with β-blockers prior to the SAH were associated with a lower risk of developing TCM [56]. In one small study (n = 18), the use of β-blockers prior to or after the diagnosis of TCM was not associated with a significant difference in neurological outcome [1]. The role of a newer inotropic agent levosimendan is more controversial, with mixed expert opinion based on preclinical and limited clinical experience [1, 55]. Future studies on the effectiveness of these drugs in prevention or treatment of TCM may be warranted in larger population.

### 4.4. TPTD-guided early goal-directed fluid management

Fluid management of peri- and postoperative SAH patients is aimed primarily at maintaining CO to increase cerebral blood flow, and at preventing hypovolemia by minimizing cardiopulmonary complications [44, 57, 58]. The practical usefulness of early goal-directed fluid therapy (EGDT) with TPTD has been proposed in SAH patients including those suffered from TCM [12, 36, 37, 41, 42, 59].

Hemodynamic stability is defined as CO ≥3 L/min/m², GEDV ≥680 mL/m², and ELWI ≤14 mL/kg (the upper limits chosen were the values associated with a higher risk of mortality in patients with pulmonary edema) [60]. If CO fell below the target value due to hypovolemia, patients received 500 mL of either crystalloid fluid or 6% hydroxyethyl starch. If this fluid loading did not increase the GEDV to above the target value, and the low CO persisted for at least 8 h, 25% albumin solution was administered. If the low CO persisted even with hypervolemia (GEDV ≥ 850 mL/m²) and fluid therapy for at least 12 h, inotropic support was initiated with dobutamine [61] or milrinone [12, 37] to maintain CO above the target value. If the patient had elevated EVLW (>14 mL/kg) and any signs of congestive heart failure or pulmonary edema (such as bilateral pulmonary infiltrates or cardiomegaly with a cardiothoracic ratio >50% on chest radiography), furosemide (5 mg bolus) was administered intravenously.

According to our institutional protocol, clinical deterioration due to DCI or evidence of cerebral vasospasm on transcranial Doppler ultrasonography (mean flow velocity in the middle cerebral artery >120 cm/s) was treated with hyperdynamic therapy with incremental doses of dobutamine (3 μg/kg/min, maximum 15 μg/kg/min) or milrinone (0.125 μg/kg/min, maximum 0.75 μg/kg/min) to raise the CO above the normal limit (>5.0 L/min/m²) or to resolve the deficit [12, 62, 63]. Recovery of RWMA [64] and the absence of LVOT obstruction were confirmed by echocardiography before the initiation of hyperdynamic therapy to avoid adverse effects due to the use of inotropic agents [27].

### 4.5. Outcome of EGDT in post-SAH TCM

In TCM patients managed with aforementioned post-SAH EGDT, multivariate logistic regression analysis showed that persisted low CFI (<4.0 per minute) for ≥4 days was independently associated with DCI (odds ratio, 1.87) and poor functional outcome at 3 months (modified Rankin Scale of 4–6: odds ratio, 1.92). In addition, coexisting pulmonary edema (EVLW > 12 mL/kg) also increased the risk of poor functional outcome at 3 months (odds ratio, 1.85). The results may have an advantage of EGDT because neither a lower LEVF nor the presence of concomitant pulmonary edema correlated with unfavorable outcomes in 30 SAH patients with TCM managed by conventional fluid management using echocardiography and standard hemodynamic parameters [10]. Furthermore, the finding that EGDT has a lower incidence of therapy-related pulmonary edema than standard care [65] may support the value of intensive hemodynamic monitoring.

## 5. Conclusion

TCM is a well-recognized neurogenic stress-induced complication early after SAH. It is a self-limiting condition but often adds an additional layer of clinical morbidity to a patient particularly suffering from DCI. Our clinical data suggest that prolonged cardiac dysfunction and concurrent pulmonary edema can increase the risk of DCI, contributing to poor functional outcome in patients with SAH complicated with TCM. Serial measurements of CFI and EVLW may provide an easy bedside method of estimating changes in LVEF in TCM and predicting the outcome, as well as detecting fluid therapy-related cardiopulmonary complications.

## Acknowledgements

The authors gratefully acknowledge the financial support of Grants: Grant-in-Aid for Scientific Research from the Japan Society for the Promotion of Science (15K10966) and Life Science Foundation of Japan.

## Author details

Tatsushi Mutoh[1,2*], Tomoko Mutoh[2], Yasuyuki Taki[2] and Tatsuya Ishikawa[1]

*Address all correspondence to: tmutoh@tiara.ocn.ne.jp

1 Research Institute for Brain and Blood Vessels-AKITA, Akita, Japan

2 Institute of Development, Aging and Cancer, Tohoku University, Sendai, Japan

## References

[1] Talahma M, Alkhachroum AM, Alyahya M, et al. Takotsubo cardiomyopathy in aneurysmal subarachnoid hemorrhage: Institutional experience and literature review. *Clin Neurol Neurosurg* 2016; 141:65–70.

[2] Kilbourn KJ, Ching G, Silverman DI, et al. Clinical outcomes after neurogenic stress induced cardiomyopathy in aneurysmal sub-arachnoid hemorrhage: A prospective cohort study. *Clin Neurol Neurosurg* 2015; 128:4–9.

[3] Lee VH, Oh JK, Mulvagh SL, et al. Mechanisms in neurogenic stress cardiomyopathy after aneurysmal subarachnoid hemorrhage. *Neurocrit Care* 2006; 5:243–249.

[4] Templin C, Ghadri JR, Diekmann J, et al. Clinical features and outcomes of Takotsubo (stress) cardiomyopathy. *N Engl J Med* 2015; 373:929–938.

[5] Dote K, Sato H, Tateishi H, et al. Myocardial stunning due to simultaneous multivessel coronary spasms: A review of 5 cases. *J Cardiol* 1991; 21:203–214.

[6] Bybee KA, Prasad A. Stress-related cardiomyopathy syndromes. *Circulation* 2008; 118:397–409.

[7] Abd TT, Hayek S, Cheng JW, et al. Incidence and clinical characteristics of Takotsubo cardiomyopathy post-aneurysmal subarachnoid hemorrhage. *Int J Cardiol* 2014; 176: 1362–1364.

[8] Roshanzamir S, Showkathali R. Takotsubo cardiomyopathy a short review. *Curr Cardiol Rev* 2013; 9:191–196.

[9] Scantlebury DC, Prasad A. Diagnosis of Takotsubo cardiomyopathy. *Circ J* 2014; 78:2129–2139.

[10] Inamasu J, Ganaha T, Nakae S, et al. Therapeutic outcomes for patients with aneurysmal subarachnoid hemorrhage complicated by Takotsubo cardiomyopathy. *Acta Neurochir (Wien)* 2016; 158:885–893.

[11] Lee VH, Connolly HM, Fulgham JR, et al. Tako-tsubo cardiomyopathy in aneurysmal subarachnoid hemorrhage: An underappreciated ventricular dysfunction. *J Neurosurg* 2006; 105:264–270.

[12] Mutoh T, Kazumata K, Terasaka S, et al. Impact of transpulmonary thermodilution-based cardiac contractility and extravascular lung water measurements on clinical outcome of patients with Takotsubo cardiomyopathy after subarachnoid hemorrhage: A retrospective observational study. *Crit Care* 2014; 18:482.

[13] Hirashima Y, Takashima S, Matsumura N, et al. Right sylvian fissure subarachnoid hemorrhage has electrocardiographic consequences. *Stroke* 2001; 32:2278–2281.

[14] Takahashi C, Hinson HE, Baguley IJ. Autonomic dysfunction syndromes after acute brain injury. *Handb Clin Neurol* 2015; 128:539–551.

[15] Naderi S, Ozguven MA, Bayhan H, et al. Evaluation of cerebral vasospasm in patients with subarachnoid hemorrhage using single photon emission computed tomography. *Neurosurg Rev* 1994; 17:261–265.

[16] Christensen TE, Bang LE, Holmvang L, et al. $^{123}$I-MIBG scintigraphy in the subacute state of Takotsubo cardiomyopathy. *JACC Cardiovasc Imaging* 2016;

[17] Aoki Y, Kodera S, Watanabe T, et al. Autopsy findings in Takotsubo cardiomyopathy with special reference to the autonomic nervous system. *Int J Cardiol* 2016; 203:236–237.

[18] van der Bilt IA, Vendeville JP, van de Hoef TP, et al. Myocarditis in patients with subarachnoid hemorrhage: A histopathologic study. *J Crit Care* 2016; 32:196–200.

[19] Goodloe AH, Evans JM, Middha S, et al. Characterizing genetic variation of adrenergic signalling pathways in Takotsubo (stress) cardiomyopathy exomes. *Eur J Heart Fail* 2014; 16:942–949.

[20] Kuo BT, Choubey R, Novaro GM. Reduced estrogen in menopause may predispose women to Takotsubo cardiomyopathy. *Gend Med* 2010; 7:71–77.

[21] Manto A, De Gennaro A, Manzo G, et al. Early endovascular treatment of aneurysmal subarachnoid hemorrhage complicated by neurogenic pulmonary edema and Takotsubo-like cardiomyopathy. *Neuroradiol J* 2014; 27:356–360.

[22] Gianni M, Dentali F, Grandi AM, et al. Apical ballooning syndrome or Takotsubo cardiomyopathy: A systematic review. *Eur Heart J* 2006; 27:1523–1529.

[23] Sharkey SW, Lesser JR, Maron BJ. Cardiology patient page. Takotsubo (stress) cardiomyopathy. *Circulation* 2011; 124:e460–462.

[24] Pilgrim TM, Wyss TR. Takotsubo cardiomyopathy or transient left ventricular apical ballooning syndrome: A systematic review. *Int J Cardiol* 2008; 124:283–292.

[25] Ahmed S, Ungprasert P, Ratanapo S, et al. Clinical characteristics of Takotsubo cardiomyopathy in North America. *N Am J Med Sci* 2013; 5:77–81.

[26] Spina R, Baron D, Wong S, et al. Severe stress (Takotsubo) cardiomyopathy following subarachnoid haemorrhage. *Int J Cardiol* 2016; 210:119–121.

[27] Zada G, Terterov S, Russin J, et al. Cerebral vasospasm and concurrent left ventricular outflow tract obstruction: Requirement for modification of hyperdynamic therapy regimen. *Neurocrit Care* 2010; 12:265–268.

[28] El Mahmoud R, Mansencal N, Pilliere R, et al. Prevalence and characteristics of left ventricular outflow tract obstruction in Tako-tsubo syndrome. *Am Heart J* 2008; 156:543–548.

[29] Jabot J, Monnet X, Bouchra L, et al. Cardiac function index provided by transpulmonary thermodilution behaves as an indicator of left ventricular systolic function. *Crit Care Med* 2009; 37:2913–2918.

[30] Lee VH, Abdelmoneim SS, Daugherty WP, et al. Myocardial contrast echocardiography in subarachnoid hemorrhage-induced cardiac dysfunction: Case report. *Neurosurgery* 2008; 62:E261–E262; discussion E262.

[31] Cinotti R, Piriou N, Launey Y, et al. Speckle tracking analysis allows sensitive detection of stress cardiomyopathy in severe aneurysmal subarachnoid hemorrhage patients. *Intensive Care Med* 2016; 42:173–182.

[32] McGowan JH, Cleland JG. Reliability of reporting left ventricular systolic function by echocardiography: A systematic review of 3 methods. *Am Heart J* 2003; 146:388–397.

[33] Merenkov VV, Kovalev AN, Gorbunov VV. Bedside lung ultrasound: A case of neurogenic pulmonary edema. *Neurocrit Care* 2013; 18:391–394.

[34] Stevens RD, Naval NS, Mirski MA, et al. Intensive care of aneurysmal subarachnoid hemorrhage: An international survey. *Intensive Care Med* 2009; 35:1556–1566.

[35] Yoneda H, Nakamura T, Shirao S, et al. Multicenter prospective cohort study on volume management after subarachnoid hemorrhage: Hemodynamic changes according to

severity of subarachnoid hemorrhage and cerebral vasospasm. *Stroke* 2013; 44:2155–2161.

[36] Mutoh T, Kazumata K, Yokoyama Y, et al. Comparison of postoperative volume status and hemodynamics between surgical clipping and endovascular coiling in patients after subarachnoid hemorrhage. *J Neurosurg Anesthesiol* 2015; 27:7–15.

[37] Mutoh T, Kazumata K, Kobayashi S, et al. Serial measurement of extravascular lung water and blood volume during the course of neurogenic pulmonary edema after subarachnoid hemorrhage: Initial experience with 3 cases. *J Neurosurg Anesthesiol* 2012; 24:203–208.

[38] Tagami T, Kuwamoto K, Watanabe A, et al. Optimal range of global end-diastolic volume for fluid management after aneurysmal subarachnoid hemorrhage: A multicenter prospective cohort study. *Crit Care Med* 2014; 42:1348–1356.

[39] Sakka SG, Reuter DA, Perel A. The transpulmonary thermodilution technique. *J Clin Monit Comput* 2012; 26:347–353.

[40] Profant M, Vyska K, Eckhardt U. The stewart-hamilton equations and the indicator dilution method. *SIAM J Appl Math* 1978; 34:666–675.

[41] Mutoh T, Kazumata K, Ishikawa T, et al. Performance of bedside transpulmonary thermodilution monitoring for goal-directed hemodynamic management after subarachnoid hemorrhage. *Stroke* 2009; 40:2368–2374.

[42] Mutoh T, Kazumata K, Ueyama-Mutoh T, et al. Transpulmonary thermodilution-based management of neurogenic pulmonary edema after subarachnoid hemorrhage. *Am J Med Sci* 2015; 350:415–419.

[43] Ritter S, Rudiger A, Maggiorini M. Transpulmonary thermodilution-derived cardiac function index identifies cardiac dysfunction in acute heart failure and septic patients: An observational study. *Crit Care* 2009; 13:R133.

[44] Suarez JI, Tarr RW, Selman WR. Aneurysmal subarachnoid hemorrhage. *N Engl J Med* 2006; 354:387–396.

[45] Vergouwen MD, Vermeulen M, van Gijn J, et al. Definition of delayed cerebral ischemia after aneurysmal subarachnoid hemorrhage as an outcome event in clinical trials and observational studies: Proposal of a multidisciplinary research group. *Stroke* 2010; 41:2391–2395.

[46] Muench E, Horn P, Bauhuf C, et al. Effects of hypervolemia and hypertension on regional cerebral blood flow, intracranial pressure, and brain tissue oxygenation after subarachnoid hemorrhage. *Crit Care Med* 2007; 35:1844–1851.

[47] Mutoh T, Ishikawa T, Yasui N. Application of the FloTrac™ arterial pressure-based continuous cardiac output monitor to dobuta-induced hyperdynamic therapy for

cerebral vasospasm after subarachnoid hemorrhage. *No Shinkei Geka* 2009; 37:1085–1093.

[48] Mori K, Arai H, Nakajima K, et al. Hemorheological and hemodynamic analysis of hypervolemic hemodilution therapy for cerebral vasospasm after aneurysmal subarachnoid hemorrhage. *Stroke* 1995; 26:1620–1626.

[49] Mittal M, Radhakrishnan M, UmamaheswaraRao GS. Management of catecholamine-induced stunned myocardium – a case report. *J Clin Anesth* 2015; 27:527–530.

[50] Saito R, Takahashi T, Noshita N, et al. Takotsubo cardiomyopathy induced by dobutamine infusion during hypertensive therapy for symptomatic vasospasm after subarachnoid hemorrhage – case report. *Neurol Med Chir (Tokyo)* 2010; 50:393–395.

[51] Al-Mufti F, Morris N, Lahiri S, et al. Use of intra-aortic-balloon pump counterpulsation in patients with symptomatic vasospasm following subarachnoid hemorrhage and neurogenic stress cardiomyopathy. *J Vasc Interv Neurol* 2016; 9:28–34.

[52] Mrozek S, Srairi M, Marhar F, et al. Successful treatment of inverted Takotsubo cardiomyopathy after severe traumatic brain injury with milrinone after dobutamine failure. *Heart Lung* 2016;

[53] Naidech A, Du Y, Kreiter KT, et al. Dobutamine versus milrinone after subarachnoid hemorrhage. *Neurosurgery* 2005; 56:21–27.

[54] Mager G, Klocke RK, Kux A, et al. Phosphodiesterase III inhibition or adrenoreceptor stimulation: Milrinone as an alternative to dobutamine in the treatment of severe heart failure. *Am Heart J* 1991; 121:1974–1983.

[55] Lyon AR, Bossone E, Schneider B, et al. Current state of knowledge on Takotsubo syndrome: A position statement from the taskforce on Takotsubo syndrome of the heart failure association of the european society of cardiology. *Eur J Heart Fail* 2016; 18:8–27.

[56] Liang CW, Chen R, Macri E, et al. Preadmission beta-blockers are associated with decreased incidence of neurogenic stunned myocardium in aneurysmal subarachnoid hemorrhage. *J Stroke Cerebrovasc Dis* 2013; 22:601–607.

[57] Rabinstein AA, Lanzino G, Wijdicks EF. Multidisciplinary management and emerging therapeutic strategies in aneurysmal subarachnoid haemorrhage. *Lancet Neurol* 2010; 9:504–519.

[58] Sen J, Belli A, Albon H, et al. Triple-H therapy in the management of aneurysmal subarachnoid haemorrhage. *Lancet Neurol* 2003; 2:614–621.

[59] Mutoh T, Kazumata K, Ajiki M, et al. Goal-directed fluid management by bedside transpulmonary hemodynamic monitoring after subarachnoid hemorrhage. *Stroke* 2007; 38:3218–3224.

[60] Kirov MY, Kuzkov VV, Bjertnaes LJ: Extravascular lung water in sepsis. In: Vincent JL, ed. Yearbook of intensive care and emergency medicine, Berlin: Springer; 2005: pp.449–461.

[61] Hadeishi H, Mizuno M, Suzuki A, et al. Hyperdynamic therapy for cerebral vasospasm. *Neurol Med Chir (Tokyo)* 1990; 30:317–323.

[62] Mutoh T, Ishikawa T, Kobayashi S, et al. Performance of third-generation FloTrac/Vigileo system during hyperdynamic therapy for delayed cerebral ischemia after subarachnoid hemorrhage. *Surg Neurol Int* 2012; 3:99.

[63] Mutoh T, Ishikawa T, Suzuki A, et al. Continuous cardiac output and near-infrared spectroscopy monitoring to assist in management of symptomatic cerebral vasospasm after subarachnoid hemorrhage. *Neurocrit Care* 2010; 13:331–338.

[64] Banki N, Kopelnik A, Tung P, et al. Prospective analysis of prevalence, distribution, and rate of recovery of left ventricular systolic dysfunction in patients with subarachnoid hemorrhage. *J Neurosurg* 2006; 105:15–20.

[65] Mutoh T, Kazumata K, Terasaka S, et al. Early intensive versus minimally invasive approach to postoperative hemodynamic management after subarachnoid hemorrhage. *Stroke* 2014; 45:1280–1284.

# Chapter 15

# Advanced Treatments and Emerging Therapies for Dystrophin-Deficient Cardiomyopathies

Jordi Camps, Enrico Pozzo, Tristan Pulinckx,
Robin Duelen and Maurilio Sampaolesi

Additional information is available at the end of the chapter

http://dx.doi.org/10.5772/65061

**Abstract**

Dystrophinopathies are characterized by skeletal and cardiac muscle complications because of a lack or shortened DYSTROPHIN protein. Ventilation assistance and corticosteroid treatment have positively affected life outcome but lead to an increased incidence of cardiomyopathy. Cardiomyopathy is now the leading cause of death in patients with dystrophinopathy. Thus, coherent guidelines for cardiac care have become essential and need to be communicated well. Progression of cardiac complications in patients with dystrophinopathy diverges from standard dilated cardiomyopathy development and monitoring and medical care for dystrophinopathy. This chapter summarizes current guidelines and recommendations for monitoring and clinical treatment of cardiac complications in patients with dystrophinopathy and provides a thorough survey of emerging therapies focusing on cardiac outcomes.

**Keywords:** dystrophin, Duchenne and Becker muscular dystrophy, dilated cardiomyopathy, symptomatic treatment, exon skipping, gene and cell therapy

## 1. Introduction

Dystrophinopathies are a group of diseases comprising Duchenne muscular dystrophy (DMD), Becker muscular dystrophy (BMD) and X-linked dilated cardiomyopathy (XLDCM), characterized by a shortened or absent *DYSTROPHIN* gene. DMD is the most prominent, with an incidence around 1:5000 live male births [1]. BMD occurs about three times less than DMD [2], while XLDCM is extremely rare [3]. *DYSTROPHIN*—part of the dystrophin-glycoprotein complex (Appendix 1)—is located on the X chromosome, and therefore, only males are affected.

The main clinical feature of patients with dystrophinopathy is an early loss of ambulation depending on the availability of DYSTROPHIN. Patients with DMD completely lack DYSTROPHIN—the pathological mechanisms are discussed in Appendix 2—and are presented with the most severe disease progression. This is indicated by a loss of ambulation around 10 years of age and consequent ventilation assistance, followed by death during the second or third decade [4]. Conversely, patients with BMD still express a truncated form of DYSTROPHIN. Although only partially functional, this still has an effect on disease progression and life expectancy, which are drastically prolonged [5]. Patients with XLDCM show the absence of DYSTROPHIN in the heart, while expression in skeletal muscles is conserved. Several hypotheses have been proposed for this peculiar genotype [3]. In patients with dystrophinopathy, the routine use of corticosteroids and nocturnal ventilation support have dramatically improved the life expectancy and its quality. Unfortunately, this brings up other complications, as the incidence of cardiomyopathy is raising and is nearly ubiquitous in older patients with DMD. In this perspective, monitoring and treatment of cardiac complications becomes more and more important.

This chapter contains an overview of the current monitoring and treatment guidelines and state-of-the-art therapies for dystrophin-deficient cardiomyopathies. The clinical features of dystrophinopathies with an emphasis on cardiac disease progression will be discussed briefly, followed by a description of the diagnostic process and current management strategies. Conclusions from recent clinical trials on current symptomatic treatments will be summarized and emerging therapies will be discussed in detail, from promising preclinical research to ongoing clinical trials.

## 2. Clinical features

### 2.1. Duchenne and Becker muscular dystrophy

Neonate boys with DMD are rarely symptomatic, and the disease will not be recognized until the second or third year of life. The patient may show evidence of mild muscle weakness before the 12th month of life (i.e., poor head control after the 6th week, mild inability to sit unsupported at the 6th month). It is possible that he achieves the motor milestones of walking (12th month) and running (2nd year) during the toddler period, but he will eventually be brought to medical attention due to being less active than expected, as well as being prone to falling [6].

One of the earliest clinical signs of DMD is pseudohypertrophy of the gastrocnemii in the calves caused by hypertrophy of muscle fibers combined with fat infiltration and proliferation of collagen. The muscles have a firm and rubbery consistency, as well as being hypotonic compared with unaffected muscles. By the age of 3–5 years, the clinical picture of DMD gradually appears and "the patient straddles as he stands and waddles as he walks". In order to rise from the ground, the typical Gowers' sign (i.e., the child first extends the arms and legs assuming a four-point position and then works each hand alternately up the corresponding thigh) is present and it is fully expressed by the age of 5 or 6 years. While standing and walking, the patient places the feet wide apart to increase the base of support, and as a result of gluteus medius weakness, there is waddling when walking [7].

The typical posture of a patient with DMD is lumbar lordosis and scoliosis (due to weakness of abdominal muscles and paravertebral muscles) with hip flexion and abduction, knee flexion and plantar flexion, as well as winging of the scapulae. Other common presentations in toddlers include falling, troubles in running or using the stairs and developmental delays [7, 8]. As the muscular wasting progresses, the weakness will spread to the muscles of the legs and forearms and patients may end up being confined to a wheelchair by 7 years of age, while other patients may continue walking with increasing difficulty until 10 years of age. Death usually occurs around the second decade of life, caused by pulmonary infections, respiratory failure, aspiration, airway obstruction or heart failure [6].

In BMD, the weakness and hypertrophy appear in the same muscles as DMD, but the onset is later (5–45 years; mean age: 12 years) with most patients losing ambulation in the third or fourth decade. However, some patients may have a milder phenotype with the onset of muscular weakness in late adulthood [6].

In both DMD and BMD groups, the median age of diagnosis of cardiac involvement is 14 years, with all patients having cardiac problems after 18 years of age [8]. While in BMD, the cardiac involvement can be the presenting symptom at diagnosis [9], and in patients with DMD, the presentation at diagnosis is usually subclinical and asymptomatic. Patients often have unspecific symptoms including fatigue, weight loss, nausea, sleep disturbance, cough, palpitations, sweating, chest and abdominal discomfort, decreased urinary output, irritability and concentration difficulties [8].

The physical examination may present some problems in patients with advanced muscular dystrophy (MD) due to scoliosis, immobility or glucocorticoid-related obesity. Tachycardia will be present, unless treated with β-blockers. Hypotension may be present—as a result of DYSTROPHIN loss in both vascular smooth muscles and low oral fluid intake—causing altered cardiac pacemaker activity, altered myocardial contractility and altered vasomotor tone. Edema is not commonly present, even in the presence of advanced right and left cardiac failure [9].

At auscultation the cardiac apex may be displaced as a result of scoliosis, with S3 gallop and S4 gallop commonly heard as a result of acute congestive heart failure and left ventricular (LV) dysfunction, respectively [9]. Moderate mitral regurgitation (due to posterior wall fibrosis and LV thinning) and moderate tricuspid regurgitation may be present [10]. Neck venous engorgement may be seen as a result of abdominal compression caused by scoliosis [8].

As dystrophy progresses, the LV function worsens, leading to the clinical picture of dilated cardiomyopathy (DCM), which can be complicated by arrhythmias. DCM is an enlargement of one or both of the ventricles combined with systolic dysfunction, usually preceding signs and symptoms of congestive heart failure. The hallmarks of DCM are decreased LV function (decreased ejection fraction), LV dilation and mitral regurgitation. The latter manifests as palpitations, vertigo, dizziness, syncope or sudden cardiac death. Moreover, in DMD, the arrhythmia occurs even in the absence of myocardial fibrosis [11]. **Table 1** provides a summary with the most important clinical characteristics for DMD, BMD and XLDCM.

| | DMD | BMD | XLDCM |
|---|---|---|---|
| **Dystrophin** | Absent | Partially functional | Absent (heart only) |
| **Incidence** | 1 : 3500–6000 male births | 1 : 18,000–19,000 male births | Very rare |
| **Myopathy onset** | 3–5 years | 12 years | Variable |
| **Loss of ambulation** | ~12 years | ~27 years | No loss |
| **Life expectancy** | Mid to late 20s | 40s | Mid to late 10s |
| **Cardiomyopathy onset** | 16–18 years | Variable, can precede skeletal muscle symptoms | Variable, from mild to severe cases |

**Table 1.** Characteristics of Duchenne muscular dystrophy (DMD), Becker muscular dystrophy (BMD) and X-linked dilated cardiomyopathy (XLDCM).

### 2.2. X-linked dilated cardiomyopathy

XLDCM is a cardio-specific dystrophinopathy presenting with congestive heart failure (CHF) due to DCM in 10- to 20-year-old patients, without the dystrophinopathy-related involvement of skeletal muscles (**Table 1**). Patients show a brisk and progressive heart failure and ventricular arrhythmias, with untreated patients that may die of congestive heart failure not long after diagnosis [3].

## 3. Diagnosis and monitoring

Dystrophinopathy is generally underdiagnosed and definitive diagnosis can even take up to 2, 5 years from the onset of symptoms [12]. The first diagnostic test performed, when dystrophinopathy is expected, is a serum creatine kinase (CK) measurement. In most cases, CK levels are elevated, around 50–100 times in DMD, while in BMD levels are lower but still higher compared to healthy patients [13]. A second level diagnostic test is a mutation analysis, which reveals the specific genetic alteration and is useful to discriminate between DMD and BMD [14]. Differences between DMD and BMD are clarified by the reading frame concept (Appendix 3) [15]. For 5% of the cases, mutation analysis is not able to diagnose for dystrophinopathy [16]. In this circumstance, a muscle biopsy is taken and the reduction or the absence of DYSTROPHIN is analyzed by tissue staining (immunohistochemistry and immunofluorescence) or immunoblot (Western blot).

Recognizing cardiac complications in patients with dystrophinopathy is challenging, especially because of physical inactivity and respiratory complications [8]. Hence, cardiomyopathies are underdiagnosed in these patients [17]. Clinical guidelines were created in 2010, recommending an echocardiogram every 2 years from the moment of diagnosis of dystro-

http://dx.doi.org/10.5772/65061

phinopathy or from the age of 6 years. From 10 years of age, a yearly screening to asses LV function is suggested [14]. Recently, it has been documented that cardiac MRI is more sensitive and can distinguish cardiac complications in an earlier stage for patients with dystrophinopathy [18]. Therefore, it is recommended to perform a cardiac MRI instead of echocardiography, also because patients with dystrophinopathy can suffer from scoliosis, which makes diagnosis with echocardiography more complicated. However, cardiac MRI can also be challenging for pediatric patients because of the need for sedation, cost and lack of accessibility. Sinus tachycardia is also known to precede any cardiac complications in patients with DMD [19].

As mentioned before, early diagnosis of cardiomyopathy onset is essential in patients with dystrophinopathy. Hence, clinical trials are still undertaken to study whether electrocardiogram (ECG), echocardiography, cardiac MRI and sera biomarkers can improve early detection of myocardial involvement and clinical outcome (NCT02020954).

## 4. Clinical management

### 4.1. Pharmacological treatment

Early diagnosis of dystrophinopathies—before the onset of cardiac complications—gives the opportunity to treat patients in a presymptomatic stage (**Figure 1**). However, for dystrophinopathy there is no general agreement on the treatment of cardiomyopathy [20]. There are some guidelines published to guide the decision-making process; however, still a huge variability in treatments exists between centers and clinicians [11].

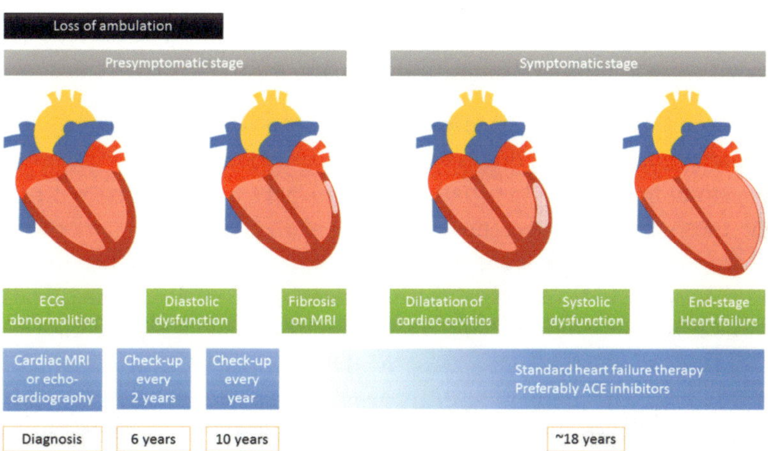


**Figure 1.** Progression of dystrophin-deficient cardiomyopathy and guidelines for monitoring and treatment. ACE, angiotensin-II-converting enzyme.

Corticosteroids improve muscle performance and delay loss of ambulation and also have beneficial effects on ventilation and scoliosis. However, this is accompanied by many side effects such as weight gain, delay of puberty, decrease of vertebral bone mass, increase of vertebral fragility, cataract formation and growth-failure [11]. Evidence exists that corticosteroids also have advantageous effects on the heart of patients with DMD, several clinical trials suggest a delayed onset of cardiomyopathy in patients with dystrophy [21]. However, these results have to be interpreted with caution; all studies were retrospective without the objective to treat for cardiomyopathic complications. In addition, corticosteroids treatment in X-linked muscular dystrophy (*mdx*) mice—an animal model for DMD with a stop codon in exon 23—led to cases of heart failure, myocardial fibrosis and sarcolemmal damage [22]. Prospective clinical trials are necessary to address the effect of corticosteroids on heart functionality. Preclinical results in dystrophic mice and hamsters are concerning, especially given the broad use of corticosteroids for treating dystrophinopathies, and reveal the gap in our understanding about effects of corticosteroids on the heart [11]. In addition, the most suitable duration of corticosteroid therapy still has to be determined.

The effect of angiotensin-converting enzyme inhibitors (ACEIs) is more clear-cut and proved to postpone cardiomyopathy onset in both preclinical animal models and patients. A three-year treatment did not show any effect among a group of DMD patients treated with perindopril and another placebo-treated group. However, after 2 additional years of perindopril treatment – in which both of these groups now received this drug - a significant reduction in LV ejection fraction was observed between the 5 year-treated and 2 year-treated group [23]. A 10-year follow-up study, observed a significantly higher survival rate in a group of DMD patients that received a presymptomatic treatment with perindopril for 3 years [24]. Current guidelines propose a start of ACEIs for DMD patients only after development of LV dysfunction [14]. However, because aforementioned results demonstrated a clear beneficial effect of presymptomatic treatment, it is now recommended to initiate treatment with ACEIs before the onset of LV dysfunction in patients with DMD [25] (**Figure 1**). In case of observed intolerance against ACEIs, angiotensin-II receptor blockers (ARBs) could be used instead, since they have been shown to be as effective as ACEIs [26].

The use of β-blockers as a combined therapy with ACEIs is common for heart failure treatment; however, for dystrophinopathies, this is not well documented. One study described improvements in LV systolic function, when patients with DMD were treated with carvedilol [27]. Unfortunately, these findings were never reproduced in dystrophic *mdx* mice [28]. Study outcomes for combined therapy were mixed and showed additional beneficial effects for β-blockers in some cases, and no additional advantageous effects in others [29]. Future clinical trials need to evaluate whether the use of β-blockers for dystrophinopathy as mono- or combination therapy have beneficial effects. At the moment, it is recommended to initiate a therapy with β-blockers in patients with dystrophinopathy that have LV dysfunction [25]. Future studies will need to assess whether therapies combining corticosteroids with β-blockers and ACEIs could be of added benefit.

Mineralocorticoid receptor antagonists are a standard heart failure therapy due to their anti-fibrotic effect in DMD and ability to attenuate cardiomyopathy [30]. In a recent randomized double-blind clinical trial, one group of DMD patients with normal LV function were treated with only ACEIs or ARBs and the other group additionally also received eplerenone (aldosterone inhibitor). Results showed a lower LV circumferential strain in both treated groups compared to control, but not between treated groups [31]. This study is the only study of mineralocorticoid-receptor antagonists on dystrophin-deficient cardiomyopathy, and although it was not able to demonstrate a significant improvement, it is essential to investigate further whether aldosterone inhibitors could be of any benefit for delaying cardiomyopathy onset.

### 4.2. Nonpharmacological treatment

Heart transplantation is the only remedy for end-stage heart failure. Some cases have been published in which patients with DMD received a successful transplantation with no significant adverse effects [25]. Heart transplantation occurs more frequently in patients with BMD because of the higher incidence of cardiomyopathy and is only recommended for patients who have end-stage heart failure [25]. A deficit in surrogate organs complicates heart transplantation; therefore, left ventricular assist devices (LVADs) are an interesting substitution, demonstrating effectiveness in DMD and BMD patients with advanced heart failure [25]. However, possible postoperative complications, such as arrhythmias, bleeding, respiratory failure, stroke and rehabilitation, need to be further addressed [25].

### 4.3. Treatments with indirect effects

Treatments that have no direct effect on the heart can also have considerable benefits on cardiac function. For example, pain reduction lowers blood levels of catecholamines, which on its turn generates no further stress on the heart.

Lung and heart function are known to affect each other. When lung function needs to be assisted by noninvasive positive pressure ventilation (NIPPV)—because of breathing difficulties—it also has favoring results on cardiac function. It leads to less strain on the heart and a correspondingly reduced heart rate. Reduced lung function is also a strong negative predictor of survival when the vital capacity hits one liter [32]. In addition, assisted ventilation increased the mean survival of DMD patients with more than 10 years; however, patients who need constant ventilation will not exceed 20 years of age [32].

Although corticosteroids treatment has positively affected the incidence of scoliosis, it still occurs that thoracolumbar surgery becomes necessary to correct the spinal curvature [33]. In this case, timing is important and certain risk factors are bound to patients with DMD that have LV dysfunction [32]. Even when surgery is undertaken, it is not certain if scoliosis will not develop. This could lead into feeding and swallowing problems [32]. When surgery is able to prevent scoliosis onset, not only does it improve positioning and pulmonary function, but it also ameliorates cardiac function [33]. It is important to note that—although spinal surgery is performed in many neurological centers—it is not uniformly supported [11]. If patients with dystrophinopathy undergo surgery, an appropriate use of anesthetics is essential and needs to be assessed and monitored carefully before, during and after surgical intervention [34]. **Table 2** gives an overview of all current clinical interventions available for the treatment of dystrophin-deficient cardiomyopathy.

| Method | Level of evidence | Recommendations | References |
|---|---|---|---|
| ***Pharmacological*** | | | |
| Corticosteroids | Mid | Initiation based on functional state and pre-existing risk factors for adverse side-effects | [14] |
| | | Be aware of controversial cardiac results in animal studies and clinical trials | [83] |
| ACEIs and ARBs | High | First-line therapy upon development of LV dysfunction | [18] |
| | | Initiate therapy from 10 years of age or earlier | [14] |
| β-Blockers | Low | Follow guidelines for adults with chronic heart failure | [84] |
| | | Variable, normally initiation after ACEIs start on the basis of ventricular dysfunction or elevated heart rate | [18] |
| Mineralocorticoid -receptor antagonists | Low | Timing not adequately addressed and variation in clinical practice | [18] |
| ***Nonpharmacological*** | | | |
| LVAD | High | Currently bridge to heart transplantation but potential for destination therapy High-risk factor: scoliosis, respiratory muscle weakness and difficulties in recovery and rehabilitation | [85] |
| Heart transplantation | High | Should be considered for patient with end-stage heart failure | [25] |
| ***Indirect effects*** | | | |
| NIPPV | High | Main need for pulmonary care is from the onset of ambulation loss. Decisions for respiratory care must be taken by a care team including a physician and skilled therapist. | [86] |
| Thoracolumbar surgery | Mid | For patients not receiving glucocorticoids: surgery warranted when spinal curvature > 20°. For patients receiving glucocorticoids: surgery warranted upon further spinal curve progression. | [33] |

ACEIs, angiotensin-converting enzyme inhibitor; ARBs, angiotensin II receptor blockers; LVAD, left ventricular assist device; NIPPV, noninvasive positive pressure ventilation.

**Table 2.** Clinical treatments of dystrophin-deficient cardiomyopathy.

# 5. Emerging therapies

## 5.1. Utrophin upregulation

In 1972, UTROPHIN—a DYSTROPHIN homolog with a shortened rod domain but many similar binding proteins—was discovered [35]. These resemblances started the speculation that UTROPHIN could partially compensate for DYSTROPHIN loss. More clarity was brought by the creation of a *DYSTROPHIN/UTROPHIN* double knockout (*mdx/utrn*$^{-/-}$) mouse model, that showed a worsened skeletal and cardiac muscle phenotype with a drastically lower life expectancy of only 2–3 months compared to *mdx* mice [36]. Several studies have been performed testing UTROPHIN upregulation in preclinical models, the most promising one coming from a small molecule screening. SMT C1100 treatment demonstrated an increase of UTROPHIN levels in *mdx* mice and improved muscle function [37]. A phase Ia and recently also a phase Ib clinical trial were completed, concluding that no serious adverse effects were accompanied by SMT C1100 treatment in healthy controls and pediatric DMD patients, respectively [38]. It is important to mention that UTROPHIN will never be able to replace symptoms of DYSTROPHIN deficiency because of its structural differences and lack of a NO binding site (Appendix 1), presuming an incomplete surrogate effect.

### 5.2. Nonsense suppression

About 10–15% of patients with DMD carry a premature stop codon that abrogates translation of *DYSTROPHIN* [39]. Aminoglycosides are mainly used as antibiotic agents but are also able to cause a ribosomal read-through—meaning it is able to ignore premature stop codons while still detecting normal stop codons—and in this way generating a shortened, although functional DYSTROPHIN protein. Although promising, clinical results have been poor with inconclusive or very low expressed DYSTROPHIN levels and major concerns about side effects caused by Gentamicin and Negamicin [40]. Henceforth, PCT124 or ataluren was discovered by another small-molecule drug screening, showing promising results in preclinical animal models without skipping normal stop codons [41]. In addition, ataluren was considered safe and showed upregulation of DYSTROPHIN in certain subgroups of patients with DMD, although nothing was mentioned about the heart [42–44]. These clinical trials confirmed the need for further understanding and a division of patients with DMD in subgroups. Currently, ataluren is involved in a randomized, double-blind and placebo-controlled phase III trial, with the primary outcome being an improvement in the 6-minute walking test (6MWT) after 48 weeks; however, cardiac function will not be monitored (NCT01826487). A search for more effective read-through compounds (RTCs) ended up with two more drugs: RTC13 and RTC14. The highest efficiency was reached by RTC13. This compound restored DYSTROPHIN levels the most in the skeletal muscle and the heart compared to gentamicin, PTC124 and RTC14. Moreover, CK levels were reduced and muscle function was improved in *mdx* mice [45].

### 5.3. Exon skipping

The idea of exon skipping originated from BMD, due to the fact that these patients express a shorter isoform of DYSTROPHIN and show a much milder phenotype [46]. Skipping the genetic alteration of *DYSTROPHIN* so that an out-of-frame shift is turned into an in-frame shift would result in the expression of a truncated DYSTROPHIN isoform such as in BMD (Appendix 2) [47]. Antisense oligonucleotides (AONs) are short, single-stranded DNA sequences that are complementary to a target pre-mRNA splice site and able to skip exons by sterically hindering splice enhancers [48]. This procedure should be able to treat 35% of patients with

DMD by targeting one exon and even 83% when two exons are simultaneously targeted [49]. The downside is that AONs can only target one exon, for this reason research currently focuses only on the most frequently involved exons [49].

There are currently two different types of AONs undergoing clinical trials: 2′O methyl phosphorothioate (2′OMePS)—also called drisapersen [50]—and phosphorodiamidate morpholino oligomers (PMO)—also known as eteplirsen [51]. Both were unable to improve DYSTROPHIN expression in the heart [52, 53]. Recently, a high degree of DYSTROPHIN rescue was achieved in the respiratory and cardiac muscles with tricyclo DNA oligomers in *mdx* mice [54]. However, these results were accomplished by multiple injections and high doses of administration (200 mg/kg per week).

Previous clinical trials picked up the inefficiency of systemic delivery of naked AONs [50, 51, 55]. For this reason, attention quickly converted toward the development of delivery methods for AONs. Systems like cell-penetrating peptides (CPPs) or encapsulation techniques such as liposomes or nanoparticles appeared. CPPs are small peptides that are conjugated to AONs. They facilitate the penetration through the plasma membrane and can be divided into three groups: arginine rich, Pip (PNA/PMO internalization peptide) or phage and chimeric peptides. Arginine-rich CPPs associated with a PMO showed the first robust cardiac DYSTROPHIN expression and an improved cardiac function [56, 57]. More recently, Pip6 conjugated with a PMO also showed cardiac Dystrophin expression and functional improvement at low doses [55] and prevented exercise-induced cardiomyopathy after long-term treatment [58]. Phage peptides were less successful with the exception of a 7-mer phage conjugated to 2′OMePS that resulted in an enhanced uptake and exon skipping in the cardiac muscle [59].

Instead of a molecular approach with AONs conjugated to CPPs, it is also possible to deliver small nuclear RNAs (snRNAs) or nucleases to the cardiac muscle. These effectors need to be incorporated into the genome; recombinant adenoviral-associated viruses (rAAVs) are the preferred choice because of their long persistence in myonuclei. However, the disadvantage is their relatively small cloning capacity (5 kb). In addition, to safely apply AAV therapy, all viral genes have to be removed except for the components necessary for replication [60].

Delivery of U7snRNA by rAAV6 has shown to restore cardiac DYSTROPHIN expression, even one year after injection higher DYSTROPHIN levels were still found [61]. The safety profile and optimal concentrations of rAAV8 U7snRNA delivery in the forelimb of a large cohort of GRMD dogs have been monitored carefully and concluded that this treatment is safe, since no adverse immunologic responses were observed [62]. Recently, an observational study was initiated, monitoring clinical and radiological changes of patients eligible for exon 53 skipping, while testing their immunization against viral serotypes (NCT01385917).

Exon skipping with nucleases such as "clustered regularly interspaced short palindromic repeats" (CRISPR) together with a Cas9 nuclease brought new insights and possibilities for gene-editing treatments. CRISPR/Cas9 is an immune protection system originating from bacteria that is able to edit the genome by introducing a double-strand break. Afterwards genomic damage is repaired by one of the two possible repair mechanisms: nonhomologous end-joining (NHEJ) or homology-directed repair (HDR). NHEJ was used as a technique for

*DYSTROPHIN* exon skipping in *mdx* mice, a CRISPR/Cas9 was designed targeting exon 23, leading into a removal of this exon by double-strand breaks where after these two ends are linked back together again by NHEJ [63]. Gene-editing components were delivered by rAAV9 through different administration routes and showed in all cases improved Dystrophin expression in the cardiac and skeletal muscle [63].

### 5.4. Gene therapy

Differently from exon skipping, it is also possible to incorporate *DYSTROPHIN* into the genome instead of designing techniques to modulate native *DYSTROPHIN*. The advantage of this therapy is that it is not patient specific, all patients can benefit from the same technique. However, due to the enormous size of *DYSTROPHIN*, it is impossible to compact it entirely into viral capsids. Because of the observation that short isoforms of only 45% of full-length DYSTROPHIN can lead to a very mild phenotype, mini- and microdystrophin were created, leaving behind redundant parts [64, 65].

Some different rAAV types have shown huge promise in delivering mini- or microdystrophin to the heart. Microdystrophin delivered by rAAV6 was able to incorporate itself in the skeletal, cardiac and respiratory muscles of *mdx* mice; however, heart function did not recover, while DYSTROPHIN was clearly expressed [66]. A subtype that has shown to be particularly efficient in transfecting the heart is rAAV9 [67]. Systemic injection of minidystrophin encapsulated in rAAV9 has shown widespread expression, also in the heart of the GRMD dogs [68].

While only one phase I clinical trial for minidystrophin has been executed [69] and another one for microdystrophin is ongoing (NCT02376816), it is clear that this field is still at its starting point. Many difficulties that need to addressed in the future are immunological responses and the necessity of high viral titers [70]. However, novel techniques like fetal transduction [71], chimeric vectors [72] and plasmapheresis [73] have already shown a drastic decrease in immunologic responses in preclinical animal models. In addition, viral gene therapy struggles with compaction size and eventually delivers smaller *DYSTROPHIN* constructs in comparison to skipped *DYSTROPHIN*. Nevertheless, full-length *DYSTROPHIN* was recently successfully incorporated into the skeletal muscle of a *mdx* mouse through the usage of three vectors carrying "intandem" sequential exonic parts of *DYSTROPHIN* [74].

### 5.5. Cell-based therapy

Cell therapy has some advantages compared to the aforementioned therapies. The idea of cell therapy is to produce healthy cells, which express full length DYSTROPHIN that are able to integrate into the tissue upon injection. In an optimal situation, these cells should also be able to repopulate the progenitor populations such as the satellite cell pool in the skeletal muscle. Many trials have been performed with adult stem cells like myoblasts, bone marrow-derived stem cells, CD133+ stem cells and mesoangioblasts (MABs). MABs are vessel-associated progenitors that are able to migrate across the vessel wall and have been shown to repopulate the skeletal muscle of GRMD dogs upon systemic injection, resulting into a variable improvement of muscle function [75]. Treatment of *mdx/utrn*$^{-/-}$ mice with aorta-derived MABs led into a delay of DCM onset and promotion of angiogenesis [76]. Recently, a completed phase I clinical trial with MABs in patients with DMD showed no sign of DYSTROPHIN expression after treatment [77]. Multiple reasons could explain this observation, such as the late age of the patients and the lengthy procedure of isolation, which does not ensure that the cells are delivered in an optimal way. However, systemic treatment with MABs has shown to be safe and efforts are being made to start a phase II clinical trial.

| Method | Phase | Model/patients | References |
|---|---|---|---|
| ***Utrophin upregulation*** | | | |
| Arginine butyrate | Preclinical | *Mdx* mice | [87] |
| SMT C1100 | I | Healthy controls | [38] |
| ***Read-through therapy*** | | | |
| Aminoglycosides | I, completed | Patients with DMD and BMD | [40] |
| Ataluren (PTC124) | III, ongoing | Patients with DMD | NCT01826487 |
| RTC13/14 | Preclinical | *Mdx* mice | [45] |
| ***Exon skipping*** | | | |
| Drisapersen (2′OMePS) | III, recruiting | Patients with DMD | [51], NCT01803412 |
| Eteplirsen (PMO) | III, recruiting | Patients with DMD | [50, 88], NCT02255552 |
| Tricyclo-DNA | Preclinical | *Mdx* mice | [54] |
| Cell-penetrating peptide/AON | Preclinical | *Mdx* mice | [55–58] |
| Phage peptide/AON | Preclinical | *Mdx* mice | [59] |
| rAAV6/U7snRNA | Preclinical | GRMD | [61] |
| rAAV9/CRISPR/cas9 | Preclinical | *Mdx* mice | [63] |
| ***Gene therapy*** | | | |
| rAAV6-microdystrophin | Preclinical | *Mdx* mice | [66] |
| rAAV9-minidystrophin | Preclinical | GRMD | [67, 89] |
| ***Cell-based therapy*** | | | |
| Mesoangioblast | Preclinical | *Mdx/utrn* mice | [76] |
| | I, completed | Patients with DMD | [77] |
| iPSC-derived cells | Preclinical | Sgcb-null mice | [78] |

*Mdx*, X-linked muscular dystrophy; DMD, Duchenne muscular dystrophy; BMD, Becker muscular dystrophy; RTC, read-through compound; AON, antisense oligonucleotide; rAAV, recombinant adenoviral-associated viruses; CRISPR, clustered regularly interspaced short palindromic repeats; GRMD, golden retriever muscular dystrophy; utrn, Utrophin; iPSC, induced pluripotent stem cell; Sgcb, sarcoglycan beta.

**Table 3.** Preclinical treatments of MD-associated cardiomyopathy.

Recently, treatments with derivatives of induced pluripotent stem cells (iPSCs) are being explored. iPSCs are basically (patient-derived) somatic cells that are reprogrammed into pluripotent stem cells that possess similar features as embryonic stem cells. These cells have been differentiated into mesodermal-like progenitors and injected directly into the skeletal and cardiac muscles of *Sgcb-null* mice, a model for limb girdle muscular dystrophy with a worsened phenotype compared to *mdx* mice. Data showed that these unique iPSC-derived myogenic progenitors are able to integrate into heart and limb muscles and functionally ameliorate both cardiac and skeletal muscles of injected dystrophic mice [78].

Another advantage of cell therapy is the possibility of correcting patient-derived cells and reinjecting them, bypassing immunological responses. Novel strategies with CRISPR/Cas9 have been developed to repair DYSTROPHIN in iPSCs, showing functional recovery upon differentiation [79]. Eventually, differentiation of iPSCs towards cardiomyocytes can also be used to set up high-throughput screenings for detecting novel patient-tailored therapeutic molecules.

Nevertheless, there are still many aspects in cell-based therapy that need to be addressed. As of yet, there is no consensus about timing of injection, which is hypothesized to be crucial. As for integration, many cell therapies suffer from extremely low integration efficiencies. Future studies should focus on tracing the injected cells, to follow their trajectory and fate during treatment [80]. **Table 3** provides an overview of all the discussed preclinical therapies.

## 6. Conclusion

Since the utilization of ventilation support and corticosteroids treatment, cardiac complications in dystrophinopathies have become more prominent, being responsible for 40% of mortality in patients with DMD [11]. Cardiomyopathy development in patients with dystrophinopathy is highly variable and can be asymptomatic for a long period of time. The earlier onset of skeletal muscle symptoms and the sequential diagnosis can be used as an advantage for cardiac treatment. At the moment, it is recommended to perform a cardiac MRI at the age of 6 or right at the time of diagnosis, followed by two-year check-ups till the age of 10 where after annual check-ups are required. Momentarily, no consensus exists about initiation of treatment. It is advised to start symptomatic treatment as soon as possible because of the beneficial effects on cardiomyopathic progression. ACEIs are the preferred choice for treatment, because of their clear and advantageous effects on cardiomyopathy in patients with dystrophinopathy. Effects of corticosteroids treatment on the heart remain distrustful and cardiac deterioration should be monitored with care, while β-blockers are shown to be effective as stand-alone therapy, but additive effects together with ACEIs are not observed. In addition, transparent results about mineralocorticoid-receptor antagonist treatment on patients with dystrophinopathy are still missing. In the case of end-stage heart failure, heart transplantation or LVADs should be considered. While treatments with indirect effects on the heart like pain reduction, NIPPV and thoracolumbar surgery could also be of added benefit for cardiac health.

Many emerging therapies exist that are being investigated in preclinical models and clinical trials. These studies aim to enhance UTROPHIN expression, read through a stop codon mutation, skip the exon—that is holding the genetic alteration in DMD to express a shorter form of DYSTROPHIN corresponding to BMD—or bring in shortened *DYSTROPHIN* variants by viral or cell-based therapy. Several of these therapies already made it into clinical trials with some undergoing phase III trials. However, as skeletal muscle complications are the most prominent, effects on the heart have not been taken up into the expected outcomes of these trials. This also because in most preclinical treatments beneficial effects on the heart were absent. Novel approaches were necessary to deliver constructs to the cardiac muscle and some preclinical studies have shown DYSTROPHIN expression in the heart together with functional improvements in small and large animal models. Emerging literature is also showing that IPSC-derived myogenic progenitors from patients with dystrophy provide an attractive model to get new insights on gene-editing treatments. This novel technology offers possibilities for autologous therapy and eventually targeting both cardiac and skeletal dystrophic muscles with a single myogenic progenitor population. It is assumed that all these preclinical therapies will make it into clinical studies and hopefully subsequently into dystrophinopathy therapies. However, many issues still exist and need to be addressed such as immunogenic reactions toward the administered cells or viruses, the need for high-dosing regimens and bodywide delivery.

## Appendix

### *Appendix 1: The dystrophin-glycoprotein complex*

DYSTROPHIN functions as a linkage rod between the actin cytoskeleton and the cell membrane, where it is connected to β-DYSTROGLYCAN, which in turn associates with the extracellular matrix via LAMININ. The SARCOGLYCAN complex is in close proximity to β-DYSTROGLYCAN and is important in signaling, which occurs through SYNTROPHIN and DYSTROBREVIN. Together these proteins are part of the dystrophin-glycoprotein complex (DGC). DYSTROPHIN also accommodates a neuronal nitric oxide synthase (nNOS)-binding site.

### *Appendix 2: The molecular mechanisms of dystrophin deficiency*

The 24 spectrin-like repeats within DYSTROPHIN neutralizes contraction-induced stress. The absence of DYSTROPHIN leads into a loss of muscle structural integrity, which generates membrane microruptures, leading to elevated CK levels in the serum and a high intracellular $Ca^{2+}$ concentration that subsequently activates calcium-dependent proteases [81]. Because of the lack of experimental proof, researchers have started questioning this theory. It became evident that activation of stretch-induced $Ca^{2+}$ channels corresponds with elevated intracellular $Ca^{2+}$ levels, although the responsible channel has still to be found [82]. Repeated contraction-induced damage leads to a continuous muscle breakdown and regeneration, with an increased build-up of fatty and fibrotic tissue, followed by an eventual loss of muscle contractility.

### *Appendix 3: The reading-frame concept*

A reading frame consists out of codons—three nucleotide-based sequences—which translate into a specific amino acid. A shift of the reading frame basically means that the reading frame

http://dx.doi.org/10.5772/65061

is altered, for example by a deletion of nucleotides. If the genetic code is extended or shortened by a multitude of "3 nucleotides", the reading frame is sustained. Therefore, this is called an "in-frame shift" resulting in a partially functional protein, which corresponds to BMD. When genetic alteration occurs by a multiplication of "1–2 nucleotides", the reading-frame shifts, leading to post-translational disintegration of DYSTROPHIN; hence, this is called an "out-of-frame shift" and corresponds to DMD.

## Acknowledgements

We would like to apologize to all authors whose work has not been reported here due to space limitations. This work has been supported with the contribution of "Opening The Future" Campaign [EJJ-OPTFUT-02010] CARIPLO 2015_0634, FWO (#G088715N, #G060612N, #G0A8813N), GOA (EJJ-C2161-GOA/11/012), IUAP-VII/07 (EJJ-C4851-17/07-P) and OT#09-053 (EJJ-C0420-OT/09/053) grants. We thank Christina Vochten and Vicky Raets for professional administrative assistance. We would also like to thank Rondoufonds voor Duchenne Onderzoek for kind donations.

## Author details

Jordi Camps[1], Enrico Pozzo[1,2], Tristan Pulinckx[1], Robin Duelen[1] and Maurilio Sampaolesi[1,2*]

*Address all correspondence to: maurilio.sampaolesi@kuleuven.be

1 Translational Cardiomyology Lab, Stem Cell Biology and Embryology Unit, Department of Development and Regeneration, KU Leuven, Leuven, Belgium

2 Division of Human Anatomy, Department of Public Health, Experimental and Forensic Medicine, University of Pavia, Pavia, Italy

## References

[1] Mendell JR, Shilling C, Leslie ND, Flanigan KM, al-Dahhak R, Gastier-Foster J, et al. Evidence-based path to newborn screening for duchenne muscular dystrophy. Ann. Neurol. 2012;71:304–13. DOI:10.1002/ana.23528

[2] Bushby KMD, Thambyayah M, Gardner-Medwin D. Prevalence and incidence of Becker muscular dystrophy. Lancet. 1991;337:1022–4. DOI:10.1016/0140-6736(91)92671-N

[3] Nakamura A. X-linked dilated cardiomyopathy: a cardiospecific phenotype of dystrophinopathy. Pharmaceuticals. 2015;8:303–20. DOI:10.3390/ph8020303

[4] Eagle M, Baudouin SV, Chandler C, Giddings DR, Bullock R, Bushby K. Survival in Duchenne muscular dystrophy: Improvements in life expectancy since 1967 and the impact of home nocturnal ventilation. Neuromuscul. Disord. 2002;12:926–9. DOI: 10.1016/S0960-8966(02)00140-2

[5] Bradley WG, Jones MZ, Mussini JM, Fawcett PR. Becker-type muscular dystrophy. Muscle Nerve. 1978;1:111–32. DOI:10.1002/mus.880010204

[6] Sarnat HB. Muscular dystrophies. In: Kliegman R, Stanton B, St. Geme J, editors. Nelson Textb. Pediatr. 19th ed. p. 2119–29. DOI:10.1016/B978-1-4377-0755-7.00601-1

[7] Ropper A, Sanuels MA. The muscular dystrophies. In: Ropper, AH, Samuels, MA, editors. Adams Victor's Princ. Neurol. 9th ed. p. 687–95. DOI:10.1055/s-0032-1329199

[8] Romfh A, McNally EM. Cardiac assessment in duchenne and becker muscular dystrophies. Curr. Heart Fail. Rep. 2010;7:212–8. DOI:10.1007/s11897-010-0028-2

[9] Spurney CF. Cardiomyopathy of duchenne muscular dystrophy: Current understanding and future directions. Muscle Nerve. 2011;44:8–19. DOI:10.1002/mus.22097

[10] Connuck DM, Sleeper LA, Colan SD, Cox GF, Towbin JA, Lowe AM, et al. Characteristics and outcomes of cardiomyopathy in children with Duchenne or Becker muscular dystrophy: a comparative study from the Pediatric Cardiomyopathy Registry. Am. Heart J. 2008;155:998–1005. DOI:10.1016/j.ahj.2008.01.018

[11] Finsterer J, Cripe L. Treatment of dystrophin cardiomyopathies. Nat. Rev. Cardiol. 2014;11:168–79. DOI:10.1038/nrcardio.2013.213

[12] Ciafaloni E, Fox DJ, Pandya S, Westfield CP, Puzhankara S, Romitti PA, et al. Delayed diagnosis in Duchenne muscular dystrophy: data from the muscular dystrophy surveillance, tracking, and research network (MD STARnet). J. Pediatr. 2009;155:380–5. DOI:10.1016/j.jpeds.2009.02.007

[13] Zatz M, Rapaport D, Vainzof M, Passos-Bueno MR, Bortolini ER, Pavanello R de CM, et al. Serum creatine-kinase (CK) and pyruvate-kinase (PK) activities in Duchenne (DMD) as compared with Becker (BMD) muscular dystrophy. J. Neurol. Sci. 1991;102:190–6. DOI:10.1016/0022-510X(91)90068-I

[14] Bushby K, Finkel R, Birnkrant DJ, Case LE, Clemens PR, Cripe L, et al. Diagnosis and management of Duchenne muscular dystrophy, part 1: diagnosis, and pharmacological and psychosocial management. Lancet Neurol. 2010;9:77–93. DOI:10.1016/S1474-4 422(09)70271-6

[15] Monaco AP, Bertelson CJ, Liechti-Gallati S, Moser H, Kunkel LM. An explanation for the phenotypic differences between patients bearing partial deletions of the DMD locus. Genomics. 1988;2:90–5. DOI:10.1016/0888-7543(88)90113-9

[16] Dent KM, Dunn DM, Von Niederhausern AC, Aoyagi AT, Kerr L, Bromberg MB, et al. Improved molecular diagnosis of dystrophinopathies in an unselected clinical cohort. Am. J. Med. Genet. 2005;134:295–8. DOI:10.1002/ajmg.a.30617

[17] Spurney C, Shimizu R, Morgenroth LP, Kolski H, Gordish-Dressman H, Clemens PR. Cooperative international neuromuscular research group duchenne natural history study demonstrates insufficient diagnosis and treatment of cardiomyopathy in duchenne muscular dystrophy. Muscle Nerve. 2014;50:250–6. DOI:10.1002/mus.24163

[18] McNally EM, Kaltman JR, Benson DW, Canter CE, Cripe LH, Duan D, et al. Contemporary cardiac issues in Duchenne muscular dystrophy. Working Group of the National Heart, Lung, and Blood Institute in collaboration with parent project muscular dystrophy. Circulation. 2015;131:1590–8. DOI:10.1161/CIRCULATIONAHA.114.015151

[19] Thomas TO, Morgan TM, Burnette WB, Markham LW. Correlation of heart rate and cardiac dysfunction in Duchenne muscular dystrophy. Pediatr. Cardiol. 2012;33:1175–9. DOI:10.1007/s00246-012-0281-0

[20] Politano L, Nigro G. Treatment of dystrophinopathic cardiomyopathy: review of the literature and personal results. Acta. Myol. 2012;31:24–30. DOI:10.1016/S0960-8966(00)00174-7

[21] Barber BJ, Andrews JG, Lu Z, West NA, Meaney FJ, Price ET, et al. Oral corticosteroids and onset of cardiomyopathy in Duchenne muscular dystrophy. J. Pediatr. 2013;163:1080–4.e1. DOI:10.1016/j.jpeds.2013.05.060

[22] Bauer R, Straub V, Blain A, Bushby K, MacGowan GA. Contrasting effects of steroids and angiotensin-converting-enzyme inhibitors in a mouse model of dystrophin-deficient cardiomyopathy. Eur. J. Heart. Fail. 2009;11:463–71. DOI:10.1093/eurjhf/hfp028

[23] Duboc D, Meune C, Lerebours G, Devaux JY, Vaksmann G, Bécane HM. Effect of perindopril on the onset and progression of left ventricular dysfunction in Duchenne muscular dystrophy. J. Am. Coll. Cardiol. 2005;45:855–7. DOI:10.1016/j.jacc.2004.09.078

[24] Duboc D, Meune C, Pierre B, Wahbi K, Eymard B, Toutain A, et al. Perindopril preventive treatment on mortality in Duchenne muscular dystrophy: 10 years' follow up. Am. Heart J. 2007;154:596–602. DOI:10.1016/j.ahj.2007.05.014.

[25] Kamdar F, Garry DJ. Dystrophin-deficient cardiomyopathy. J. Am. Coll. Cardiol. 2016;67:2533–46. DOI:10.1016/j.jacc.2016.02.081

[26] Allen HD, Flanigan KM, Thrush PT, Dvorchik I, Yin H, Canter C, et al. A randomized, double-blind trial of lisinopril and losartan for the treatment of cardiomyopathy in Duchenne muscular dystrophy. PLoS. Curr. 2013;5. DOI:10.1371/currents.md.2cc69a1dae4be7dfe2bcb420024ea865

[27] Kwon HW, Kwon BS, Kim GB, Chae JH, Park JD, Bae EJ, et al. The effect of enalapril and carvedilol on left ventricular dysfunction in middle childhood and adolescent

patients with muscular dystrophy. Korean Circ. J. 2012;42:184–91. DOI:10.4070/kcj.2012.42.3.184

[28] Blain A, Greally E, Laval SH, Blamire AM, MacGowan GA, Straub VW. Absence of cardiac benefit with early combination ACE inhibitor and beta blocker treatment in mdx mice. J. Cardiovasc. Transl. Res. 2015;8:198–207. DOI:10.1007/s12265-015-9623-7

[29] Viollet L, Thrush PT, Flanigan KM, Mendell JR, Allen HD. Effects of angiotensin-converting enzyme inhibitors and/or beta blockers on the cardiomyopathy in Duchenne muscular dystrophy. Am. J. Cardiol. 2012;110:98–102. DOI:10.1016/j.amjcard.2012.02.064

[30] Rafael-Fortney JA, Chimanji NS, Schill KE, Martin CD, Murray JD, Ganguly R, et al. Early treatment with lisinopril and spironolactone preserves cardiac and skeletal muscle in Duchenne muscular dystrophy mice. Circulation. 2011;124:582–8. DOI:10.1161/CIRCULATIONAHA.111.031716

[31] Raman S V, Hor KN, Mazur W, Halnon NJ, Kissel JT, He X, et al. Eplerenone for early cardiomyopathy in Duchenne muscular dystrophy: a randomised, double-blind, placebo-controlled trial. Lancet. Neurol. 2015;14:153–61. DOI:10.1016/S1474-4422(14)70318-7

[32] Wollinsky KH, Kutter B, Geiger PM. Long-term ventilation of patients with Duchenne muscular dystrophy: Experiences at the Neuromuscular Centre Ulm. Acta Myol. 2012;31:170–8.

[33] Bushby K, Finkel R, Birnkrant DJ, Case LE, Clemens PR, Cripe L, et al. Diagnosis and management of Duchenne muscular dystrophy, part 2: implementation of multidisciplinary care. Lancet. Neurol. 2010;9:177–89. DOI:10.1016/S1474-4422(09)70272-8

[34] Cripe LH, Tobias JD. Cardiac considerations in the operative management of the patient with Duchenne or Becker muscular dystrophy. Paediatr. Anaesth. 2013;23:777–84. DOI:10.1111/pan.12229

[35] Tinsley JM, Blake DJ, Roche A, Fairbrother U, Riss J, Byth BC, et al. Primary structure of dystrophin-related protein. Nature. 1992;360:591–3. DOI:10.1038/360591a0

[36] Deconinck AE, Rafael JA, Skinner JA, Brown SC, Potter AC, Metzinger L, et al. Utrophin-dystrophin-deficient mice as a model for Duchenne muscular dystrophy. Cell. 1997;90:717–27. DOI:10.1016/S0092-8674(00)80532-2

[37] Tinsley JM, Fairclough RJ, Storer R, Wilkes FJ, Potter AC, Squire SE, et al. Daily treatment with SMTC1100, a novel small molecule utrophin upregulator, dramatically reduces the dystrophic symptoms in the mdx mouse. PLoS One. 2011;6:e19189. DOI:10.1371/journal.pone.0019189

[38] Ricotti V, Spinty S, Roper H, Hughes I, Tejura B, Robinson N, et al. Safety, tolerability, and pharmacokinetics of SMT C1100, a 2-arylbenzoxazole utrophin modulator, following single- and multiple-dose administration to pediatric patients with Duch

enne muscular dystrophy. PLoS One. 2016;11:e0152840. DOI:10.1371/journal.pone.0152840

[39] Finkel RS. Read-through strategies for suppression of nonsense mutations in Duchenne/Becker muscular dystrophy: aminoglycosides and ataluren (PTC124). J. Child Neurol. 2-010;25:1158–64. DOI:10.1177/0883073810371129

[40] Malik V, Rodino-Klapac LR, Viollet L, Wall C, King W, Al-Dahhak R, et al. Gentamicin-induced readthrough of stop codons in Duchenne muscular dystrophy. Ann. Neurol. 2010;67:771–80. DOI:10.1002/ana.22024

[41] Welch EM, Barton ER, Zhuo J, Tomizawa Y, Friesen WJ, Trifillis P, et al. PTC124 targets genetic disorders caused by nonsense mutations. Nature. 2007;447:87–91. DOI: 10.1038/nature05756

[42] Hirawat S, Welch EM, Elfring GL, Northcutt VJ, Paushkin S, Hwang S, et al. Safety, tolerability, and pharmacokinetics of PTC124, a nonaminoglycoside nonsense mutation suppressor, following single- and multiple-dose administration to healthy male and female adult volunteers. J. Clin. Pharmacol. 2007;47:430–44. DOI:10.1177/0091270006297140

[43] Finkel RS, Flanigan KM, Wong B, Bönnemann C, Sampson J, Sweeney HL, et al. Phase 2a study of ataluren-mediated dystrophin production in patients with nonsense mutation Duchenne muscular dystrophy. Sawada H, editor. PLoS One. 2013;8:e81302. DOI:10.1371/journal.pone.0081302

[44] Bushby K, Finkel R, Wong B, Barohn R, Campbell C, Comi GP, et al. Ataluren treatment of patients with nonsense mutation dystrophinopathy. Muscle Nerve. 2014;50:477–87. DOI:10.1002/mus.24332

[45] Kayali R, Ku JM, Khitrov G, Jung ME, Prikhodko O, Bertoni C. Read-through compound 13 restores dystrophin expression and improves muscle function in the mdx mouse model for Duchenne muscular dystrophy. Hum. Mol. Genet. 2012;21:4007–20. DOI:10.1093/hmg/dds223

[46] Hoffman EP, Fischbeck KH, Brown RH, Johnson M, Medori R, Loike JD, et al. Characterization of dystrophin in muscle-biopsy specimens from patients with Duchenne's or Becker's muscular dystrophy. N. Engl. J. Med. 1988;318:1363–8. DOI:10.1056/NEJM198805263182104

[47] Wilton SD, Lloyd F, Carville K, Fletcher S, Honeyman K, Agrawal S, et al. Specific removal of the nonsense mutation from the mdx dystrophin mRNA using antisense oligonucleotides. Neuromuscul. Disord. 1999;9:330–8. DOI:10.1016/S0960-8966(99)00010-3

[48] Cartegni L, Chew SL, Krainer AR. Listening to silence and understanding nonsense: exonic mutations that affect splicing. Nat. Rev. Genet. 2002;3:285–98. DOI:10.1038/nrg775

[49] Aartsma-Rus A, Fokkema I, Verschuuren J, Ginjaar I, van Deutekom J, van Ommen GJ, et al. Theoretic applicability of antisense-mediated exon skipping for Duchenne muscular dystrophy mutations. Hum. Mutat. 2009;30:293–9. DOI:10.1002/humu.20918

[50] Mendell JR, Goemans N, Lowes LP, Alfano LN, Berry K, Shao J, et al. Longitudinal effect of eteplirsen versus historical control on ambulation in Duchenne muscular dystrophy. Ann. Neurol. 2016;79:257–71. DOI:10.1002/ana.24555

[51] Voit T, Topaloglu H, Straub V, Muntoni F, Deconinck N, Campion G, et al. Safety and efficacy of drisapersen for the treatment of Duchenne muscular dystrophy (DEMAND II): an exploratory, randomised, placebo-controlled phase 2 study. Lancet. Neurol. 2014;13:987–96. DOI:10.1016/S1474-4422(14)70195-4

[52] Malerba A, Thorogood FC, Dickson G, Graham IR. Dosing regimen has a significant impact on the efficiency of morpholino oligomer-induced exon skipping in mdx mice. Hum. Gene Ther. 2009;20:955–65. DOI:10.1089/hum.2008.157

[53] Malerba A, Boldrin L, Dickson G. Long-term systemic administration of unconjugated morpholino oligomers for therapeutic expression of dystrophin by exon skipping in skeletal muscle: implications for cardiac muscle integrity. Nucleic Acid Ther. 2011;21:293–8. DOI:10.1089/nat.2011.0306

[54] Goyenvalle A, Griffith G, Babbs A, El Andaloussi S, Ezzat K, Avril A, et al. Functional correction in mouse models of muscular dystrophy using exon-skipping tricyclo-DNA oligomers. Nat. Med. 2015;21:270–5. DOI:10.1038/nm.3765

[55] Betts C, Saleh AF, Arzumanov AA, Hammond SM, Godfrey C, Coursindel T, et al. Pip6-PMO, A new generation of peptide-oligonucleotide conjugates with improved cardiac exon skipping activity for DMD treatment. Mol. Ther. Nucleic Acids. 2012;1:e38. DOI: 10.1038/mtna.2012.30

[56] Wu B, Moulton HM, Iversen PL, Jiang J, Li J, Li J, et al. Effective rescue of dystrophin improves cardiac function in dystrophin-deficient mice by a modified morpholino oligomer. Proc. Natl. Acad. Sci. 2008;105:14814–9. DOI:10.1073/pnas.0805676105

[57] Yin H, Moulton HM, Seow Y, Boyd C, Boutilier J, Iverson P, et al. Cell-penetrating peptide-conjugated antisense oligonucleotides restore systemic muscle and cardiac dystrophin expression and function. Hum. Mol. Genet. 2008;17:3909–18. DOI:10.1093/hmg/ddn293

[58] Betts CA, Saleh AF, Carr CA, Hammond SM, Coenen-Stass AML, Godfrey C, et al. Prevention of exercised induced cardiomyopathy following Pip-PMO treatment in dystrophic mdx mice. Sci. Rep. 2015;5:8986. DOI:10.1038/srep08986

[59] Jirka SMG, Heemskerk H, Tanganyika-de Winter CL, Muilwijk D, Pang KH, de Visser PC, et al. Peptide Conjugation of 2′-O-methyl phosphorothioate antisense oligonucleotides enhances cardiac uptake and exon skipping in mdx mice. Nucleic Acid Ther. 2014;24:25–36. DOI:10.1089/nat.2013.0448

[60] Scott JM, Li S, Harper SQ, Welikson R, Bourque D, DelloRusso C, et al. Viral vectors for gene transfer of micro-, mini-, or full-length dystrophin. Neuromuscul. Disord. 2002;12:S23–9. DOI:10.1016/S0960-8966(02)00078-0

[61] Bish LT, Sleeper MM, Forbes SC, Wang B, Reynolds C, Singletary GE, et al. Long-term restoration of cardiac dystrophin expression in golden retriever muscular dystrophy following rAAV6-mediated exon skipping. Mol. Ther. 2012;20:580–9. DOI:10.1038/mt.2011.264

[62] Le Guiner C, Montus M, Servais L, Cherel Y, Francois V, Thibaud J-L, et al. Forelimb treatment in a large cohort of dystrophic dogs supports delivery of a recombinant AAV for exon skipping in Duchenne patients. Mol. Ther. 2014;22:1923–35. DOI:10.1038/mt.2014.151

[63] Long C, Amoasii L, Mireault AA, McAnally JR, Li H, Sanchez-Ortiz E, et al. Postnatal genome editing partially restores dystrophin expression in a mouse model of muscular dystrophy. Science. 2015;351:400–3. DOI:10.1126/science.aad5725

[64] England SB, Nicholson L V, Johnson MA, Forrest SM, Love DR, Zubrzycka-Gaarn EE, et al. Very mild muscular dystrophy associated with the deletion of 46% of dystrophin. Nature. 1990;343:180–2. DOI:10.1038/343180a0

[65] Koenig M, Beggs AH, Moyer M, Scherpf S, Heindrich K, Bettecken T, et al. The molecular basis for Duchenne versus Becker muscular dystrophy: correlation of severity with type of deletion. Am. J. Hum. Genet. 1989;45:498–506.

[66] Gregorevic P, Allen JM, Minami E, Blankinship MJ, Haraguchi M, Meuse L, et al. rAAV6-microdystrophin preserves muscle function and extends lifespan in severely dystrophic mice. Nat. Med. 2006;12:787–9. DOI:10.1038/nm1439

[67] Bostick B, Shin JH, Yue Y, Duan D. AAV-microdystrophin therapy improves cardiac performance in aged female mdx mice. Mol. Ther. 2011;19:1826–32. DOI:10.1038/mt.2011.154

[68] Kornegay JN, Li J, Bogan JR, Bogan DJ, Chen C, Zheng H, et al. Widespread muscle expression of an AAV9 human mini-dystrophin vector after intravenous injection in neonatal dystrophin-deficient dogs. Mol. Ther. 2010;18:1501–8. DOI:10.1038/mt.2010.94

[69] Bowles DE, McPhee SWJ, Li C, Gray SJ, Samulski JJ, Camp AS, et al. Phase 1 gene therapy for Duchenne muscular dystrophy using a translational optimized AAV vector. Mol. Ther. 2012;20:443–55. DOI:10.1038/mt.2011.237

[70] Mendell JR, Rodino-Klapac L, Sahenk Z, Malik V, Kaspar BK, Walker CM, et al. Gene therapy for muscular dystrophy: lessons learned and path forward. Neurosci. Lett. 2012;527:90–9. DOI:10.1016/j.neulet.2012.04.078

[71] Hayashita-Kinoh H, Yugeta N, Okada H, Nitahara-Kasahara Y, Chiyo T, Okada T, et al. Intra-amniotic rAAV-mediated microdystrophin gene transfer improves canine X-

linked muscular dystrophy and may induce immune tolerance. Mol. Ther. 2015;23:627–37. DOI:10.1038/mt.2015.5

[72] Foster H, Sharp PS, Athanasopoulos T, Trollet C, Graham IR, Foster K, et al. Codon and mRNA sequence optimization of microdystrophin transgenes improves expression and physiological outcome in dystrophic mdx mice following AAV2/8 gene transfer. Mol. Ther. 2008;16:1825–32. DOI:10.1038/mt.2008.186

[73] Chicoine L, Montgomery C, Bremer W, Shontz K, Griffin D, Heller K, et al. Plasmapheresis eliminates the negative impact of AAV antibodies on microdystrophin gene expression following vascular delivery. Mol. Ther. 2014;22:338–47. DOI:10.1038/mt.2013.244

[74] Koo T, Popplewell L, Athanasopoulos T, Dickson G. Triple trans-splicing adeno-associated virus vectors capable of transferring the coding sequence for full-length dystrophin protein into dystrophic mice. Hum. Gene Ther. 2014;25:98–108. DOI:10.1089/hum.2013.164

[75] Sampaolesi M, Blot S, D'Antona G, Granger N, Tonlorenzi R, Innocenzi A, et al. Mesoangioblast stem cells ameliorate muscle function in dystrophic dogs. Nature. 2006;444:574–9. DOI:10.1038/nature05282

[76] Chun JL, O'Brien R, Song MH, Wondrasch BF, Berry SE. Injection of vessel-derived stem cells prevents dilated cardiomyopathy and promotes angiogenesis and endogenous cardiac stem cell proliferation in mdx/utrn$^{-/-}$ but not aged mdx mouse models for duchenne muscular dystrophy. Stem. Cells. Transl. Med. 2013;2:68–80. DOI:10.5966/sctm.2012-0107

[77] Cossu G, Previtali SC, Napolitano S, Cicalese MP, Tedesco FS, Nicastro F, et al. Intra-arterial transplantation of HLA-matched donor mesoangioblasts in Duchenne muscular dystrophy. EMBO Mol. Med. 2015;7:1513–28. DOI:10.15252/emmm.201505636

[78] Quattrocelli M, Swinnen M, Giacomazzi G, Camps J, Barthélemy I, Ceccarelli G, et al. Mesodermal iPSC-derived progenitor cells functionally regenerate cardiac and skeletal muscle. J. Clin. Invest. 2015;125:4463–82. DOI:10.1172/JCI82735

[79] Young CS, Hicks MR, Ermolova N V, Nakano H, Jan M, Younesi S, et al. A single CRISPR-Cas9 deletion strategy that targets the majority of DMD patients restores dystrophin function in hiPSC-derived muscle cells. Cell. Stem. Cell. 2016;18:533–40. DOI:10.1016/j.stem.2016.01.021

[80] Holvoet B, Quattrocelli M, Belderbos S, Pollaris L, Wolfs E, Gheysens O, et al. Sodium iodide symporter PET and BLI noninvasively reveal mesoangioblast survival in dystrophic mice. Stem. Cell. Rep. 2015;5:1183–95. DOI:10.1016/j.stemcr.2015.10.018

[81] Petrof BJ. Molecular pathophysiology of myofiber injury in deficiencies of the dystrophin-glycoprotein complex. Am. J. Phys. Med. Rehabil. 2002;81:S162–74. DOI:10.1097/01.PHM.0000029775.54830.80

[82] van Westering TLE, Betts CA, Wood MJA. Current understanding of molecular pathology and treatment of cardiomyopathy in duchenne muscular dystrophy. Molecules. 2015;20:8823–55. DOI:10.3390/molecules20058823

[83] Hoffman EP, Reeves E, Damsker J, Nagaraju K, McCall JM, Connor EM, et al. Novel approaches to corticosteroid treatment in Duchenne muscular dystrophy. Phys. Med. Rehabil. Clin. N. Am. 2012;23:821–8. DOI:10.1016/j.pmr.2012.08.003

[84] Hunt SA. ACC/AHA 2005 Guideline update for the diagnosis and management of chronic heart failure in the adult: a report of the American College of Cardiology/ American Heart Association Task Force on Practice Guidelines (Writing Committee to Update the 2001 Guideli. Circulation. 2005;112:e154–235. DOI:10.1161/CIRCULATIO-NAHA.105.167586

[85] Geller G, Harrison KL, Rushton CH. Ethical challenges in the care of children and families affected by life-limiting neuromuscular diseases. J. Dev. Behav. Pediatr. 2012;33:548–61. DOI:10.1097/DBP.0b013e318267c62d

[86] Finder JD, Birnkrant D, Carl J, Farber HJ, Gozal D, Iannaccone ST, et al. Respiratory care of the patient with Duchenne muscular dystrophy. Am. J. Respir. Crit. Care. Med. 2004;170:456–65. DOI:10.1164/rccm.200307-885ST

[87] Vianello S, Yu H, Voisin V, Haddad H, He X, Foutz AS, et al. Arginine butyrate: A therapeutic candidate for Duchenne muscular dystrophy. FASEB J. 2013;27:2256–69. DOI:10.1096/fj.12-215723

[88] Mendell JR, Rodino-Klapac LR, Sahenk Z, Roush K, Bird L, Lowes LP, et al. Eteplirsen for the treatment of Duchenne muscular dystrophy. Ann. Neurol. 2013;74:637–47. DOI: 10.1002/ana.23982

[89] Bostick B, Yue Y, Lai Y, Long C, Li D, Duan D. Adeno-associated virus serotype-9 microdystrophin gene therapy ameliorates electrocardiographic abnormalities in mdx mice. Hum. Gene. Ther. 2008;19:851–6. DOI:10.1089/hum.2008.058.

Chapter 16

# Cardiomyopathies in Sub-Saharan Africa: Hypertensive Heart Disease (Cardiomyopathy), Peripartum Cardiomyopathy and HIV-Associated Cardiomyopathy

Okechukwu S. Ogah and Ayodele O. Falase

Additional information is available at the end of the chapter

http://dx.doi.org/10.5772/67023

**Abstract**

Cardiomyopathy is an important cause of cardiac-related morbidity and mortality in sub-Saharan Africa. Dilated cardiomyopathy is responsible for 20–30% of adult heart failure (HF) in the region. It is only second to hypertensive heart disease as etiological risk factor for HF in many parts of the continent. The aim of the chapter is to review the current epidemiology, clinical features, management, and prognosis of hypertensive heart disease, peripartum cardiomyopathy, and HIV-associated cardiomyopathy in sub-Saharan Africa.

**Keywords:** cardiomyopathy, heart muscle disease, hypertensive heart disease, peripartum cardiomyopathy, HIV-associated cardiomyopathy, heart failure

## 1. Introduction

Cardiomyopathies are common in Africa. Common causes of myocardial diseases in the region are hypertensive heart disease, endemic cardiomyopathies such as dilated cardiomyopathy, endomyocardial fibrosis, and peripartum cardiomyopathy and most recently heart diseases due to HIV/AIDS and ischemic cardiomyopathy. They are often associated with high morbidity and mortality due to late presentation, lack of modern day treatment available in high-income countries, as well poverty, which limits access to healthcare. **Figure 1** shows the common causes of heart failure (HF) in sub-Saharan Africa (SSA) based on a recent survey of acute HF in the region [1]. The chapter deals with hypertensive heart disease (hypertensive cardiomyopathy) peripartum cardiomyopathy and HIV-associated cardiomyopathy.

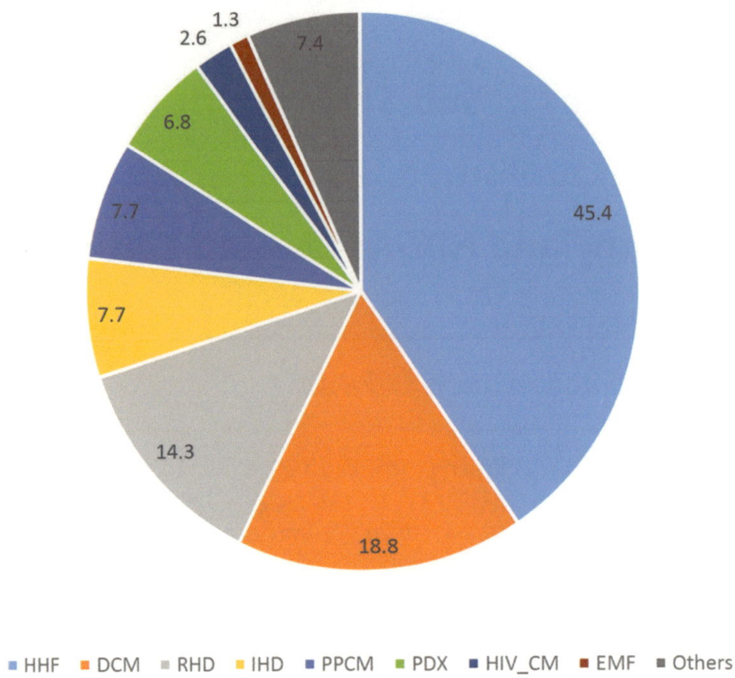


**Figure 1.** Etiological risk factors for heart failure in sub-Saharan Africa. (Adapted from Damasceno et al. HHF = Hypertensive heart failure, DCM = Dilated cardiomyopathy, RHD = Rheumatic heart disease, IHD = Ischemic heart disease, PPCM = Peripartum cardiomyopathy, PDX = Pericardial diseases, HIV_CM = HIV associated cardiomyopathy, EMF = Endomyocardial fibrosis.

## 2. Hypertensive heart disease (hypertensive cardiomyopathy)

### 2.1. Epidemiology

More than 30% of adults in SSA have hypertension. The prevalence rate is among the world highest. Worse still, the region has some of the world's lowest rates of hypertension awareness, treatment, and control. About 66% of the people are not aware, 82% are not treated and 93% are uncontrolled. In the year 2010, the age standardized prevalence of hypertension in adults aged 20-years and above was estimated as 36.9 and 36.3% for men and women, respectively (this is compared to 20.9 and 20.3%, 10 years earlier). This translates to 64.8 and 63.8 million men and women with elevated blood pressure in 2010 (compared to 25.5 and 24.9 million hypertensive men and women in the year 2000).

In a recent systematic analysis of population-based studies of hypertension in SSA, the pooled prevalence in the region rose from 19.7% in 1990 to 30.8% in 2010. It is estimated that there were about 54.6 million people with hypertension in Africa in 1990. This rose to 130.2 million cases in 2010. It is also projected that by the year 2030, there will be about 216.8 million cases of hypertension in the region [2].

Hypertension is the commonest and strongest risk factor for cardiovascular disease (CVD) in SSA [3]. It is also the commonest cause of disability and death from non-communicable diseases (NCDs) in the region [4]. The condition often manifests in young and middle aged adults in their productive years [4]. It is estimated to cause over 500,000 adult deaths annually and about 10-million years of life lost. Over 50% of heart disease and HF in the region is attributed to elevated blood pressure.

According to the African Union, hypertension is one of the greatest health challenges in adults in Africa after HIV/AIDS [4]. Recent data indicate that hypertension is rising in SSA at a faster rate compared to other regions of the world [5, 6]. This has been attributed to that adoption of western lifestyle, diet and culture, urbanization, urban migration from rural areas, ageing of the population, and increasing use of cigarettes and alcohol [3, 5–7].

It has been demonstrated that a chronic hyperadrenergic state is common among African hypertensives and may be responsible for the high prevalence of hypertension observed in Africans [8].

### 2.2. Clinical features

Heart disease secondary to elevated blood pressure (hypertensive heart disease), which may manifest in the following ways:

#### *2.2.1. LV diastolic dysfunction*

LV diastolic dysfunction is common in hypertensive subjects in the region [9–12]. About 62% of hypertensive individuals have various degrees of LV diastolic dysfunction compared to 12% of normal subjects [9, 13]. Diastolic dysfunction is worse in those with concentric LV geometry [9] as well as in individuals at risk of obstructive sleep apnea [14]. Diastolic dysfunction also occurs in offspring of hypertensive subjects [15–17].

#### *2.2.2. RV diastolic dysfunction*

Right ventricular systolic dysfunction has been reported in about 62% of a cohort of hypertensive patients [18, 19]. RV diastolic dysfunction may be an early clue to the development of hypertensive heart disease in Africans [19].

#### *2.2.3. Atrial function and dysfunction*

Absolute and indexed left atrial diameter, area, or volume is increased in African hypertensive subjects [20, 21]. Compared to their age- and sex-matched controls, hypertensive Africans show statistically significant left atrial structural and functional alterations [21].

### 2.3. Left ventricular hypertrophy

Electrocardiographic LVH occurs in 18–56% of hypertensive Africans depending on the criteria employed for the diagnosis. Sokolow-Lyon criteria appear to have the best sensitivity, while Estes score and Cornell criteria have the best specificity. Some workers in the region have proposed new criteria for ECG diagnosis of LVH in Africans especially in obese subjects [22–28]. ECG LVH with strain pattern is associated with worse LV structure and function in hypertensive Africans [29, 30].

The prevalence of echocardiographic LVH ranges from 30.9 to 74%. This, however, depends on the threshold used for the indexation of LV mass. Adebiyi et al. report 61–74% prevalence of abnormal LV geometry in hospital patients at the University College Hospital, Ibadan, Nigeria [31].

In a similar study in Northern Tanzania [32], 70% of the hypertensive subjects have abnormal LV geometry. The distribution of the abnormal LV geometric patterns is 19.8, 28.2, and 22% for concentric remodeling, concentric hypertrophy, and eccentric LVH, respectively. The best yield appears to be when LV mass is indexed to height raised to the power of 2.7 (allomeric growth rate of the heart). Age, systolic blood pressure, and duration of hypertension are independent predictors of LVH.

#### *2.3.1. LV systolic dysfunction*

LV systolic dysfunction (LVSD) occurs in 18.1% (9.6, 3.7, and 4.8% for mild, moderate, and severe LVSD, respectively) of hypertensive Africans [33]. The independent predictors of LVSD are LV mass, body mass index, and male gender. Ojji et al. [34] report LVSD in 6.7% (mild—3.5%, moderate—2.3%, and severe—0.9%) of 1943 hypertensive subjects and LV dysfunction is associated with older age, male sex, presence of diabetes mellitus, and some indices of the LV structure.

The Tei index (index of global myocardial performance) is significantly higher in hypertensive Africans compared to controls. The index increases with severity of LVSD. It is negatively related to the LVEF.

#### *2.3.2. RV systolic dysfunction*

RV systolic dysfunction occurs in about in 32% of hypertensive subjects seen in tertiary centers in the region [18, 35, 36]. RVSD is worse in subjects with eccentric LV geometry. LVEF appears to be the main determinant of RVSD. Recently, Ojji et al. [37] reported RVSD in 44.5% of 611 hypertensive subjects. RVSD estimated by TAPSE <15mm is associated with worse prognosis. LVEF and right atrial area are the main determinants of RVSD.

### 2.4. Hypertensive heart failure

Hypertensive HF (HHF) is a common and major form of presentation of HF in Africa. **Table 1** shows the contribution of hypertension in the etiology of HHF in SSA. In the Heart of Soweto study [38], 54% of hypertensive patients visit the hospital on account of this disorder. This devastating form of HHD is often associated with concurrent LVH, renal dysfunction, and anemia. In a study of 180 HHF patients in Ghana, the mean age of presentation is 63.6 years (range-24–88 years) and seen more often in women. The mean systolic blood pressure at presentation is 162.4 mmHg. Shortness of breath, easy fatigability, and palpitation are common symptoms while pulmonary edema and displaced apex beat are the common signs.

http://dx.doi.org/10.5772/67023

| S. No. | Author/Publication Year | Country | HHF (%) |
|---|---|---|---|
| 1 | Damasceno [1], 2012 | 9 countries | 45.4 |
| 2 | Stewart [41], 2008 | South Africa (Soweto) | 33.3 |
| 3 | Ojji [42], 2009 | Nigeria(Abuja) | 62.6 |
| 4 | Ojji [43], 2013 | Nigeria(Abuja) | 60.6 |
| 5 | Ogah [44], 2014 | Nigeria(Abeokuta) | 78.5 |
| 6 | Karaye [45], 2008 | Nigeria(Kano) | 57 |
| 7 | Laabes [46], 2008 | Nigeria(Jos) | 44.1 |
| 8 | Onwuchekwa [47], 2009 | Nigeria(Port-Harcourt) | 56.3 |
| 9 | Adewuya [48], 2006 | Nigeria(Ile-Ife) | 54 |
| 10 | Yonga [49], 2010 | Kenya | 64 |
| 11 | Kingue [50], 2005 | Cameroon (Urban) | 54.5 |
| 12 | Tantchou [51], 2011 | Cameroon (rural) | 15 |
| 13 | Soliman [52], 2008 | Malawi | 24 |
| 14 | Kuule [53], 2009 | Uganda | 24.2 |
| 15 | Okello [54], 2014 | Uganda | 9.1 |
| 17 | Owusu [55], 2013 | Ghana (Outpatients-Kumasi) | 45 |
| 18 | Owusu [56], 2006 | Ghana (In-patients-Kumasi) | 42.6 |
| 19 | Soliman [52], 2011 | Sudan | 28 |
| 20 | Habte [57], 2010 | Ethiopia | 24.2 |
| 21 | Makubi [58], 2014 | Tanzania | 45 |

**Table 1.** Summary of contribution of hypertension to HF in recent SSA studies.

Cardiomegaly on chest radiography is present in 75.6%. ECG-LVH or ECHO-LVH occur in 75.6 and 83.3%, respectively. About 62% have heart failure with preserved ejection fraction HFpEF [39].

In Nigeria, HHF is more common in men (56%). The mean age of presentation is 58.4 and 60.6 years in men and women, respectively. Over 80% present in NYHA class III and IV. HFpEF is present in about 35% of cases. The median length of hospital stay is about 9-days while 3.4% die while on admission. A 30-, 90-, and 180-day mortality rates of 0.9, 3.5, and 11.7%, respectively have been reported. Renal dysfunction appears to be the main independent predictor of mortality [40].

**Table 2** shows the characteristics of African patients with HHF compared with similar patients in other parts of the world.

### 2.5. Possible pathophysiologic mechanism of hypertensive heart disease in SSA

Hypertension is a common cause of pressure overload of the left ventricle. LVH develops as an adaptation to this overload. Hypertensive patient with ECG LVH has 10-fold higher risk

| Characteristics | Ogah et al. [40] ($n$ = 320) | Stewart et al. [41] ($n$ = 281) | Nieminen et al. [59] ($n$ = 200) | Spinar et al. [60] ($n$ = 179) | Venskutonyte et al. [61] ($n$ = 65) |
|---|---|---|---|---|---|
| Female (%) | 42.5 | 61 | 39.6 | 65.4 | 33.3 |
| Mean age (yrs) | 59.3 | 61 | 69.8 | 74.8 | 65.5 |
| Denovo HF (%) | 85.6 | NA | 37.3 | 74.3 | 66.7 |
| NYHA III+IV (%) | 82.2 | 29 | NA | 34.0 | NA |
| Previous history of hypertension (%) | 90.6 | 100 | 94.6 | 94.3 | 100 |
| Diabetes mellitus (%) | 12.2 | 14 | 34.5 | 43.1 | 33.3 |
| Previous MI or CAD (%) | 0.3 | 1.0 | 53.8 | 26.4 | 46.7 |
| COPD (%) | 2.5 | NA | 18.0 | 17.8 | 26.7 |
| Stroke or TIA in history (%) | 0.3 | 12 | 16.0 | 26.4 | 20 |
| Atrial fibrillation (%) | 12.8 | 9 | 37.7 | 19.0 | 46.7 |
| Mean systolic BP(mmHg) | 144 | 140 | NA | 198 | NA |
| Mean diastolic BP(mmHg) | 91 | 80 | NA | 100 | NA |
| Heart rate (beats/min) | 96 | NA | NA | 93 | NA |
| Body mass index (kg/m$^2$) | 24.2 | NA | NA | 28.0 | 33.9 |
| Hospitalization for HF within last 12 months (%) | 82.2 | NA | NA | 45.1 | 46.6 |
| Renal failure (%) | 14.4 | 27 | 18.7 | NA | NA |
| Anemia (%) | 11.5 | 10 | 11.3 | NA | NA |
| Infection (%) | 63.4 | NA | 15.6 | NA | 13.3 |
| Noncompliance with therapy (%) | 74.1 | NA | 21.9 | NA | 66.7 |
| ACE inhibitors (%) | 99.1 | NA | NA | 71.3 | NA |
| Beta-blockers (%) | 2.7 | NA | NA | 77.0 | NA |
| Calcium antagonists (%) | 30.6 | NA | NA | 51.1 | NA |
| Diuretics (%) | 86.9 | NA | NA | 88.5 | NA |
| Spironolactone (%) | 81.3 | NA | NA | 36.2 | NA |
| Digoxin (%) | 73.1 | NA | NS | 13.8 | NA |
| LVEDD (mm) | 55 | 46 | 56 | NA | 50* |
| Mean ejection fraction | 42.7 | 53 | 44 | 55 | 50.5 |
| LA (mm) | 47 | NA | 45 | NA | 42* |
| Mitral regurgitation (%) | 79.1 | 7 | 77.6 | NA | 100 |
| Tricuspid regurgitation (%) | 60.8 | 6 | 53.7 | NA | 93.3 |
| LOS days, median | 9 | NA | 8 | NA | 13 |
| Intrahospital mortality (%) | 3.4 | NA | 1.5 | 2.2 | 6.6 |

Abbreviation: HOS = Heart of Soweto Study, EHFS II = European Heart Failure Survey II, AHEAD = Acute Heart Failure Database, HF = Heart Failure, NYHA = New York Heart Association, MI = Myocardial Infarction, CAD = Coronary Artery Disease, COPD = Chronic Obstructive Pulmonary Disease, TIA = Transient Ischemic Attack, BP = Blood Pressure, LVEDD = Left Ventricular End-Diastolic Diameter, LA = Left Atrium, LOS = Length of Hospital Stay

**Table 2.** Comparison of our findings with similar studies in other parts of the world.

of developing HF [41]. There is increased wall thickness at the expense of chamber volume in LVH due to hypertrophy of the myocyte and by a parallel alignment of the sarcomere [42]. Specific hypertensive cardiomyopathy has been proposed. This cardiomyopathy has been divided into four stages: in stage 1, there is diastolic dysfunction, which is present in 20–30% of patients. This is common in elderly women, hypertensive diabetics, and ischemic heart disease patients [43]. LV diastolic dysfunction precedes systolic HF and is therefore a more common mechanism of HF in hypertension. Stage 2 is hypertension with impaired LV relaxation abnormalities, while grade 4 is dilated cardiomyopathy with LV systolic dysfunction. It has been shown that apoptosis may be responsible for the reduction of myocyte mass that accompanies progression from compensated hypertrophy to HF.

Several theories have been proposed to explain the relationship between LVH and HF. This includes changes in the coronary microcirculation, which leads to poor myocardial perfusion, impaired cardiac function, loss of contractile protein, and thus reduced cardiac contractility [44]. The second theory is increased LV pressure overload, which leads to ventricular dilatation and reduced cardiac output [45].

Finally, LVH in hypertension is governed by different loading conditions, which involve both hormonal and paracrine factors such as the sympathetic nervous system and renin-angiotensin-aldosterone axis [46].

## 3. Peripartum cardiomyopathy (PPCM)

### 3.1. Definition

Peripartum cardiomyopathy (PPCM) is a form of heart disease characterized by "the development of HF in the last month of pregnancy or within the first 5 months postpartum in the absence of any other determinable cause for cardiac failure and in the absence of demonstrable heart disease before the last month of pregnancy, and bears echocardiographic evidence of left ventricular systolic dysfunction" [62]. In addition, the diagnosis of the condition requires evidence of impaired LV systolic function by echocardiography (LVEF < 45% or LVFS < 30%). LV dilation is common although in some patients, LV dimension may be normal but the LV systolic function is impaired [62, 63].

### 3.2. Epidemiology

In terms of epidemiology, PPCM is common in developing and poor communities. The incidence is 1/1000 in most parts of low- and middle-income countries [64]. However, very high incidence has been reported from Northern Nigeria (1/100 live births) [65–69] and Haiti (1/300 live births) [70, 71]. The incidence in high-income countries is in the range of 1/3000–1/4000 deliveries [64]. There has been an increase in the awareness of the disease worldwide with the establishment of a global registry.

PPCM is responsible for about 1.5% cases of HF in the Heart of Soweto study [41], 1.3% in the Abeokuta HF registry [44] and 3.2% in the Abuja Heart Study [42]. It is still the most prevalent form of cardiomyopathy (54.6%) in Northern Nigeria [45].

### 3.3. Risk factors

Risk factors for the development of this cardiac disorder include low socioeconomic status, women of African descent (although PPCM is a global disease), young pregnant women, multiparity, multiple pregnancy, and longer period of breast feeding [64]. However, recent prospectively collected data on PPCM do not support strong association with older age of pregnancy, multiparity, twin pregnancy, gestational hypertension, and the use of tocolytic agents [72].

### 3.4. Clinical features

Shortness of breath is common form of presentation. Other common clinical features include, cardiomegaly, tachycardia, pulmonary rales, high blood pressure and dysrhythmias. Dyspnea, cough, orthopnea, palpitation, hemoptysis, chest pain, and abdominal pain are other common features. Most patients in SSA present in NYHA class III/IV [68, 72]. Thromboembolic complications are common in the form of pulmonary embolism and stroke from mural thrombus [73, 74].

There are some differences between PPCM and hypertensive heart failure of pregnancy (HHFP). Patients with HHFP are more likely to present in the last trimester, while PPCM patients are more likely to present within the first month of the postpartum period. Family history of hypertension and history of hypertension in previous pregnancy is commoner in HHFP. Twin pregnancy and presence of leg edema are more common in PPCM. Blood pressures are generally higher in HHFP and they are also more likely to have basal rales. Furthermore, functional murmurs (tricuspid and mitral regurgitation) occur more often in PPCM compared to HHFP [75].

### 3.5. Laboratory findings

Arrhythmias are also common. In severe cases, anemia and renal dysfunction may be present. The liver enzymes may be normal or mildly raised from hepatic congestion. Some authors in Benin republic, Mali and Nigeria have reported the association of PPCM with micronutrient deficiencies, e.g., selenium, ceruloplasmin [76–78]. LV function and mortality in PPCM patients with HIV infection and those without have been found not to differ significantly [79].

The 12-leads ECG often show sinus rhythm, ST-T changes are common, which resolves after the postpartum. Ventricular arrhythmia occurs in about 20% [80–83].

Echocardiography is the diagnostic procedure of choice. Useful for the evaluation of LV systolic function ($EF < 45\%$), and diastolic function as well as assessment for presence of intramural thrombus formation. The mean LV internal dimension in diastole is often about 6 cm; however, some patients have nondilated LV. Where available in SSA, magnetic resonance imaging helps in the detection of myocardial fibrosis with late enhancement imaging. It also helps in the assessment function, shape, size, as well as contents. Immunohistochemistry of biopsy specimen from patient with PPCM is not different from that of idiopathic DCM. Similar viral particles, e.g., coxsackie, encephalomyelocarditis, parvovirus B19, adenoviruses, herpes simplex virus, Ebstein-Burr virus, and cytomegalovirus DNA. Inflammatory markers such as tumor necrosis factor alpha (TNF-alpha) and C-reactive protein levels are raised in both conditions and cannot be used to differentiate one from the other. However, peculiar to PPCM are some immune activation processes, e.g., elevated levels of marker of apoptosis-FAS/APO 1. This has been shown to predict prognosis [84].

### 3.6. Recent advances in the pathophysiology

More recently, Sliwa and her colleagues have shown the role of cleavage of prolactin in the pathogenesis of PPCM. A 16-KDa fragment of prolactin may induce myocardial damage [85]. This has provided a new option of blocking prolactin secretion with bromocriptine in the treatment of PPCM.

### 3.7. Prognosis

Full recovery of LV function occurs in about half of PPCM patients [72]. About 25% recover by the end of 6 months and around 10–15% die within 6 months. Long-term prospective follow-up studies show that overall recovery occurs in about 25% of patients and this mostly occurs in the first 18–24 months of diagnosis [79].

In recent time, there has been an increased awareness of this condition, and it has been recognized in the guidelines of the American College of Cardiology and European Society of Cardiology. Large global or continental registries of PPCM exist and many centers in SSA are participating. The European society of Cardiology has recently released a position paper on the disorder [62].

## 4. HIV-associated cardiomyopathy

### 4.1. Prevalence

SSA contributes about 69 and 90% of the global adult and childhood HIV/AIDS burden. HIV-associated cardiomyopathy is therefore a significant contributor to CVD morbidity and mortality in the region [86, 87].

The true prevalence of HIV-associated cardiomyopathy is unknown. The prevalence of HIV-associated cardiomyopathy in the pre-HAART era was about 50%. The incidence of any cardiac abnormality in HIV-infected individuals was 55% over a 7-year period [88–90]. It was common in young persons with CD4 count of <100 cells/mm$^3$, lower socioeconomic class, longer duration of the infection, higher viral load, and advanced stage of the disease [89, 91]. In-hospital mortality was 15% [89].

Because of the availability of HAART, the prevalence has reduced by about 50% in high-income countries [92]. However, in low-income countries (where most of the countries in SSA belong to), the prevalence of the condition has increased by 32% due to poor and limited access to HAART as well the impact of malnutrition [93].

Echocardiographic studies have reported prevalence ranging from 5% (in Nigeria) to 57% in Burkina Faso [89, 91, 94]. Differences may be due to study design and lack of common definition of the disorder [95].

In the Heart of Soweto study, about 9.7% of the cohort were HIV infected, 54% of who were on HAART [41, 81]. They were younger, had lower blood pressure and body mass index, and higher heart rate compared to the general cohort. HIV associated HF was the commonest diagnosis. The mean LVEF was 46% and common in women who were also about 6-years younger than the men. HIV patients who had HF had lower CD4 count compared to those who did not have. They were also more likely to have right-heart failure and valve dysfunction [96].

About 2.6% of HF cases in the THESU-HF survey were due to HIV infection. They were younger by 10–15 years and were less often smokers, hypertensive, or diabetic. They had larger LV dimensions but had similar LVEF compared to the general cohort [1]. The findings from the Heart of Soweto and the THESUS-HF survey are similar to more recent observational studies in the region. The prevalence is in the range of 1–5% [67, 73, 74]. It is often diagnosed in the third decade of life and more often in women. Both systolic and diastolic HF are common (about 30%).

### 4.2. Pathophysiologic mechanism

The proposed mechanism in the pathogenesis of HIV-associated cardiomyopathy include the direct myocardial invasion by the HIV, post-viral autoimmunity, immune system dysregulation, adverse effect of the viral protein, endothelial dysfunction, transcriptional activation of cellular genes, and beta-adrenergic dysregulation. Others include HIV-immunosuppression-related myocarditis due to opportunistic infection with toxoplasmosis, cryptococcus, and mycobacteria. Myocardial dysfunction as a result of systemic effects of sepsis may also play a role. Some of the anti-retroviral medications may play a role in the pathogenesis. Nucleoside reverse transcriptase inhibitors cause mitochondrial damage by inhibiting mitochondrial DNA polymerase. Zalcitabine is thought to exhibit the greatest toxicity among this group [97]. Zidovudine causes cardiac and skeletal myopathy [98].

Malnutrition especially selenium deficiency is another possible mechanism. Selenium has an antioxidant property and protects against endothelial dysfunction. Its deficiency is associated with cardiac dysfunction. Due to soil composition and agricultural practices in the region, selenium deficiency is common and 285 of the SSA population are at risk of selenium deficiency. Selenium deficiency has been demonstrated in HIV patients [99]. Selenium supplementation has also been shown to improve cardiac function in some studies [100].

Heavy alcohol use and smoking have also been implicated especially in high-income countries [101]. This was not demonstrated in a Rwandan study [101].

The role of genetic factor has not been demonstrated in Africa. " The mitochondrial DNA T16189C polymorphism, with a homopolymeric C-tract of 10-12 cystosines—a putative genetic risk factor for idiopathic dilated cardiomyopathy in the African and British populations—was not associated with HIV-associated cardiomyopathy in a South-African case control study" [102].

http://dx.doi.org/10.5772/67023

## Author details

Okechukwu S. Ogah* and Ayodele O. Falase

*Address all correspondence to: osogah56156@gmail.com

Division of Cardiology, Department of Medicine, University College Hospital, Ibadan, Nigeria

## References

[1] Damasceno A, Mayosi BM, Sani M, Ogah OS, Mondo C, Ojji D, et al. The causes, treatment, and outcome of acute heart failure in 1006 Africans from 9 countries: results of the sub-Saharan Africa survey of heart failure. Archives of Internal Medicine. 2012;172 (18):1386–94.

[2] Adeloye D, Basquill C. Estimating the prevalence and awareness rates of hypertension in Africa: a systematic analysis. PLoS One. 2014;9(8):e104300.

[3] Organization WH. A global brief on hypertension: silent killer, global public health crisis. World. 2016.

[4] WHO RO for Africa. The health of the people: the African regional health report. World Health Organization. 2006.

[5] Lawes CM, Vander Hoorn S, Law MR, Elliott P, MacMahon S, Rodgers A. Blood pressure and the global burden of disease 2000. Part 1: estimates of blood pressure levels. Journal of Hypertension. 2006;24(3):413–22.

[6] Lawes CM, Vander Hoorn S, Law MR, Elliott P, MacMahon S, Rodgers A. Blood pressure and the global burden of disease 2000. Part II: estimates of attributable burden. Journal of Hypertension. 2006;24(3):423–30.

[7] Beaglehole R, Bonita R, Alleyne G, Horton R, Li L, Lincoln P, et al. UN high-level meeting on non-communicable diseases: addressing four questions. The Lancet. 2011;378(9789):449–55.

[8] Adebiyi AA, Akinosun OM, Nwafor CE, Falase AO. Plasma catecholamines in Nigerians with primary hypertension. Ethnicity & Disease. 2011;21(2):158–62.

[9] Adamu UG, Kolo PM, Katibi IA, Opadijo GO, Omotosho AB, Araoye MA. Relationship between left ventricular diastolic function and geometric patterns in Nigerians with newly diagnosed systemic hypertension. Cardiovascular Journal of Africa. 2009;20(3):173–7.

[10] Adebiyi AA, Aje A, Ogah OS, Ojji DB, Oladapo OO, Falase AO. Left ventricular diastolic function parameters in hypertensives. Journal of the National Medical Association. 2005;97(1):41–5.

[11] Akintunde AA, Familoni OB, Akinwusi PO, Opadijo OG. Relationship between left ventricular geometric pattern and systolic and diastolic function in treated Nigerian hypertensives. Cardiovascular Journal of Africa. 2010;21(1):21–5.

[12] Ike SO, Onwubere JC. For the patient. Poor diastolic function and blood pressure in Blacks. Ethnicity & Disease. 2003;13(4):547.

[13] Adebayo AK, Oladapo OO, Adebiyi AA, Ogunleye OO, Ogah OS, Ojji DB, et al. Characterisation of left ventricular function by tissue Doppler imaging technique in newly diagnosed, untreated hypertensive subjects. Cardiovascular Journal of Africa. 2008;19(5):259–63.

[14] Akintunde A, Kareem L, Bakare A, Audu M. Impact of obstructive sleep apnea and snoring on left ventricular mass and diastolic function in hypertensive Nigerians. Annals of Medical and Health Sciences Research. 2014;4(3):350–4.

[15] Adeoye AM, Adebiyi AA, Oladapo OO, Ogah OS, Aje A, Ojji DB, et al. Early diastolic functional abnormalities in normotensive offspring of Nigerian hypertensives. Cardiovascular Journal of Africa. 2012;23(5):255–9.

[16] Kolo P, Sanya E, Ogunmodede J, Omotoso A, Soladoye A. Normotensive offspring of hypertensive Nigerians have increased left ventricular mass and abnormal geometric patterns. The Pan African Medical Journal. 2012;11:6.

[17] Kolo PM, Sanya EO, Omotoso AB, Soladoye A, Ogunmodede JA. Left ventricular hypertrophy is associated with diastolic filling alterations in normotensive offspring of hypertensive Nigerians. ISRN Cardiology. 2012;2012:256738.

[18] Karaye KM, Habib AG, Mohammed S, Rabiu M, Shehu MN. Assessment of right ventricular systolic function using tricuspid annular-plane systolic excursion in Nigerians with systemic hypertension. Cardiovascular Journal of Africa. 2010;21(4):186–90.

[19] Akintunde AA, Akinwusi PO, Familoni OB, Opadijo OG. Effect of systemic hypertension on right ventricular morphology and function: an echocardiographic study. Cardiovascular Journal of Africa. 2010;21(5):252–6.

[20] Adebiyi AA, Aje A, Ogah OS, Ojji DB, Dada A, Oladapo OO, et al. Correlates of left atrial size in Nigerian hypertensives. Cardiovascular Journal of South Africa: Official Journal for Southern Africa Cardiac Society [and] South African Society of Cardiac Practitioners. 2004;16(3):158–61.

[21] Adebayo AK, Oladapo OO, Adebiyi AA, Ogunleye OO, Ogah OS, Ojji DB, et al. Changes in left atrial dimension and function and left ventricular geometry in newly diagnosed untreated hypertensive subjects. Journal of Cardiovascular Medicine. 2008;9(6):561–9.

[22] Jaggy C, Perret F, Bovet P, van Melle G, Zerkiebel N, Madeleine G, et al. Performance of classic electrocardiographic criteria for left ventricular hypertrophy in an African population. Hypertension. 2000;36(1):54–61.

[23] Huston SL, Bunker CH, Ukoli FA, Rautaharju PM, Kuller LH. Electrocardiographic left ventricular hypertrophy by five criteria among civil servants in Benin City, Nigeria: prevalence and correlates. International Journal of Cardiology. 1999;70(1):1–14.

[24] Lodha SM, Makene WJ. Electrocardiographic changes in systemic hypertension. (A study of Tanzanian Africans). East African Medical Journal. 1976;53(8):424–34.

[25] Maunganidze F, Woodiwiss AJ, Libhaber CD, Maseko MJ, Majane OH, Norton GR. Left ventricular hypertrophy detection from simple clinical measures combined with electrocardiographic criteria in a group of African ancestry. Clinical Research in Cardiology. 2014;103(11):921–9.

[26] Maunganidze F, Woodiwiss AJ, Libhaber CD, Maseko MJ, Majane OH, Norton GR. Obesity markedly attenuates the validity and performance of all electrocardiographic criteria for left ventricular hypertrophy detection in a group of black African ancestry. Journal of Hypertension. 2013;31(2):377–83.

[27] Sliwa K, Ojji D, Bachelier K, Bohm M, Damasceno A, Stewart S. Hypertension and hypertensive heart disease in African women. Clinical Research in Cardiology. 2014; 103(7):515–23.

[28] Robinson C, Woodiwiss AJ, Libhaber CD, Norton GR. Novel approach to the detection of left ventricular hypertrophy using body mass index–corrected electrocardiographic voltage criteria in a group of African ancestry. Clinical Cardiology. 2016;39(9):524–30.

[29] Ogah O, Oladapo O, Adebiyi A, Salako B, Falase A, Adebayo A, et al. Electrocardiographic left ventricular hypertrophy with strain pattern: prevalence, mechanisms and prognostic implications. Cardiovascular Journal of Africa. 2008;19(1):39.

[30] Ogah O, Adebiyi A, Oladapo O, Aje A, Ojji D, Adebayo A, et al. Association between electrocardiographic left ventricular hypertrophy with strain pattern and left ventricular structure and function. Cardiology. 2006;106(1):14–21.

[31] Adebiyi AA, Ogah OS, Aje A, Ojji DB, Adebayo AK, Oladapo OO, et al. Echocardiographic partition values and prevalence of left ventricular hypertrophy in hypertensive Nigerians. BMC Medical Imaging. 2006;6(1):1.

[32] Silangei LK, Maro VP, Diefenthal H, Kapanda G, Dewhurst M, Mwandolela H, et al. Assessment of left ventricular geometrical patterns and function among hypertensive patients at a tertiary hospital, Northern Tanzania. BMC Cardiovascular Disorders. 2012;12:109.

[33] Ogah OS, Akinyemi RO, Adegbite GD, Udofia OI, Udoh SB, Adesina JO, et al. Prevalence of asymptomatic left ventricular systolic dysfunction in hypertensive Nigerians: echocardiographic study of 832 subjects. Cardiovascular Journal of Africa. 2011;22(6):297–302.

[34] Ojji D, Atherton J, Sliwa K, Alfa J, Ngabea M, Opie L. Left ventricular systolic dysfunction in asymptomatic black hypertensive subjects. American Journal of Hypertension. 2015;28(7):924–9.

[35] Karaye KM. Relationship between Tei Index and left ventricular geometric patterns in a hypertensive population: a cross-sectional study. Cardiovascular Ultrasound. 2011;9:21.

[36] Karaye KM, Sai'du H, Shehu MN. Right ventricular dysfunction in a hypertensive population stratified by patterns of left ventricular geometry. Cardiovascular Journal of Africa. 2012;23(9):478–82.

[37] Ojji DB, Lecour S, Atherton JJ, Blauwet LA, Alfa J, Sliwa K. Right ventricular systolic dysfunction is common in hypertensive heart failure: a prospective study in sub-Saharan Africa. PLoS One. 2016;11(4):e0153479.

[38] Stewart S, Libhaber E, Carrington M, Damasceno A, Abbasi H, Hansen C, et al. The clinical consequences and challenges of hypertension in urban-dwelling black Africans: insights from the Heart of Soweto Study. International Journal of Cardiology. 2011;146(1):22–7.

[39] Owusu IK, Adu-Boakye Y, Tetteh LA. Hypertensive heart failure in Kumasi, Ghana. Open Science Journal of Clinical Medicine. 2014;2(1):39–43.

[40] Ogah OS, Sliwa K, Akinyemi JO, Falase AO, Stewart S. Hypertensive heart failure in Nigerian Africans: insights from the Abeokuta Heart Failure Registry. Journal of Clinical Hypertension. 2015;17(4):263–72.

[41] Stewart S, Wilkinson D, Hansen C, Vaghela V, Mvungi R, McMurray J, et al. Predominance of heart failure in the Heart of Soweto Study cohort: emerging challenges for urban African communities. Circulation. 2008;118(23):2360–7.

[42] Ojji DB, Alfa J, Ajayi SO, Mamven MH, Falase AO. Pattern of heart failure in Abuja, Nigeria: an echocardiographic study. Cardiovascular Journal of Africa. 2009;20(6):349–52.

[43] Ojji D, Stewart S, Ajayi S, Manmak M, Sliwa K. A predominance of hypertensive heart failure in the Abuja Heart Study cohort of urban Nigerians: a prospective clinical registry of 1515 de novo cases. European Journal of Heart Failure. 2013;15(8):835–42.

[44] Ogah OS, Stewart S, Falase AO, Akinyemi JO, Adegbite GD, Alabi AA, et al. Contemporary profile of acute heart failure in Southern Nigeria: data from the Abeokuta Heart Failure Clinical Registry. JACC Heart Failure. 2014;2(3):250–9.

[45] Karaye KM, Sani MU. Factors associated with poor prognosis among patients admitted with heart failure in a Nigerian tertiary medical centre: a cross-sectional study. BMC Cardiovascular Disorders. 2008;8:16.

[46] Laabes EP, Thacher TD, Okeahialam BN. Risk factors for heart failure in adult Nigerians. Acta Cardiologica. 2008;63(4):437–43.

[47] Onwuchekwa AC, Asekomeh GE. Pattern of heart failure in a Nigerian teaching hospital. Vascular Health Risk Management. 2009;5:745–50.

[48] Adewuya AO, Ola BA, Ajayi OE, Oyedeji AO, Balogun MO, Mosaku SK. Prevalence and correlates of major depressive disorder in Nigerian outpatients with heart failure. Psychosomatics. 2006;47(6):479–85.

[49] Prevalence, causes and risk factors for left ventricular dysfunction and heart failure in Kenya population [Internet]. 2009 [cited 14 Dec 2014]. Available from: http://spo.escardio.org/eslides/view.aspx?eevtid=40&fp=3567.

[50] Kingue S, Dzudie A, Menanga A, Akono M, Ouankou M, Muna W. [A new look at adult chronic heart failure in Africa in the age of the Doppler echocardiography: experience of the medicine department at Yaounde General Hospital]. In Annales de cardiologie et d'angeiologie 2005 Sep;54(5):276–283.

[51] Tantchou Tchoumi JC, Ambassa JC, Kingue S, Giamberti A, Cirri S, Frigiola A, et al. Occurrence, aetiology and challenges in the management of congestive heart failure in sub-Saharan Africa: experience of the Cardiac Centre in Shisong, Cameroon. The Pan African Medical Journal. 2011;8:11.

[52] Soliman EZ, Juma H. Cardiac disease patterns in northern Malawi: epidemiologic transition perspective. Journal of Epidemiology/Japan Epidemiological Association. 2008;18(5):204–8.

[53] Kuule JK, Seremba E, Freers J. Anaemia among patients with congestive cardiac failure in Uganda—its impact on treatment outcomes. South African Medical Journal = Suid-Afrikaanse tydskrif vir geneeskunde. 2009;99(12):876–80.

[54] Okello S, Rogers O, Byamugisha A, Rwebembera J, Buda AJ. Characteristics of acute heart failure hospitalizations in a general medical ward in Southwestern Uganda. International Journal of Cardiology. 2014;176(3):1233–4.

[55] Owusu IK, Boaky Y. Prevalence and aetiology of heart failure in patients seen at a Teaching Hospital in Ghana. Journal of Cardiovascular Diseases & Diagnosis. 2013;1:131.

[56] Owusu IK. Causes of heart failure as seen in Kumasi, Ghana. Internet J Third world med. 2007;5:201–14.

[57] Habte B, Alemseged F, Tesfaye D. The pattern of cardiac diseases at the cardiac clinic of Jimma University specialised hospital, South West Ethiopia. Ethiopian Journal of Health Sciences. 2010;20(2):99–105.

[58] Makubi A, Hage C, Lwakatare J, Kisenge P, Makani J, Ryden L, et al. Contemporary aetiology, clinical characteristics and prognosis of adults with heart failure observed in a tertiary hospital in Tanzania: the prospective Tanzania Heart Failure (TaHeF) study. Heart. 2014;100(16):1235–41.

[59] Nieminen MS, Brutsaert D, Dickstein K, Drexler H, Follath F, Harjola VP, et al. EuroHeart Failure Survey II (EHFS II): a survey on hospitalized acute heart failure patients: description of population. European Heart Journal. 2006;27(22):2725–36.

[60] Sato N, Kajimoto K, Asai K, Mizuno M, Minami Y, Nagashima M, et al. Acute decompensated heart failure syndromes (ATTEND) registry. A prospective observational multicenter cohort study: rationale, design, and preliminary data. American Heart Journal. 2010;159(6):949–55 e1.

[61] Venskutonyte L, Molyte I, Ablonskyte-Dudoniene R, Mizariene V, Kavoliuniene A. Characteristics and management of acute heart failure patients in a single university hospital center. Medicina. 2009;45(11):855–70.

[62] Sliwa K, Hilfiker-Kleiner D, Petrie MC, Mebazaa A, Pieske B, Buchmann E, Regitz-Zagrosek V, Schaufelberger M, Tavazzi L, Veldhuisen DJ, Watkins H. Current state of knowledge on aetiology, diagnosis, management, and therapy of peripartum cardiomyopathy: a position statement from the Heart Failure Association of the European Society of Cardiology Working Group on peripartum cardiomyopathy. European journal of heart failure. 2010 Aug 1;12(8):767–78.

[63] Pearson GD, Veille J-C, Rahimtoola S, Hsia J, Oakley CM, Hosenpud JD, et al. Peripartum cardiomyopathy: national heart, lung, and blood institute and office of rare diseases (national institutes of health) workshop recommendations and review. Journal of the American Medical Association. 2000;283(9):1183–8.

[64] SliwaK, FettJ, ElkayamU. Peripartum cardiomyopathy. The Lancet. 2006;368(9536):687–93.

[65] Ford L, Abdullahi A, Anjorin FI, Danbauchi SS, Isa MS, Maude GH, et al. The outcome of peripartum cardiac failure in Zaria, Nigeria. QJM. 1998;91(2):93–103.

[66] Abengowe CU. Cardiovascular disease in Northern Nigeria. Tropical & Geographical Medicine. 1979;31(4):553–60.

[67] Abengowe CU, Das CK, Siddique AK. Cardiac failure in pregnant Northern Nigerian women. International Journal of Gynaecology & Obstetrics: the Official Organ of the International Federation of Gynaecology and Obstetrics. 1980;17(5):467–70.

[68] Isezuo SA, Abubakar SA. Epidemiologic profile of peripartum cardiomyopathy in a tertiary care hospital. Ethnicity & Disease. 2007;17(2):228–33.

[69] Ladipo GO, Froude JR, Parry EH. Pattern of heart disease in adults of the NigerianwSavanna: a prospective clinical study. African Journal of Medicine and Medical Sciences. 1977;6(4):185–92.

[70] Fett JD. Peripartum cardiomyopathy. Insights from Haiti regarding a disease of unknown etiology. Minnesota Medicine. 2002;85(12):46–8.

[71] Fett JD, Carraway RD, Dowell DL, King ME, Pierre R. Peripartum cardiomyopathy in the Hospital Albert Schweitzer District of Haiti. American Journal of Obstetrics & Gynecology. 2002;186(5):1005–10.

[72] Blauwet LA, Libhaber E, Forster O, Tibazarwa K, Mebazaa A, Hilfiker-Kleiner D, et al. Predictors of outcome in 176 South African patients with peripartum cardiomyopathy. Heart. 2013;99(5):308–13.

[73] Isezuo SA, Njoku CH, Airede L, Yaqoob I, Musa AA, Bello O. Case report: acute limb ischaemia and gangrene associated with peripartum cardiomyopathy. Nigerian Postgraduate Medical Journal. 2005;12(3):237–40.

[74] Talle MA, Buba F, Anjorin CO. Prevalence and aetiology of left ventricular thrombus in patients undergoing transthoracic echocardiography at the University of Maiduguri Teaching Hospital. Advances in Medicine. 2014;2014:731936.

[75] Ntusi NB, Badri M, Gumedze F, Sliwa K, Mayosi BM. Pregnancy-associated heart failure: a comparison of clinical presentation and outcome between hypertensive heart failure of pregnancy and idiopathic peripartum cardiomyopathy. PLoS One. 2015;10(8):e0133466

[76] Cenac A, Simonoff M, Moretto P, Djibo A. A low plasma selenium is a risk factor for peripartum cardiomyopathy. A comparative study in Sahelian Africa. International Journal of Cardiology. 1992;36(1):57–9.

[77] Cenac A, Toure K, Diarra MB, Sergeant C, Jobic Y, Sanogo K, et al. Plasma selenium and peripartum cardiomyopathy in Bamako, Mali. Medecine Tropicale (Mars). 2004; 64(2):151–4.

[78] Cenac A, Sacca-Vehounkpe J, Poupon J, Dossou-Yovo-Akindes R, D'Almeida-Massougbodji M, Tchabi Y, et al. [Serum selenium and dilated cardiomyopathy in Cotonou, Benin]. Medecine Tropicale (Mars). 2009;69(3):272–4.

[79] Sliwa K, Forster O, Tibazarwa K, Libhaber E, Becker A, Yip A, et al. Long-term outcome of peripartum cardiomyopathy in a population with high seropositivity for human immunodeficiency virus. International Journal of Cardiology. 2011;147(2):202–8.

[80] Karaye KM, Lindmark K, Henein MY. Electrocardiographic predictors of peripartum cardiomyopathy. Cardiovascular Journal of Africa. 2015;27(2):66–70.

[81] Sliwa K, Wilkinson D, Hansen C, Ntyintyane L, Tibazarwa K, Becker A, et al. Spectrum of heart disease and risk factors in a black urban population in South Africa (the Heart of Soweto Study): a cohort study. The Lancet. 2008;371(9616):915–22.

[82] Karaye KM. Clinical characteristics and prognosis of Peripartum Cardiomyopathy. Print and Media, Umea University, 2016.

[83] Tibazarwa K, Mayosi B, Sliwa K, Carrington M, Stewart S, Lee G. The 12-lead ECG in peripartum cardiomyopathy. Cardiovascular Journal of Africa. 2012;23(6):322–9.

[84] Sliwa K, Forster O, Libhaber E, Fett JD, Sundstrom JB, Hilfiker-Kleiner D, et al. Peripartum cardiomyopathy: inflammatory markers as predictors of outcome in 100 prospectively studied patients. European Heart Journal. 2006;27(4):441–6.

[85] Hilfiker-Kleiner D, Sliwa K. Pathophysiology and epidemiology of peripartum cardiomyopathy. Nature Reviews Cardiology. 2014;11(6):364–70.

[86] WHO. Global update on HIV treatment 2013: results, impact and opportunities. 2013.

[87] HIV/AIDS JUNPo. Global AIDS response progress reporting 2013: construction of core indicators for monitoring the 2011 UN Political Declaration on HIV. AIDS. 2013.

[88] Hakim J, Matenga J, Siziya S. Myocardial dysfunction in human immunodeficiency virus infection: an echocardiographic study of 157 patients in hospital in Zimbabwe. Heart. 1996;76(2):161–5.

[89] Niakara A, Drabo Y, Kambire Y, Nebie L, Kabore N, Simon F. [Cardiovascular diseases and HIV infection: study of 79 cases at the National Hospital of Ouagadougou (Burkina Faso)]. Bulletin de la Societe de Pathologie Exotique (1990). 2002;95(1):23–6.

[90] Longo-Mbenza B, Seghers K, Phuati M, Bikangi FN, Mubagwa K. Heart involvement and HIV infection in African patients: determinants of survival. International Journal of Cardiology. 1998;64(1):63–73.

[91] Twagirumukiza M, Nkeramihigo E, Seminega B, Gasakure E, Boccara F, Barbaro G. Prevalence of dilated cardiomyopathy in HIV-infected African patients not receiving HAART: a multicenter, observational, prospective, cohort study in Rwanda. Current HIV Research. 2007;5(1):129–37.

[92] Patel K, Van Dyke RB, Mittleman MA, Colan SD, Oleske JM, Seage III GR. The impact of HAART on cardiomyopathy among children and adolescents perinatally infected with HIV-1. AIDS (London, England). 2012;26(16):2027.

[93] Barbaro G. WJC. World. 2010;2(3):53–7.

[94] Olusegun-Joseph DA, Ajuluchukwu JN, Okany CC, Mbakwem AC, Oke DA, Okubadejo NU. Echocardiographic patterns in treatment-naive HIV-positive patients in Lagos, south-west Nigeria. Cardiovascular Journal of Africa. 2012;23(8):e1–6.

[95] Ntsekhe M, Mayosi BM. Cardiac manifestations of HIV infection: an African perspective. Nature Clinical Practice Cardiovascular Medicine. 2009;6(2):120–7.

[96] Sliwa K, Carrington MJ, Becker A, Thienemann F, Ntsekhe M, Stewart S. Contribution of the human immunodeficiency virus/acquired immunodeficiency syndrome epidemic to de novo presentations of heart disease in the Heart of Soweto Study cohort. European Heart Journal. 2012;33(7):866–74.

[97] Currie PF, Jacob AJ, Foreman AR, Elton RA, Brettle RP, Boon NA. Heart muscle disease related to HIV infection: prognostic implications. BMJ. 1994;309(6969):1605–7.

[98] Nzuobontane D, Blackett K, Kuaban C. Cardiac involvement in HIV infected people in Yaounde, Cameroon. Postgraduate Medical Journal. 2002;78(925):678–81.

[99] Look M, Rockstroh J, Rao G, Kreuzer K, Barton S, Lemoch H, et al. Serum selenium, plasma glutathione (GSH) and erythrocyte glutathione peroxidase (GSH-Px)-levels in asymptomatic versus symptomatic human immunodeficiency virus-1 (HIV-1)-infection. European Journal of Clinical Nutrition. 1997;51(4):266–72.

[100] Kavanaugh-Mchugh AL, Ruff A, Perlman E, Hutton N, Modlin J, Rowe S. Selenium deficiency and cardiomyopathy in acquired immunodeficiency syndrome. Journal of Parenteral and Enteral Nutrition. 1991;15(3):347–9.

[101] Mondy KE, Gottdiener J, Overton ET, Henry K, Bush T, Conley L, et al. High prevalence of echocardiographic abnormalities among HIV-infected persons in the era of highly active antiretroviral therapy. Clinical Infectious Diseases. 2011;52(3):378–86.

[102] Hsue PY, Deeks SG, Hunt PW. Immunologic basis of cardiovascular disease in HIVinfected adults. Journal of Infectious Diseases. 2012;205(suppl 3):S375–82.

Chapter 17

# Cardiomyopathies in Animals

Kazumasu Sasaki, Tatsushi Mutoh, Kinji Shirota and
Ryuta Kawashima

Additional information is available at the end of the chapter

http://dx.doi.org/10.5772/65060

**Abstract**

A wide variety of animal models in cardiomyopathy have been established for the discovery of pathophysiological mechanisms, diagnosis, and treatment of human myocardial disease. Experimentally, several species including rodents, rabbit, canine, pig, and sheep have been involved in the fundamental research in medical field. However, knowledge about naturally occurring myocardial disease in animals is limited in the veterinary medicine. Among small and large animals that develop myocardial disease, to the best of authors' knowledge, naturally occurring cardiomyopathy in canine and feline is commonly encountered in veterinary clinical setting. Their pathophysiology is not fully described; specific pathophysiology is documented in both species, which resembles those of humans. These conditions are hypertrophic cardiomyopathy (HCM) in feline and dilated cardiomyopathy (DCM) in canine. Each has distinct etiology and pathophysiology. In order to translate new findings from naturally occurring cardiomyopathies in small and large animals into medical applications, knowledge gained through animals with cardiomyopathies becomes a necessary approach. The purpose of this chapter is to introduce the overview of findings on small and large animals with naturally occurring cardiomyopathies already investigated.

**Keywords:** animal model, canine dilated cardiomyopathy, feline hypertrophic cardiomyopathy, naturally occurring cardiomyopathies

## 1. Introduction

Several animal models in cardiomyopathy have been established for the discovery of pathophysiological mechanisms, diagnosis, and treatment of human myocardial disease. Experimentally, rodents, rabbit, canine, pig, sheep, and other species have been involved in the fundamental research in medical field [1–7]. Although anatomic and biochemical differences between species are critical, each experimentally induced animal model plays an important role for translation to clinical practice in human. In addition to experimentally induced animal models, naturally occurring cardiomyopathies in small and large animals offer an excellent opportunity to evaluate novel therapies for those of human. However, knowledge about naturally occurring myocardial disease in animals is limited in the veterinary medicine. Among animals that develop myocardial disease, to the best of authors' knowledge, cardiomyopathy in canine and feline is commonly encountered in veterinary clinical setting [8–12]. Their pathophysiology is not always clearly described yet; however, specific features are documented in both canine and feline. Briefly, naturally occurring myocardial disease is one of the most common heart diseases in canine and feline. A number of remarkable similarities have been reported between these animals and humans [13, 14]. Several causes concerning genetic, metabolic, inflammatory, nutritional, infectious, and drug-induced myocardial disease have been reported as canine and feline idiopathic or secondary myocardial disease [15, 16]. Generally speaking, treatment strategy of these naturally occurring diseases in veterinary clinical setting is based on those of humans. Therefore, this chapter provides pathophysiological aspects of these diseases.

Dilated cardiomyopathy (DCM) was first reported in 1970, as congestive heart failure (CHF). It is characterized by chamber dilation and myocardial systolic and diastolic dysfunction. DCM appears to be common in canine, which has been suspected to be inherited defects and mainly affects the certain large- to giant-sized pure-bred such as English Cocker Spaniels, Doberman Pinschers, Irish Wolfhounds, Newfoundlands, Boxers, German Short-haired Pointers, Portuguese Water Dog, Airedale Terriers, St. Bernards, Standard Poodles, Scottish Deerhounds, Afghan Hounds, and other breeds [8, 15–17]. Myocardial dysfunction results from ischemia, tachycardia, and trauma in canine myocardial disease. An underlying disease associated with neoplasia, renal disease, immune-mediated hemolytic anemia, acute pancreatitis, disseminated intravascular coagulopathy (DIC), myocardial infarction, mitral insufficiency, and other disease results in ischemic myocardial disease. Atrioventricular nodal-reciprocating tachycardias can lead to the tachycardia-induced cardiomyopathy in several breeds. However, hypertrophic cardiomyopathy (HCM) occurs less often in canine [15–17].

On the other hand, HCM is being the most commonly diagnosed cardiomyopathy in feline [10, 18, 19]. It is prevalent in certain populations. The disease is known to be inherited in some breeds, most notably The Domestic Shorthair, Turkish Van, Maine Coon, Persian, Ragdoll, Sphynx, Scottish Fold Cats, Chartreux, British Shorthair, Norwegian Forest Cat, Persian, and other breeds [14–16, 18]. The pathogenic mechanisms responsible for the development of HCM remain unclear; however, causal genetic mutations in genes encoding the sarcomere protein myosin-binding protein C (MYBPC3) have been identified in specific breeds such as Maine Coons and Ragdolls [14, 19–21].

Limited information exists on naturally occurring cardiomyopathies in large animals such as swine, cattle, and other species. Generally, these large animals are classified as farm animals and treated under group control. Compared with small animal veterinary practice, which mainly treats canine and feline, large animals are not potentially therapeutic objectives. From this circumstance, few opportunities exist for veterinarian to treat the disease. Even though numerous anatomic and biochemical differences exist, naturally occurring disease in large animal species can provide significant advantages for understanding those human conditions.

## 2. Canine DCM

### 2.1. Etiology and pathogenesis

The canine DCM can be divided into two categories: idiopathic and secondary (**Table 1**). The exact underlying molecular and biochemical mechanisms for canine DCM are generally not established in all cases. However, the etiology concerning genetic, nutritional, infectious, metabolic, inflammatory, drug- or toxin-induced myocardial hypokinesis have been proposed in canine DCM [17]. In idiopathic cases, genetic basis is thought to exist especially in certain breeds with high prevalence or familial occurrence of disease [15–17]. Large and giant breeds such as Great Danes, Scottish Deerhounds, Boxers, St. Bernards, Newfoundlands, Dalmatians, Doberman Pinschers, Irish Wolfhounds, and other breeds have been documented [8, 15, 16]. Newfoundlands, Irish Wolfhounds, Boxers, and Doberman Pinschers appear to have an autosomal dominant mode of transmission pattern of inheritance [8, 22, 23]. An autosomal recessive transmission has been documented in the inherited form of DCM in juvenile Portuguese Water Dogs [24, 25]. The disease is rapidly progressive and fatal in puppies. In some German Short-haired Pointer littermates, DCM appears to be an X-linked disorder caused by mutations in the Duchenne muscular dystrophy (DMD) gene [8, 26]. This gene codes for dystrophin, which is thought to strengthen muscle fiber membranes.

Myocardial function can impair result from a variety of causes including infections, inflammation, nutritional deficiencies, metabolic abnormalities, certain drugs, and other factors. These factors can lead to canine secondary myocardial disease. The antineoplastic drug doxorubicin and ethyl alcohol can cause severe myocardial damage and death. Plant toxins (e.g., *Taxus*, foxglove, black locust, buttercup, gossypol), cocaine, cobalt, catecholamines, and anesthetic drug can also affect the myocardial function [8, 15–17]. Carnitine and taurine deficiencies have been described in canine DCM [8]. L-Carnitine deficiency is not a primary cause of canine DCM; however, in Boxers, Doberman Pinschers, American Cocker Spaniels, Irish Wolfhounds, Newfoundlands, and Great Danes, low myocardial L-carnitine concentration has been reported [15]. L-Carnitine is an essential component of the long-chain fatty acids, which is an important energy-producing substrate of the myocardium. Taurine is known to regulate calcium influx across membranes in heart muscle. However, most cases with canine DCM are not taurine deficient; a reversible canine DCM associated with low plasma taurine concentration was reported in Cocker Spaniels [27]. Low plasma taurine level has also been described in Golden Retrievers, Labrador Retrievers, St. Bernards, Dalmatians, and other breeds with DCM.

| Etiology/pathogenesis | Breed | References |
|---|---|---|
| **Idiopathic DCM** | | |
| *Genetic disorder* | | |
| Dystrophin | German Short-haired Pointers | Schatzberg et al. [47] |
| Desmin | Doberman Pinschers | Stabej et al. [48] |
| Titin-cup | Irish Wolfhounds | Philipp et al. [49] |
| α-actinin | Doberman Pinschers | O'Sullivan et al. [50] |
| Striatin | Boxers | Cattanach et al. [51] |
| **Secondary DCM** | | |
| *Nutritional disorder* | | |
| L-Carnitine | Doberman Pinschers, Boxers | Keene et al. [52] |
| | American Cocker Spaniels | Kittleson et al. [53] |
| *Metabolic disorder* | | |
| Thyroid hormone | Great Dane | Phillips and Harkin [54] |
| | Alaskan Malamute | Flood and Hoover [55] |
| | Doberman Pinschers | Beier et al. [56] |
| *Immunological disorder* | | |
| Anti-mitochondrial antibodies | English Cocker Spaniel | Day [57] |
| Canine adenovirus type 1 | Crossed breed | Maxson et al. [58] |

**Table 1.** Possible factors of naturally occurring canine DCM.

### 2.2. Pathophysiology

Dilation of all cardiac chambers is typical in canine DCM [8, 15, 16, 28]. Decreased ventricular contractility is the major functional defect. Compensatory mechanisms become activated as progressive cardiac chamber dilation and remodeling develop as cardiac output worsens. Development of higher end-diastolic pressure, venous congestion, and congestive heart failure occurs in response to increased diastolic stiffness. Valve insufficiency also occurs because of cardiac enlargement and papillary muscle dysfunction. Arterial fibrillation (AF) is typical in canine DCM [15].

### 2.3. Histologic description

Gross anatomically, canine idiopathic DCM reveals marked dilation of all four cardiac chambers and/or predominantly dilation of the left chambers [8, 29–31]. Generally, myocardial hypertrophy is evident in the lesion. Distinct two histological forms of canine DCM have been reported: the fatty infiltration-degenerative type observed in specific breeds such as Boxers and Doberman Pinschers, and the attenuated wavy fiber type reported in medium-, large-, and giant-sized breed (**Table 2**). Histological forms such as vacuolar degeneration of myofib-

http://dx.doi.org/10.5772/65060

ers, atrophic myofibers, lipid deposits, and fatty infiltration replacing myofibers are evident for the fatty infiltration-degenerative type. On the other hand, the attenuated wavy fiber type seems to be a major histological form of canine DCM. The myofibers are stretched and thinner than normal with wavy appearance. The morphological alterations including myofiber atrophy, impairing wavy appearance to the fibers, and diffuse infiltration of subendocardial fibrosis were reported [8]. These lesions were most abundant in the lateral wall of the left ventricle (LV) [32, 33].

| References | Breed |
|---|---|
| **Fatty infiltration-degenerative type** | |
| Calvert et al. [59] | Doberman Pinschers |
| Harpster et al. [34] | Boxers |
| Hazlet et al. [60] | Doberman Pinschers |
| Tidholm and Jünsson [61] | Newfoundland |
| Calvert et al. [62] | Doberman Pinschers |
| Dambach et al. [25] | Portuguese Water Dogs |
| Everett et al. [63] | Doberman Pinschers |
| Vollmar et al. [64] | Doberman Pinschers |
| Lobo et al. [65] | Estrela Mountain Dogs |
| **Attenuated wavy fiber type** | |
| Tilley and Liu [66] | Great Dane, Doberman Pinschers, Irish Wolfhound |
| Sandusky et al. [67] | Afghan Hound, Doberman Pinschers, Great Dane |
| Tidholm et al. [33] | Large- and medium-size breeds |
| Dambach et al. [25] | Portuguese Water Dogs |
| Tidholm et al. [32] | Newfoundlands |
| Alroy et al. [68] | Portuguese Water Dogs |
| Vollmar et al. [69] | Doberman Pinschers |
| Sleeper et al. [24] | Portuguese Water Dogs |

**Table 2.** Two distinct histological forms of canine idiopathic DCM.

### 2.4. Survival and prognosis

Prognosis in canine DCM varies from weeks to several years. Sudden death may occur before the development of disease. Survival rate of Doberman Pinschers with fatty infiltration-degenerative type of DCM is shorter than attenuated wavy fiber type of those with DCM [8].

## 3. Cardiomyopathy in Boxers

Inherited cardiomyopathy in Boxers has similar features to arrhythmogenic right ventricular cardiomyopathy (ARVC) [15, 23]. Three forms were originally described by Harpster in 1983 including the cases with asymptomatic arrhythmias, ventricular tachyarrhythmias, cardiac arrhythmias, and congestive heart failure [34]. The disease appears to have an autosomal dominant inherited pattern. The Boxers with cardiac arrhythmias and congestive heart failure is considered to be a form of canine DCM, which is characterized by left and right ventricular myocardial systolic dysfunction [15, 23]. Histologic form of the disease includes myofibers atrophy, fibrosis, and fatty infiltration in the right ventricular wall. Deletion in the desmosomal striatin gene is associated with the disease developed in Boxer with ARVC [23]. The prognosis is varied in the forms of disease but survival is less than 6 months in case of CHF. Sudden death is common in asymptomatic cases.

## 4. Feline HCM

### 4.1. Etiology and pathogenesis

Recent report suggested that feline cardiomyopathy may be classified as HCM, hypertrophic obstructive cardiomyopathy (HOCM), restrictive cardiomyopathy (RCM), dilated cardiomyopathy, arrhythmogenic right ventricular cardiomyopathy, and unclassified cardiomyopathy (UCM) based on echocardiography and other factors [12]. However, diagnosis is quite challenging because of complexity of the disease. Feline idiopathic HCM is the most commonly diagnosed heterogeneous disease, which is transmitted in autosomal dominant trait in some specific breeds [15]. The disease is more frequent in male than in female. Genetic mutations in gene encoding in sarcomere protein myosin-binding protein C (MYBPC3) is associated with the development of disease in Manine Coon Cats (A31P mutation) and Ragdoll Cats (R820W mutation) [18]. Other breeds including Domestic Short Hair, Norwegian Forest Cats, Sphinx, Bengals, Chartreux, British Shorthairs, European, Scottish Folds, Cornish Rex, and Persian breeds are also high in disease prevalence but causative mutations associated with disease have yet to be documented [11, 15, 16]. In addition to specific gene mutation, feline myocardial hypertrophy results from possible causes such as an excessive production of catecholamines, myocardial ischemia, fibrosis, primary collagen abnormality, and abnormalities in myocardial calcium-handling process [15].

### 4.2. Pathophysiology

The disease is characterized by papillary muscle and LV hypertrophy, systolic anterior motion (SAM) of the mitral valve, diastolic dysfunction, end-systolic cavity obliteration, and enlargement of the left atrium [14, 35]. Abnormal sarcomere function results from myocyte hypertrophy and increased collagen synthesis. Asymmetric or symmetric LV free-wall concentric hypertrophy with interventricular septum is the characteristic form of the disease [36]. Some have limited abnormality in the basal septum and/or papillary muscles. These different patterns of hypertrophy may be caused by different phenotypic expression between different breeds.

Myocardial hypertrophy and reduced ventricular distensibility result in increased diastolic pressure and LV filling accompanying increased left arterial (LA) and pulmonary venous pressure. Secondary right-sided congenital heart failure (CHF) may occur in response to prolonged pulmonary vasoconstriction and increased pulmonary arterial pressure. LV outflow obstruction accompanying ejection murmur results from LV papillary muscle hypertrophy. Several factors contribute to myocardial ischemia, which leads to fibrosis, arrhythmias, and other complications. CHF, arterial thromboembolism (ATE), and sudden cardiac death are common clinical manifestation in end-stage feline HCM [15].

### 4.3. Histologic description

Gross anatomy is characterized by moderate to severe papillary muscle and LV concentric hypertrophy (**Figure 1**). Histologic findings based on hematoxylin and eosin (HE) staining and other specific markers revealed several abnormalities including multifocal myocardial interstitial fibrosis, myofiber disarray, diffuse myocyte hypertrophy with or without scattered individual cell necrosis, and arteriosclerosis in papillary muscles in the LV wall, interventricular septum, and intramural coronary artery [10, 37]. Recent evidence showed remodeling of the myofibrils and interfibrillar mitochondria, sarcolemmal remodeling with depletion of the subsarcolemmal mitochondria, changes of Z-disc morphology, myofibrillar degeneration, and endomysial fibrosis based on electron microscopic examination [10].

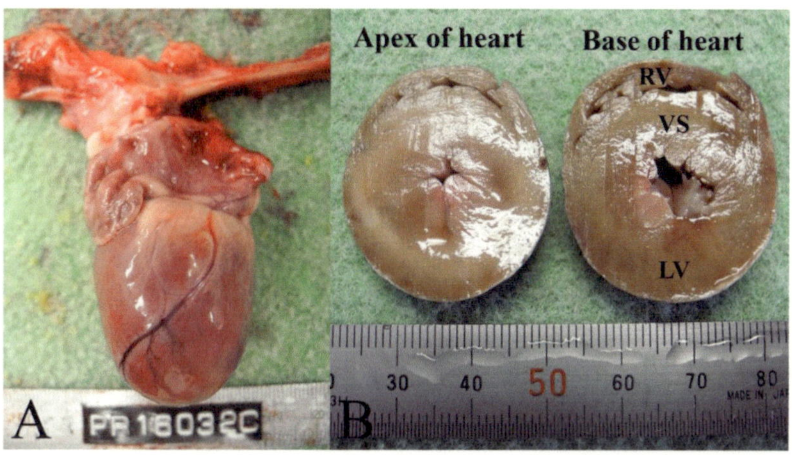


**Figure 1.** Gross morphologic features of heart from feline with HCM. (A) Overview of the heart from feline HCM. (B) Hypertrophy of ventricular septum (VS) in relation to left ventricular (LV) free wall. RV = right ventricle. Images courtesy of Prof. Kinji Shirota.

### 4.4. Survival and prognosis

Some prognostic factors such as heart rate and LA size are associated with survival time [12]. The prognosis is worse in case with ATE and/or CHF. Restrictive cardiomyopathy may be a consequence of the end stage of myocardial failure and infarction caused by HCM. Several factors cause a secondary RCM including tumor and infectious disease that were documented [15]. The prognosis is poor for feline with RCM accompanied by heart failure.

## 5. Other species

### 5.1. Swine

Experimentally induced porcine model of cardiomyopathy is widely used for medical applications [2, 38]. On the other hand, we have limited knowledge about naturally occurring swine cardiomyopathies. To date, naturally occurring porcine HCM and DCM have been described [39–41]. In addition to experimentally induced animal models, characteristics of naturally occurring affected pigs would be useful for translational research.

Several findings from swine HCM resemble those of humans with HCM. Higher incidence of specific breeds such as Landrace, Yorkshire, and Duroc were reported [39]. Pathological findings including increased number of mitochondria contained in the LV, increased amount of collagen matrix and abnormality in intramural coronary arteries, alternation of endogenous antioxidant enzymes, and decreased $Ca^{2+}$-ATPase activity in the LV are identical to those found in humans [39]. Histological abnormalities in swine HCM including abnormal intramural coronary arteries, subendocardial fibrosis in the ventricular septum, myocardial fibrosis, abnormalities in matrix connective tissue in myocardium, increased perimysial coil, and weave fibers of matrix connective tissue space between myocytes were documented [41, 42].

Recently, the case of spontaneous DCM was recognized in Yorkshire-Landrace crossbred [40]. The postmortem investigation after sudden death of this case revealed marked dilated ventricles and thinned ventricular walls and interventricular septum. Characteristics of gross anatomy and histological findings including multifocal myofiber attenuation and loss of myofiber cross striations supported the diagnosis of swine DCM. Cardiac lesions observed in the reported case were consistent with DCM as recognized in other species.

### 5.2. Cattle

Few reports on cardiomyopathies in cattle were descried [43, 44]. Hereditary cardiomyopathy in cattle has been described in some breeds including Japanese Black Calves, Holstein-Friesian-Cattle, Simmental/Red and White Holstein crossbreds, and Polled Hereford Calves [44, 45]. Recently, evidence suggested that specific breeds appear to have an autosomal dominant mode of transmission pattern of inheritance [45]. However, limited information exists about pathophysiological features compared with those of canine and feline. Affected cattle had multifocal myocardial degeneration and necrosis under histological investigation [46].

## 6. Conclusion

Naturally occurring inherited canine DCM and feline HCM are well-recognized myocardial disease in veterinary clinical setting. Although anatomic and biochemical differences between species are critical, reported findings resemble those of human disease condition. Little is known about naturally occurring cardiomyopathies in large animals but evidence suggested that they also develop spontaneous myocardial disease, which resembles those of other species

http://dx.doi.org/10.5772/65060

including human. Given the similarities of cardiomyopathies in both human and other species, the knowledge of naturally occurring myocardial disease in small and large animals may help expand the understanding of disease pathophysiology.

## Acknowledgements

The authors gratefully acknowledge the financial support: Sendai Animal Care and Research Center Foundation of Japan.

## Author details

Kazumasu Sasaki[1,2*], Tatsushi Mutoh[3,4], Kinji Shirota[5] and Ryuta Kawashima[6]

*Address all correspondence to: kazumasu.sasaki.d8@tohoku.ac.jp

1 Department of Functional Brain Imaging and Preclinical Evaluation, Institute of Development, Aging and Cancer, Tohoku University, Sendai, Japan

2 Sendai Animal Care and Research Center, Sendai, Japan

3 Department of Nuclear Medicine and Radiology, Institute of Development, Aging and Cancer, Tohoku University, Sendai, Japan

4 Department of Surgical Neurology, Research Institute for Brain and Blood Vessels-AKITA, Akita, Japan

5 Department of Veterinary Pathology, School of Veterinary Medicine, Azabu University, Kanagawa, Japan

6 Department of Functional Brain Imaging, Institute of Development, Aging and Cancer, Tohoku University, Sendai, Japan

## References

[1] Sirasaka T, Miyagawa S, Fukushima S, et al. Skeletal myoblast cell sheet implantation ameliorates both systolic and diastolic cardiac performance in canine dilated cardiomyopathy model. *Transplantation*. 2016;100:295–302.

[2] Lacroix D, Gluais P, Marquié C, et al. Repolarization abnormalities and their arrhythmogenic consequences in porcine tachycardia-induced cardiomyopathy. *Cardiovasc Res.* 2002;54:42–50.

[3] Mittal A, Sharma R, Prasad R, et al. Role of cardiac TBX20 in dilated cardiomyopathy. *Mol Cell Biochem.* 2016;414:129–36.

[4] Wilder T, Ryba DM, Wieczorek DF, et al. N-acetylcysteine *reverses* diastolic dysfunction and hypertrophy in familial hypertrophic cardiomyopathy. *Am J Physiol Heart Circ Physiol.* 2015;309:1720–1730.

[5] Frey N, Franz WM, Gloeckner K, et al. Transgenic rat hearts expressing a human cardiac troponin T deletion reveal diastolic dysfunction and ventricular arrhythmias. *Cardiovascular Res.* 2000;47:254–264.

[6] Sanbe A, James J, Tuzcu V, et al. Transgenic rabbit model for human troponin I-based hypertrophic cardiomyopathy. *Circulation.* 2005;111:2330–2338.

[7] Geens JH, Trenson S, Rega FR, et al. Ovine models for chronic heart failure. *Int J Artif Organs.* 2009;32:496–506.

[8] Tidholm A, Jünsson L. Histologic characterization of canine dilated cardiomyopathy *Vet Pathol.* 2005;42:1–8.

[9] Martin MW, Stafford Johnson MJ, Strehlau G, et al. Canine *dilated* cardiomyopathy: a retrospective study of prognostic findings in 367 clinical cases. *J Small Anim Pract.* 2010;51:428–436.

[10] Christiansen LB, Prats C, Hyttel P, Koch J. Ultrastructural myocardial changes in seven cats with spontaneous hypertrophic cardiomyopathy. *J Vet Cardiol.* 2015;17: 220–232.

[11] Maron BJ, Fox PR. Hypertrophic cardiomyopathy in man and cats. *J Vet Cardiol.* 2015;17:6–9.

[12] Ferasin L. Feline myocardial disease 2: *diagnosis*, prognosis and clinical management. *J Feline Med Surg.* 2009;11:183–194.

[13] Simpson S, Edwards J, Ferguson-Mignan TF, et al. Genetics of human and canine dilated cardiomyopathy. *Int J Genomics.* 2015;2015:204823.

[14] Kitteleson MD, Meurs KM, Harris SP. The genetic basis of hypertrophic cardiomyopathy in cats and humans. *J Vet Cardiol.* 2015;17:53–73.

[15] Nelson RW, Couto CG., editors. Small animal internal medicine. St. Louis, MO: Elsevier Mosby; 2014.

[16] Tilley LP, Smith, Jr FWK, Oyama MA, Sleeper MM. Manual of canine and feline cardiology. St. Louis, MO: Saunders Elsevier; 2008.

[17] Tidholm A, Häggstrüm J, Borgarelli M, et al. Canine idiopathic dilated cardiomyopathy. Part I: aetiology, clinical characteristics, epidemiology and pathology. *Vet J.* 2001;162:92–107.

[18] Longeri M, Ferrari P, Knafelz P, et al. Myosin-binding protein C DNA variants in domestic cats (A31P, A74T, R820W) and their association with hypertrophic cardiomyopathy. *J Vet Intern Med.* 2013;27:275–285.

[19] Häggstrüm J, Luis Fuentes V, Wess G. Screening for hypertrophic cardiomyopathy in cats. *J Vet Cardiol.* 2015;17:134–149.

[20] Meurs KM, Norgard MM, Ederer MM, et al. A substitution mutation in the myosin binding protein C gene in ragdoll hypertrophic cardiomyopathy. *Genomics.* 2007;90:261–264.

[21] Meurs KM, Sanchez X, David RM, et al. A cardiac myosin binding protein C mutation in the Maine Coon cat with familial hypertrophic cardiomyopathy. *Hum Mol Genet.* 2005;14:3587–3593.

[22] Meurs KM, Fox PR, Norgard M, et al. A prospective genetic evaluation of familial dilated cardiomyopathy in the Doberman Pinscher. *J Vet Intern Med.* 2007;21:1016–1020.

[23] Meurs KM, Stern JA, Sisson DD, et al. Association of dilated cardiomyopathy with the striatin mutation genotype in boxer dogs. *J Vet Intern Med.* 2013;27:1437–1440.

[24] Sleeper MM, Henthorn PS, Vijayasarathy C, et al. Dilated cardiomyopathy in juvenile Portuguese Water Dogs. *J Vet Intern Med.* 2002;16:52–62.

[25] Dambach DM, Lannon A, Sleeper MM, et al. Familial dilated cardiomyopathy of young Portuguese water dogs. *J Vet Intern Med.* 1999;13:65–71.

[26] Towbin JA, Hejtmancik JF, Brink P, et al. X-linked dilated cardiomyopathy. Molecular genetic evidence of linkage to the Duchenne muscular dystrophy (dystrophin) gene at the Xp21 locus. *Circulation.* 1993;87:1854–1865.

[27] Gavaghan BJ, Kittleson MD. Dilated cardiomyopathy in an American cocker spaniel with taurine deficiency. *Aust Vet J.* 1997;75:862–868.

[28] Borgarelli M, Tarducci A, Tidholm A, et al. Canine idiopathic dilated cardiomyopathy. Part II: pathophysiology and therapy. *Vet J.* 2001;162:182–195.

[29] Liu SK, Roberts WC, Maron BJ. Comparison *of morphologic* findings in spontaneously occurring hypertrophic *cardiomyopathy in* humans, cats and dogs. *Am J Cardiol.* 1993;72:944–951.

[30] Legge CH, López A, Hanna P, *et al. Histolog*ical characterization of dilated cardiomyopathy in the juvenile toy Manchester terrier. *Vet Pathol.* 2013;50:1043–1052.

[31] Janus I, Noszczyk-Nowak A, Nowak M, et al. A comparison of the histopathologic pattern of the left atrium in canine dilated cardiomyopathy and chronic mitral valve disease. *BMC Vet Res.* 2016;12:3.

[32] Tidholm A, Häggstrüm J, Jünsson L. Detection of attenuated wavy fibers in the myocardium of Newfoundlands without clinical or echocardiographic evidence of heart disease. *Am J Vet Res.* 2000;61:238–241.

[33] Tidholm A, Häggstrüm J, Jünsson L. Prevalence of attenuated wavy fibers in myocardium of dogs with dilated cardiomyopathy. *J Am Vet Med Assoc.* 1998;212:1732–1734.

[34] Harpster N. Boxer cardiomyopathy. *Vet Clin North Am Small Anim Pract.* 1991;21:989–1004.

[35] Granstrüm S, Godiksen MT, Christiansen M, et al. Prevalence of hypertrophic cardiomyopathy in a cohort of British Shorthair cats in Denmark. *J Vet Intern Med.* 2011;25:866–871.

[36] Gundler S, Tidholm A, Häggstrüm J. Prevalence of myocardial hypertrophy in a population of asymptomatic Swedish Maine coon cats. *Acta Vet Scand.* 2008;50:22.

[37] Cesta MF, Baty CJ, Keene BW, et al. Pathology of end-stage remodeling in a family of cats with hypertrophic cardiomyopathy. *Vet Pathol.* 2005;42:458–467.

[38] Saito Y, Suzuki Y, Kondo N, et al. Direct epicardial assist device using artificial rubber muscle in a swine model of pediatric dilated cardiomyopathy. *Int J Artif Organs.* 2015;38:588–594.

[39] Lin JH, Huang SY, Lee WC, et al. Echocardiographic features of pigs with spontaneous hypertrophic cardiomyopathy. *Comp Med.* 2002;52:238–242.

[40] Collins DE, Eaton KA, Hoenerhoff MJ. Spontaneous dilated cardiomyopathy and right-sided heart failure as a differential diagnosis for hepatosis dietetica in a production pig. *Comp Med.* 2015;65:327–332.

[41] Shyu JJ, Cheng CH, Erlandson RA, et al. Ultrastructure of intramural coronary arteries in pigs with hypertrophic cardiomyopathy. *Cardiovasc Pathol.* 2000;11:104–111.

[42] Liu SK, Chiu YT, Shyu JJ, et al. Hypertrophic cardiomyopathy in pigs: quantitative pathologic features in 55 cases. *Cardiovasc Pathol.* 1994;3:261–268.

[43] Horiuchi N, Kumagai D, Matsumoto K, et al. Detection of the nonsense mutation of OPA3 gene in Holstein Friesian cattle with dilated cardiomyopathy in Japan. *J Vet Med Sci.* 2015;77:1281–1283.

[44] Van Vleet JF, Ferrans VJ. Myocardial diseases of animals. *Am J Pathol.* 1986;124:98–178.

[45] Owczarek-Lipska M, Plattet P, Zipperle L, et al. A nonsense mutation in the optic atrophy 3 gene (OPA3) causes dilated cardiomyopathy in Red Holstein cattle. *Genomics.* 2011;97:51–57.

[46] Furuoka H, Yagi S, Murakami A, et al. Hereditary dilated cardiomyopathy in Holstein-Friesian cattle in Japan: association with hereditary myopathy of the diaphragmatic muscles. *J Comp Pathol.* 2001;125:159–165.

[47] Schatzberg SJ, Olby NJ, Breen M, et al. Molecular analysis of a spontaneous dystrophin 'knockout' dog. *Neuromuscul Disord.* 1999;9:289–295.

[48] Stabej P, Imholz S, Versteeg SA, et al. Characterization of the canine desmin (DES) gene and evaluation as a candidate gene for dilated cardiomyopathy in the Doberman. *Gene.* 2004;340:241–249.

[49] Philipp U, Vollmar A, Distl O. Evaluation of the titin-cap gene (TCAP) as candidate for dilated cardiomyopathy in Irish wolfhounds. *Anim Biotechnol.* 2008;19:231–236.

[50] O'Sullivan ML, O'Grady MR, Pyle WG, Dawson JF. Evaluation of 10 genes encoding cardiac proteins in Doberman Pinschers with dilated cardiomyopathy. *Am J Vet Res.* 2011;72:932–939.

[51] Cattanach BM, Dukes-McEwan J, Wotton PR, et al. A pedigree-based genetic appraisal of Boxer ARVC and the role of the Striatin mutation. *Vet Rec.* 2015;176:492.

[52] Keene BW, Panciera DP, Atkins CE, et al. Myocardial L-carnitine deficiency in a family of dogs with dilated cardiomyopathy. *J Am Vet Med Assoc.* 1991;198:647–650.

[53] Kittleson MD, Keene B, Pion PD, et al. Results of the multicenter spaniel trial (MUST): taurine- and carnitine-responsive dilated cardiomyopathy in American cocker spaniels with decreased plasma taurine concentration. *J Vet Intern Med.* 1997;11:204–211.

[54] Phillips DE, Harkin KR. Hypothyroidism and myocardial failure in two Great Danes. *J Am Anim Hosp Assoc.* 2003;39:133–137.

[55] Flood JA, Hoover JP. Improvement in myocardial dysfunction in a hypothyroid dog. *Can Vet J.* 2009;50:828–34.

[56] Beier P, Reese S, Holler PJ, et al. The role of the hypothyroidism in the etiology and progression of dilated cardiomyopathy in Doberman Pinschers. *J Vet Intern Med.* 2015;29:141–149.

[57] Day MJ. Inheritance of serum autoantibody, reduced serum IgA and autoimmune disease in a canine breeding colony. *Vet Immunol Immunopathol.* 1996;53:207–219.

[58] Maxson TR, Meurs KM, Lehmkuhl LB, et al. Polymerase chain reaction analysis for viruses in paraffin-embedded myocardium from dogs with dilated cardiomyopathy or myocarditis. *Am J Vet Res.* 2001;62:130–135.

[59] Calvert CA, Chapman WL, Toal RL. Congestive cardiomyopathy in Doberman Pinscher dogs. *J Am Vet Med Assoc.* 1982;181:598–602.

[60] Hazlett MJ, Maxie MG, Allen DG, et al. A retrospective study of heart disease in Doberman Pinscher dogs. *Can Vet J.* 1983;24:205–210.

[61] Tidholm A, Jünsson L. Dilated cardiomyopathy in the Newfoundland: a study of 37 cases (1983–1994). *J Am Anim Hosp Assoc.* 1996;32:465–470.

[62] Calvert CA, Pickus CW, Jacobs GJ, et al. Signalment, survival and prognostic factors in Doberman Pinschers with end-stage cardiomyopathy. *J Vet Intern Med.* 1997;11:323–326.

[63] Everett RM, McGann J, Wimberly HC, et al. Dilated cardiomyopathy of Doberman Pinschers: retrospective histomorphologic evaluation of heart from 32 cases. *Vet Pathol.* 1999;36:221–227.

[64] Vollmar AC, Fox PR, Meurs KM, et al. Dilated cardiomyopathy in juvenile Doberman Pinscher dogs. *J Vet Cardiol.* 2005;5:23–27.

[65] Lobo L, Carvalheira J, Canada N, et al. Histologic characterization of dilated cardiomyopathy in Estrela mountain dogs. *Vet Pathol.* 2010;47:637–642.

[66] Tilley LP, Liu S-K. Cardiomyopathy in the dog. *Recent Adv Stud Cardiac Struct Metab.* 1975;10:641–653.

[67] Sandusky GE, Capen CC, Kerr KM. Histological and ultrastructural evaluation of cardiac lesions in idiopathic cardiomyopathy in dogs. *Can J Comp Med.* 1984;48:81–86.

[68] Alroy J, Rush JE, Freeman L, et al. Inherited infantile dilated cardiomyopathy in dogs: genetic, clinical, biochemical, and morphologic findings. *Am J of Med Genet.* 2000;95:57–66.

[69] Vollmar AC, Fox PR, Meurs KM, et al. Dilated cardiomyopathy in juvenile Doberman Pinscher dogs. *J Vet Cardiol.* 2005;5:23–27.

Section 5

# Diagnosis and Invasive Treatments

# Chapter 18

# Cardiac Magnetic Resonance T1 Mapping in Cardiomyopathies

Christian R. Hamilton-Craig, Mark W. Strudwick and Graham J. Galloway

Additional information is available at the end of the chapter

http://dx.doi.org/10.5772/65327

**Abstract**

Cardiac magnetic resonance (CMR) imaging has been widely used to assess myocardial perfusion and scar and is the noninvasive reference standard for identification of focal myocardial fibrosis. However, the late gadolinium enhancement (LGE) technique is limited in its accuracy for absolute quantification and assessment of diffuse myocardial fibrosis by technical and pathophysiological features. CMR relaxometry, incorporating T1 mapping, has emerged as an accurate, reproducible, highly sensitive, and quantitative technique for the assessment of diffuse myocardial fibrosis in a number of disease states. We comprehensively review the physics behind CMR relaxometry, the evidence base, and the clinical applications of this emerging technique.

**Keywords:** cardiac magnetic resonance, T1 mapping, myocardial fibrosis, cardiomyopathy

## 1. Introduction

Cardiac Magnetic Resonance (CMR) imaging has been used widely to assess myocardial perfusion and scar [1–5]. It is the noninvasive reference standard for left and right ventricular quantitation, as well as the assessment and quantitation of focal myocardial fibrosis (after infarction or due to other causes of cellular injury). Myocardial necrosis causes high signal on late gadolinium enhancement (LGE) inversion recovery T1-weighted images with excellent signal-noise ratios, and this has become the reference standard for noninvasive scar imaging in cardiomyopathies of various causes [1–4]. However, LGE is limited in its ability to assess and quantitate diffuse (nonfocal) myocardial injury and fibrosis. LGE is affected by inconsistencies in acquisition parameters, such as choice inversion time, and in postprocessing when signal intensity thresholds may be arbitrarily applied to distinguish normal myocardium from fibrotic tissue [6, 7]. Moreover, the critical issue with LGE is that signal intensity is expressed on an arbitrary scale (*relative* signal intensity compared with "nulled" normal myocardium). Detection of myocardial fibrosis using *relative* differences between scar and normal myocardium tissue is therefore *qualitative*. Thus, in nonischemic cardiomyopathies, such as hypertension or diabetes, LGE CMR is unable to detect signal differential where the collagen deposition is diffuse and widespread throughout the myocardium [8].

## 2. CMR relaxometry

CMR is an evolving technique, providing valuable and comprehensive data on the anatomy and functional integrity of both the heart and coronary blood vessels. Currently, CMR is performed at magnetic field strengths of 1.5 or 3 T.

## 3. T1 mapping with Look–Locker

The initial technique to measure spin–lattice T1 relaxation time values was the eponymously named "Look–Locker" sequence (also known as "TI scout"). It has been widely used to estimate the optimal inversion time for assessment of myocardial LGE [9, 10]. It was originally proposed by Look and Locker in 1968 and analyzed more fully in 1970 [11] and consists of an initial inversion pulse, followed by a train of pulses with a constant, limited flip angle (7–15°).

The development of LL technique is summarized in **Table 1**.

The LL sequence has been widely applied in CMR due to its fast acquisition with minimal breath-hold requirements. The LL sequence has been used to measure T1 values in patients with myocardial fibrosis [9]. However, it suffers from significant limitations: low flip angle RF pulse exciting the magnetization and the two RR intervals in the LL sequence are not sufficient for the magnetization to return to equilibrium. This causes *underestimation* of true T1 values using LL. Furthermore, the LL T1 images with different TIs are acquired at different cardiac phases. Therefore, images are "cine" with cardiac motion effect, which requires tedious manual tracking of the myocardial borders for each phase, a labour-intensive and error-prone process, which is challenging in clinical practice. The drawing of regions of interest "ROI" in myocardial segments requires adjusting for cardiac motion, which results in including blood pool (partial volume averaging) and artificially increasing the measured T1 [12].

To address these shortcomings, several myocardial T1 mapping sequences have been created, including modified Look-Locker inversion (MOLLI) recovery.

http://dx.doi.org/10.5772/65327

| Author | Year | Summary of research findings |
|---|---|---|
| Look & Locker | 1968 | Initial proposition of Look–Locker technique |
| Look & Locker | 1970 | Fully analyzed NMR pulse sequence to measure a spin–lattice T1 relaxation time |
| Kaptein et al. | 1976 | LL was co-opted to quickly sample the recovery after a preparation pulse during the recovery period |
| Gerumann | 1987 | T1 by Multiple Readout Pulses (TOMROP) was proposed through which the multiple samples of a particular recovery after RF preparation each correspond to a separate image |
| Hinson and Sobol | 1988 | LL method was applied without preparation pulse |
| Crawley and Henkelman | 1988 | Compared (LL, saturation recovery, inversion recovery, and stimulated echo) and concluded that LL was almost as efficient |
| Brix et al. | 1990 | TMPROP was used with 32 gradient echoes in a total acquisition time of 4 min |
| Kay | 1991 | LL single-shot IR method has been optimized and refined |
| Gowland | 1992 | LL single-shot IR method has been optimized and refined |
| Been et al. | 1988 | Improved RF preparation pulses |
| Gowland et al. | 1989 | Improved RF preparation pulses |
| Ordidge et al. | 1990 | Echo-planar imaging (EPI) was incorporated into the inversion recovery LL-based method |
| Gowland and Mansfield | 1993 | EPI was applied in vivo in less than 3 s |
| Freeman et al. | 1998 | An entire image was acquired at each point on a single recovery of longitudinal magnetization after a saturation pulse |
| Karlsson and Nordell | 1999 | EPI- with LL method has found application in pharmacokinetic modeling in the head |
| Daniel et al. | 2004 | Modified Look–Locker inversion recovery is proposed to overcome the limitations of the conventional LL approach for cardiac applications |
| Daniel et al. | 2006 | Studied the single breath-hold myocardial MR T1 mapping with MOLLI technique with high spatial resolution at 1.5 T MR-reproducibility study |
| Daniel et al. | 2007 | Investigated optimization and validation of a fully integrated pulse sequence for (MOLLI) T1 mapping of the heart |
| Iles et al. | 2008 | Evaluation of diffuse myocardial fibrosis in heart failure with cardiac magnetic resonance contrast-enhanced T1 mapping |

**Table 1.** Summary of development of Look–Locker technique.

## 4. T1 mapping with Modified Look-Locker Inversion "MOLLI" recovery

Currently, the most evaluated sequence for myocardium T1 mapping is a modified Look-Locker inversion recovery (MOLLI) sequence [13, 14]. The T1 mapping identifies a significant variation between normal and abnormal myocardium. It demonstrates the myocardial fibrosis among different myocardial disorders include ischemia [15], acute/chronic infraction [16], amyloidosis [17], diabetic [18], dilated and hypertrophic cardiomyopathy [19], and heart failure [8].

MOLLI is a CMR pulse sequence that is used for accurate T1 mapping of myocardium with high spatial resolution. MOLLI is an ECG-gated pulse sequence scheme and uses three prepared Look–Locker experiments consecutively within one breath-hold over 17 heartbeats to reconstruct 11 images with different inversion times. Three successive ECG-triggered LL experiments (LL**1**, LL**2**, and LL**3**) are carried out with three, three, and five single-shot readouts, respectively, at end diastole of consecutive heartbeats to sample the recovery of longitudinal magnetization after the inversion pulse. MOLLI pulse sequence scheme is illustrated in **Figure 1**. T1 maps can be generated any time before or after contrast agent (e.g., gadolinium) administration [12].

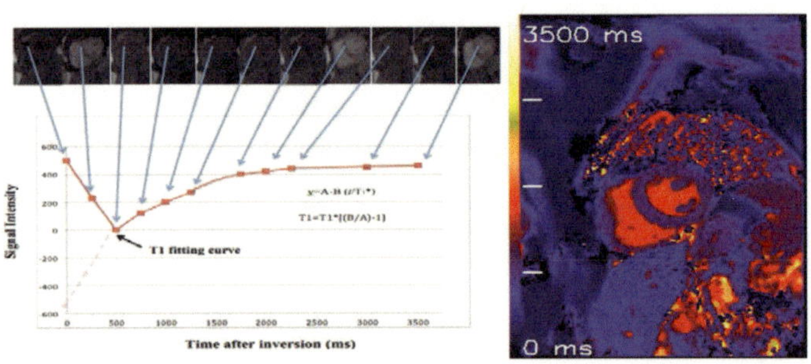


**Figure 1. T1 map of a healthy volunteer**: Using 17 heartbeats to reconstruct 11 images with different inversion times at end of diastole phase. By merging these images into one data set, T1 values are computed for every pixel with three parameters curve fitting. A reconstructed T1 map with parametric color scale is produced for these pixel values and the segmental and global T1 times can be estimated.

The MOLLI sequence has been described, optimized, tested, and retested in phantoms and in large cohorts of healthy volunteers [12, 14] as well as being applied in cardiomyopathies [8, 15, 17, 19, 20]. In addition, the T1 mapping with MOLLI has been validated against histopathology for assessment of myocardial fibrosis. It demonstrated that the precontrast "native T1" has a linear correlation with the percentage of myocardial fibrosis as measured histologically on invasive myocardial biopsy. T1 times postcontrast administration (10–15 min) had an inverse linear relationship with collagen content in myocardial fibrosis subjects [8, 21, 22].

- Precontrast "Native" T1 = predominant signal from *myocytes* (replacement fibrosis or intracellular accumulation, e.g., Fabry disease)
- Postcontrast T1 = predominant signal from *interstitial* space (interstitial fibrosis)

http://dx.doi.org/10.5772/65327

T1 mapping can be generated for different segments of the myocardium (base, mid-cavity, and apex) within a single breath-hold of about 15–20 s. However, the apex T1 values with MOLLI are slightly higher than basal and mid-cavity. The increasing in T1 values may be caused by partial volume effect and some degree of overestimation effect in apical level of left ventricle [23–25].

T1 mapping with MOLLI has a greater reproducibility, accuracy, and an excellent overall inter- and intra-observer agreement over a wide range of TIs as compared with the traditional LL sequence [13, 14].

However, the T1 mapping with MOLLI sequence is sensitive to extremes of heart rate (bradycardia or tachycardia) [14] leading to a slight underestimation of T1 values. This may be corrected though *heart rate correction* by changing the timing of the readouts with respect to the inversion pulses at different heart rates.

Moreover, MOLLI is also limited by long breath-hold for about 15–20 s (17 heartbeats to acquire the final T1 maps). This may be difficult for elderly and pulmonary compromised patients and generates respiratory and motion artifacts [26]. Modern in-line processing provides registration tools to reduce motion artifacts before the computation of final T1 maps (motion-corrected or "MoCo MOLLI") [27]. A shortened Modified Look-Locker inversion recovery (*shMOLLI*) with shorter breath-holds has been validated and recently applied for cardiomyopathies [28, 29].

## 5. MRI field strength

At 1.5 T, the pre- and postcontrast (10 mins) T1 times of normal myocardium are 980 ± 53 ms and 470 ± 26 ms, respectively [14]. Precontrast T1 values of myocardial fibrosis (Infarction scar) are significantly longer than those of normal myocardium (1060 ± 61 ms vs. 987 ± 34 ms) [20]. The postcontrast T1 times (10 mins) were significantly shorter in chronic infarct scar compared with normal myocardium at 0.15 mmol/kg (390 ± 20 ms vs. 483 ± 23 ms, respectively) [20].

**3 T**: T1 mapping at higher magnetic field (3 T) has been reported in a few studies of interstitial myocardial fibrosis, but minimal data exist for ultra-high field at 7 T. 3 T data are similar to 1.5 T, the precontrast T1 was longer, and postcontrast T1 was shorter in myocardial fibrosis patients compared with normal myocardium. Puntmann et al. [30] reported higher precontrast T1 values for hypertrophic and nonischemic dilated cardiomyopathies at 3 T compared with controls (Hypertrophic 1.254 ± 43 ms, and nonischemic dilated cardiomyopathy 1.239 ± 57 ms vs. healthy 1.070 ± 55 ms). Also, the postcontrast T1 values (10 mins) at 3 T were shorter in hypertrophic and dilated cardiomyopathies compared with healthy (hypertrophic: 307 ± 47 ms, dilated cardiomyopathies: 296 ± 43 ms vs. controls: 402 ± 58 ms) [30].

There are studies published for normal and diffuse myocardial fibrosis of myocardium T1 values, as described comprehensively in **Tables 2** and **3**:

| First author (Ref.#) | Sample size | T1/T2* mapping sequence | Result of T1 or T2* mapping (ms) |
|---|---|---|---|
| Wacker et al. [31] | 5 | srTFL, segmented T2* gradient echo pulse | T1 = 1219 ± 72 ms<br>T2* = 35 ± 3 ms |
| Sebastian et al. [32] | 12 | LL | T1 = 1033 ± 126 ms<br>T2* = NA |
| Messroghli et al, [33] | 15 | MOLLI | T1 = 980 ± 53 ms<br>T2* = NA |
| Messroghli et al. [34] | 20 | MOLLI | T1 = 939 ± 63 ms<br>T2* = NA |
| Sparrow et al, [35] | 15 | MOLLI | T1 = 980 ± 53 ms<br>T2* = NA |
| Iles et al. [8] | 20 | VAST | T1 = 975 ± 62 ms<br>T2* = NA |
| Li et al. [36] | 13 | 2 echo times GRE | T1 = NA<br>T2* = 33 ± 6.5 ms |
| Reeder et al. [37] | 5 | Multi echo GRE | T1 = NA<br>T2*= 38 ± 6 ms |
| Anderson et al. [38] | 15 | Multi echo GRE | T1 = NA<br>T2*= 52 ± 16 ms |
| Positano et al. [39] | 15 | Multi echo GRE | T1 = NA<br>T2* = 38 ± 9.2 ms in endocardial sectors, and 33.1 ± 8.4 ms in epicardial sectors |
| Messroghli et al. [40] | 20 | Multi echo GRE | T1 = NA<br>T2* = 27.9 ± 3.4 ms in anteroseptal and 23.1 ± 5.2 ms in inferolateral |
| Piechnik et al. [28] | 342 | shMOLLI | T1 = 962 ± 25 ms<br>T2* = NA<br>Heart rate only physiologic factors effect on myocardial T1 values |

Note: NA, not applicable; srTFL, saturation recovery turboFLASH; LL, Look-Locker; MOLLI, modified Look–Locker inversion recovery sequence; VAST, inversion recovery gradient echo sequence with Variable Sampling of the k-space in Time; GRE, gradient pulse sequence; shMOLLI, short modified Look-Locker sequence.

**Table 2.** Healthy clinical studies using T1 and T2*.

http://dx.doi.org/10.5772/65327

| First author (Ref. #) | Cardiac disease category | Patient sample size | T1 mapping method | Summary of findings |
|---|---|---|---|---|
| Franck Thuny | Systemic sclerosis | 37 | MOLLI | LV diastolic dysfunction had a shorter 15 min postcontrast T1 time (ms) than those with a normal diastolic function (431 ± 7 vs. 464 ± 8, $p = 0.01$). |
| Helene Thibault | Type II diabetic patient | 24 | MOLLI | Mean myocardial T1 relaxation time was significantly shorter in diabetic patients than in volunteers both at 5 (312 ± 5 vs. 361 ± 6 milliseconds, respectively, $p < 0.001$) and 15 min (405 ± 6 vs. 456 ± 5 milliseconds, respectively, $p < 0.001$) after gadolinium injection. |
| Andris H Ellims | Hypertrophy cardiomyopathy | 51 | VAST | Postcontrast myocardial T1 time was significantly shorter in patients with HCM compared with controls, consistent with diffuse myocardial fibrosis (498 ± 80 ms vs. 561 ± 47 ms, $p < 0.001$). |
| Beatrice A Marzluf | Patients with $NH_2$-terminal portion of the precursor of brain natriuretic peptide (NT-proBNP) | 37 | N/A | In patients with NT-proBNP levels >400 pg/ml mean T1 was significantly shorter than in patients with NT-proBNP <400 pg/ml (374.6 ± 51.1 vs. 404.6 ± 34.4 ms, $p = 0.042$) and controls (509.4 ± 46.5 ms, p < 0.001). |
| Christopher T Sibley | Nonischemic cardiomyopathy | 73 | LL | 47 patients had a focal myocardial scar and 26 without scar tissue. The midwall circumferential strain (Ecc) was reduced (−13.0 +/− 5.4%) and mean T1 time was 478 +/ − 70 ms in patients with no scar tissue. |
| Jellis et al. [18] | Type II diabetic patients | 67 | VAST | Subjects has a shorter post contrast T1 = 434 ± 20 ms. Postcontrast T1 was associated with Echocardiography diastolic dysfunction (Em $r = 0.28$, $p = 0.020$; E/Em $r = -0.24$, $p = 0.049$). |
| Messroghli et al. [13] | Acute myocardial infarction | 8 | Inversion recovery (IR)-prepared fast gradient echo sequence | T1 precontrast value of the infarcted myocardium was significantly prolonged compared with noninfarcted normal myocardium (+18 ± 7%). T1 10-min postcontrast value of the infarct was significantly reduced compared with normal myocardium (−27 ± 4%). |
| Messroghli et al. [20] | Acute and chronic myocardial infarction | 24 | MOLLI | In chronic MI, the precontrast T1 relaxation time of hyper-enhanced areas was higher than T1 of remote areas (1060 ± 61 vs. 987 ± 34 ms, $p < 0.0001$). In acute MI, the precontrast T1 value of hyper-enhanced areas was higher |

| First author (Ref. #) | Cardiac disease category | Patient sample size | T1 mapping method | Summary of findings |
|---|---|---|---|---|
| | | | | than remote areas (1197 ± 76 vs. 1011 ± 66). The hyper-enhanced in acute is higher than chronic infarction. |
| Flacke and Sebastian [32] | Acute and chronic myocardial infarction | 10 | LL | Mean T1 values of the normal myocardium postcontrast was 536 ± 66 ms, chronically infracted precontrast and postcontrast was 1000 ± 67 ms and 408 ± 43 ms, respectively. |
| Sparrow et al. [35] | Myocardial Fibrosis in Chronic Aortic Regurgitation | 8 | Molli | There is a significant difference in segmental averaged T1 relaxation between in abnormal wall motion vs. Normal control segments in 10, 15, and 20 min after administration Gd: (510 vs. 476 ms, 532 vs 501 ms, and 560 vs. 516 ms, respectively). |
| Iles et al. [8] | Chronic heart failure | 25 | VAST | Postcontrast myocardial T1 times were shorter in heart failure subjects than in controls (383 ± 17 ms vs. 564 ± 23 ms) even when excluding areas of regional fibrosis. T1 15-min postcontrast values correlated significantly with collagen volume fraction on myocardial biopsies ($R = -0.7$). |
| Maceira 2005 | Cardiac amyloidosis | 22 | Segmented inversion recovery sequence | Subendocardial T1 in amyloid patients was shorter than in controls (at 4 min: 427 ± 73 vs. 579 ± 75 ms; $p < 0.01$). |

**Table 3.** Clinical studies using T1 mapping for myocardial diffuse fibrosis in clinical patients.

## 6. Limitations of T1 mapping

Challenges remain with myocardial relaxometry for T1 mapping. These include technical challenges such as variations of T1 times at different field strength and across different vendors, and the rapidity in growth of pulse sequences being released as product and as works-in-progress (WIP), calling into question both the inherent accuracy and the level agreement between these techniques. Furthermore, the variations in T1 relaxometry values with different contrast doses and image timing require further investigation to establish the test–retest and intersite reproducibility of this technique. Next, the challenges to application of T1 mapping to clinical practice include establishment of robust normal ranges in large cohorts across multiple ethnic groups and the observation that T1 mapping appears to be a highly sensitive technique, with the ability to discriminate healthy normal myocardium and identify very early changes in substrate. However, this technique lacks specificity; a wide variety of conditions prolong native T1 and/or shorten postcontrast myocardial T1. Therefore, further clinical data are required in order to establish the use of these parameters in relation to disease (e.g., early

http://dx.doi.org/10.5772/65327

detection of target organ damage in systemic conditions such as hypertension or diabetes), to inform treatment decisions, and their ability to predict or alter clinical outcomes.

## 7. Conclusions

Myocardial T1 mapping using quantitative relaxometry is an emerging and important tool in the assessment of global myocardial fibrosis. It is a highly sensitive marker of disease, but is not specific, with changes in myocardial T1 occurring in many different conditions. Nevertheless, the high sensitivity and excellent reproducibility of the technique offer a tool for the early detection of myocardial damage, over-and-above techniques such as the CMR LGE technique and other modalities such as speckle tracking echocardiography, pulse wave velocity, and tissue tagging. Native T1 mapping is proving to be a robust indicator of early myocardial disease in many conditions, and normal ranges and guidelines for postprocessing have been published by the Society of Cardiovascular Magnetic Resonance [41]. Myocardial T1 mapping is a rapidly evolving technique, now with longitudinal prognostic data emerging, and normal ranges established at 1.5 and 3.0 T in healthy humans and in aging persons. Further questions remain as to the standardization of pulse sequences across field strengths and between vendors, the affect of contrast type, dose and timing, the postprocessing software, and the interpretation of T1 mapping results to inform clinical practice.

## Acknowledgements

The author acknowledges the contribution of Dr Qurain Alshammari's to the background work.

### Abbreviations

| | |
|---|---|
| CMR | cardiac magnetic resonance |
| LL | Look- Locker |
| LGE | late gadolinium enhancement |
| LV | left ventricle |
| MOLLI | modified Look-Locker inversion recovery |
| MRI | magnetic resonance imaging |
| ROI | regions of interest |
| RV | right ventricle |
| *sh*MOLLI | shortened modified Look-Locker inversion recovery |

## Author details

Christian R. Hamilton-Craig[1,2*], Mark W. Strudwick[3] and Graham J. Galloway[1,4]

*Address all correspondence to: c.hamiltoncraig@uq.edu.au

1 Centre for Advanced Imaging, University of Queensland, Brisbane, Australia

2 Department of Radiology, University of Washington, Seattle, WA, USA

3 Medical Imaging and Radiation Science, Monash University, Australia

4 Translational Research Institute, Brisbane, Australia

## References

[1] Croisille P, Revel D, Saeed M. Contrast agents and cardiac MR imaging of myocardial ischemia: from bench to bedside. European Radiology 2006;16:1951–1963.

[2] Judd RM, Atalay MK, Rottman GA, Zerhouni EA. Effects of myocardial water exchange on T1 enhancement during Bolus administration of MR contrast agents. Magnetic Resonance in Medicine 1995;33:215–223.

[3] Lima JAC. Myocardial viability assessment by contrast-enhanced magnetic resonance imaging. Journal of the American College of Cardiology 2003;42:902–904.

[4] Kim RJ, Chen E-L, Lima JoAC, Judd RM. Myocardial Gd-DTPA kinetics determine MRI contrast enhancement and reflect the extent and severity of myocardial injury after acute reperfused infarction. Circulation 1996;94:3318–3326.

[5] Mahrholdt H, Wagner A, Judd RM, Sechtem U, Kim RJ. Delayed enhancement cardiovascular magnetic resonance assessment of non-ischaemic cardiomyopathies. European Heart Journal 2005;26:1461–1474.

[6] Simonetti OP, Kim RJ, Fieno DS et al. An improved MR imaging technique for the visualization of myocardial infarction. Radiology 2001;218:215–223.

[7] Spiewak M, Malek LA, Misko J et al. Comparison of different quantification methods of late gadolinium enhancement in patients with hypertrophic cardiomyopathy. European Journal of Radiology 2010;74:e149–e153.

[8] Iles L, Pfluger H, Phrommintikul A et al. Evaluation of diffuse myocardial fibrosis in heart failure with cardiac magnetic resonance contrast-enhanced T1 mapping. Journal of the American College of Cardiology 2008;52:1574–1580.

http://dx.doi.org/10.5772/65327

[9] Amano Y, Takayama M, Kumita S. Contrast-enhanced myocardial T1-weighted scout (Look–Locker) imaging for the detection of myocardial damages in hypertrophic cardiomyopathy. Journal of Magnetic Resonance Imaging 2009;30:778–784.

[10] Karlsson M, Nordell B. Analysis of the Look-Locker T1 mapping sequence in dynamic contrast uptake studies: simulation and in vivo validation. Magnetic Resonance Imaging 2000;18:947–954.

[11] Look DC, Locker DR. Time saving in measurement of NMR and EPR relaxation times. The Review of scientific Instruments 1970;41:250–251.

[12] Messroghli DR, Radjenovic A, Kozerke S, Higgins DM, Sivananthan MU, Ridgway JP. Modified Look-Locker inversion recovery (MOLLI) for high-resolution T1 mapping of the heart. Magnetic Resonance in Medicine 2004;52:141–146.

[13] Messroghli DR, Niendorf T, Schulz-Menger J, Dietz R, G. FM. T1 Mapping in patients with acute myocardial infarction. Journal of Cardiovascular Magnetic Resonance 2003;5:353–359.

[14] Messroghli DR, Plein S, Higgins DM et al. Human myocardium: single-breath-hold MR T1 mapping with high spatial resolution—reproducibility study. Radiology 2006;238:1004–1012.

[15] Goldfarb JW, Arnold S, Han J. Recent Myocardial infarction: assessment with unenhanced T1-weighted MR imaging1. Radiology 2007;245:245–250.

[16] Messroghli DR, Greiser A, Fröhlich M, Dietz R, Schulz-Menger J. Optimization and validation of a fully-integrated pulse sequence for modified look-locker inversion-recovery (MOLLI) T1 mapping of the heart. Journal of Magnetic Resonance Imaging 2007;26:1081–1086.

[17] Karamitsos TD, Piechnik SK, Banypersad SM et al. Noncontrast T1 mapping for the diagnosis of cardiac amyloidosis. Journal of American College of Cardiology: Cardiovascular Imaging 2013;6:488–497.

[18] Jellis C, Wright J, Kennedy D et al. Association of imaging markers of myocardial fibrosis with metabolic and functional disturbances in early diabetic cardiomyopathy. Circulation: Cardiovascular Imaging 2011;4:693–702.

[19] Dass S, Suttie JJ, Piechnik SK et al. Myocardial tissue characterization using magnetic resonance non-contrast T1 mapping in hypertrophic and dilated cardiomyopathy. Circulation: Cardiovascular Imaging 2012.

[20] Messroghli DR, Walters K, Plein S et al. Myocardial T1 mapping: application to patients with acute and chronic myocardial infarction. Magnetic Resonance in Medicine 2007;58:34–40.

[21] Sibley CT, Noureldin RA, Gai N et al. T1 mapping in cardiomyopathy at cardiac MR: comparison with endomyocardial biopsy. Radiology 2012;256:724–732.

[22] Bull S, White SK, Piechnik SK et al. Human non-contrast T1 values and correlation with histology in diffuse fibrosis. Heart 2013;99:923–927.

[23] Lima JAC, Jeremy R, Guier W et al. Accurate systolic wall thickening by nuclear magnetic resonance imaging with tissue tagging: correlation with sonomicrometers in normal and ischemic myocardium. Journal of the American College of Cardiology 1993;21:1741–1751.

[24] Forbat SM, Karwatowski SP, Gatehouse PD, Firmin DN, Longmore DB, Underwood SR. Rapid measurement of left ventricular mass by spin echo magnetic resonance imaging. British Journal of Radiology 1994;67:86–90.

[25] Aurigemma G, Davidoff A, Silver K, Boehmer J, Pattison N. Left ventricular mass quantitaton using single-phase cardiac magnetic resonance imaging. The American Journal of Cardiology 1992;70:259–262.

[26] Solano JP, Gomes B, Higginson IJ. A comparison of symptom prevalence in far advanced cancer, AIDS, heart disease, chronic obstructive pulmonary disease and renal disease. Journal of Pain and Symptom Management 2006;31:58–69.

[27] Messroghli DR, Rudolph A, Abdel-Aty H et al. An open-source software tool for the generation of relaxation time maps in magnetic resonance imaging. BMC Medical Imaging 2010:10–16.

[28] Piechnik S, Ferreira V, Lewandowski A et al. Normal variation of magnetic resonance T1 relaxation times in the human population at 1.5 T using ShMOLLI. Journal of Cardiovascular Magnetic Resonance 2013;15:13.

[29] Piechnik S, Ferreira V, Dall'Armellina E et al. Shortened Modified Look-Locker Inversion recovery (ShMOLLI) for clinical myocardial T1-mapping at 1.5 and 3 T within a 9 heartbeat breathhold. Journal of Cardiovascular Magnetic Resonance 2010;12:69.

[30] Puntmann VO, Voigt T, Chen Z et al. Native T1 mapping in differentiation of normal myocardium from diffuse disease in hypertrophic and dilated cardiomyopathy. JACC: Cardiovascular Imaging 2013;6:475–484.

[31] Wacker CM, Bock M, Hartlep AW et al. Changes in myocardial oxygenation and perfusion under pharmacological stress with dipyridamole: assessment using T*2 and T1 measurements. Magnetic Resonance in Medicine 1999;41:686–695.

[32] Sebastian J. Flacke SEF, and Christine H. Lorenz measurement of the Gadopentetate Dimeglumine partition coefficient in human myocardium in vivo: normal distribution and elevation in acute and chronic infarction. Radiology 2001;218:703–710.

[33] Messroghli DR, Plein S, Higgins DM et al. Human myocardium: single-breath-hold MR T1 mapping with high spatial resolution-reproducibility study. Radiology 2006;238:1004–1012.

[34] Messroghli DR, Greiser A, Frohlich M, Dietz R, Schulz-Menger J. Optimization and validation of a fully-integrated pulse sequence for modified look-locker inversion-

http://dx.doi.org/10.5772/65327

recovery (MOLLI) T1 mapping of the heart. Journal of Magnetic Resonance Imaging 2007;26:1081–1086.

[35] Sparrow P, Messroghli DR, Ridgway SP, Bainbridge G, Sivanthan MU. Myocardial T1 mapping for detection of left ventricular myocardial fibrosis in chronic aortic regurgitation: pilot study. American Journal of Roentgenology 2006;187:630–635.

[36] Li D, Dhawale P, Rubin PJ, Haacke EM, Gropler RJ. Myocardial signal response to dipyridamole and dobutamine: Demonstration of the BOLD effect using a double-echo gradient-echo sequence. Magnetic Resonance in Medicine 1996;36:16–20.

[37] Reeder SB, Faranesh AZ, Boxerman JL, McVeigh ER. In vivo measurement of T2 star and field inhomogeneity maps in the human heart at 1.5 T. Magnetic Resonance in Medicine 1998;39:988–998.

[38] Anderson LJ, Holden S, Davis B et al. Cardiovascular T2-star (T2*) magnetic resonance for the early diagnosis of myocardial iron overload. European Heart Journal 2001;22:2171–2179.

[39] Positano V, Pepe A, Santarelli MF, Scattini B, De Marchi D, et al. Standardized T2* map of normal human heart in vivo to correct T2* segmental artefacts. NMR in Biomedicine 2007;20:578–590.

[40] Messroghli DR, Wassmuth R, Zagrosek A, Rudolph A, Schulz-Menger J. Assessment of myocardial T2* from pixel-by-pixel maps on a clinical MR system. Journal of Cardiovascular Magnetic Resonance 2008;10(Suppl 1):A240.

[41] Moon JC, Messroghli DR, Kellman P et al. Myocardial T1 mapping and extracellular volume quantification: a Society for Cardiovascular Magnetic Resonance (SCMR) and CMR Working Group of the European Society of Cardiology consensus statement. Journal of Cardiovascular Magnetic Resonance 2013;15.

# Chapter 19

# Hypertrophic Cardiomyopathy: Treatment, Risk Stratification, and Implantable Defibrillators

Peter Magnusson

Additional information is available at the end of the chapter

http://dx.doi.org/10.5772/65392

**Abstract**

Hypertrophic cardiomyopathy (HCM) affects 1:500 individuals, and in majority of cases, a mutation in sarcomere proteins can explain the disease. Phenotype is heterogeneous and thus the prognosis. Many patients suffer from dyspnoea, especially at exercise. Unfortunately, sudden cardiac death (SCD) does occur at all ages and is a major cause of death in young adults. There is no proven pharmacological treatment to reduce hypertrophy or fibrosis, but beta-blockers are first-line treatment. In patients with obstruction, myectomy is preferred in the young, but in older patients, alcohol septal ablation is tried to reduce symptoms and possibly prognosis. Risk stratification of sudden cardiac death is challenging. The major established risk factors are extreme myocardial thickness, non-sustained ventricular tachycardia, unexplained syncope, abnormal exercise blood pressure response, and family history of sudden cardiac death. In 2014, a novel risk calculator was developed that also takes age, outflow gradient, and left atrial seize into account. Implantable defibrillator treatment is effective in HCM, but complications requiring surgery and inappropriate shocks remain a problem.

**Keywords:** complications, hypertrophic cardiomyopathy, implantable defibrillator, inappropriate shock, risk stratification, risk markers, sudden cardiac death

## 1. Diagnosis

Hypertrophic cardiomyopathy (HCM) implies increased ventricular thickness that is not only a response to hypertension, aortic stenosis, or any other loading condition with abnormal loading of the ventricle [1]. In adults, a wall thickness of ≥15 mm is typically required for diagnosis. In borderline cases (≥13 mm), a thorough evaluation including family history is needed [1, 2]. In siblings, parents or children of a HCM patient, 13-mm thickness is enough for diagnosis [1, 2]. In children and adolescents, a wall thickness more than two standard deviations in the corresponding age group should raise suspicion of the diagnosis of HCM [3]. An ultrasound of the heart, echocardiography, typically reveals the diagnosis of HCM. Echocardiography is usually readily available, but occasionally other imaging techniques are needed. Cardiac magnetic resonance (CMR), computed tomography (CT) or rarely positron emission tomography (PET) is sometimes used for diagnostic purposes or to gain additional information for optimal disease management [4]. The hypertrophied segment is almost always affecting the left ventricle even though right wall involvement does occur [1, 2]. Typically, the septal part is enlarged, either the basal part or the middle part, but could affect lateral, posterior and apical part, or a combination thereof [1]. A concentric hypertrophic is often associated with secondary causes of hypertrophy but does occur as HCM entity. If an isolated hypertrophy solely involves the basal part of the septal wall in an elderly and no other signs or family history of HCM is found, often an explanation such as hypertension is the major cause [1, 2]. Even though the diagnosis of most cases of HCM is straight forward, careful attention to other causes and robust imaging techniques, including a cardiologist with expertise in the field, is warranted. Because HCM is a life-long disease with consequences not only for the patient but also for relatives, a correct diagnosis is indeed important.

## 2. Symptoms and signs

Dyspnoea is the predominant symptom of HCM that leads to evaluation with an echocardiogram. Shortness of breath is pronounced at exertion due to relaxation disturbance of the left ventricle during diastole and/or outflow tract obstruction. This latter form is called hypertrophic obstructive cardiomyopathy, and the obstruction is often dynamic with regard to filling pressure, heart rate and body position and affected by medications with effect on the cardiovascular system. Often the patient has an adopted life style to decreased physical stamina, and often the diagnostic presentation is rather vague including tiredness. The HCM diagnosis is often delayed or sometimes misclassified from the initial diagnostic work-up.

A progressive HCM may sometimes lead to deterioration of the systolic function of the left ventricle. The ventricle dilates and hypertrophic segments remodel into dilatation, which sometimes can make it difficult to discern from other cardiomyopathies with dilated morphology. This condition is called end stage and indicates a worse prognosis [5–8].

Chest pain without coronary disease may also lead the physician to evaluate alternative diagnosis, and sometimes HCM is revealed. Microvascular dysfunction and fibrosis are part of the disease progression; biopsies show myocardial disarray, and modern PET imaging techniques confirm structural and functional abnormalities, which explain symptoms. However, biopsies are not indicated as part of routine evaluation as the same information would be gained non-invasively [2, 4]. Syncope evaluation is sometimes the initial work-up that leads to the diagnosis of HCM. The mechanisms could be either hemodynamic or cardiac

http://dx.doi.org/10.5772/65392

arrhythmias [9]. Less specific symptoms such as pre-syncope, near-syncope or vertigo will often include ECG and that in turn will lead to suspicion of morphological disease.

Atrial fibrillation is common among HCM, and thus, the risk of embolization stroke warrants effective anticoagulants even without other risk factors [10, 11]. The CHADSVASC score is not validated for HCM patients, and current guidelines recommend warfarin/dual oral anticoagulants if no contraindication is present [2].

Unfortunately, the first manifestation of HCM could be sudden cardiac death (SCD). In such cases, the autopsy confirms or at least suspects HCM even though the microscopy and post-mortem genetic evaluation will aid. A conclusive diagnosis of HCM is of uttermost importance because of the inheritance pattern and relatives need to be evaluated.

## 3. Inheritance

In more than half of the HCM cases, modern genetic panels can explain the cause of HCM and partly predict the outcome [12–14]. Of all mutations associated with HCM, the vast majority affects myosin proteins: beta-myosin heavy chain (MYH7) and myosin-binding protein (MYBPC3). Other components of the actin-myosin filaments, such as troponins or tropomyosin, rarely explain disease [2]. However, there is a steady increase in disease causing mutations due to increased research activities and widened genetic panels in everyday practise.

The mutations of HCM are autosomal dominant with the exception of the X-linked Danon disease due to lysosome-associated membrane protein 2 [15]. The most common metabolic disease causing hypertrophy of the heart is Anderson-Fabry, which is a storage dysfunction of the lysosomes. In children, hypertrophy of the heart is part of a syndrome, and constellations of malformations may lead suspicion towards Noonans disease, LEOPARD or even more rare diseases. In adults, amyloidosis should be part of the differential diagnosis. A correct molecular diagnosis can sometimes provide clinicians with specific treatment options and thus improve prognosis for the individual.

Family-history taking is a compulsory part of the initial evaluation of a patient with a suspected or conformed hypertrophy. The clinician should systematically document the patients' report on family members who died suddenly or suffered from unexplained syncope or other symptoms suggesting an inheritance. This history taking may include not only first or secondary degree relatives and but also often tedious and administrative efforts to search for older documents, medical records, military service tests like ECG and autopsy protocols. In families who have members who moved to other regions or emigrated from the country, this can be especially challenging. A portion of detective abilities and a critical approach to information from historical medical records or a patients' explanation to a sudden death may be unmasked by a pedigree of suspected HCM. In these efforts, a specialized health care provider trained in history taking, administrative paths and updated knowledge of genetic counselling including bioinformatics will be valuable in conjunction with the cardiologist.

## 4. Epidemiology

Since the first descriptions of hypertrophy of the heart, numerous labels have been used [2, 16]. Still hypertrophic *obstructive* cardiomyopathy is frequently used, sometimes to stress that an individual patient is symptomatic due to obstructive. While this can be illustrative in a case eligible for septal reductive procedures such as myectomy or alcohol ablation, it can often confuse health care providers, patients and relatives. Furthermore, since the dynamic state of the disease, it can be difficult to assess even though guidelines provide support for establishing degree of obstruction using pharmacological and physiological provocations of obstructiveness. Nowadays, guidelines recommend the usage of HCM and avoid former nomenclature [2].

In echocardiographic studies of populations in the USA, the prevalence of HCM is 1:500, which has been confirmed in other geographical parts of the world with highly available resources of diagnostic tools [17, 18]. Interestingly, also if patients without hypertrophy (phenotype) but who have mutations associated with HCM (genotype), the prevalence is 1:350 [19]. This makes HCM the most prevalent inherited myocardial disease. Because of the high prevalence, a basic knowledge about the disease is needed among a broad spectrum of heath care providers and managers.

The public awareness of HCM has been increased. This is probably due the journalistic attention to sudden death among young people especially during sport activities. In fact, in some countries and certain sport associations, screening of members of athletes is established. However, the approach to screening has been a matter of controversies and the benefits questioned and criticism of the resources it takes and the number of borderline cases that has to be evaluated and managed [20–23].

Nevertheless, HCM or at least unexplained post-mortem left ventricular hypertrophy is considered the most common cause of sudden cardiac death among sport persons younger than 35 years of age; HCM accounts for a half of the cases [24]. A historical perspective on this topic found HCM as a major cause of sudden death in the young [25]. A recent study in Denmark of all cases of SCD in the country reported a lower number [26]. From this Danish cohort, the cases of HCM were further analysed with regard to medical attention before death and about half of the cases had been evaluated for symptoms associated with HCM [26]. This stresses the importance of a qualified disease management including risk stratification of sudden cardiac death.

## 5. Pharmacological treatment

Recommendations of pharmacological treatment are based on smaller trials or empirical findings on HCM patients or evidence from other patient groups. No drug has been proven to reverse disease progression, but reduction in symptoms can often be achieved. Treatment strategies are based on whether the patient suffers from left ventricular outflow tract obstruc-

http://dx.doi.org/10.5772/65392

tion or not. A peak gradient of ≥30 mmHg is considered as obstruction, but one should bear in mind that this varies over time due to the hemodynamic situation [2].

The principle behind treatment options in patients with obstruction is to avoid severe dehydration with risk of low filling pressures, which could be deleterious for certain patients. Therefore, dehydration, drugs with vessel dilatation actions, or increase in heart rate is disadvantageous. Atrial arrhythmias are frequently encountered in HCM, and often a trigger of unbearable symptoms leads the patient to hospitalization. If the patient is admitted within 48 hours or properly anticoagulated, direct electrical conversion is preferred. However, this is often not the case. In such circumstances, beta-blockers are the drug of choice and digoxin should be avoided due to inotropic increase in myocardium [2].

The first-line treatment option is beta-blocking agents [2]. Notably, the beta-blocker carvedilol exerts vaso-dilating effects and should be avoided. Historically, propranolol was used, but nowadays metoprolol is often the drug of choice. Unfortunately, beta-blockers commonly imply side effects like cognitive impairment and exercise intolerance. This limit dosage titration and compliance to the drug may be questioned. It is important to recognize side effects and discuss alternatives rather than prompt withdrawal, which could possibly provoke worsening of symptoms and cause arrhythmias due to rebound effects on beta-receptors.

The calcium channel antagonist verapamil is often the drug of choice when beta-blockers are not reducing symptoms enough or not tolerated due to side effects. Diltiazem is an alternative choice but not dihydropyridine calcium antagonists because of their vascular effects. Contraindications of verapamil are systolic heart failure and conduction disturbances, i.e., bundle branch block.

The class 1A drug disopyramide has been studied in HCM cohorts and may relieve obstructive symptoms and are considered safe with regard to risk of ventricular arrhythmias. It can be prescribed in addition to beta-blockers. In practise, intolerance is frequent due to anticholinergic side effects (dry mucous membrane, urinary retention, and obstipation), and in some countries, it is not available.

In patients without obstructive component of HCM, the same principle to diminish relaxation disturbance of the left ventricle holds true. Loop diuretics and thiazides can be used without the same precautions as in HCM with obstruction. If disease progression reaches the crossroad with decreased systolic function with ejection fraction below 50%, treatment options include the same drugs as in heart failure due to other causes: beta-blockers, ACE/ARB-inhibitors, aldosterone receptor blockers, and diuretics.

## 6. Septal reduction therapy

In patients with symptoms due to pronounced obstruction (≥50 mmHg) despite pharmacological treatment, invasive options remain. Myectomy requires open-heart surgery and can be performed concomitant mitral plasty or replacement [27]. The incision is typically up to 70 mm and provides long-term success even though complications, i.e., atrioventricular block, aortic valve insufficiency, septal shunts occur. Perioperative death is 1–4% and increase with age, left atrial size, and female sex [28].

Alcohol septal ablation implies injection in an arterial branch with resulting necrosis and decreased obstruction. It is less invasive but requires careful judgement of the targeted vessel and still AV-block complications in up to 20% of patients in some series and overall mortality comparable to myectomy. Typically, alcohol ablation is the preferred method for older patients and can be performed multiple times in the same patient. It is important to stress that the decision to performed either alcohol septal ablation or myectomy should be done in centres with expertise in the field and adequate volumes.

There has been a preference of myectomy over alcohol ablation in the USA compared to Europe. The low number of myectomies in Europe has been criticized by experts [29].

Moreover, both myectomy and alcohol septal ablation result in scarring tissue, which have been reported to be a substrate for ventricular arrhythmias have been a matter of debate. However, in larger series, both methods seem to be safe at middle or long-term follow-ups even if individual risk stratification is important even after successful septum reduction procedure [30].

## 7. Pacemaker therapy

A pacemaker protects from bradycardia and is indicated in high degree AV-block, tachy-brady, and occasionally to reduce outflow gradients in patient where options are not suitable [2, 31]. Ventricular pacing from the right apical part may relieve obstruction by an electrical dyssynchrony between septal and lateral segments of the left ventricle. Earlier studies showed promising results, but current guidelines have constrained indications to include selected patients described above [2, 31, 32]. In the case of indication of an implantable cardioverter defibrillator (ICD) in patients with obstruction, patients should be considered for a dual chamber system for this reason.

Cardiac resynchronization therapy (CRT) has evaluated in smaller observational trial of HCM patients [33]. The experience is that it provides improved exercise capacity, functional class and ejection fraction, and biomarker levels. The vast experience and solid scientific ground of CRT treatment in patients with functional class II–IV, EF ≤ 35% despite optimal pharmacological treatment in left bundle branch block gives a rationale for usage in HCM patients with end-stage heart failure [31, 34, 35].

## 8. End-stage heart failure

Lowering EF is a predictor of worse outcome and is sometimes called 'burned-out HCM.' It is important to recognize the beginning of this stage and take prompt action including optimal pharmacologic treatments and device therapy. Notably, many patients have supernormal EF

http://dx.doi.org/10.5772/65392

for several years, and when EF is below 50%, this is a turning point. An EF < 50% also predicts risk of life threatening ventricular arrhythmias. This marks a risk for appropriate ICD therapy and should thus imply consideration for preventing sudden cardiac death [34, 35].

If not CRT is enough in end-stage heart failure due to HCM, the same approach as in life threatening heart failure should apply. Rarely, very small left ventricular chamber cavity or intractable ventricular arrhythmia situation without systolic dysfunction may be an indication. Totally, 1–7% of all transplants have HCM as the indication [36]. Left ventricular assist devices may be an option, and continuous axial flow assist therapy has shown promising results in a small series [37].

## 9. Risk assessment

HCM is heterogeneous disease in many aspects including the risk of sudden cardiac death. The combined risk of cardiovascular mortality is estimated to 6% per year [2]. The cardiovascular mortality constitutes heart failure, sudden cardiac death, and stroke. Many HCM cohorts from highly specialized centres do not necessarily reflect the mortality of the whole HCM population. In fact, a report with less selection bias reported a mortality of 2% [2]. In elderly patients, above 65 years old, the mortality is similar to age- and sex-matched population according to US data [2]. However, sudden cardiac death does occur at all ages and is notably high in early adulthood when sudden cardiac death otherwise is rare.

Survivors of cardiac arrest due to spontaneous ventricular fibrillation or sustained ventricular tachycardia with hemodynamic compromise have 33% mortality at seven years or 41% appropriate ICD therapy at five years [2, 38]. The survival after a cardiac arrest is approximately 10% in the general population. Because of the low chance of survival of cardiac arrest, these patients need an ICD. Thus, these patients are eligible for ICDs as secondary prevention of SCD, and the decision to implant is usually straight forward.

In patients who had not experienced a life threatening ventricular arrhythmia (primary prevention), the decision to implant an ICD requires careful judgement of clinical risk markers and consideration of comorbidities and risk of complications.

There have been three guidelines covering the complex task of ICD as primary prevention of SCD; a joint guideline between the American College of Cardiology/American Heart Association and European Society of Cardiology from 2003, an updated guideline 2011 from ACC/AHA and an ESC guideline launched in August 2014 [2, 39, 40]. The 2003 and 2011 guidelines provide readily evaluated risk factors from history taking, echocardiography and exercise test. Often, one risk factor is considered enough for offering an ICD, but there are differences between countries and centres. It has also not been conclusive if more than risk factor actually correlates with increased risk of appropriate ICD therapy even though more recent studies point in that direction. In addition, possible risk markers have been suggested based on observational studies on ICD cohorts or case reports or expert opinions.

According to guidelines from 2003 and 2011, five major risk factors are established: nonsustained ventricular tachycardia (NSVT), family history of sudden cardiac death (FHSCD), abnormal blood pressure response (ABPRE), unexplained syncope, and MWT 30 mm. A meta-analysis from 2010 based on 30 articles confirmed these risk factors [41]. From this meta-analysis, the presence of left ventricular outflow tract obstruction showed convincing evidence to support in association with SCD. There also seemed to be higher risk for younger patients even though there is no age above which could be safe, but SCD occurs at all ages in HCM [2]. Atrial dilatation and subsequent atrial fibrillation also correlated with SCD in some studies [2]. In patients with concomitant coronary ischemic disease, there was possibly an additional risk as well as in the small subset of patients with left ventricular apical aneurysms [2]. Genetic factors are indirectly included because of the risk factor FHSCD but guideline stress phenotype on an individual level; however, the presence of certain mutations, especially in the cases of double or multiple mutations, there seemed to be an increased risk. ECG is abnormal in 90% of HCM patients, and efforts have been made to correlate abnormalities to risk of SCD suggesting QRS amplitudes and/or fragmentation as risk markers [2]. However, ECG pattern has not been part of guidelines. SCD in athletes due to HCM is well known, and 2003 guideline considered intense (competitive) physical exertion a possible risk factor [39]. Fibrosis assessed on CMR has been studied is advocated as risk factor but is not yet part of guidelines [42, 43].

The evolving criticism on guidelines resulted in a completely new algorithm to assess 5-year risk of SCD in HCM [44]. The article preceding the guidelines change in August 2014 argued that previous guideline considered the clinical parameters left ventricular hypertrophy as binary (30 mm), and in the new guideline, it is treated as continuous [2]. They also included age as the validation work was based on cohorts where risk was higher in the young. Atrial enlargement was again considered a risk factor and included in the algorithm are treated as a continuous variable. The new European algorithm is based on 3,675 patients from six centres and follow-up time of more than 24,000 patient years. One of the centres constituted an external validation. Since the introduction of the 2014 ESC guidelines, external validation work has been published [45]. These two reports support for using the new guidelines. The sophisticated statistics behind the new guideline resulting in a formula with a prognostic index as an exponential function have been overcome by an open access link where a clinician within a few minutes can calculate 5-year risk in an individual patient [2, 46]. However, one should consider the aim of the new guidelines carefully and recognize its limitations. The authors of the new algorithm considered the rationale for the new approach because previous guideline would lead to overuse of ICD; many patients would experience harm of the ICD and never have benefit of the device. One should bear in mind that the underlying patient cohorts were adults and risk stratification in children and adolescent should be used with caution. Hypertrophic as part of metabolic disease or syndromes were not part of study base. Paradoxically, extreme left myocardial thickness 35 mm had low SCD risk, but this subset of patient was few and the model does not seem to cover all ranges. Furthermore, the model does not take into account the obstruction only at exercise but at rest.

Even though the new model has been widely recognized, it is still unclear to what degree it is actually used globally. Recently, an independent assessment of the ESC risk model concluded

http://dx.doi.org/10.5772/65392

that the model was unreliable because many patients with SCD or appropriate ICD therapy had a low risk score. The implementation of new guidelines may take time or require further refinement. Probably it will not replace previous strategies completely but serve as important tool. Risk stratification is and will always be a complex task.

## 10. Age and gender

Most studies found no significant association with age and sudden death in HCM cohorts, but these studies are typically ICD populations selected from tertiary centres [47]. Furthermore, usually these studies do not take age- and sex-matched comparison with general population into account. Many studies on ICD cohorts lack statistical power to detect differences at different age strata. In two studies, there was an inverse relationship between age and sudden cardiac death, but in the majority of studies, no association was demonstrated [2]. In a recently published nationwide Swedish study without selection, bias age was not significantly associated with appropriate ICD therapy [34, 35]. In American guidelines, age is not part of risk stratification, whereas in the European guidelines, age is part of the equation based on validation of cohorts, which showed an increased risk in younger patients [2]. The association between age and other risk factors is quite complicated, but there seems to be data supporting the rationale for offering ICDs with NSVT, severe left ventricular hypertrophy (LVH) and unexplained syncope in younger patients [2]. Age is further complicated by the individual comorbidities and the discrepancy between biological and calendric age. From other guidelines on general ICD candidates, guidelines state at least 2 years of life expectancy to be eligible for an ICD. An experienced clinician may reflect about age in the individual case but cannot neglect local resources and risk of complications in addition to effective patient communication on prognosis.

Most HCM cohorts have a majority of males. In the six cohorts in the ESC risk algorithm, the proportion of males ranged from 59 to 72% (mean 64%) [2]. This pattern is also seen in several ICD cohorts [34, 35, 47]. However, there does not seem to be a significant difference with regard to risk of appropriate ICD therapy in these cohorts. It is important to recognize the individual risk factor profile rather than gender itself. Neither previous nor current guidelines use gender as part of risk stratification. Notably, females may have a higher risk for complications related to the ICD system [47].

## 11. Nonsustained ventricular tachycardia (NSVT)

The presence of NSVT has been part on guidelines since it first appeared in 2003 after several reports on the association to sudden cardiac death in HCM. This is in contrast to general ICD population with ischemic or dilated CM with low EF in which NSVT is not part of guidelines The definition of NSVT is at least three beats in a row of ventricular origin but varies with regard to cycle length; the formal cut-off of 100 bpm is seldom used, and 120 or 150 bpm is typically used [2]. The association of life threatening arrhythmias does not seem to vary with length or cycle length. The maximal duration of NSVT is 30 seconds while longer duration is called sustained ventricular tachycardia. The diagnosis of NSVT could be from an ambulatory monitor such as Holter for 24–48 hours as prescribed in the evaluation of HCM patients. However, sometimes NSVT is detected from telemetry in the ward or from a cardiac device, i.e., a pacemaker EGM or implantable loop recorder. Interestingly, NSVT seems to be quite common in ICD recipients. Thus, the more often a HCM patient is monitored for NSVT, the higher the likelihood for detecting the risk factor NSVT. Prolonged monitoring with implantable devices or non-invasive ECG patches is currently not indicated without a history of syncope but remains to be evaluated in the future.

## 12. Syncope

Syncope deserves special attention when it comes to interviewing the patient about the actual episode. This includes observations from witness about duration (which often may be overestimated) and signs before or after the loss of consciousness. Certain situations may be typical for vaso-vagal syncope (i.e., defection, micturition), situational or orthostatic hypotension. Carotid sinus mechanism for syncope can sometimes be reproduced. The body position and activity may aid important clues. If exercise-induced syncope is experienced, this should imply prompt evaluation because a malignant cause is likely. Notably, tiredness and seizure may indicate epilepsy but do not rule out cardiac causes as severe cerebral hypoxia mimics the clinical scenario. In some studies, unexplained syncope within six months seems to predict worse outcome to higher extent [2]. Nevertheless, a syncopal episode suggestive or arrhythmic cause independent of when it happened should warrant careful evaluation.

## 13. Family history

A family history of SCD is a dramatic event. Relatives of the victim have to deal with their own attitude and subsequent risk assessment beside emotional impact of the lost relative. Unfortunately, not every physician is aware of the inheritance component in family of SCD or the family does not seek medical advice due to this. Documentation from possibly related HCM is often lacking, misinterpreted or unavailable. Current European guidelines state SCD in the first-degree relative before the age of 40, but no age cut-off when SCD can be attributed to HCM [2]. The underlying studies are quite heterogeneous using different age limit. This risk factor is further complicated as it does not take into account second- or third-degree relatives nor the number of siblings in a family. It is understandable that the motivation for patient and clinicians is usually high when there is case of SCD in the family. However, the scientific basis is less strong than for NSVT, unexplained syncope, or MWT, based on three studies, whereas several other studies could not prove an association [2, 48]. If this inability is due to power problems of studies because of the limited number of patients included and/or few outcome of events, is difficult to judge. The heterogeneity of definitions and relative short follow-up time may

http://dx.doi.org/10.5772/65392

also influence the results. Statistical methods often account for uni- and multi-variable influence of risk factors but have difficulties to prove interaction between risk factors in smaller samples with few events.

## 14. Wall thickness

In patients with a ≥30 mm maximal wall thickness, there was a three-fold increased risk, which makes it a comparatively strong risk factor. Later analyses suggest a U-shaped correlation to sudden cardiac death [49]. As mentioned above, this risk factor has been treated as binary risk factor previously, at least theoretically, but in practise, it is likely that number patients have been offered an ICD even if they did not fulfil this criterion formally. For example, in a 25-year-old patient with otherwise long-life expectancy, a 29 mm thickness would probably be enough for most clinicians. Another limit is the fact that hypertrophy can be more or less unevenly distributed, and it is not known if this influences risk. Moreover, echocardiography does not always provide accurate estimations and certain parts, i.e., apical parts may be difficult to trace. Other imaging techniques may resolve this problem in individuals. The progression of disease is difficult to predict, but in a young patient, it is more likely and effect of hypertensive disease is more easy to rule out. Future validation work on this risk factor will hopefully elucidate this factor better. Here, CMR and PET may add important knowledge of not only structural findings but also functional and metabolic disturbances associated with risk of arrhythmia.

## 15. Exercise blood pressure response

The assessment of this risk factor requires referral for ergometer bicycle test or any other exercise test. In series of HCM patients, one third of patients show abnormal blood pressure response [2, 50]. The definition of abnormal blood pressure response varies, but with regard to risk stratification, a failure to increase systolic pressure at least 20 mmHg or a fall of 20 mmHg from peak pressure is considered relevant [2]. This risk factor seems to be more pronounced in patients younger than 40 years old. In some studies, this risk factor has not been analysed because not all patients were systematically assessed. This is understandable as if a clinician already has data enough to support the decision to implant an ICD, there is a rationale for omitting this test as is does not add clinical insight for further management of the individual patient. In the new guidelines, the authors took the decision to abandon exercise test as part of risk stratification, and it remains to be seen if upcoming guidelines will stick to this policy.

## 16. Atrial fibrillation and left atrial diameter

The increased filling pressures of the left ventricle will result in wall stress of left atrium and risk of dilatation. There is a well-known risk of atrial fibrillation and a dilated left atrium, and this in turn increases risk of embolic events. In a recent study, AF was a stronger risk factor than the established five major risk factors in both univariable and multivariable analyses in HCM-ICD cohort [34, 35]. AF should be considered as a sole factor for risk stratification and lead to an ICD, but in patients implanted based on the five major risk factors, AF predicted high probability of appropriate ICD therapy [2, 34, 35].

Left atrial diameter is assessed by echocardiography using a parasternal projection and is now part of the risk model algorithm [46]. It is handled as a continuous variable, but it does not take into account the different shapes of the atrium as some patients have elongated atrium mostly visualized in an apical four-chamber view. Neither is the volume calculated, but a simple diameter in one projection sometimes allows inter-user variability and anatomical variation difficult to standardize.

## 17. LVOT obstruction

The outflow gradient of the left chamber may vary and change with exercise or can be provoked by drugs. In the meta-analysis, they concluded that LVOT gradient should be reassessed as a risk factor based on evidence from numerous observational studies [41, 51, 52]. This also holds true when developing the new algorithm and was then included and treated as a continuous variable.

## 18. CMR, CT and PET

Cardiac magnetic resonance using a contrast-enhanced technique has demonstrated association with arrhythmias, and substantial amount of fibrosis may be suggestive increased risk for SCD [53]. The accurate delineation and spatial resolution of CMR may aid in cases where echocardiography is inadequate. However, to assess association between CMR-derived baseline data and outcome such as SCD or appropriate ICD therapy will follow-up time and large cohorts with enough events to prove association. Therefore, CMR has been included in the first prospective registry on HCM patients, and this will hopefully provide gain of insight in this matter. CMR uses magnetic fields instead of ionizing radiation, but contraindication needs to be considered. Notably, ICD patients should be assessed before a device is implanted even though newer ICD model may allow CMR at least 1.5 Tesla investigations but gives rise to artefacts. PET can be used in conjunction within either CT or CMR and is a promising field for research with functional, structural and metabolic assessment, which is available.

## 19. Driving

While most HCM patients have no driving restrictions, patients with ICD devices need special considerations. This advice needs to be in harmony with national laws besides checking

http://dx.doi.org/10.5772/65392

international guidelines that provide update recommendation on this topic. A survivor of cardiac arrest should not drive for the first six months after the event, and careful assessment of cognitive function is then advised. The same considerations should be made after stroke, epilepsy, diabetes and other medical conditions. The risk after an arrhythmic event is highest in the first few months, which makes six-month restriction reasonably. In primary prevention of ICD patients, there is no restriction except for unexplained syncope with a typical restriction in the first 6 months. Professional driving (buss, truck, taxi) is not accepted for ICD carriers, independent of indication (primary or secondary) in most countries. Other vehicles, including trains and aeroplanes, need to be considered and legal actions taken.

## 20. Pregnancy

Pregnancy implies increased loading pressures, and in last semester, a cardiovascular demand may increase risk. HCM is a heterogeneous disease, and risk of SCD during pregnancy needs to be addressed based on individual factors. Few women need to give up a wish to become a biological mother; however, there are fatal cases reported, but these have been in patients with a known high risk. Because of the non-negligible risk, females are advised to plan pregnancy and counselling should be offered during the pregnancy and delivery by a multidisciplinary team. In the rare case of need for ICD implant during pregnancy, efforts need to be taken to provide protection from radiation or using echocardiography to assess position of leads.

## 21. Combinations of risk markers and modifiers

The new algorithm takes several risk factors into account and weights them using a formula [46]. But even this method has the same lack of accurate estimation of mediating or possibly protective interaction between markers. All markers are somewhat surrogates and life-time risk can never be exactly assessed in the individual. Long-term follow-up in all studies is actually typically less than 10 years for the majority of the patient, and risk is not linear. Besides, risk markers are assessed at the time for decision to implant and may change during the course and should therefore be re-assessed every 1–3 years. Again, a multicentre, international, prospective registry will provide more insights in the challenge to stratify risk in HCM.

## 22. Children

Risk stratification in children equals adult strategy in many ways, but primary prevention is typically based on two or more risk factors rather than one. Historically, epicardial lead has been used in a growing child, but nowadays subcutaneous ICD may be a more attractive option. A single device (ICD-VVI) is usually sufficient as pacing indication is rare in the young, and this approach seems to limit complications.

## 23. ICD therapy

ICD is an effective way to prevent sudden cardiac death in HCM. The landmark trial by Maron et al. demonstrated 11% annual rate in secondary and 5% annual rate in primary prevention [54]. Several studies have confirmed the usefulness on ICD in HCM [47]. Schinkel et al. performed a meta-analysis of 2,190 patients from 16 cohorts (mean age 42 years, 62% males) with 83% primary prevention indication [47]. The summary estimate for appropriate ICD therapy was 3.3% per year (95% confidence interval 2.2–4.4%). A later nationwide ICD cohort of unselected patients reported 4.5% appropriate ICD therapy in primary prevention and 7.0% in secondary prevention [34, 35].

It should be noted that *not* every appropriate ICD therapy is indeed lifesaving. A ventricular arrhythmia can self-terminate, which can lead to an overestimation of benefit of ICD. Therefore, it is important to programme a number of intervals to at least 30 before therapy. The detection zones should be carefully considered, and antitachycardia pacing (ATP) should be used to avoid unnecessary shocks. However, the risk of a sustained ventricular below detection zone could lead to fatal hemodynamic collapse including pulseless electrical tachycardia or recurrent ventricular fibrillation when ventricles are finally exhausted. Patients on amiodarone are known to have a slower rate than otherwise [2]. Earlier there have been worries about the efficacy in hypertrophic heart due to increased myocardial mass to discharge, but large series of a patient show efficacy of ICD discharges with very few exceptions. The discussion on DFT testing preoperatively could be extended to HCM populations, but the trend to induce patients more rarely, if at all, will continue for HCM patients. One may argue that induction is not without risk; devices have high voltage and sufficient margin, and the clinical situation is not exactly the same as during implant. Moreover, it may be advisable to choose a type and brand of ICD device capable of wave form optimization and to deliver high voltage discharges. Different devices offer different solutions to avoid T-wave oversense, which should be reflected upon. A T-wave oversense leads to double counting and will deliver inappropriate shocks. Technical failure of lead, fracture and insulation defects, or external noise could lead inappropriate shocks. The overall annual risk of inappropriate shocks is 4.8% in a meta-analysis [47] and confirmed in later analyses of unselected populations [55]. Hopefully, with programming optimization, this could likely be reduced. The most common cause of inappropriate shocks is atrial arrhythmias, predominantly. In addition to programming longer duration, longer cycle length, discrimination algorithm should be considered such as interval stability, but one should neglect the risk of misdiagnosis simultaneous ventricular arrhythmias that need appropriate therapy. Furthermore, other actions to avoid atrial tachycardia and to reduce rapid atrioventricular conduction are needed: beta-blockers, antiarrhythmics, and occasionally His-ablation.

Compared to other ICD populations where ATP is effective in a vast majority of cases, the proportion of ATP success was less in HCM-ICD cohorts. This has been seen in other HCM trials, and HCM possibly carries an increased risk of rapid ventricular tachycardia or ventricular fibrillation to a larger extent than other ICD groups.

ICD systems offer an alert function for the patient if technical failure or essential clinical episode takes place. Remote monitoring of ICD devices is standard, and this increases safety

http://dx.doi.org/10.5772/65392

as it detects technical problems between follow-ups in clinic or detects atrial fibrillation, which implies decision to anticoagulated.

## 24. Death despite ICD

The efficacy of ICDs to prevent sudden cardiac death leads to a swift in cases of death. The vast majority of death in the ICD population dies because of progressive heart failure. The standardized mortality was 3.4 (95% confidence interval 2.4–4.5) compared to general population [56]. This implies that heart failure care needs to be addressed if improved survival should be achieved. Importantly, a holistic approach to device patient is warranted, and one should not just focus on the prevention of arrhythmia death.

## 25. Implant procedure

The procedure to implant an ICD in a HCM patient is essentially the same as in other indication. The vascular access is typically from the left side either through cephalic cut-down or punctures of the axillary or subclavian vein. The ventricular lead is implanted in the apical region of the right ventricle if R-waves and thresholds are acceptable in this position. It is important to check for T-wave oversensing before deciding the final position of the lead. In obstructive HCM, it is of special importance to implant the lead in apex as this could facilitate reduction in outflow gradient if AV-pacing is tried. For the same reason, an atrial lead (ICD-DR) is often preferred. Furthermore, many HCM patients have high beta-blocking dosage, conduction defects or paroxysmal atrial fibrillation with the help of AV synchronous pacing. The ventricle lead could be either single or dual coil. There is a tendency to increased use of single-coil system as possible defibrillation threshold difference is negligible, easier to implant and extract. The device could be implanted subcutaneously or intramuscular. As described above, less number of patients is induced nowadays. The typical procedure time is less than 1 hour, and the patient can often be discharged the same day. The battery of an ICD in a modern system lasts for 8–10 years, depending on amount pacing and, in few cases, the demand of therapies. CRT system in end-stage HCM has been tried with preliminary promising results.

## 26. Health-related quality of life

In a British study from 1995 on HCM patients, health-related quality of life was decreased [57]. Since then, improvement of health care has been made, and there may be different outcomes in a HCM population that is not selected from a specialized centre. Recently, a study on HCM patients with ICDs confirmed poor quality of life, regardless of sex, age, or primary/secondary indication [58]. Instead, atrial fibrillation and systolic heart failure are determinants of poor quality of life, especially physical aspects. Notably, inappropriate, but appropriate therapies are associated with poorer mental health. To further address quality of life issues, qualitative studies may provide valuable insights.

## 27. S-ICD

An subcutaneous-ICD (S-ICD) system contains a subcutaneously implanted lead (in an L-configuration) connected to a device inserted subcutaneously, or preferably intramuscular. It effectively terminates ventricular arrhythmias and can offer supportive post-chock pacing. Current devices cannot be used in patients who need permanent pacing, but technical solutions are developed to combine a leadless pacemaker system communicating with an S-ICD system. This is beneficial in patients with abnormal vascular anatomy, i.e., malformations or vessel occlusions. But, in young patient, there is an increasing interest in S-ICD to save vessels for future interventions and avoid short-term and long-term vessel-related complications. S-ICD has been used in HCM, but careful pre-operative assessment of possibly risk of T-wave oversense is of importance in this group. The cost of S-ICD device is currently much larger than for transvenous device, but this probably diminishes. Studies so far have shown a promising short-term use of S-ICD among HCM patients [59].

## 28. Future perspectives

There remain many challenges in the field of HCM. A detailed understanding of pathophysiologic mechanism of disease progression, arrhythmia substrate and triggers and molecular-genetic base of the heterogeneous disease is crucial. This could lead to improvement in the therapeutic arsenal, but this development relies on scientific progress in the field of cardiology and basic sciences. Multicentre, prospective registries and other international collaborations to evaluate outcome and refine risk stratification are promising [60, 61].

## Author details

Peter Magnusson

Address all correspondence to: peter.magnusson@regiongavleborg.se

1 Cardiology Research Unit, Department of Medicine, Karolinska Institute, Karolinska University Hospital, Solna, Stockholm, Sweden

2 Centre for Research and Development, Uppsala University/Region Gävleborg, Gävle, Sweden

## References

[1] Elliott P, Andersson B, Arbustini E, Bilinska Z, Cecchi F, Charron P, Dubourg O, Kühl U, Maisch B, McKenna WJ, Monserrat L, Pankuweit S, Rapezzi C, Seferovic P, Tavazzi L, Keren A. Classification of the cardiomyopathies: a position statement from the European Society of Cardiology Working Group on Myocardial and Pericardial Diseases. Eur Heart J. 2008;29(2):270-6. DOI: 10.1093/eurheartj/ehm342

[2] Elliott PM, Anastasakis A, Borger MA, Borggrefe M, Cecchi F, Charron P, Hagege AA, Lafont A, Limongelli G, Mahrholdt H, McKenna WJ, Mogensen J, Nihoyannopoulos P, Nistri S, Pieper PG, Pieske B, Rapezzi C, Rutten FH, Tillmanns C, Watkins H. 2014 ESC Guidelines on diagnosis and management of hypertrophic cardiomyopathy: the Task Force for the Diagnosis and Management of Hypertrophic Cardiomyopathy of the European Society of Cardiology (ESC). Eur Heart J. 2014;35(39):2733-79. DOI: 10.1093/eurheartj/ehu284

[3] Kampmann C, Wiethoff CM, Wenzel A, Stolz G, Betancor M, Wippermann CF, Huth RG, Habermehl P, Knuf M, Emschermann T, Stopfkuchen H. Normal values of M mode echocardiographic measurements of more than 2000 healthy infants and children in central Europe. Heart. 2000;83(6):667-72. DOI: 10.1136/heart.83.6.667

[4] Cardim N, Galderisi M, Edvardsen T, Plein S, Popescu BA, D'Andrea A, Bruder O, Cosyns B, Davin L, Donal E, Freitas A, Habib G, Kitsiou A, Petersen SE, Schroeder S, Lancellotti P, Camici P, Dulgheru R, Hagendorff A, Lombardi M, Muraru D, Sicari R. Role of multimodality cardiac imaging in the management of patients with hypertrophic cardiomyopathy: an expert consensus of the European Association of Cardiovascular Imaging Endorsed by the Saudi Heart Association. Eur Heart J Cardiovasc Imaging. 2015;16(3):280. DOI: 10.1093/ehjci/jeu291

[5] Kawarai H, Kajimoto K, Minami Y, et al. Risk of sudden death in end-stage hypertrophic cardiomyopathy. J Card Fail. 2011;17:459-64.

[6] Biagini E, Coccolo F, Ferlito M, et al. Dilated-hypokinetic evolution of hypertrophic cardiomyopathy: prevalence, incidence, risk factors, and prognostic implications in pediatric and adult patients. J Am Coll Cardiol. 2005;46:1543-50.

[7] Harris KM, Spirito P, Maron MS, et al. Prevalence, clinical profile, and significance of left ventricular remodeling in the end-stage phase of hypertrophic cardiomyopathy. Circulation. 2006;114:216-25.

[8] Melacini P, Basso C, Angelini A, et al. Clinicopathological profiles of progressive heart failure in hypertrophic cardiomyopathy. Eur Heart J. 2010;31:2111-23.

[9] Williams L, Frenneaux M. Syncope in hypertrophic cardiomyopathy: mechanisms and consequences for treatment. Europace. 2007;9(9):817-22. DOI: 10.1093/europace/eum093

[10] Guttmann OP, Rahman MS, O'Mahony C, Anastasakis A, Elliott PM. Atrial fibrillation and thromboembolism in patients with hypertrophic cardiomyopathy: systematic review. Heart. 2014;100(6):465-72. DOI: 10.1136/heartjnl-2013-304276

[11] Guttmann OP, Pavlou M, O'Mahony C, Monserrat L, Anastasakis A, Rapezzi C, Biagini E, Gimeno JR, Limongelli G, Garcia-Pavia P, McKenna WJ, Omar RZ, Elliott PM, Hypertrophic Cardiomyopathy Outcomes Investigators. Prediction of thrombo-embolic risk in patients with hypertrophic cardiomyopathy (HCM Risk-CVA). Eur J Heart Fail. 2015;17(8):837-45. DOI: 10.1002/ejhf.316.

[12] Lopes LR, Rahman MS, Elliott PM. A systematic review and meta-analysis of genotype-phenotype associations in patients with hypertrophic cardiomyopathy caused by sarcomeric protein mutations. Heart. 2013;99(24):1800-11. DOI: 10.1136/heartjnl-2013-303939.

[13] Morita H, Nagai R, Seidman JG, et al. The impact of genetic testing on hypertrophic cardiomyopathy and heart failure. J Cardiovasc Transl Res. 2010;3:297-303.

[14] Bos JM, Towbin JA, Ackerman MJ, et al. Diagnostic, prognostic, and therapeutic implications of genetic testing for hypertrophic cardiomyopathy. J Am Coll Cardiol. 2009;54:201-11.

[15] Sébillon P, Bouchier C, Bidot LD, Bonne G, Ahamed K, Charron P, Drouin-Garraud V, Millaire A, Desrumeaux G, Benaïche A, Charniot JC, Schwartz K, Villard E, Komajda M. Expanding the phenotype of LMNA mutations in dilated cardiomyopathy and functional consequences of these mutations. J Med Genet. 2003;40(8):560-7.

[16] Teare D. Asymmetrical hypertrophy of the heart in young adults. Br Heart J. 1958;20:1-18.

[17] Maron BJ, Gardin JM, Flack JM, Gidding SS, Kurosaki TT, Bild DE. Prevalence of hypertrophic cardiomyopathy in a general population of young adults. Echocardio-graphic analysis of 4111 subjects in the CARDIA study. Coronary artery risk develop-ment in (Young) adults. Circulation. 1995;92(4):785-9.

[18] Corrado D, Basso C, Schiavon M, Thiene G. Screening for hypertrophic cardiomyop-athy in young athletes. N Engl J Med. 1998;339(6):364-9.

[19] Semsarian C, Ingles J, Maron MS, Maron BJ. New perspectives on the prevalence of hypertrophic cardiomyopathy. J Am Coll Cardiol. 2015;65(12):1249-54. DOI: 10.1016/j.jacc.2015.01.019.

[20] Caselli S, Maron MS, Urbano-Moral JA, Pandian NG, Maron BJ, Pelliccia A. Differen-tiating left ventricular hypertrophy in athletes from that in patients with hypertrophic cardiomyopathy. Am J Cardiol. 2014;114(9):1383-9. DOI: 10.1016/j.amjcard.2014.07.070

[21] Ostman-Smith I. Sudden cardiac death in young athletes. Open Access J Sports Med. 2011;2:85-97. DOI: 10.2147/OAJSM.S10675.

[22] Maron BJ, Haas TS, Doerer JJ, Thompson PD, Hodges JS. Comparison of U.S. and Italian experiences with sudden cardiac deaths in young competitive athletes and implications for preparticipation screening strategies. Am J Cardiol. 2009;104(2):276-80. DOI: 10.1016/j.amjcard.2009.03.037

[23] Pelliccia A, Zipes DP, Maron BJ. Bethesda Conference #36 and the European Society of Cardiology Consensus Recommendations revisited a comparison of U.S. and European criteria for eligibility and disqualification of competitive athletes with cardiovascular abnormalities. J Am Coll Cardiol. 2008;52(24):1990-6. DOI: 10.1016/j.jacc.2008.08.055

[24] Maron BJ, Epstein SE, Roberts WC. Hypertrophic cardiomyopathy: a common cause of sudden death in the young competitive athlete. Eur Heart J. 1983;4 (Suppl F):135-44.

[25] Maron BJ. Historical perspectives on sudden deaths in young athletes with evolution over 35 years. Am J Cardiol. 2015;116(9):1461-8. DOI: 10.1016/j.amjcard.2015.07.072.

[26] Lynge TH, Risgaard B, Jabbari R, Glinge C, Bundgaard H, Maron B, Haunsø S, Winkel BG, Tfelt-Hansen J. Cardiac symptoms before sudden cardiac death caused by hypertrophic cardiomyopathy: a nationwide study among the young in Denmark. Europace. 2016 Jan 27. pii: euv403. [Epub ahead of print]

[27] Yu EH, Omran AS, Wigle ED, Williams WG, Siu SC, Rakowski H. Mitral regurgitation in hypertrophic obstructive cardiomyopathy: relationship to obstruction and relief with myectomy. J Am Coll Cardiol. 2000;36(7):2219-25

[28] Desai MY, Bhonsale A, Smedira NG, Naji P, Thamilarasan M, Lytle BW, Lever HM. Predictors of long-term outcomes in symptomatic hypertrophic obstructive cardiomyopathy patients undergoing surgical relief of left ventricular outflow tract obstruction. Circulation. 2013;128(3):209-16. DOI: 10.1161/CIRCULATIONAHA

[29] Maron BJ, Yacoub M, Dearani JA. Controversies in cardiovascular medicine. Benefits of surgery in obstructive hypertrophic cardiomyopathy: bring septal myectomy back for European patients. Eur Heart J. 2011;32(9):1055-8. DOI: 10.1093/eurheartj/ehr006.

[30] Jensen MK, Prinz C, Horstkotte D, van Buuren F, Bitter T, Faber L, Bundgaard H. Alcohol septal ablation in patients with hypertrophic obstructive cardiomyopathy: low incidence of sudden cardiac death and reduced risk profile. Heart. 2013;99(14):1012-7. DOI: 10.1136/heartjnl-2012-303339.

[31] Brignole M, Auricchio A, Baron-Esquivias G, Bordachar P, Boriani G, Breithardt OA, Cleland J, Deharo JC, Delgado V, Elliott PM, Gorenek B, Israel CW, Leclercq C, Linde C, Mont L, Padeletti L, Sutton R, Vardas PE. 2013 ESC guidelines on cardiac pacing and cardiac resynchronization therapy: the task force on cardiac pacing and resynchronization therapy of the European Society of Cardiology (ESC). Developed in collaboration with the European Heart Rhythm Association (EHRA). Europace. 2013;15(8):1070-118. DOI: 10.1093/europace/eut206.

[32] Jurado Román A, Montero Cabezas JM, Rubio Alonso B, García Tejada J, Hernández Hernández F, Albarrán González-Trevilla A, Velázquez Martín MT, Coma Samartín R,

Rodríguez García J, Tascón Pérez JC. Sequential atrioventricular pacing in patients with hypertrophic cardiomyopathy: an 18-year experience. Rev Esp Cardiol (Engl Ed). 2016;69(4):377-83. DOI: 10.1016/j.rec.2015.08.023.

[33] Rogers DP, Marazia S, Chow AW, Lambiase PD, Lowe MD, Frenneaux M, et al. Effect of biventricular pacing on symptoms and cardiac remodelling in patients with end-stage hypertrophic cardiomyopathy. Eur J Heart Fail. 2008;10:507-13.

[34] Ponikowski P, Voors AA, Anker SD, Bueno H, Cleland JG, Coats AJ, Falk V, González-Juanatey JR, Harjola VP, Jankowska EA, Jessup M, Linde C, Nihoyannopoulos P, Parissis JT, Pieske B, Riley JP, Rosano GM, Ruilope LM, Ruschitzka F, Rutten FH, van der Meer P; Authors/Task Force Members; Document Reviewers. 2016 ESC Guidelines for the diagnosis and treatment of acute and chronic heart failure: the Task Force for the diagnosis and treatment of acute and chronic heart failure of the European Society of Cardiology (ESC). Developed with the special contribution of the Heart Failure Association (HFA) of the ESC. Eur J Heart Fail. 2016;18(8):891-975. DOI: 10.1002/ejhf.592.

[35] Magnusson P, Gadler F, Liv P, Mörner S. Risk markers and appropriate implantable defibrillator therapy in hypertrophic cardiomyopathy. Pacing Clin Electrophysiol. 2016;39(3):291-301. DOI: 10.1111/pace.12801

[36] Kato TS, Takayama H, Yoshizawa S, Marboe C, Schulze PC, Farr M, Naka Y, Mancini D, Maurer MS. Cardiac transplantation in patients with hypertrophic cardiomyopathy. Am J Cardiol. 2012;110(4):568-74. DOI: 10.1016/j.amjcard.2012.04.030. Epub 15 May 2012.

[37] Wynne E, Bergin JD, Ailawadi G, Kern JA, Kennedy JL. Use of a left ventricular assist device in hypertrophic cardiomyopathy. J Card Surg. 2011;26(6):663-5. DOI: 10.1111/j.1540-8191.2011.01331.x.

[38] Maron BJ, Spirito P, Shen WK, Haas TS, Formisano F, Link MS, Epstein AE, Almquist AK, Daubert JP, Lawrenz T, Boriani G, Estes NA 3rd, Favale S, Piccininno M, Winters SL, Santini M, Betocchi S, Arribas F, Sherrid MV, Buja G, Semsarian C, Bruzzi P. Implantable cardioverter-defibrillators and prevention of sudden cardiac death in hypertrophic cardiomyopathy. JAMA. 2007;298(4):405-12

[39] Maron BJ, McKenna WJ, Danielson GK, et al. American College of Cardiology/European Society of Cardiology clinical expert consensus document on hypertrophic cardiomyopathy. A report of the American College of Cardiology Foundation Task Force on clinical expert consensus documents and the European Society of Cardiology Committee for practice guidelines. J Am Coll Cardiol. 2003;42:1687-713.

[40] Gersh BJ, Maron BJ, Bonow RO, et al. 2011 ACCF/AHA Guideline for the diagnosis and treatment of hypertrophic cardiomyopathy: a report of the American College of Cardiology Foundation/American Heart Association Task Force on Practice Guidelines developed in collaboration with the American Association for Thoracic Surgery, American Society of Echocardiography, American

Society of Nuclear Cardiology, Heart Failure Society of America, Heart Rhythm Society, Society for Cardiovascular Angiography and Interventions, and Society of Thoracic Surgeons. J Am Coll Cardiol. 2011;58:e212-60.

[41] Christiaans I, van Engelen K, van Langen IM, et al. Risk stratification for sudden cardiac death in hypertrophic cardiomyopathy: systematic review of clinical risk markers. Europace. 2010;12:313-21.

[42] Bruder O, Wagner A, Jensen CJ, et al. Myocardial scar visualized by cardiovascular magnetic resonance imaging predicts major adverse events in patients with hypertrophic cardiomyopathy. J Am Coll Cardiol. 2010;56:875-87.

[43] Chan RH, Maron BJ, Olivotto I, Pencina MJ, Assenza GE, Haas T, et al. Prognostic value of quantitative contrast-enhanced cardiovascular magnetic resonance for the evaluation of sudden death risk in patients with hypertrophic cardiomyopathy. Circulation. 2014;130:484-95.

[44] O'Mahony C, Jichi F, Pavlou M, Monserrat L, Anastasakis A, Rapezzi C, Biagini E, Gimeno JR, Limongelli G, McKenna WJ, Omar RZ, Elliott PM, Hypertrophic Cardiomyopathy Outcomes Investigators. A novel clinical risk prediction model for sudden cardiac death in hypertrophic cardiomyopathy (HCM risk-SCD). Eur Heart J. 2014;35(30):2010-20. DOI: 10.1093/eurheartj/eht439.

[45] Vriesendorp PA, Schinkel AFL, Liebregts M, Willems R, Ten Cate FJ, Van Cleemput J, et al. Independent validation of the novel clinical risk prediction model for sudden cardiac death in hypertrophic cardiomyopathy (HCM Risk-SCD). Eur Heart J. 2014;35(Suppl 1):210.

[46] European Society of Cardiology. HCM Risk-SCD Calculator. 2014. Available at: www.doc2do.com/hcm/webHCM.html

[47] Schinkel AF, Vriesendorp PA, Sijbrands EJ, Jordaens LJ, ten Cate FJ, Michels M. Outcome and complications after implantable cardioverter defibrillator therapy in hypertrophic cardiomyopathy: systematic review and meta-analysis. Circ Heart Fail. 2012;5(5):552-9

[48] Watkinson OT, Elliott PM. A family history of sudden death should not be a primary indication for an implantable cardioverter defibrillator in hypertrophic cardiomyopathy. Can J Cardiol. 2015;31(11):1407-9. DOI: 10.1016/j.cjca.2015.07.724

[49] O'Mahony C, Jichi F, Monserrat L, Ortiz-Genga M, Anastasakis A, Rapezzi C, Biagini E, Gimeno JR, Limongelli G, McKenna WJ, Omar RZ, Elliott PM, Hypertrophic Cardiomyopathy Outcomes Investigators. Inverted U-shaped relation between the risk of sudden cardiac death and maximal left ventricular wall thickness in hypertrophic cardiomyopathy. Circ Arrhythm Electrophysiol. 2016 Jun;9(6). pii: e003818. doi: 10.1161/CIRCEP.115.003818.

[50] Coats CJ, Rantell K, Bartnik A, Patel A, Mist B, McKenna WJ, Elliott PM. Cardiopulmonary exercise testing and prognosis in hypertrophic cardiomyopathy. Circ Heart Fail. 2015;8(6):1022-31. DOI: 10.1161/CIRCHEARTFAILURE.

[51] Elliott PM, Gimeno JR, Tomé MT, Shah J, Ward D, Thaman R, et al. Left ventricular outflow tract obstruction and sudden death risk in patients with hypertrophic cardiomyopathy. Eur Heart J. 2006;27:1933-41.

[52] Autore C, Bernabò P, Barillà CS, et al. The prognostic importance of left ventricular outflow obstruction in hypertrophic cardiomyopathy varies in relation to the severity of symptoms. J Am Coll Cardiol. 2005;45:1078-80.

[53] Ismail TF, Jabbour A, Gulati A, Mallorie A, Raza S, Cowling TE, Das B, Khwaja J, Alpendurada FD, Wage R, Roughton M, McKenna WJ, Moon JC, Varnava A, Shakespeare C, Cowie MR, Cook SA, Elliott P, O'Hanlon R, Pennell DJ, Prasad SK. Role of late gadolinium enhancement cardiovascular magnetic resonance in the risk stratification of hypertrophic cardiomyopathy. Heart. 2014;100(23):1851-8. DOI: 10.1136/heartjnl-2013-305471.

[54] Maron BJ, Shen WK, Link MS, Epstein AE, Almquist AK, Daubert JP, Bardy GH, Favale S, Rea RF, Boriani G, Estes NA 3rd, Spirito P. Efficacy of implantable cardioverter-defibrillators for the prevention of sudden death in patients with hypertrophic cardiomyopathy. N Engl J Med. 2000;342(6):365-73.

[55] Magnusson P, Gadler F, Liv P, Mörner S. Hypertrophic cardiomyopathy and implantable defibrillators in Sweden: inappropriate shocks and complications requiring surgery. J Cardiovasc Electrophysiol. 2015;26(10):1088-94. DOI: 10.1111/jce.12750.

[56] Magnusson P, Gadler F, Liv P, Mörner S. Causes of death and mortality in hypertrophic cardiomyopathy patients with implantable defibrillators in Sweden. J Cardiovasc Med (Hagerstown). 2016;17(7):478-84. DOI: 10.2459/JCM.0000000000000359.

[57] Cox S, O'Donoghue AC, McKenna WJ, Steptoe A. Health related quality of life and psychological wellbeing in patients with hypertrophic cardiomyopathy. Heart. 1997;78(2):182-7.

[58] Magnusson P, Mörner S, Gadler F, Karlsson J. Health-related quality of life in hypertrophic cardiomyopathy patients with implantable defibrillators. Health Qual Life Outcomes. 2016;14:62. DOI: 10.1186/s12955-016-0467-x.

[59] Weinstock J, Bader YH, Maron MS, Rowin EJ, Link MS. Subcutaneous implantable cardioverter defibrillator in patients with hypertrophic cardiomyopathy: an initial experience. J Am Heart Assoc. 2016 Feb 12;5(2). pii: e002488. doi: 10.1161/JAHA.115.002488.

[60] Kramer CM, Appelbaum E, Desai MY, Desvigne-Nickens P, DiMarco JP, Friedrich MG, Geller N, Heckler S, Ho CY, Jerosch-Herold M, Ivey EA, Keleti J, Kim DY, Kolm P, Kwong RY, Maron MS, Schulz-Menger J, Piechnik S, Watkins H, Weintraub WS, Wu P, Neubauer S.Hypertrophic cardiomyopathy registry: the rationale and design of an

international, observational study of hypertrophic cardiomyopathy. Am Heart J. 2015;170(2):223-30. DOI: 10.1016/j.ahj.2015.05.013.

[61] Elliott P, Charron P, Blanes JR, Tavazzi L, Tendera M, Konté M, Laroche C, Maggioni AP; EORP Cardiomyopathy Registry Pilot Investigators. European cardiomyopathy pilot registry: EURObservational Research Programme of the European Society of Cardiology. Eur Heart J. 2016;37(2):164-73. DOI: 10.1093/eurheartj/ehv497

Chapter 20

# Electrical Devices (Resynchronization and Defibrillators) in the Treatment of Cardiomyopathies: Indications, Present and Future of these Therapies

Miguel Ángel García García,
María de los Ángeles Rosero Arenas,
Alfonso Martínez Cornejo,
Marta Bertolo Domínguez and
Vicente Miranda Gozalvo

Additional information is available at the end of the chapter

http://dx.doi.org/10.5772/65317

**Abstract**

Cardiomyopathies are heart diseases involving high risk of heart failure and sudden cardiac death. In this chapter, we review the use of electrical devices (cardiac resynchronization therapy and implantable cardioverter defibrillator) to reduce the progression of heart failure and prevent arrhythmogenic sudden death in patients affected with these pathologies. The future of these therapies is a more appropriate indication for primary prevention of sudden death (defibrillator) and treatment of heart failure in a broader spectrum of patients (resynchronization).

**Keywords:** cardiac resynchronization therapy, implantable cardioverter defibrillator, cardiomyopathy, heart failure, sudden death

## 1. Introduction

Cardiomyopathies (CMP) are a group of diseases that affect the cardiac muscle associated with myocardial dysfunction and can be caused by known disorders such as hypertension, ischemic heart disease, valvular disease, and so on. Other causes, such as genetic illnesses, inflammatory processes, metabolic, or toxic diseases, may also be responsible for this pathology. Its origin could also be primary, i.e., not known cause. One simple and initial classification of the CMP divides them into ischemic and nonischemic ones. In 1995, the World Health Organization (WHO)/International Society and Federation of Cardiology (ISFC) Task Force on the Definition and Classification of the Cardiomyopathies classified them into dilated, hypertrophic, restrictive, arrhythmogenic right ventricular dysplasia, and other [1]. Since these diseases can have mechanical and/or electrical dysfunction, in this chapter, we review the usefulness of electrical therapies (cardiac resynchronization therapy or/and implantable cardioverter defibrillator) to treat heart failure and arrhythmogenic sudden cardiac death associated with these diseases.

The etiology of heart failure may be predictive of long-term outcome: survival of peripartum CMP was better; medium in hypertension, myocarditis, sarcoidosis, and substance abuse; and worse in infiltrative myocardial disease –amyloidosis and hemochromatosis-, HIV disease, chemotherapy with doxorubicin, ischemic heart disease, or connective tissue disease. And in all of them, the added presence of diabetes involves an increased risk of mortality.

Heart failure is a complex clinical syndrome that causes inadequate systemic perfusion to meet the body's metabolic demands with usually increased left ventricular filling pressures. The two leading causes of death in patients with heart failure are arrhythmic or sudden cardiac death and progressive pump failure [2]. Life-threatening ventricular arrhythmias are common in patients with heart failure and CMP, and unexpected sudden cardiac death and sudden cardiac death during episodes of clinical worsening of heart failure each account for approximately one-third of deaths. Management of patients with heart failure includes several strategies: controlling contributing factors, lifestyle modification, pharmacological therapy, rehabilitation, preventive care, and electrical devices if indicated. The mode of death in patients with heart failure is more likely to be "sudden" in patients with New York Heart Association (NYHA) II-III classes and related to pump failure in patients with NYHA IV class [3].

Ventricular arrhythmias are common in heart failure and CMP. The prognosis of these arrhythmias depends on the cause of the CMP [4]. There is no preventive drug therapy to treat ventricular arrhythmias (i.e., amiodarone). However, those patients with nonsustained ventricular tachycardia may be candidates (with preliminary electrophysiological study) to an implantable cardioverter defibrillator. Patients with spontaneous sustained ventricular tachycardia are at high risk for sudden cardiac death; patients with heart failure or CMP who are survivors of sudden cardiac death due to ventricular tachycardia or ventricular fibrillation must be treated with implantable cardioverter defibrillator for secondary prevention [4, 5] (**Figure 1**).

A pacemaker placed in right ventricle can exacerbate heart failure by several mechanisms: firstly, contraction of the right ventricle before the left ventricle (interventricular dyssynchrony), and secondly the "left bundle branch block effect" causing that septum contracts before the lateral wall (intraventricular dyssynchrony); the final outcome of both phenomena results in a reduced efficiency of cardiac pump. It is likely that a pacemaker placed in right atrium and right ventricle provides benefit in heart failure, but DAVID trial, which included patients with left ventricular ejection fraction ≤40% and without indication for bradycardia showed that pacing with DDD function (dual, atrial and ventricular, pacing and sensing, and also dual, triggered and inihibited, response to sensing, according to accepted international code accepted in 2002) [6] can worsen heart failure. The same concept could be generalized to patients with CMP [7].

Therapy known as cardiac resynchronization can optimize cardiac function, symptoms, and survival in patients with heart failure with left ventricular dysfunction (with left ventricular

http://dx.doi.org/10.5772/65317

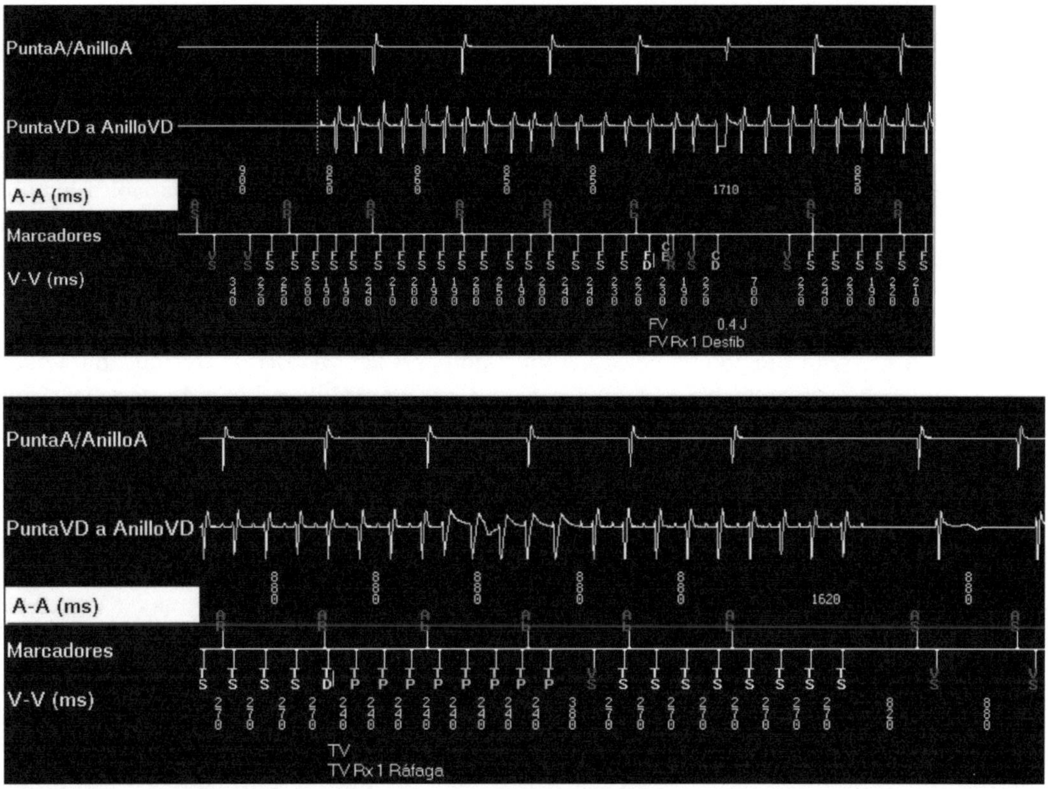


**Figure 1.** Endocavitary registry of two ventricular arrhythmias: ventricular tachycardia, treated with anti-tachycardia pacing (ATP), and ventricular fibrillation, treated with defibrillation (0.4 J).

ejection fraction ≤35% and wide QRS with left bundle branch block), added to optimal medical treatment. On the other hand, implantable cardioverter defibrillator can abort sudden arrhythmic deaths, thus prolonging survival in patients with cardiac disease and that patients may progress in later stages to more advanced heart failure.

## 2. Ischemic CMP

Risk stratification of a patient who has an acute myocardial infarction and ischemic CMP should include: identification of risk for recurrent ischemic events and identification of high risk of death (arrhythmic or non-arrhythmic of origin). Postinfarction mortality has decreased by optimizing the initial therapy (reperfusion) and secondary prevention measures [4].

### 2.1. Role of implantable cardioverter defibrillator

Several works (VALIANT [8]) described an increased risk of sudden cardiac death in patients with postinfarction left ventricular failure; the rate of sudden cardiac death or resuscitated cardiac arrest was 1.4 % in the first month, with a rate of 2.3% if left ventricular ejection fraction <30%), but the frequency of use of reperfusion therapy and beta-blockers was low. Two studies

(DINAMIT [9] and IRIS [10]) showed no improvement in survival after implantable cardioverter defibrillator placement between 31 and 40 days post infarction. Several risk factors are associated with threatening arrhythmia: low ejection fraction of left ventricle or history of heart failure, ventricular tachycardia induced in the electrophysiologic study, spontaneous ventricular premature beats and nonsustained ventricular tachycardia seen in the 24-hour Holter, and other. On the other hand, reperfusion therapy has decreased the predictive value of these variables. Finally, implantable cardioverter defibrillator should be recommended in patients with a left ventricular ejection fraction ≤30% (MADIT II criteria) or with ischemic CMP, left ventricular ejection fraction ≤35%, and NYHA II or III heart failure (SCD-HEFT criteria) [11] (**Figure 2**). In recent guidelines [12, 13], implantable cardioverter defibrillator is an effective therapy to reduce sudden cardiac death in patients with previous myocardial infarction and left ventricular dysfunction, which have hemodynamically unstable sustained ventricular tachycardia, and in patients with recurrent ventricular tachycardia and normal/near normal left ventricular function.

### 2.2. Role of cardiac resynchronization therapy

The usefulness of resynchronization is demonstrated in patients with ischemic CMP. In several pivotal studies, which demonstrated the utility of resynchronization (CARE-HF, COMPANION, etc), there was a significant percentage of patients with ischemic CMP. In other old studies [14], patients with ischemic CMP may respond less favorably to resynchronization compared with patients with idiopathic dilated CMP. In recent years, studies comparing the effectiveness of this therapy in ischemic vs dilated CMP have been developed [15]; estimated survival at 4 years were 55% for ischemic and 77% for dilated CMP, and no significant difference was found in the incidence of inappropriate implantable cardioverter defibrillator shocks between both groups. Patients with implantable cardioverter defibrillator functionality remained at higher risk for death after controlling for pre-implant variables (hazard ratio (HR), 1.6). So, patients with dilated CMP experienced greater improvement in left ventricular systolic function and reverse remodeling than those with ischemic CMP, which means sustaining a greater survival benefit.

Another study [16] showed that after atrioventricular node ablation along with biventricular pacemaker placement, in patients with heart failure and refractory atrial fibrillation, echocardiographic reverse remodeling was lower in patients with ischemic compared with dilated CMP [16], with a greater number of hospitalizations due to heart failure in this first group and less improvement of left ventricular ejection fraction.

Finally, a combination of resynchronization + surgery in dilated ischemic CMP could be useful: optimization of ventricular function by myocardial revascularization with synchronized contraction of papillary muscle by biventricular pacing could improve the abnormal conformation/shape of the left ventricle, responsible for the functional mitral regurgitation. Therefore, preoperative assessment of myocardial viability and synchronism of the papillary muscles is the key to the success of this intervention.

Recent clinical guidelines [17] show greater benefit of CRT in several subgroups: women, QRS ≥150 ms, and nonischemic CMP. Despite the lower efficacy against nonischemic patients, the implant in these patients is recommended.

http://dx.doi.org/10.5772/65317

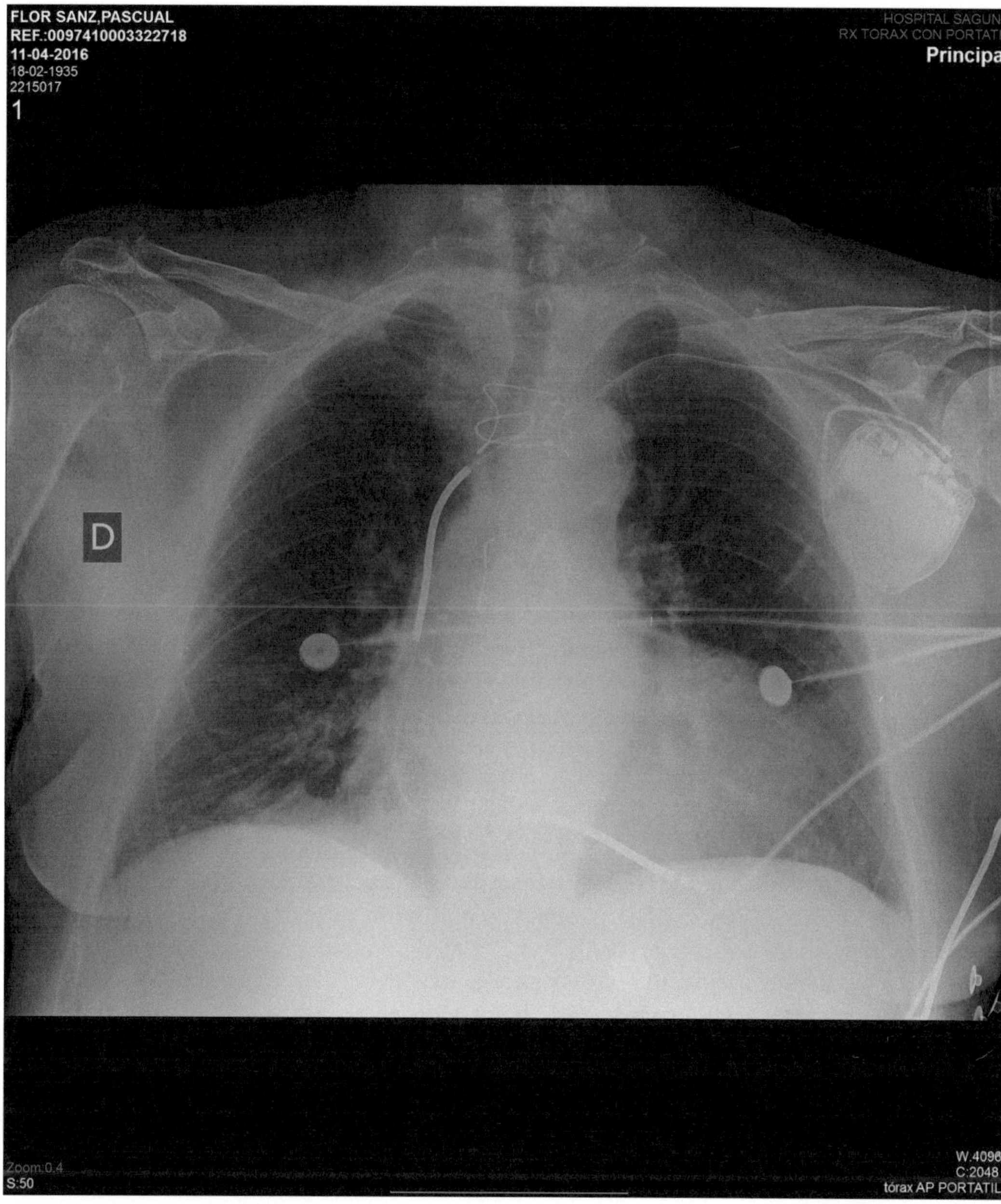


**Figure 2.** Monocameral implantable cardioverter defibrillator in a patient with ischemic dilated cardiomyopathy.

## 3. Myocarditis

It is an inflammatory disease of the myocardium, characterized from a histopathologic point of view by inflammatory infiltrates within the myocardium associated with degeneration and necrosis, with a nonischemic origin. The most common etiology is infectious, followed by immune (drugs, autoimmune diseases, etc) and toxic (drugs, metals, radiation, etc). Acute myocarditis can lead to chronic myocarditis or dilated CMP up to 10% of cases [18, 19]. In patients with sudden cardiac death, sustained ventricular tachycardia, ventricular fibrillation, and/or dilated CMP with ventricular dysfunction, the decision to implant and implantable cardioverter defibrillator should be based on the same indications as in other CMP, according to clinical practice guidelines [13]. It seems reasonable to delay the placement of an implantable cardioverter defibrillator until the resolution of the acute episode, meanwhile can be raised using a vest defibrillator as a bridge in high-risk patients [20]. Once dilated CMP has been developed, implantation of a cardiac resynchronization therapy device is recommended in patients with severe depression of left ventricular systolic function (<35%) and left bundle block in functional class II–IV [21].

In clinical guidelines [12, 13], implantable cardioverter defibrillator is indicated if inflammatory infiltrates persist in biopsies and if there is abnormal fibrosis in magnetic resonance; these elements are risk factors for sudden cardiac death.

## 4. Hypertrophic CMP

Patients with hypertrophic CMP can develop left ventricle outflow tract gradient/obstruction, diastolic dysfunction, myocardial ischemia, mitral regurgitation, and systolic dysfunction (in advanced stages) [22]. Therapeutic options to decrease the pressure gradient are as follows: drugs (beta-blockers or calcium antagonists), septal resection surgery, septal percutaneous reduction with ablation with alcohol, and atrial ventricular permanent pacing.

### 4.1. Role of cardiac resynchronization therapy

The aim consists of reducing the left ventricular outflow tract gradient, probably related with heart failure, classically using DDD pacemaker, and more recently with cardiac resynchronization therapy. In several works (1970s and 1980s), right atrial and right ventricular pacing, with short auricular-ventricular interval is performed, with positive effects: pre-excitation from right ventricular apex—with paradoxical septal movement and ejection speed reduction, delayed septal contraction—with systolic anterior motion of mitral valve improvement, and reduction of mitral regurgitation and subaortic gradient; a critical issue is to maintain constant ventricular and auricular capture. However, the success of the therapy lies in optimized individual programming of stimulation parameters to maintain atrial ventricular synchrony. The maintained benefit in functional status of sequential atrial ventricular pacing has been demonstrated in long series of cases (median follow-up of 8.5 years) [23]. Lenarczyk et al. [24] shows in his preliminary study a decrease in outflow tract gradient and improvement of the functional status. In several series, we can see a symptomatic benefit and an improvement of exercise capacity, although evolution is erratic. In recent guidelines for the treatment of hypertrophic CMP [25], cardiac resynchronization therapy is recommended in the following situations: sequential conventional pacing for reducing gradient or facilitating medical treatment if gradient ≥50 mmHg, sinus rhythm and refractory symptoms to medical treatment with contraindication to myectomy or septal ablation, with high risk to develop atrial ventricular block after it; resynchronization is also indicated in patients who meet indications of bicameral implantable cardioverter defibrillator to make sequential pacing.

We are waiting for the results of the study TRICHAMPION (clinicaltrials.gov NCT01614717): triple chamber pacing in hypertrophic obstructive cardiomyopathy patients. This is a prospective, randomized, single blind trial including N = 80 patients with atrial pacing only in back-up versus atrial biventricular pacing for 1 year. Expected preliminary results will be in 2016.

Recent clinical guidelines [17] show, in the absence of current clinical trials, the option of considering cardiac resynchronization therapy in individual patients with left ventricular failure data and asynchrony. And for patients with left ventricular outflow tract obstruction and treated with dual chamber pacemaker or implantable cardioverter defibrillator, you must schedule a short atrial ventricular interval for maximum apical right ventricle pre-excitation without altering left ventricle diastolic filling.

### 4.2. Role of implantable cardioverter defibrillator

Hypertrophic CMP is the most frequent cause of sudden cardiac death in adults under 35 years; annual mortality is 1% and half of it is sudden cardiac death [26, 27]. In the Spanish Implantable Cardioverter Defibrillator registry [28], 6% of carriers of this device had a previous diagnosis of hypertrophic CMP. Unfortunately, sudden cardiac death could be the first manifestation of this entity, so it is necessary a risk stratification. However, although implantable cardioverter defibrillator is recommended for high-risk patients with hypertrophic CMP, there is no agreement on its general use. In European centers, a conservative approach has been adopted: in primary prevention, there is indication to implant an implantable cardioverter defibrillator if at least two risk factors are present [27]; but that does not mean it is accompanied by theoretical high risk. It can be seen at an annual rate of 11.1% adequate treatment in secondary prevention and 1.6% in primary prevention.

In several series [29], differences are observed in the placement criteria (**Table 1**) between hospitals and even populations of each center. It is remarkable that patients with an episode of resuscitated sudden cardiac death or sustained ventricular tachycardia had fewer risk factors than those with implantable cardioverter defibrillator for primary prevention (1.94 vs 2.96). The main factors associated with appropriate therapies were history of resuscitated sudden death and sustained ventricular tachycardia. These data reflect the difficulty in identifying patients at risk and make adequate primary prevention. The history of sustained ventricular tachycardia or ventricular fibrillation makes unnecessary to look for other risk factors. On the other hand, the presence of ventricular aneurysm, myocardial infarction, or systolic dysfunction may indicate the need for this therapy.

The current selection criteria do not predict in a reliable manner the occurrence of sudden cardiac death or ventricular arrhythmias. On the other hand, the quantification of fibrosis or genetic study may help proper selection of candidates for implantable cardioverter defibrillator for primary prevention. This becomes more important if we consider the associated complications in the primary prevention group (unnecessary electric shocks, battery replacements, etc). A new algorithm [30] can give greater discriminatory power than previous ones.

| |
|---|
| • Resuscitated SD |
| • Sustained VT |
| • Family history of SD |
| • Causeless recurrent syncope (without apparent cause) |
| • Ventricular hypertrophy (≥30 mm) |
| • Subaortic gradient (left ventricular outflow tract, LVOT >30 mmHg at rest) |
| • Abnormal response to exertion in less than 45 years (inability to increase 25 mmHg systolic arterial pressure) |
| • NSVT in Holter ECG (three or more ventricular beats, followed by more than 120 beats/min and less than 30 s in length) |

**Table 1.** Checked risk factors of sudden death. SD, sudden death. VT, ventricular tachycardia. NSVT, non sustained VT.

Recent clinical guidelines [12, 13] recommend, in the absence of clinical trials, the use of implantable cardioverter defibrillator for secondary prevention in patients with aborted cardiac arrest or sustained ventricular tachycardia associated with a high risk of subsequent lethal arrhythmia. Also, recommendations for implantable cardioverter defibrillator therapy for primary prophylaxis are based on the 5-year SCD risk calculated using the HCM Risk-SCD model and taking into account the age and general health of the patient.

## 5. Dilated MCP

The etiology of this CMP is varied: idiopathic 50% (**Figure 3**), myocarditis 9%, ischemic CMP 7%, infiltrative disease 5%, and other (peripartum, arterial hypertension, treatment with doxorubicin, etc.

*Chagas disease*: It is a protozoal infection due to *Tripanosoma cruzi*. It is the leading cause of dilated CMP in Central/South America and is the leading cause of cardiovascular death in patients between 30 and 50 years old. Cardiac involvement is manifested as arrhythmias, heart failure, and thromboembolic phenomena. In these countries it is a major cause of sudden cardiac death. Nonsustained ventricular tachycardia, NYHA functional class, and left ventricular ejection fraction are predictors of mortality, with a 16% survival at 36 months in patients with NYHA class IV and left ventricular ejection fraction <35% despite optimal medical treatment [31]. With similar indications to previous trials (severe heart failure despite optimal medical treatment, QRS > 120 ms, left ventricular ejection fraction <35%, and left ventricular end-diastolic diameter >55 mm assessed by Doppler echocardiography), improved NYHA functional status is obtained, with increase in left ventricular ejection fraction and reduction in left ventricular end diastolic diameter; 33% of patients do not respond to cardiac resynchronization therapy, probably by the advanced NYHA class.

Pharmacological treatment has little benefit, and recurrence rates of severe arrhythmia are close to 100%. Mortality is high—40% at 1 year, with frequent need for implantable cardioverter defibrillator implantation when evolves to dilated CMP [32]. Recent guidelines

http://dx.doi.org/10.5772/65317

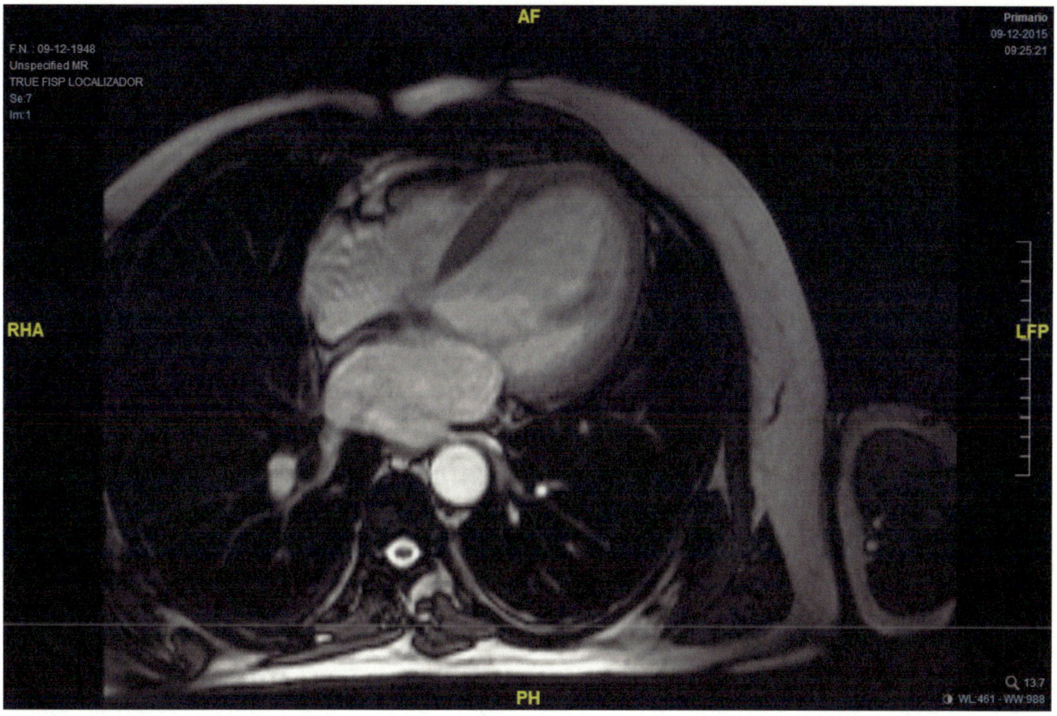


**Figure 3.** MR image of a patient with idiopathic dilated cardiomyopathy, with increased ventricular dimensions with a homogeneous myocardial uptake signal.

[11, 12] say that implanted cardioverter defibrillator should be considered in patients with left ventricular ejection fraction <40% when they are expected to survive >1 year with good functional status

*Stress CMP* (*takotsubo*) does not seem to be an indication for treatment with cardiac resynchronization therapy even in cases with refractory heart failure (usual indication of these devices in ambulatory patients).

Cardiac involvement in *Becker muscular dystrophy* varies from myocardial hypertrophy with preserved systolic function to severe left ventricular dilatation with anomalies in contractility by anomalies in contractility and severe depression of systolic function. Cardiac resynchronization therapy implantation depends on the baseline condition and comorbidities of patients. Few cases have been described [33].

*Peripartum*: It is a rare form of nonischemic CMP defined as heart failure secondary to left ventricular systolic dysfunction with a left ventricular ejection fraction <45% toward the end of pregnancy or in the months following delivery, where no other cause of heart failure can be found. The treatment of peripartum CMP is similar to that employed for other types of heart failure with left ventricular dysfunction; however, modifications to standard therapy are often necessary to ensure the safety of the mother and the unborn or breastfeeding child. The time to potential recovery from severe remodeling of ventricular function is difficult to predict [34]. In general, severely reduced left ventricular ejection fraction is linked to a higher risk of life-threatening ventricular tachyarrhythmic events, and implantation of a defibrillator is often recommended. An alternative for these patients can be the wearable cardioverter/defibrillator, with temporary protection during a phase of high arrhythmic risk [35]. An elevated incidence of ventricular fibrillation episodes during an early phase of peripartum CMP in patients with severely reduced left ventricular ejection fraction and heart failure symptoms and uninterrupted vest defibrillator wearing for up to 6 months can protect these young mothers from dying suddenly and yield important information about a potential permanent risk that will indicate implantable cardioverter defibrillator implantation. Recent guidelines [12, 13] point that implantation of an implantable cardioverter defibrillator in patients with ventricular arrhythmia or low left ventricular ejection fraction should follow standard guidelines; the high rate of spontaneous recovery of dilated CMP after delivery must be considered when decisions are made.

*Amyloid CMP*: The efficacy and safety of implantable cardioverter defibrillator are uncertain. Sudden cardiac death is common in patients with cardiac amyloidosis, but electromechanical dissociation seems to be a significant cause of sudden death [36]. In recent guidelines [12, 13], implantable cardioverter defibrillator should be considered in patients with ventricular arrhythmia causing hemodynamic instability who are expected to survive >1 year with good functional status.

*Idiopathic dilated CMP*: Several observational registries [37] show that early diagnosis and tailored medical therapy are independent protectors against pump-failure death/heart transplant, and lower left ventricular ejection fraction is a predictor of sudden death, while implantable cardioverter defibrillator has a protective role.

Any observational study [38] shows the usefulness of cardiac resynchronization therapy in patients with *dilated CMP of valvular origin after corrective valve surgery* (an underrepresented population in randomized controlled trials). In patients with left bundle branch block, wide QRS (161 ms), and advanced functional class (III 82% - IV), there is a functional improvement in class and better data in left ventricular remodelation and asynchrony.

### 5.1. Role of cardiac resynchronization therapy

The usefulness of resynchronization has been recorded in clinical trials that included patients with severe depression of left ventricular systolic function, complete left bundle brain block, and heart failure syndrome. One important issue has been described recently: the relationship between QRS duration and left ventricular remodelation. Several factors that help to predict response to cardiac resynchronization replacement have been identified: systolic pulmonary artery pressure, renal function, left ventricular dyssynchrony, inappropriate left ventricular electrode position, ischemia, and 6-minute walking distance; but it remains unclear if QRS duration, measured before cardiac resynchronization therapy, can predict its effectiveness (conflicting results, with data pointing to one direction and to the opposite [39]). And patients with nonischemic CMP are more likely to benefit from cardiac resynchronization therapy compared to patients with ischemic CMP. According to the reduction of left ventricular end-diastolic diameter 6 months after cardiac resynchronization therapy, patients were divided into responder and nonresponder; measured parameters were not statistically different before resynchronization. After 6 months, responders exhibited significant reversal of their left ventricular remodeling, with improved left ventricular ejection fraction and exercise tolerance, and a shorter QRS compared to nonresponders; the preoperative parameters were not predictive of the ultimate response of patients to resynchronization. Zhang [39] also shows that QRS duration change correlated with reduction in left ventricular end-diastolic diameter; QRS duration that can easily measured before and after resynchronization may be a predictive factor of response to cardiac resynchronization therapy in patients with heart failure due to dilated CMP. In a Spanish work, it is exposed that early normalization of ejection fraction after resynchronization is long-term maintained and identify better clinical and arrhythmic prognosis [40].

Cardiac resynchronization therapy is not strongly recommended for patients with narrow QRS. There are some described cases of CRT implant in patients with dilated CMP and narrow QRS in which it was obtained a dramatic response optimizing the atrioventricular delay, remembering the importance of atrioventricular optimization for successful resynchronization.

In addition, early normalization of left ventricular function in idiopathic dilated CMP is held long term after resynchronization device implant and indicates an improvement in prognosis from clinical and arrhythmic points of view. A decrease in cardiovascular mortality is observed, and also there is a decrease of arrhythmic events; this finding is consistent as described by García Lunar et al. [41]. The question is whether resynchronization device must be associated with implantable cardioverter defibrillator over time or even this mixed device (resynchronization + defibrillator) must be replaced by a resynchronization device only, especially if patient has inappropriate therapies.

It is stated in clinical guidelines [17] that the benefit is greater in patients with wider QRS and left bundle branch block and in women and non-ischemic cardiomyopathy, intermediate in men with ischemic cardiomyopathy; and lesser, or even non-responsive, in patients with narrow QRS and without left bundle block.

### 5.2. Role of implantable cardioverter defibrillator

Life-threatening ventricular arrhythmias are common in patients with heart failure and CMP, and their presence may lead to sudden death. These devices may have a primary and secondary indication. Secondary prevention with implantable cardioverter defibrillator is planned in patients with heart failure and CMP, also dilated CMP, who survive to an episode of sudden cardiac death. This indication is based on the results of several studies, AVID (entry criteria: left ventricular ejection fraction <40%), CASH, and CIDS. Some studies show a greater benefit of defibrillators in younger patients [42], whereas other studies did not found such differences [43, 44]. Also, there are studies focused on primary prevention in nonischemic dilated CMP; the trials CAT [45] and AMIOVIRT [46] showed a nonsignificant trend to decreased mortality, due to its methodological limitations. Other trials (DEFINITE, SCD-HeFT y COMPANION) did show reduction in mortality. At the view of these results and the results of a recent meta-analysis, primary prevention with implantable cardioverter defibrillator in patients with dilated CMP, left ventricular ejection fraction ≤35%, and NYHA II-III is recommended. The ability to induce ventricular arrhythmias is not predictive of sudden cardiac death in patients with nonischemic CMP; thus, electrophysiology testing does not have a role in risk stratification of these patients [5] (**Figure 4**).

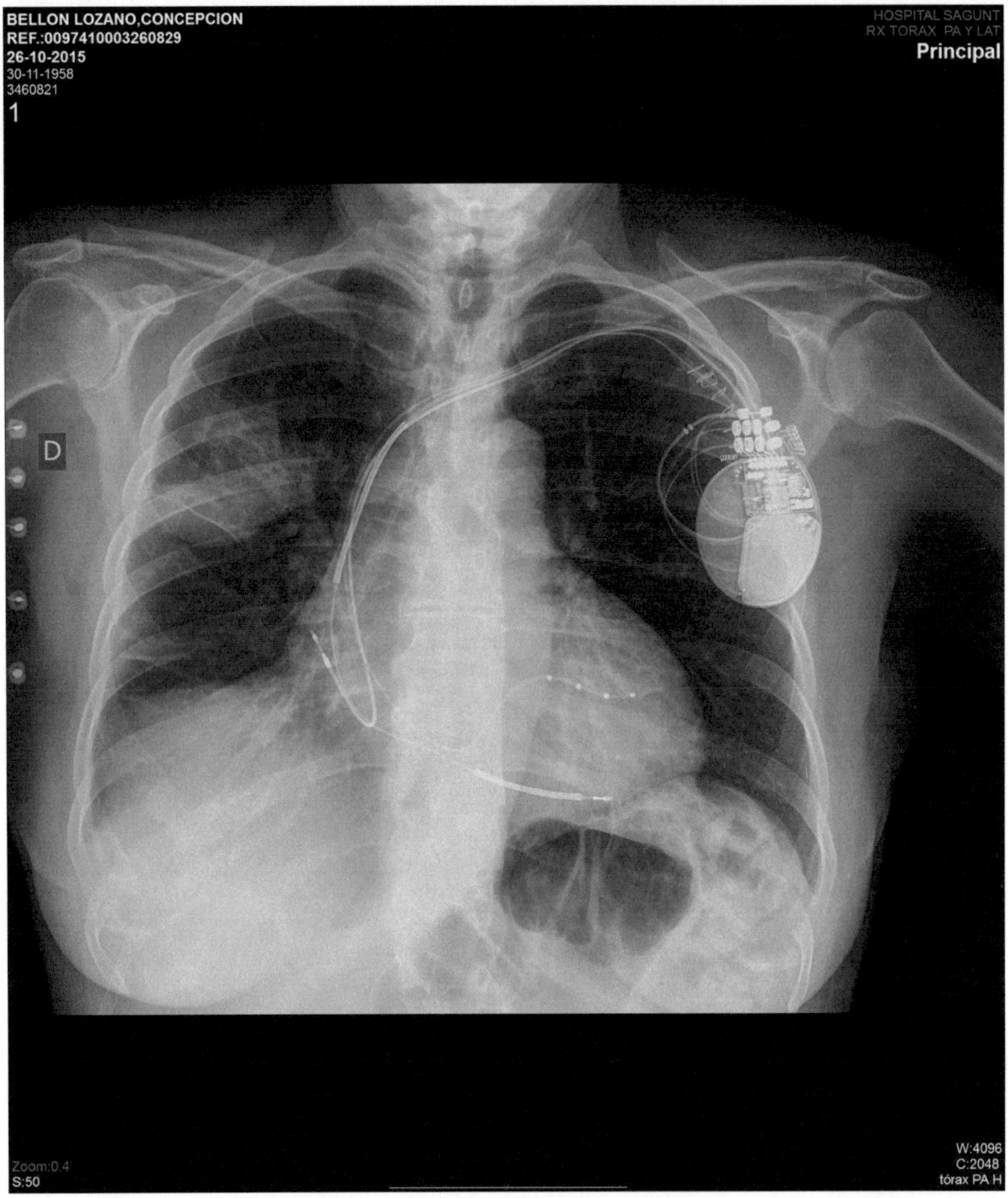


**Figure 4.** Cardiac resynchronization therapy in the same patient with idiopathic dilated cardiomyopathy. An alveolar condensation in the medium lobe compatible with nosocomial pneumonia (coincident with device implantation) can be seen.

http://dx.doi.org/10.5772/65317

As we have said before, in recent guidelines [12, 13], implantable cardioverter defibrillator is recommended, as secondary prophylaxis, in patients with hemodynamically nontolerated ventricular tachycardia/ventricular fibrillation, who are expected to survive for >1 year with good functional status. And for primary prophylaxis, defibrillator is recommended in patients with symptomatic heart failure (NYHA class II–III) and left ventricular ejection fraction ≤35% despite ≥3 months of treatment with optimal medical treatment who are expected to survive for >1 year with good functional status.

## 6. Restrictive CMP

This is the least frequent in the group of CMP and the only one for which the WHO/ISFC Task Force 81 does not offer specific diagnostic criteria. The diagnosis is based on clinical signs of heart failure due to a restriction on the diastolic filling of the heart with preserved systolic function and in the absence of hypertrophy or ventricular dilation. Amyloidosis, mucopolisacaridosis, and Löeffler's endocarditis are the more frequent causes. Treatment does not follow standard treatment guidelines as in other cases of cardiomyopathies and is based on a careful management of diuretics and vasodilators. The management of restrictive CMP is difficult because the underlying processes usually do not respond to intervention and is mostly palliative. In several cases, there has been an indication of implantable cardioverter defibrillator to prevent sudden cardiac death in high-risk patients; recent guidelines [12, 13] make a similar recommendation to other diseases with poor prognosis and state that defibrillators are recommended in patients with sustained ventricular arrhythmia causing hemodynamic instability who are expected to survive >1 year with good functional status to reduce the risk of sudden cardiac death. In relation to its pathophysiology, there is no indication to resynchronization. In most cases of restrictive CMP, caused by amyloidosis or other infiltrative diseases, there is a very poor prognosis, except in the case that the patient will receive a heart transplant. In patients with sarcoidosis, defibrillator implantation is recommended if left ventricular ejection fraction is <35%, maintained after a period of immunosuppression, and considered in patients with induced ventricular tachycardia in electrophysiology test and with late gadolinium enhancement in cardiac gammagraphy, although the left ventricular function is normal [47].

## 7. Arrhythmogenic right ventricular cardiomyopathy (ARVC)

It is a CMP, a hereditary disease of the desmosomal proteins, and is associated with sudden cardiac death; there is a fibrofatty replacement of the right ventricle myocardium that initially produces typical regional wall motion abnormalities that later become global and finally leads to right ventricular dilatation [48]. Its mechanism is re-entrant arrhythmias.

### 7.1. Role of implantable cardioverter defibrillator

Selection of patients for defibrillator is controversial. Natural history of the disease suggests several risk factors for sudden cardiac death: marked right ventricle dilatation, left ventricular involvement with left ventricular reduced function, occurrence of prior hemodynamically unstable rapid sustained monomorphic ventricular tachycardia or ventricular fibrillation, and history of syncope; T-wave inversions could be a predictor of any ventricular arrhythmia in follow-up and a younger age; probably, the major risk for death was reduced left ventricular function [49]. Inducible sustained monomorphic ventricular tachycardia did not predict the presence of the same arrhythmia in the follow-up (although Bhonsale et al. found a relationship in their work [50]). When defibrillator is placed, anti-tachycardia pacing is highly successful in terminating sustained monomorphic ventricular tachycardia and should be programmed for all sustained monomorphic ventricular tachycardia, regardless of heart rate. Some authors comment that defibrillator implant with primary prevention has an excessively low rate of appropriate therapies, and the criteria for risk stratification have little predictive power; for these reasons, there should be revised. New genetic techniques help us to classify left ventricular hypertrophy in some patients as Fabry disease or other metabolopathies, with different prognosis and risk of sudden death than primary hypertrophic CMP. In addition, some registries have short (3.3 years) follow-up, and there have been appropriate therapies 9–10 years after the implant; given the youth of these patients and the long at-risk period, it is

| **Predictor variable** | **Definition** | **Coding** |
|---|---|---|
| Age | Age at evaluation [30] | Continuous, years |
| Family history of SCD | History of sudden cardiac death in one or more first degree relatives under 40 years of age or SCD in a first degree relative with confirmed HCM at any age (post-or ante-mortem diagnosis) [13, 22, 28, 29] | Binary (yes = 1/no = 0) |
| Maximal wall thickness | The greatest thickness in the anterior septum, posterior septum, lateral wall, and posterior wall of the LV, measured at the level of the mitral value, papillary muscles, and apex using parasternal short-axis plane using 2D echocardiography at the time of evaluation [15, 17, 20, 23, 24, 26] | Continuous, mm |
| Fractional shortening | (LV end-diastolic dimension-LV end-systolic dimension)/LV end-diastolic dimension measured by M-Mode or 2D echocardiography at time of evaluation [23] | Continuous, % |
| Left atrial diameter | Left atrial diameter determined by M-Mode or 2D echocardiography in the parasternal long-axis plane at the time of evaluation [30] | Continuous, mm |
| Maximal left ventricular outflow tract gradients | The maximum LV outflow gradient determined at rest and with Valsalva provocation (irrespective of concurrent medical treatment) using pulsed and continuous wave Doppler from the apical three- and five-chamber views. Peak outflow tract gradients were determined using the modified Bernoulli equation: Gradient = 4$V$ [2], where $V$ is the peak aortic outflow velocity [13, 18, 22, 27, 28] | Continuous, mmHg |
| Nonsustained ventricular tachycardia | ≥3 consecutive ventricular beats at a rate of ≥120 bpm and <30 s in duration on Holter monitoring (minimum duration 24 hours) at or prior to evaluation [13, 17, 28, 29] | Binary (yes = 1/no = 0) |
| Unexplained syncope | History of unexplained syncope at or prior to evaluation [13, 20, 25, 28, 30] | Binary (yes = 1/no = 0) |

**Table 2.** HCM Risk-SCD tool. HCM, hypertrophic CMP. SCD, sudden cardiac death. LV, left ventricle.

http://dx.doi.org/10.5772/65317

very important to perform long follow-up periods. The number of inappropriate therapies can decrease with better diagnostic algorithms. Recent guidelines for management of this disease [51] highlight several elements; the most important, little usefulness of algorithms based on binary variables that do not take into account the magnitude of each risk factor, with poor discriminatory power between high and low risk. Therefore, it is recommended to use the HCM Risk-SCD tool (**Table 2**) [30]. Recent guidelines [12, 13] state that defibrillator implantation is recommended in patients with a history of aborted sudden cardiac death and hemodynamically poorly tolerated ventricular tachycardia (secondary prevention) and should be considered in patients who have hemodynamically well-tolerated sustained Ventricular tachycardia or have one or more recognized risk factors for ventricular arrhythmia with a life expectancy >1 year.

### 7.2. Role of cardiac resynchronization therapy

It has been described as any case of mixed defibrillator-resynchronization device in special circumstances. In advanced cases of this disease, with low voltages in electrical signal from right ventricle, there can be difficult to detect ventricular tachyarrhythmias. The advanced degree of atrioventricular block indicates permanent cardiac pacing. There must be a catheter in coronary sinus for sensing and pacing, and another catheter in right ventricle as backup if left ventricle catheter capture fails, taking into account the high degree of atrioventricular block.

## Acknowledgements

The authors thank Leyre Cendrero and Omar Ferrús, technical consultants of Medtronic Company; Ricardo Ruiz and Francisco Javier Chorro, from Cardiology Department of Hospital Clínico, Valencia; and Vicent López and all staff in Intensive Care Unit of Hospital Sagunto, for their help in the preparation of this work.

## Author details

Miguel Ángel García García[1]*, María de los Ángeles Rosero Arenas[2], Alfonso Martínez Cornejo[1], Marta Bertolo Domínguez[3] and Vicente Miranda Gozalvo[4]

*Address all correspondence to: mangelesymangel@hotmail.com

1 Intensive Care Unit, Sagunto Hospital, Valencia, Spain

2 Centro de Salud (Health Facility) Cheste, Valencia, Spain

3 Radiology Department, Sagunto Hospital, Valencia, Spain

4 ERESA/Radiology Department, Sagunto Hospital, Valencia, Spain

## References

[1] Richardson P, McKenna W, Bristow M et al. Report of the 1995 World Health Organization/International Society and Federation of Cardiology Task Force on the Definition and Classification of Cardiomyopathies. Circulation. 1996; 93: 841–842.

[2] The SOLVD Investigators. Effect of enalapril on survival in patients with reduced left ventricular ejection fractions and congestive heart failure. N Engl J Med 1991; 325: 293–302.

[3] Marine JE, Russo AM. Primary prevention of sudden cardiac death in heart failure and cardiomyopathy. In: UpToDate, Post TW(Ed), UpToDate, Waltham, MA. (Accessed on April 07, 2016).

[4] Podrid PJ, Ganz LI. Incidence of and risk stratification for sudden cardiac death after acute myocardial infarction.

[5] Podrid PJ. Ventricular arrhythmias in heart failure and cardiomyopathy. In: UpToDate, Post TW(Ed), UpToDate, Waltham, MA. (Accessed on April 18, 2016).

[6] Bernstein AD, Daubert JC, Fletcher RD et al. The revised NASPE/BPEG generic code for antibradycardia, adaptative-rate, and multisite pacing. North American Society of Pacing and Electrophysiology/British Pacing and Electrophysiology Group. Pacing Clin Electrophysiol 2002; 25: 260–264.

[7] Saxon LA. Overview of cardiac pacing in heart failure. In: UpToDate, Post TW(Ed), UpToDate, Waltham, MA. (Accessed on April 18, 2016).

[8] Pfeffer MA, McMurray JJ, Velazquez EJ et al. Valsartan, captopril, or both in myocardial infarction complicated by heart failure, left ventricular dysfunction or both. N Engl J Med 2003; 349: 893–906.

[9] Höhnloser SH, Kuck KH, DorianP et al. Prophylactic use of an implantable cardioverter-defibrillator after acute myocardial infarction. N Engl J Med 2004; 351: 2481–2488.

[10] Steinbeck G, Andresen D, SeidlK et al. Defibrillator implantation early after myocardial infarction. N Engl J Med 2009; 361: 1427–1436.

[11] Bardy GH, Lee KL, Mark DB et al. Amiodarone or an implantable cardioverter-defibrillator for congestive heart failure. N Engl J Med 2004; 352: 225.

[12] Zipes DP, Camm AF, Borggrefe M et al. ACC/AHA/ESC 2006 Guidelines for management of patients with ventricular arrhythmias and the prevention of sudden cardiac death. J Am Coll Cardiol 2006; 48: e247–e346.

[13] Priori SG, Blomström-Lundqvist C, Mazzanti A et al. 2015 ESC Guidelines for the management of patients with ventricular arrhythmias and the prevention of sudden cardiac death. Eur Heart J 2015; 36:2793–2867.

[14] Molhoek SG, Bax JJ, van ErvenL et al. Comparison of benefits from cardiac resynchronization therapy in patients with ischemic cardiomyopathy versus idiopathic dilated cardiomyopathy. Am J Cardiol 2004; 93: 860–863.

[15] McLeod CJ, Shen WK, Rea RF et al. Differential outcome of cardiac resynchronization therapy in ischemic cardiomyopathy and idiopathic dilated cardiomyopathy. Heart Rhythm 2011; 8: 377–382.

[16] Sohinki D, Ho J, Srinivasan N et al. Outcomes after atrioventricular node ablation and biventricular pacing in patients with refractory atrial fibrillation and heart failure: a comparison between non-ischaemic and ischaemic cardiomyopathy. Europace 2014; 16: 880–886.

[17] The Task Force on cardiac pacing and resynchronization therapy of the European Society of Cardiology (ESC). Developed in collaboration with the European Heart Rhythm Association (EHRA), Brignole M, Auricchio A, Baron-Esquivias et al. 2013 ESC Guidelines on cardiac pacing and cardiac resynchronization therapy. Rev Esp Cardiol (Engl Ed). 2014 Jan;67(1):58.

[18] Baughman KL. Diagnosis of myocarditis: death of Dallas criteria. Circulation 2006; 113: 593–595.

[19] D'Ambrosio A, Patti G, Manzoli A et al. The fate of acute myocarditis between spontaneous improvement and evolution to dilated cardiomyopathy: a review. Heart 2001; 85: 499–504.

[20] Chung MK. The role of the wearable cardioverter defibrillator in clinical practice. Cardiol Clin 2014; 32: 253–270.

[21] Dickstein K, Vardas PE, Auricchio A et al. 2010 Focused update of ESC guidelines on device therapy in heart failure: an update of the 2008 ESC guidelines for the diagnosis and treatment of acute and chronic heart failure and the 2007 ESC guidelines for cardiac and resynchronization therapy. Eur J Heart Fail 2010; 12: 1143–1153.

[22] Maron MS. Hypertrophic cardiomyopathy: clinical manifestations, diagnosis and evaluation. In: UpToDate, Post TW (Ed), UpToDate, Waltham, MA. (Accessed on April 07, 2016).

[23] Jurado Román A, Montero Cabezas JM, Rubio Alonso B et al. Sequential Atrioventricular Pacing in Patients With Hypertrophic Cardiomyopathy: An 18-year Experience. Rev Esp Cardiol(Engl Ed). 2016 Apr;69 (4):377-83.

[24] Lenarczyk R, Wozniak R, Kowalski O et al. Effect of cardiac resynchronization on gradient reduction in patients with obstructive hypertrophic cardiomyopathy: preliminary study. Pacing Clin Electrophysiol 2011; 34: 1544–1552.

[25] Authors/Task Force members, Elliott PM, Anastasakis A, Borger MA et al. 2014 ESC Guidelines on diagnosis and management of hypertrophic cardiomyopathy: the Task Force for the Diagnosis and Management of Hypertrophic Cardiomyopathy of the European Society of Cardiology (ESC). Eur Heart J. 2014 Oct 14;35(39):2733-79.

[26] Maron BJ. Prevention of sudden death with the implantable defibrillator in hypertrophic cardiomyopathy. Rev Esp Cardiol. 2006 Jun;59:527-30.

[27] Maron BJ. Hypertrophic cardiomyopathy: a systematic review. JAMA. 2002 Mar 13;287:1308-20.

[28] Peinado R, Arenal A, Arribas F et al. Spanish implantable cardioverter-defibrillator registry. First official report of the spanish society of cardiology working group on implantable cardioverter-defibrillators (2002-2004). Rev Esp Cardiol. 2005;58:1435-49.

[29] Marín F, Gimeno JR, Payá E et al. The implantable cardioverter-defibrillator and hypertrophic cardiomyopathy. Experience at three centers. Rev Esp Cardiol. 2006 Jun;59(6):537-44.

[30] O'Mahony C, Jichi F, Pavlou M et al. A novel clinical risk prediction model for sudden cardiac death in hypertrophic cardiomyopathy (HCM Risk-SCD). Eur Heart J 2014; 35: 2010–2020.

[31] Rassi A Jr, Rassi A, Rassi SG et al. Predictors of mortality in chronic Chagas disease: a systematic review of observational studies. Circulation 2007; 115: 1101–1108.

[32] Muratore C, Rabinovich R, Iglesias R et al. Implantable cardioverter defibrillators in patients with Chagas' disease: Are they different from patients with coronary disease? Pacing Clin Electrophysiol 1997; 20: 194–197.

[33] Andrikopoulos G, Kourouklis S, Trika C et al. Cardiac resynchronization therapy in Becker muscular dystrophy. Hellenic J Cardiol 2013; 54: 227–229.

[34] Tsang W, Bales AC, Lang RM. Peripartum cardiomyopathy: treatment and prognosis. In: UpToDate, Post TW(Ed), UpToDate, Waltham, MA. (Accessed on April 07, 2016).

[35] Duncker D, Haghikia A, Konig T et al. Risk for ventricular fibrillation in peripartum cardiomyopathy with severely reduced left ventricular function value of the wearing cardioverter/defibrillator. Eur J Heart Fail 2014; 16: 1331–1336.

[36] McKenna WJ. Treatment of amyloid cardiomyopathy. In: UpToDate, Post TW(Ed), UpToDate, Waltham, MA. (Accessed on April 07, 2016).

[37] Merlo M, Pivetta A, Pinamonti B et al. Long-term prognostic impact of therapeutic strategies in patients with idiopathic dilated cardiomyopathy: Changing mortality over the last 30 years. Eur J Heart Fail 2014; 16: 317–324.

[38] Macías A, Gavira JJ, Castaño S et al. Cardiac resynchronization therapy and valvular cardiomyopathy after corrective surgery. Rev Esp Cardiol 2008; 61: 1088–1091.

[39] Zhang J, Zhang Y, Zhou X et al. QRS duration shortening predicts left ventricular reverse remodeling in patients with dilated cardiomyopathy after cardiac resynchronization therapy. Acta Cardiol 2015; 70: 307–313.

[40] Cabrera-Bueno F, Alzueta J, Fernández-Pastor J et al. Premature normalizing of ejection fraction after resynchronization inidiopathic dilated cardiomyopathy is maintained long-term and identifies the best clinical arrhythmic prognosis Cardiocore 2015; 50: 71–75.

[41] García Lunar I, Castro Urda V, Toquero Ramos J et al. Ventricular arrhythmias in super-responders to cardiac resynchronization therapy. Rev Esp Cardiol (Engl Ed). 2014;67:883-9.

[42] Healey JS. Hallstrom AP, Kuck KH et al. Role of the implantable defibrillator among elderly patients with a history of life-threatening ventricular arrhythmias. Eur Heart J 2007; 28: 1746 - 9.

[43] Huang DT, Sesselberg HW, McNittS et al. Improved survival associated with prophylactic implantable defibrillators in elderly patients with prior myocardial infarction and depressed ventricular function: a MADIT-II substudy. J Cardiovasc Electrophysiol 2007; 18: 833 – 8.

[44] Duray G, Richter S, Manegold J et al. Efficacy and safety of ICD therapy in a population of elderly patients treated with optimal background medication. J Interv Card Electrophysiol 2005; 14: 169 - 73.

[45] Strickberger SA, Hummel JD, Bartlett TG et al. Amiodarone versus implantable cardioverter-defibrillator: randomized trial in patients with nonischemic dilated cardiomyopathy and asymptomatic nonsustained ventricular tachycardia—AMIOVIRT. J Am Coll Cardiol 2003; 41: 1707 - 12.

[46] Bänsch D, Antz M, Boczor S et al. Primary prevention of sudden cardiac death in idiopathic dilated cardiomyopathy: the Cardiomyopathy Trial (CAT). Circulation 2002; 105: 1453 – 8.

[47] Birnie DH, Sauer WH, Bogun F et al. Diagnosis and management of arrhythmias associated with cardiac sarcoidosis. Heart Rhythm 2014; 11: 1304–1323.

[48] McKenna WJ. Clinical manifestations and diagnosis of arrhythmogenic right ventricular cardiomyopathy. In: UpToDate, Post TW(Ed), UpToDate, Waltham, MA. (Accessed on April 07, 2016).

[49] Link MS, Laidlaw D, Polonsky B et al. Ventricular arrhythmias in the North American Multidisciplinary Study of Arrhythmogenic right ventricular cardiomyopathy. Predictors, characteristics and treatment. J Am Coll Cardiol 2014; 64: 119 - 25.

[50] Bohnsale A, James CA, Tichnell C et al. Incidence and predictors of implantable cardioverter-defibrillator therapy in patients with arrhythmogenic right ventricular dysplasia/cardiomyopathy undergoing implantable cardioverter-defibrillator implantation for primary prevention. J Am Coll Cardiol 2011; 58: 1485 - 96.

[51] McKenna WJ. Arrhythmogenic right ventricular cardiomyopathy: treatment and prognosis. In: UpToDate, Post TW(Ed), UpToDate, Waltham, MA. (Accessed on April 07, 2016).

# Chapter 21

# Invasive Treatment in Advanced (Stage-D) Heart Failure

Kaan Kırali, Özge Altaş Yerlikhan and Hakan Hançer

Additional information is available at the end of the chapter

http://dx.doi.org/10.5772/67455

**Abstract**

Heart failure is a complex, true pandemic clinical syndrome and is responsible for 5% of hospitalizations globally. Severe heart failure can manifest as two lethal clinical entities: (1) acute cardiac decompensation with cardiogenic shock after large acute myocardial infarction with mortality rates approaching 50% or after cardiac surgery with mortality rates higher than 65% and (2) chronic destructive cardiac remodeling or acute decompensative exacerbations of cardiomyopathies with one-year mortality of approximately 80% (worse than most types of cancer). Interventional therapies aim first to improve symptoms and life expectancy in patients with severe heart failure syndrome, second to prevent left ventricular remodeling, and third to bridge patients to long-term mechanical circulatory support or transplantation. Several treatment options can be used to stabilize patients. In particular, new percutaneous mitral valve interventions and short-term circulatory support devices open up a new temporary treatment area in symptomatic Stage-D heart failure. The durable or curable surgical destination treatment will be only permanent ventricular assist devices or heart transplantation. This chapter focuses on the treatment steps and new approaches in hospitalized Stage-D heart failure patients.

**Keywords:** heart failure, heart transplantation, ventricular assist device, ECMO, ECLS

At end-stage, any type of cardiomyopathy (CMP) causes a complex clinical heart failure (HF) syndrome, which results from structural and/or functional impairment of ventricular filling or ejection. This dire clinical situation can cause an adverse vicious cycle that is ultimately fatal if not treated by pharmacological or invasive mechanical support or heart transplantation (HTx). Left ventricular functional abnormalities range from normal-sized left ventricle (LV) with preserved left ventricular ejection fraction (LVEF) to severe left ventricular dilatation (LVD) with markedly reduced LVEF. Reduced LVEF is defined as the clinical diagnosis of HF and LVEF ≤40%, which means a clinic and functional association of systolic and/or diastolic LVD.

Abnormal systolic and/or diastolic functions impair left ventricular contractile and relaxation functions that result in increasing left ventricular end-diastolic volume (LVEDV) and left ventricular end-systolic volume (LVESV), as well as left ventricular end-diastolic diameter (LVEDD) and left ventricular end-systolic diameter (LVESD), with the alteration of the left ventricular shape from conical form to spherical form. Adverse elevation of preload and afterload results in increasing left ventricular end-diastolic pressure (LVEDP) and left ventricular end-systolic pressure (LVESP). Inadequate unloading is the primary cause of diastolic LVD due to left ventricular overloading, and ineffectual ejection is the primary cause of systolic LVD due to left ventricular overstretching. This LVD induces overpressure behind the LV, which is initially transient but becomes permanent over time. Increasing left atrial pressure (LAP) in acute decompensation of LVD results in pulmonary congestion and pulmonary edema; however, chronic overload causes increasing pulmonary vascular resistance (PVR) and pulmonary hypertension (PHT). Decompensation of the LV and increased right ventricular afterload also impairs the right ventricle (RV) over time. Both preload pressures defined as pulmonary capillary wedge pressure (PCWP) and central venous pressure (CVP) increase during cardiac failure and cause pulmonary and systemic symptoms. Sympathetic stimulation causes a rise of systemic vascular resistance (SVR) that worsens cardiac decompensation due to increased left ventricular afterload. The goals of HF therapy are decreasing both preloads to prevent tissue-congestion, increasing cardiac output (CO) via lowering both afterloads, and improving contractility of both ventricles to increase blood oxygenation and tissue perfusion.

Clinical appearance depends on systolic and/or diastolic ventricular dysfunction, and all treatment strategies are designed according to the HF-classification from Stage-A to Stage-D (**Table 1**). In the twenty-first century, new treatment options have facilitated delay or interruption of this cardiac deterioration and even enabled functional recovery and structural regeneration through corrective anatomic, functional, hemodynamic, and mechanical interventions and clinical medical improvement (**Figure 1**) [1]. Therapeutic and curative percutaneous or surgical treatments should be performed to rescue the damaged heart, and in this way, to recovery the deterioration of the heart and to prevent the development of HF. So, by definition, of left ventricular recovery presupposes that the patient can tolerate a moderate myocardial dysfunction and remain clinically and hemodynamically stable thereafter. Preinvasive therapy is usually implemented in Stage-C HF and consists of medical treatment, home rest, physical activity restriction, and closer medical follow-up.

Stage-D, advanced, end-stage, or refractory HF are various terms used to describe very sick patients (**Table 2**) [2]. Patients with decompensated Stage-D HF should be hospitalized for invasive, aggressive, effective, and interventive treatment combinations [3]. There are clinical clues that may assist clinicians in identifying patients who are progressing toward advanced HF (**Table 3**) [4]. Stage-D patients are those with truly refractory HF who might be eligible for specialized, advanced treatment strategies including mechanical circulatory support (MCS), procedures to facilitate fluid removal, continuous inotropic infusions, other innovative or experimental surgical procedures, or for end-of-life care, such as hospice [5]. After patients' clinical status improves, they will be bridged to destination treatment or HTx. The Interagency Registry for Mechanically Assisted Circulatory Support (INTERMACS) has developed seven

| AHA/ACC | Stage-A | Stage-B | Stage-C | Stage-D (end-stage) | | |
|---|---|---|---|---|---|---|
| NYHA class | | I | II III-A III-B | IV | | |
| INTERMACS | | | 7 | 6 5 4 | 3 2 | 1 |
| STATUS | | | | 2 | 1-B | 1-A |

**Stage-A:** At high risk for developing HF without structural heart disease

**Stage-B:** Asymptomatic HF with structural heart disease, but without signs or symptoms of HF

**Stage-C:** Symptomatic HF with structural heart disease with prior or current symptoms of HF

**Stage-D:** Refractory end-stage HF despite maximal medical therapy, requiring specialized interventions

**Class I:** No limitation of physical activity. Ordinary physical activity does not cause symptoms of HF.

**Class II:** Slight limitation of physical activity. Comfortable at rest, but ordinary physical activity (e.g., long-distance walking, climbing two flights of stairs) results in symptoms of HF.

**Class III:** Marked limitation of physical activity. Comfortable at rest, but less than ordinary activity (e.g., short-distance walking, climbing one flights of stairs) causes symptoms of HF.

*B:* *LVEF* ≤ *30%* and *LVEDD* ≥ *60 mm* and *peak oxygen uptake <20 mL/min/kg* and *stable > 2 months*

**Class IV:** Unable to carry on any physical activity without symptoms of HF, or symptoms of HF at rest.

**INTERMACS 1:** Cardiogenic shock

**INTERMACS 2:** High dose intravenous inotropic support with/without t-MCS in instable condition

**INTERMACS 3:** Low dose inotropic support with stable hemodynamics

**INTERMACS 4–6:** Stable hemodynamics without intravenous inotropic support

**INTERMACS 7:** Clinical stable

**STATUS 1A:** On the intravenous inotropic and mechanical circulatory support for acute hemodynamic decompensation with/without mechanical ventilation following by continuous monitoring of both ventricular filling pressures, and recertification every 7th day

**(a)** Ventricular assist device (left, right, biventricular) <30 days

**(b)** Total artificial heart

**(c)** Extracorporeal circulatory support with/without oxygenator

**(d)** Counterpulsatile balloon pumping (intra-, extra-, para-aortic)

**STATUS 1B:** On the intravenous inotropic support or ventricular assist device >30 days

**STATUS 2:** Do not meet above criteria (patients on non-intravenous medical treatment at home)

HF = heart failure; LVEDD = left ventricular end-diastolic diameter; LVEF = left ventricular ejection fraction.

**Table 1.** Classification and interrelation of HF.

profiles that further stratify patients with advanced HF, who will be treated with a destination therapy (**Table 4**) [6]. All other causes, which can manifest in severe cardiac decompensation, should be ruled out during diagnosis.

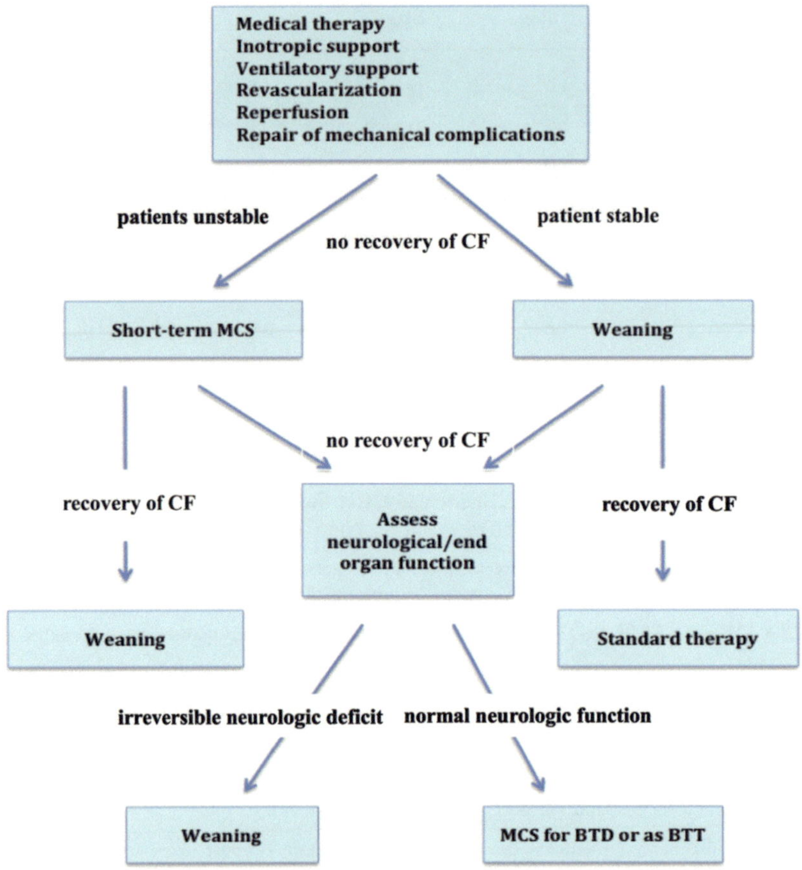


**Figure 1.** Management algorithm for Stage-D heart failure. BTD = bridge to destination; BTT = bridge to transplantation; CF = cardiac function; MCS = mechanical circulatory support.

Invasive treatments against HF depend on the nature and type of cardiac pathology; however, the systematic approach to their application is well defined (**Table 5**). The first step is to stabilize the patient's hemodynamics using pharmacological hemodynamic support (PHS), with full intravenous medication including inotropics, vasodilatators, inodilatators, diuretics, etc. Management of total fluid volume (1.5–2 L/day) and sodium restriction are essential to reduce congestive symptoms, although it is important to avoid hyponatremia by maintaining sodium above 132 mEq/L. Full and continuous monitoring of pre- and afterload (central venous and pulmonary artery catheterization) and CO measurements, echocardiographic examinations (transthoracic and/or transesophageal), and laboratory findings should be implemented in the intensive care unit (ICU). The second step is to carry out any percutaneous interventional support required to eliminate anatomorphologic pathologies (coronary artery stenosis, fibrotic valvular stenosis, etc.) for the purpose of maintaining the satisfactory filling pressures, myocardial contractility, and forward ejection in both circulations. The third and fourth steps apply to patients that are provided with electrical resynchronization and/or mechanical ventilatory support as needed to relieve the negative effects of electromechanical

http://dx.doi.org/10.5772/67455

1. Severe symptoms of HF with dyspnea and/or fatigue at rest or with minimal exertion (NYHA class III or IV)
2. Episodes of fluid retention (pulmonary and/or systemic congestion, peripheral edema) and/or reduced cardiac output at rest (peripheral hypoperfusion)
3. Objective evidence of severe cardiac dysfunction shown by at least one of the following:
   a. LVEF < 30%
   b. Pseudonormal or restrictive mitral flow pattern
   c. Mean PCWP > 16 mmHg and/or RAP >12 mmHg by pulmonary artery catheterization
   d. High BNP or NT-proBNP plasma levels in the absence of noncardiac causes
4. Severe impairment of functional capacity shown by one of the following:
   a. Inability to exercise
   b. 6-minute walk distance ≤ 300 m
   c. Peak $Vo_2$ < 12 to 14 mL/kg/min
5. History of ≥ 1 HF hospitalization in past 6 months
6. Presence of all the previous features despite "attempts to optimize" therapy, including diuretics and GDMT, unless these are poorly tolerated or contraindicated, and CRT when indicated

BNP = B-type natriuretic peptide; CRT = cardiac resynchronization therapy; GDMT = guideline-directed medical therapy; HF = heart failure; LVEF = left ventricular ejection fraction; NT-proBNP = N-terminal pro-B-type natriuretic peptide; NYHA = New York Heart Association; PCWP = pulmonary capillary wedge pressure; RAP = right atrial pressure.

**Table 2.** Definition of advanced heart failure.

- Repeated (≥2) hospitalizations or emergency department visits for HF in the past year
- Progressive deterioration in renal function (e.g., rise in BUN and creatinine)
- Weight loss without other cause (e.g., cardiac cachexia)
- Intolerance to ACE inhibitors due to hypotension and/or worsening renal function
- Intolerance to beta blockers due to worsening HF or hypotension
- Frequent systolic blood pressure <90 mmHg
- Persistent dyspnea with dressing or bathing requiring rest
- Inability to walk 1 block on the level ground due to dyspnea or fatigue
- Recent need to escalate diuretics to maintain volume status, often reaching daily furosemide equivalent dose >160 mg/d and/or use of supplemental metolazone therapy
- Progressive decline in serum sodium, usually to <133 mEq/L
- Frequent ICD shocks

ACE = angiotensin-converting enzyme; BUN = blood urea nitrogen; HF = heart failure; ICD = implantable cardioverter defibrillator.

**Table 3.** Clinical events and findings for identifying patients with advanced HF.

| Profile | Profile description | Shorthand | Features | IABP | t-MCS* | Hospitalization | Life expectancy | p-MCS** | Timing |
|---|---|---|---|---|---|---|---|---|---|
| 1 | Critical cardiogenic shock | Crash and burn | Life-threatening hypotension and excessive inotropic/ vasopressor support, critical organ hypoperfusion, often worsening acidosis and lactate levels | Yes | Yes | Yes (ICU) | Hours | Emergent (Rescue) | <7 days |
| 2 | Progressive decline | Sliding fast | Dependent on inotropic support with/without continuing nutritional depletion, worsening renal function, inability to restore volume balance, or other major status indicator. | Yes | Yes | Yes (ICU/Ward) | Days to weeks | Urgent (salvage) | <30 days |
| 3 | Stable, but inotrope-dependent | Dependent stability | Stable blood pressure, organ function and nutrition on mild-moderate doses of continuous intravenous inotropic support after repeated documentation of failure to wean without symptomatic hypotension, worsening symptoms, or progressive organ dysfunction (usually renal). | Yes/ no | Yes/no | Yes (Ward) | Few weeks | Elective (destination) | <90 days |
| 4 | Recurrent advanced HF | Frequent flyer | Resting and/or daily living activities (dressing or bathing) symptoms of congestion (orthopnea, abdominal discomfort, nausea, poor appetite, disabling ascites, or severe lower-extremity edema), on oral therapy at home, | No | No | No | Weeks to months | Elective (destination) | >90 days |
| 5 | Exertion intolerant | House-bound | Comfortable at rest, but unable to engage in any activity, living predominantly within the house or housebound | No | No | No | Weeks to months | Yes/no | ? |
| 6 | Exertion limited | Walking wounded | Comfortable at rest without evidence of fluid overload and able to do some mild activity, daily living are comfortable and minor activities outside the home, but fatigue results within a few minutes or with any meaningful physical exertion. | No | No | No | Months | Yes/no | No |
| 7 | NYHA class III B | | Clinically stable with a reasonable level of comfortable activity, despite a history of previous decompensation that is not recent, able to walk more than a block. | No | No | No | | No | No |

*t-MCS includes IABP, ECMO, ECCS, and others;
**p-MCS includes LVAD, TAH.
HF = heart failure; ICU = intensive care unit; p-MCS = permanent mechanical circulatory support; t-MCS = temporary mechanical circulatory support; NYHA = New york Heart Association.

**Table 4.** INTERMACS profiles.

http://dx.doi.org/10.5772/67455

**(I)** Pharmacological hemodynamic support (PHS)

**(II)** Percutaneous interventional support (PIS)

- **1.** Coronary revascularization
  - **a.** Angioplasty
  - **b.** Coronary artery bypass grafting on the beating heart (CABG-BH)
    - **i.** Off-pump
    - **ii.** On-pump
- **2.** Mitral valve repair
  - **a.** Percutaneous
  - **b.** Surgical neo-chordae

**(III)** Electrical resynchronizational support (ERS)

**(IV)** Mechanical ventilatory support (MVS)

**(V)** Mechanical counterpulsatile hemodynamic support (MCHS)

- **1.** Intraaortic counterpulsatile support (IACP)
  - **a.** Intraaortic balloon pump (IABP)
- **2.** Extraaortic counterpulsatile support (EACP)
  - **a.** Extra-aortic balloon pump (EABP)
- **3.** Paraaortic counterpulsatile circulation (PACP)
  - **a.** Paraaortic circulatory device (PACD)
  - **b.** Pressure-unload left ventricular assist device (PULVAD)
  - **c.** Kantrowitz CardioVAD (KCV)
  - **d.** Symphony

**(VI)** Mechanical circulatile support (MCS)

- **1.** Temporary mechanical cardiopulmonary support (t-MCPS)
  - **a.** Cardiopulmonary bypass (CPB)
  - **b.** Extracorporeal cardiopulmonary support (ECCPS) or Extracorporeal life support (ECLS)
- **2.** Temporary mechanical circulatory support (t-MCS)
  - **a.** Extracorporeal circulatory support (ECCS)
  - **b.** Intracorporeal circulatory support (ICCS)
- **3.** Permanent mechanical circulatory support (p-MCS)
  - **a.** Ventricular assist device (VAD)
  - **b.** Total artificial heart (TAH)

**(VII)** Heart transplantation

- **1.** Isolated

| | | | | |
|---|---|---|---|---|
| | **2.** | Heart and lung transplantation | | |
| **(VIII)** | Left ventricular structural restoration | | | |
| | **1.** | Aneurysmectomy | | |
| | **2.** | Cardiomyoplasty | | |
| | **3.** | Reshaping | | |
| | | **a.** | Intracardiac | |
| | | **b.** | Extracardiac | |
| | | | **i.** | CorCap Cardiac Support Device |
| | | | **ii.** | Paracor HeartNet Device |

**Table 5.** Invasive treatment sequences of the severe end stage heart failure.

dyssynchrony and poor systemic oxygenation. The fifth step entails provision of hemodynamic supports using temporary mechanical circulatory support (t-MCS) devices such as counter-pulsatile circulatory support (CPCS), extracorporeal cardiopulmonary support (ECCPS), or extracorporeal circulatory support (ECCS) to maintain adequate CO for sufficient body perfusion without any congestive sign of the left and/or right HF. The sixth step consists a long-term circulatory support to obtain adequate left with or without right heart circulation for bridging to a destination therapy. The left ventricular assist device (LVAD) and total artificial heart (TAH) are permanent mechanical circulatory support (p-MCS) devices, and for the time being represent the last and best chance to bridge patients to transplantation or destination therapy. The last step is HTx with or without lung(s), which is considered the gold standard for the treatment of refractory Stage-D HF.

## 1. Pharmacological hemodynamic support (PHS)

Decompensation of Stage-D HF should be treated in hospital immediately, medically, aggressively, intravenously, and with a multidisciplinary approach. Nowadays, we have a lot of pharmacological treatment weapons with contractor, vasodilator, vasopressor, and inactivator effects [7]. Diuretics for congestion, antiarrhythmics for dysrhythmia, anticoagulations for thrombosis, and digoxin for right heart failure are integral parts of medical treatment (**Figure 2**). With the advent of neurohormonal blockade, tremendous progress has been made in the medical treatment of the advanced HF. Treatment of comorbid conditions such as diabetes and iron deficiency can aid clinical recovery.

**Inotropic or inodilator therapy** is the initial pharmacological strategy to improve myocardial contractility, increase heart rate, reduce afterload through peripheral vasodilatation, and augment CO. Dobutamine and dopamine (inotropic), and milrinone (inodilator) are the three most commonly used intravenous agents.

*Dobutamine* (2–20 μg/kg/min) is the most used sympathomimetic agent, and its inotropic and chronotropic effects derive from direct stimulation of $\beta_1$ adrenergic receptors, which are

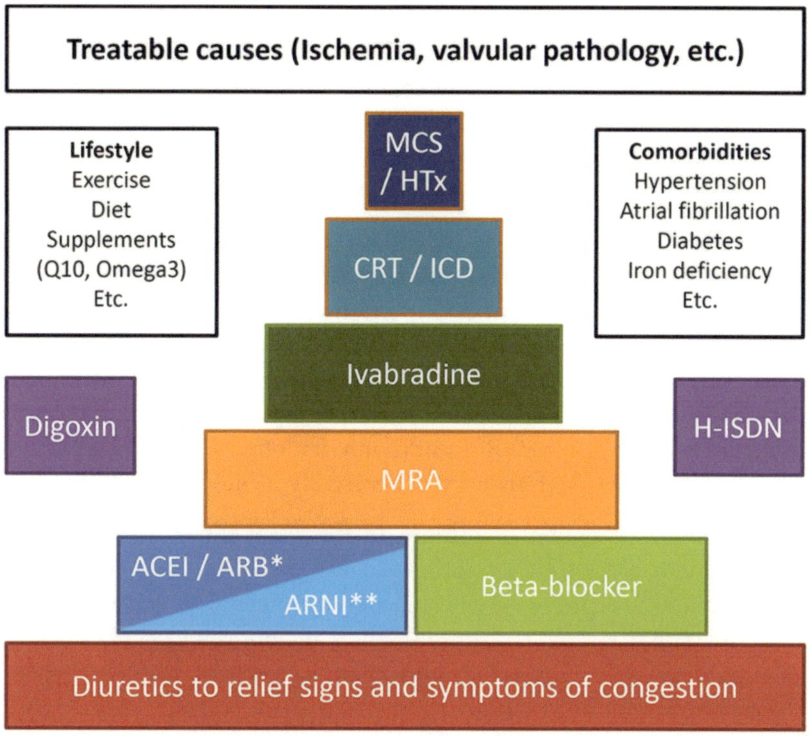


**Figure 2.** Current therapies for end-stage heart failure. *An ARB is recommended when an ACEI is not tolerated. **An ARNIs is recommended when both RAAS inhibitors are ineffective. ACEI = angiotensin converting-enzyme inhibitor; ARB = angiotensin receptor blocker; ARNI = angiotensin receptor neprilysin inhibitor; CRT = cardiac resynchronization therapy; ICD = implantable cardioverter defibrillator; H-ISDN = hydralazine-isosorbide dinitrate; HTx = heart transplantation; MCS = mechanical circulatory support; MRA= mineralocorticoid antagonist; omega3 = omega-3 polyunsaturated fatty acids; Q10 = coenzyme Q10.

mostly downregulated in end-stage HF patients. The main effect is inotropic, and it may increase coronary blood flow, but myocardial oxygen consumption can increase if dobutamine induces tachycardia. Tachycardia depends more on dobutamine-related cardiac output than on infusion level.

*Dopamine* stimulates different receptors depending on dose level: in low (diuretic) doses (0.5–3 μg/kg/min) dopaminergic receptors in the renal, mesenteric, and coronary arterial beds are stimulated; in moderate (inotropic) doses (3–10 μg/kg/min), nonselective adrenergic receptors are activated; in high (vasoconstrictive) doses (>10 μg/kg/min), especially $\alpha$-adrenergic receptors are induced.

*Milrinone* (0.25–0.75 μg/kg/min) acts by a nonadrenergic mechanism, increasing c-AMP via phosphodiesterase III inhibition. It is preferred mostly in patients with increased PVR and/or SVR due to better vascular vasodilation than dobutamine. It is crucial to be aware of the risk of systemic hypotension, for which concomitant vasopressors should be added. Milrinone increases CO without increasing overall myocardial oxygen consumption, but does improve myocardial diastolic relaxation (lusitropic effect).

**Vasopressor therapy** is necessary to increase SVR, blood pressures, and mean arterial pressure, when the low cardiac output syndrome (LCOS) is serious with fairly lower systemic blood pressure. *Adrenalin* (2–10 μg/min or 0.01–0.4 μg/kg/min) is used primarily to maintain cardiac contractility and CO by counteracting bradycardia and hypocontractility. *Noradrenalin* (2–16 μg/min or 0.01–0.3 μg/kg/min) is used primarily to maintain mean systemic arterial pressure by controlling hypotension, severe vasodilatation, or vasoplegia syndrome. It is also an integral part of inodilator treatment modality to prevent systemic vasodilatation.

**Vasodilator therapy** is needed in most HF patients to decrease SVR and also PVR. Nitroglycerin (10–500 μg/min) and nitroprusside (10–500 μg/min) are the most commonly-used agents in cardiac surgery, but prostaglandins and nitric oxide (NO) more specifically decrease PVR and right ventricular afterload in patients with end-stage HF due to the improvement of the right ventricular dysfunction (RVD) and CO. Long-term therapy with sildenafil has demonstrated better hemodynamics in lowering PVR. In addition, endothelin receptor antagonists, such as bosentan, can also be used although they are not currently included in treatment guidelines.

**Diuretics** restrict the reabsorption of sodium in the renal tubes, increase urinary sodium excretion, and decrease congestive symptoms in HF patients. Loop diuretics (furosemide, bumetanide, torsemide) are preferred pharmacological agents in hospitalized patients and used intravenously. The first goal is to resolve fluid retention and congestive signs (edema, hepatomegaly, pulmonary edema, etc.), and then to prevent the recurrence of volume overload. The most common side effects of excessive diuretic usage include fluid depletion, hypokalemia, hypomagnesaemia, and azotemia. Furosemide is the most common used loop diuretic, the dose and frequency should be increased until the adequate diuresis and weight loss is maintained. Low-dose dopamine (2 μg/kg/min) infusion can improve diuresis and better preserve renal function. If the diuretic strategy is unsatisfactory or ineffective due to renal failure, ultrafiltration to remove water and small- to medium-weight solutes may be considered as a primary volume-removal therapy. After acute decompensation caused by volume overload resolves, oral diuretic therapy is started with furosemide and/or thiazides and spironolactone combination. Daily recording of body weight is the best parameter to follow diuretic treatment's effectiveness and to adjust dosage.

**Renin-angiotensin-aldosterone system (RAAS)** is at the core of the pathophysiology of HF, and its modulation is central to altering the disease process in HF with reduced LVEF. Blockade of RAAS can be provided by an angiotensin-converting enzyme inhibitor (ACEI), angiotensin-receptor blocker (ARB), or mineralocorticoid receptor antagonist (MRA). This inhibition can reduce blood pressure in hypertensive patients, prevent target organ damage in diabetes, and improve outcomes in HF patients [8]. This hormone system regulates protective acute stress response through inflammatory and proliferative mechanisms; however, chronic stimulation has detrimental effects including vasoconstriction, sodium and water retention, vascular smooth muscle proliferation, endothelial dysfunction, inflammation, fibrosis, and thrombosis [9]. The RAAS cascade begins with renin secretion by renal juxtaglomerular cells, continues with the conversion of hepatic angiotensinogen to the inactive angiotensin I, and finishes with conversion of angiotensin I to angiotensin II by angiotensin-converting enzyme (ACE). Angiotensin II is the strongest mediator to promote all effects above mentioned, and it stimulates the

http://dx.doi.org/10.5772/67455

secretion of aldosterone from adrenal cortex and arginine vasopressin from posterior pituitary. Blockade of the RAAS with ACEIs has been a cornerstone of HF therapy for over 20 years, so that ACEIs decrease the formation of angiotensin II and inhibit the breakdown of bradykinin with the formation of NO and other vasodilators. Additionally, further blockade of RAAS with aldosterone antagonists and ARBs has increased the efficiency, so that ARBs bind competitively to and dissociate slowly from angiotensin type-1 receptors and blockade aldosterone secretion. MRAs cover mineralocorticoid receptors for competitive inhibition. The direct renin inhibitor (DRI) agents blockade the RAAS at the most proximal step via the inhibition of angiotensinogen conversion.

**Natriuretic peptide system (NPS)** counter regulates the detrimental effects of the up-regulation of RAAS, inhibits secretion of arginine vasopressin, modulates the autonomic nervous system, and antagonizes their vasopressor effects in HF [10]. There are three peptides: atrial natriuretic peptide (ANP), brain natriuretic peptide (BNP), and endothelial cell natriuretic peptide (CNP). Both ANP and BNP have similar structural, hypotensive, natriuretic, and diuretic properties. Distension of the atria and ventricles due to cardiac injury and/or overload, ventricular dysfunction, and HF stimulates the expression of ANP from atria and BNP from brain and ventricles with several effects: (1) activation of membrane-bound natriuretic peptide receptors-A leading to vasorelaxation, natriuresis, and diuresis; (2) inhibition of RAAS due to blocked of renin secretion and associated aldosterone production; (3) reduction in adverse cardiovascular changes via remodeling, apoptosis, ventricular hypertrophy, and fibrosis; and (4) enhanced myocardial relaxation. On the other hand, CNP extracted from endothelial cells and brain acts only as a vasodilator without potent diuretic and natriuretic effects. Measurements of peptides ANP, BNP, and its inactive precursor N-terminal fragment of pro-B-type natriuretic peptide (NT-proBNP) are useful in prognosis assessment and antifailure therapy monitoring, but CNP is not measurable due to low concentrations in circulating blood. Natriuretic peptides are removed from circulation through two mechanisms: clearing by natriuretic peptide clearance receptor (NPRC and NPRC3) or inactivating by a degrading enzyme. The endothelial enzyme *neprilysin* hydrolyzes ANP rapidly and also degrades a large number of other vasodilators and vasoconstrictors although BNP is relatively resistant to its digestion. Inhibition of neprilysin (NEPi) with *sacubitril* (1) increases concentrations of circulating vasodilators (ANP, adrenomedullin, and bradykinin), but also circulating vasopressors (angiotensin II, endothelin I); (2) augments plasma ANP and BNP levels leading to enhanced natriuretic-diuretic-vasodilator effects, lower preloads, and inhibition of fibrosis; (3) inhibits renin secretion and angiotensin I to II conversion, but that is not a complete inhibition effect on the RAAS. However, blocking neprilysin alone does not effect a complete inhibition of RAAS, which is stimulated by the activated sympathetic nervous system (SNS) leading to increasing renin secretion and ACE activation of angiotensin I to II. These opposing effects neutralize each other and therefore NPS inhibitors alone exert little effect on hemodynamics. This problem is solved by dual blockade of RAAS by ARB and NPS by NEPi. The combined molecule of sacubitril (NEPi) and valsartan (ARB) is a first drug (LCZ696) in class angiotensin receptor neprilysin inhibitor (ARNi), and represents a new treatment modality by blocking the angiotensin type-1 receptor and inhibiting the natriuretic peptide system concurrently [11]. Valsartan does not inhibit the breakdown of bradykinin, with decreasing angioedema risk; however, inhibition of angiotensin II action prevents vasopressor effects. This combination favors NPS activation and RAAS blockade, as well as residual angiotensin II effects from the SNS [12].

**Digoxin** is the oldest cardiac drug still in contemporary use, and can be useful in patients with persistent severe end-stage HF (LVEF <25%, cardiothoracic ratio >55%, New York Heart Association (NYHA) class III or IV) undergoing guideline-directed medical therapy, and especially symptomatic patients being treated with neurohormonal antagonists [13]. Digoxin has been used as the first line of pharmacological treatment for HF until the understanding of HF pathophysiology changed in recent decades, which leads to the shift from inotropic support to neurohormonal modulation [14]. The effect is regardless of the rhythm, etiology of HF, or concomitant therapy. Digoxin binds for the sarcolemmal $Na^+$-$K^+$-ATPase pump to blocking and impeding $Na^+$ extrusion outside, accumulated intracellular $Na^+$ decreases the transmembrane sodium gradient, and as a consequence suppresses the activity of the $Na^+$-$Ca^{++}$-exchanger, raising the intracellular $Ca^{++}$ concentration and effecting more forceful contraction. Digoxin is the only inotrope known to improve LVEF and CO and also to reduce PCWP without tachycardia and/or hypotension. The beneficial effect of the drug occurs even at low maintenance dosage (serum digoxin concentration 0.5–0.9 ng/mL; 0.125 mg/day) with positive inotropic but negative chronotropic (4–7 beats/min in sinus rhythm) properties. The hemodynamic effects of digoxin are not attenuated by chronic administration, because $Na^+$-$K^+$-ATPase is not upregulated. In noncardiac tissue, digoxin acts as a neurohormonal modulator by increasing parasympathetic tone and dampening activation of the SNS (sympatholytic) and RAAS.

## 2. Percutaneous interventional support (PIS)

Cardiac decompensation is usually a consequence of myocardial ischemia and/or mechanical complications, or chronic remodeling. Acute HF develops after ischemic damage or acute hemodynamic compromise of chronic HF with well-known structural pathologies during medical follow-up. These patients may not improve with medical therapy; however, correction of underlying pathologies such as coronary artery disease, valvular stenosis, or regurgitation can result in significant improvement in functional status. Before mechanical circulatory treatments, all applicable interventional therapies must be evaluated and performed confidentially. First of all, percutaneous revascularization is the initial step in managing inadequate oxygen delivery due to stenotic or occluded coronary arteries, and that must be followed by percutaneous palliative mitral valve repair if it is necessary. Significant mitral regurgitation (MR) resulting in inadequate forward ejection of the LV can cause intractable left heart failure (LHF), even if total stroke volume seems enough to produce adequate CO. The goal of palliative percutaneous interventions for these pathologies is to maintain and sustain adequate left ventricular filling and forward ejection. If these treatment strategies are successful, patients have the chance to get better and postpone mechanical hemodynamic and/or circulatory support; however, inoperable or untouchable patients should be considered for destination therapy.

### 2.1. Coronary revascularization

Ischemic myocardium or acute coronary syndrome decreases significantly ventricular contractile function due to oxygen supply/demand imbalance. Hibernating, stunning, or infarction reduces LVEF, causes left ventricular remodeling, and exacerbates mitral valve dysfunction. Coronary angiography shows stenotic or occluded coronary territory, but stress echocardiography, nuclear imaging, and magnetic resonance imaging examinations show whether there are viable tissues and/or valvular dysfunction requiring corrective interventions, as well as for surgical treatment despite higher procedural risks. Coronary revascularization can salvage and improve the myocardium histologically and functionally, but these strategies usually fail to improve myocardial recovery due to nonviable myocardium.

#### 2.1.1. Angioplasty

Any severe atherosclerotic plaque, plaque rupture, or thrombotic occlusion reduces oxygen delivery to the myocardium, which results acute LHF. Persistent angina is also a common symptom (approximately 30%) in patients with ischemic CMP despite medical therapy, which increases major cardiac events by one third [15]. Percutaneous coronary intervention via balloon angioplasty associated with or without stent implantation is the first-stage therapy for coronary artery disease causing severe cardiac decompensation due to massive ischemia in high-risk patients with well-known compensated HF associated with or without mechanical complications of myocardial infarction, particularly MR. Coronary revascularization could aid in recovery of myocardial dysfunction if the affected myocardium consists of viable tissue, and MR may also be improved. Myocardial reserve after angioplasty also results in contractile improvement and favorable left ventricular remodeling in patients with LVD, and it also decreases HF symptoms (angina, functional class, BNP levels) [16, 17]. Partially or fully viability or transmural scar within the infarct should be identified by any test (scintigraphy, magnetic resonance, etc.) in this group of patients, because improvement in oxygen supply will abate ischemia burden [18, 19]. Transmural distribution of the postinfarction scar, which spreads from the subendocardium to the subepicardium without intermittent viability, does not provide any benefit by angioplasty. Although surgical coronary revascularization is superior to medical therapy in patients with HF [20], there is no real superiority of surgery over angioplasty [21]. Contrarily, the positive benefit of percutaneous revascularization of the viable region is a significant improvement in the LVEF and LVESV in the LHF patients. New designed clinical trials will give more detailed results regarding angioplasty performed in HF [22]. Unstable or hemodynamically instable patients with significant HF symptoms must be undertaken in catheter laboratory with a t-MCS to prevent sudden decompensation or cardiac arrest. The most preferable device to maintain adequate CO during percutaneous procedures is intraaortic balloon pump (IABP), which can be supported or replaced by a percutaneous temporary device (Impella, TandemHeart, etc.).

#### 2.1.2. Coronary artery bypass grafting

Patients with severe HF and coronary artery disease suitable for coronary artery bypass grafting (CABG) are at higher risk for surgical morbidity and mortality. Paradoxically, those patients who derive the greatest clinical benefit from CABG and are also at the greatest operative risk, which leads clinicians to hesitate to refer these patients for CABG [23]. Despite the fact that bypass surgery can create potential risks for HF patients, significantly viable tissue should be revascularized by on- or off-pump CABG [24]. Minimal invasive CABG procedures are an option, but dilated left ventricular cavity with or without right ventricular enlargement complicates off-pump CABG due to hemodynamic instability during the elevation of the heart for circumflex or right coronary artery anastomoses [25]. Single vessel bypass to the dominant left anterior descending territory can be useful in symptomatic multivessel disease patients, and this approach can cause a limited improvement in the LVEF and clinical status [26]. But, in the case of unsuitable pathology and anatomic structure of the coronary artery territory, viable tissue should be identified before surgery. Single coronary artery revascularization could be performed percutaneously or off-pump surgically [27]. On-pump CABG could be more harmful due to aortic cross clamping, but enrichment of cardioplegia with different agents may be protective [28].

### 2.2. Mitral valve repair

Functional MR due to LVD and remodeling is a common complication in dilated or ischemic CMPs, and severe symptomatic MR requires an invasive corrective intervention to prevent poor prognosis and to improve clinical status. However, the effectiveness of repair of MR in these situations is often compromised because it does not reverse the underlying cause of the CMP. While surgical mitral valve repair is the conventional treatment for MR, it is controversial in end-stage HF patients due to high surgical risk and lack of randomized trials about survival benefit. Because severe functional MR clearly increases the mortality as an independent predictor but mitral valve repair does not improve mid- and long-term survival in patients with end-stage HF, most major guidelines recommend against isolated mitral valve surgery in these patients, although surgery is generally recommended if aortic valve or coronary artery bypass graft surgery is also being performed [29]. Ideal candidates should have less fibrotic spherical ventricle with more contractile reserve, patients with irreversible pulmonary hypertension and severe right ventricle dysfunction would be unlikely to benefit from intervention [30]. Transcatheter mitral valve repair or implantation alternatives are currently preferred in high-risk patients not eligible for surgery [31]. Percutaneous mitral valve implantation seems to be the best solution to eliminate MR in end-stage HF patients with significant MR caused by severe annular enlargement [32].

#### *2.2.1. Percutaneous mitral valve repair*

Newly developed percutaneous mitral valve repair techniques can be useful in patients, who cannot be referred for surgical therapy (**Table 6**) [33]. In contrast to the positive effect of percutaneous mitral valve repair techniques in patients with severe MR-associated nonfailed hearts, mitral valve repairing is offered without targeting of full coaptation of mitral valve in end-stage HF patients. It is usually anatomically impossible to fully repair the mitral valve completely due to severe annular enlargement and/or thethering of the leaflets caused by left

| Percutaneous mitral valve repair | |
|---|---|
| **Leaflet** | |
| Edge-to-edge (leaflet plication) | MitraClip |
| | MitraFlex |
| Space occupier (leaflet coaptation) | Percu-Pro |
| Leaflet ablation | Thermocool |
| **Annulus** | |
| *Indirect approaches* | |
| Coronary sinus annuloplasty | Carillon |
| | Monarc |
| | Viacor |
| Asymmetrical approach | St Jude annulus reshaping device |
| | NIH-cerclage technology |
| *Direct approaches* | |
| Percutaneous mechanical cinching | Mitralign suture-based plication |
| | Accucinch GDS millipede ring system |
| Percutaneous energy-mediated cinching | QuantumCor |
| | ReCor |
| Hybrid | Mitral solution |
| | MiCardia |
| **Chordal implants** | |
| Transapical artificial chord | NeoChord |
| | MitraFlex |
| Transapical-Transseptal | Babic |
| **Left ventricle** | |
| LV remodelling | Mardil-BASE |
| | iCoapsys |
| **Percutaneous mitral valve implantation** | |
| Right mini-thoracotomy | Endovalve-Herrmann prosthesis |
| Transapical | Lutter prosthesis |
| Transseptal | CardiaQ prosthesis |

**Table 6.** Percutaneous mitral interventions.

ventricular enlargement, as well as it can be very devastating for failed hearts. Therefore, percutaneous mitral valve repair techniques are palliative, but also preparative interventions to improve patients' clinical status and hemodynamics before destination therapies like LVAD or HTx.

**The MitraClip** is a a novel technology for percutaneous treatment of MR, although its utility in patients with end-stage HF is somewhat limited [34]. This leaflet plication technology is based on the surgical Alfieri technique, which brings the anterior and posterior leaflets together with a suture, creating a "double orifice" mitral valve. The device is inserted by way of the femoral vein and utilizes a 24F guidewire to gain transseptal access to the left atrium (LA). It is essential to place the V-shaped clip at the main MR site between the anterior and posterior leaflet with the guidance of transesophageal echocardiography. The first clip may not solve the problem, but decreases degree of regurgitation from massive to severe or moderate-severe, and additional clip(s) could be applied to significantly reduce degree of regurgitation to moderate or lower. At least 50% reduction in the MR performed by mitral clips could be accepted as a successful procedure, while more than 75% without mitral stenosis could cause effective correction. This new device has shown benefit in outcomes for patients without HF, but it is unable to improve the clinical course in end-stage HF patients due to an immediate deterioration of left ventricular function, further aggravation of afterload mismatch, and progressive LHF [35]. MitraClip is a good alternative to surgery in functional MR refractory to medical and/or resynchronization therapy in patients with adequate anatomy, but not in patients who are considered inoperable due to high surgical risks [36]. It can be considered an important clinical option in the multidisciplinary treatment of HF, but postprocedural MR increases midterm cardiac mortality [37]. To increase utilization of the MitraClip treatment, this new approach must be used in selective cases or as an earlier step before the destination therapy. The first 30 days have an acceptable course, but after that the frequency of adverse events increases, especially early recurrence/persistence of MR [38].

**The Carillon** is a percutaneous coronary sinus-based mitral annuloplasty device designed to treat functional MR in end-stage HF patients [39]. This device consists of self-expandable nitinol distal and proximal anchors connected by a nitinol bridge, which are placed in the great cardiac vein and proximal coronary sinus located behind the posterior mitral annulus. Tension applied on the system results in cinching of the posterior periannular tissue, and displacement of the posterior mitral leaflet toward the anterior leaflet to reduce anterior-posterior (septal-lateral) dimension improves their coaptation and reduces functional MR [40]. Residual MR is not frequently observed in patients without HF, and it can decrease significantly in the first 3 months [41]. However, LVD associated with significant mitral annular enlargement results in significant MR, but also, mitral valve thethering complicates MR. This pathologic course could not be reversed completely by percutaneous mitral annuloplasty devices. This technique reduces functional MR significantly, increases functional capacity and quality of life, as well as induces improvement of left ventricular remodeling [42]. The major limitations to use this kind of devices are the significant distance between coronary sinus and mitral annulus, closed anatomic neighborhood of coronary arteries, and annular calcifications.

### *2.2.2. Surgical mitral valve repair*

Surgical mitral valve correction is seldom preferred because of the high risks associated with the operation. On-pump surgery is usually not recommended, and severe MR with clinical deterioration can be the first indication for LVAD implantation. Transapical

http://dx.doi.org/10.5772/67455

correction using NeoChord has been popularized in degenerative MR, and the new devices facilitate transapical implantation of neo-chordae on the beating heart without cardiopulmonary bypass (CPB) [43]. This approach is useful in isolated mitral valve leaflet(s) prolapse with lower operative risk [44]. However, no high-quality studies have investigated the possibility of implantation in severe HF situations with LVD and mitral leaflet thethering. This approach could be preferred in severe MR caused by chordal rupture without adding of ring annuloplasty. However, patients with a LVD and a significant MR have significant mitral annular dilatation without mitral valve prolapses, and in such cases MR can be corrected only via a prosthetic ring percutaneously. Otherwise, severe HF associated with significant MR is one of the best candidates for LVAD destination therapy.

## 3. Electrical resynchronizational support (ERS)

Electromechanical dyssynchrony is common in end-stage HF patients and can be found at different levels within the heart. Electrical dyssynchrony is evidenced by QRS prolongation (≥120 ms) and has a prevalence of 15–30% in HF population. Electrical dyssynchrony, and the subsequent abnormal mechanical activation, results in cellular, structural, hemodynamic, and ultimately clinical adverse effects [45]. Left bundle branch block results in a shorter diastolic time interval and longer isovolumetric contraction and relaxation times, which impair pump function because of abnormal electrical and mechanical properties, as well as functional MR. These effects can be ameliorated by resynchronizing the failing heart by means of pacing in the right atrium (RA) and both ventricles (biventricular pacing). Cardiac resynchronization therapy restores the appropriate timing of the cardiac contraction pattern and thereby not only reduces cellular, hemodynamic, and structural maladaptations to dyssynchrony, but also ultimately improves functional status, reduces hospitalization, and improves survival.

## 4. Mechanical ventilatory support (MVS)

Even when cardiac dysfunction is the only reason for HF syndrome, increased PVR raises respiratory effort and increased SVR reduces systemic output, decreasing pre- and afterload and increasing oxygenation, which results hemodynamic stability. The most common supportive approach in end-stage HF patients with respiratory failure is mechanical ventilation under general anesthesia. Intubation is usually the first step to maintain hemodynamic stability through decreased respiratory effort and adrenergic stimulation. Increasing oxygenation and use of vasodilator inhalation decrease adverse responses and PVR, which is the main treatment strategy for the right ventricular failure (RVF). Supportive mechanical hemodynamic approaches prevent unnecessary and prolonged mechanical ventilation, which can be a significant risk factor for ventilator-dependent infections. Elective intubation is also required for percutaneous mitral valve repair.

## 5. Mechanical counterpulsatile hemodynamic support (MCHS)

In severe cases of decompensated HF, pharmacological hemodynamic support cannot usually achieve complete hemodynamic stability and maintain adequate blood supply to end-organs and tissues in the decompensated HF. End-stage HF patients with severe ventricular decompensation are frequently referred to ICUs for hemodynamic support. After full monitoring and assessment of hemodynamic parameters, the required appropriate medications are used to solve symptoms and signs of LCOS; however, full medication can heal patients for once, but then healing degrades and pharmacologic bridge to transplantation cannot stabilize patients, and hence mechanical counterpulsatile hemodynamic support (MCHS) becomes necessary.

### 5.1. Intraaortic counterpulsatile support (IACPS)

Counterpulsatile devices for MHS improve patient status by same physiologic effects, but with different mechanisms (**Table 7**) [46]. The principle of counterpulsation is to produce diastolic augmentation. Prediastolic inflation coincided with T-P interval on electrocardiogram provides increase in peak diastolic aortic pressure (aortic uploading) to enhance coronary perfusion during ventricular relaxation and filling. Presystolic deflation coincided with QRS-T interval on electrocardiogram, which is always triggered by R wave, assures decreasing in end-diastolic aortic pressure (aortic unloading) to facilitate intraaortic impedance reduction during ventricular contraction and ejection. These devices are usually used for short-term supportive therapy in early postoperative period to wean patients from CPB. There are several positive effects of counterpulsation on systemic hemodynamics and left ventricular mechanoenergetics, but the main goal is to increase CO without bypassing the heart or the related ventricle [47]. Second application area in end-stage HF patients is to stabilize hemodynamics and to gain time for keeping patients alive or bridging to a more durable therapy. The first step

| | Intraaortic | Paraaortic |
|---|---|---|
| Insertion | Percutaneously | Surgically |
| Incision | Sliding technique or local incision | Intraoperatively or left thoracotomy |
| Placement way | Peripheral | Semicentral |
| Placement area | Suprarenal thoracoabdominal aorta | Thoracal descending aorta |
| Capacity | 30–50 mL | 20–100 (or more) mL |
| Working principle | Volumetric | Circulatory |
| Working space | Intraluminal | Extraluminal |
| Working risk | Systolic occlusive | Nonocclusive |
| Inflation/deflation | Diastole/systole | Diastole + systole |
| Coronary perfusion | Optimum/steal | Optimum |
| Stroke work | Decreasing (+) | Decreasing (+++) |
| Cardiac output | Increasing | Increasing |

**Table 7.** Comparison of counterpulsatil devices.

http://dx.doi.org/10.5772/67455

is to stabilize the end-stage HF patients using IABP for up to 2 weeks and if the patients are hemodynamically stabilized (no need for inotropes, no peripheral organ malfunction, CVP ≤ 10 mmHg, mean arterial pressure ≥ 65 mmHg) but could not wean from IABP, then they can be transitioned to a more effective counterpulsatile or t-MCS devices as a bridge to recovery or to end-stage therapy (p-MCS device or HTx).

**Intraaortic balloon pump (IABP)** is the most preferred, well-tolerated, and most cost-efficient method among mechanical supportive approaches with significant hemodynamic improvements in patients with unstable hemodynamic status (**Table 8**) [48]. But the frequency of IABP

- **(I)** Therapeutic
  - **A.** Preoperatively
    - **1.** Unstable myocardial ischemia
      - **a.** acute coronary syndrome
      - **b.** intractable coronary ischemia
      - **c.** severe left main disease
      - **d.** malign ventricular arrhythmia
    - **2.** Cardiogenic shock
      - **a.** myocardial infarction
      - **b.** mechanical complications of AMI (MR, VSD, LVR)
      - **c.** myocarditis
      - **d.** sepsis
    - **3.** Cardiomyopaties
    - **4.** Procedural support during coronary angiography
    - **5.** Stabilization for surgery
      - **a.** cardiac surgical patients (LCOS, VSD, severe MR)
      - **b.** noncardiac surgical patients
  - **B.** Intraoperatively
    - **1.** Off-pump CABG
    - **2.** On-pump CABG on the beating heart
    - **3.** LVAD implantation
  - **C.** Postoperatively
    - **1.** Failure to separate from CPB
    - **2.** LCOS
- **(II)** Bridging
  - **A.** Heart transplantation
  - **B.** Left ventricular assist device

| | | |
|---|---|---|
| | **C.** | Total artificial heart |
| **(III)** | Diagnostic | |
| | **A.** | Reversibility of pulmonary (PAH, PVR) |

AMI = acute myocardial infarction; CABG = coronary artery bypass grafting; CPB = cardiopulmonary bypass; IABP = intraaorrtic balloon pump; LCOS = low cardiac output syndrome; LVAD = left ventricular assist device; LVR = left ventricular rupture; MR = mitral regurgitation; PAH = pulmonary arterial hypertension; PVR = pulmonary vascular resistance; VSD = ventricular septal defect.

**Table 8.** Indications for IABP.

usage in the end-stage HF patients has broadened in last decade due to the increase in the usage of t-MCS devices to bridge to HTx or LVAD implantation. The main indications for IABP are to increase myocardial perfusion in critical uncontrolled coronary artery stenosis preoperatively and to improve CO in severe LHF postoperatively [49]. The purpose of this indication is to decrease afterload and consequently to facilitate unloading of the LV, especially LHF complicated with significant MR. Intraaortic balloon pumping relies on the principle of diastolic counterpulsation, which causes a reduction in left ventricular afterload and an increase in aortic diastolic and consequently coronary artery perfusion pressures. Because the descending aorta has a particular diameter the balloon catheter should have a limited volume, which are two types for adults: 40 mL (26 cm length and 1.5 cm diameter) and 50 mL (27 cm length and 1.8 cm diameter). Even the hemodynamic effect of this capacity affects the myocardial oxygen supply/demand ratio favorably due to the decreasing peak systolic wall stress and contractile work of the LV, the net effect will be an increase in forward LVEF, CI, and CO (**Table 9**). However, when IABP support has only limited positive impact on cardiac hemodynamics, it cannot maintain adequate cardiac output in patients with decompensated severe left HF or reduce clinical symptoms and hemodynamic signs. In such cases, this hemodynamic supportive strategy must be complemented by more advanced MCS devices [50].

Therapeutic usage of IABP is well known and accepted treatment strategy to reverse or prevent moderate LCOS owing to hibernating or stunned myocardium after acute coronary syndrome, during percutaneous cardiac interventions, along malign ventricular arrhythmias, and after mechanical complications of myocardial infarction [51]. High-risk patients undergoing cardiac operations may be also protected against adverse outcomes [52, 53]. Pharmacological and mechanical hemodynamic supports remedies pre- and afterload deterioration through improved CO, coronary perfusion, and improved end-organ perfusion. The latter effect is the main curative treatment strategy to terminate and reverse organ dysfunctions, which increase pre- and postoperative mortality and morbidity. The significant life-saving benefit of IABP support on the early mortality is well known; however, the benefit on either 30-day or 1-year all-cause mortality is dubious in end-stage HF patients due to insufficiency to achieve and sustain adequate CO. Therefore, a more effective MCS device should be utilized if IABP could not achieve adequate CO in a couple of days (<7 days) or immediately when any decompensation develops on the IABP treatment.

Prophylactic long-term usage of counterpulsation to optimize cardiac output and RV function as a bridge to HTx or long-term LVAD implantation is a growing area of application (**Table 10**) [54].

http://dx.doi.org/10.5772/67455

| | |
|---|---|
| **Decrease** | |
| Systolic blood pressure | up to 10% |
| Presystolic aortic pressure (afterload) | up to 30% |
| LV systolic pressure (wall tension) | up to 20% |
| Isometric phase of LV contraction | |
| LV energy utilization (myocardial oxygen consumption; TTI) | |
| LVEDV + LVEDP (preload) | |
| PCWP | |
| **Increase** | |
| Diastolic blood pressure | |
| LV mechanical performance | |
| EF | up to 5% |
| CI | up to 20% |
| CO | up to 30% (0.5-1 L/min) |
| LV energy obtainment (myocardial oxygen supply; DPTI) | |
| Endocardial Viability Ratio improvement | DPTI/TTI > 1 |
| *(<0.7 indicates severe myocardial ischemia)* | |
| LV contractility and active relaxation | |
| Coronary blood flow | |
| Cerebral, renal, mesenteric, and pulmonary blood flow | |
| Mean arterial pressure (in shock) | |

CI = cardiac index; CO = cardiac output; DPTI = diastolic pressure time index; EF = ejection fraction; LV = left ventricular; LVEDP = left ventricular end-diastolic pressure; LVEDV = left ventricular end-diastolic volume; PCWP = pulmonary capillary wedge pressure; SV = stroke volume; TTI = tension time index.

**Table 9.** Effects of counterpulsation on hemodynamics mechanoenergetics.

Predestinative usage of IABP improves and stabilizes clinical status of potential recipients suffering from multi-organ hypoperfusion and ischemia, which are significant predictors for adverse outcome after HF surgery, to obtain good postoperative results [55]. Prophylactic IABP implementation decreases left ventricular preload and therefore RV upload, which could

| Outcome | Recovery | Destination |
|---|---|---|
| Bridge to recovery (BTR) | Biventricular or left ventricular | Discharge |
| Bridge to candidacy (BTC) | Bi- or univentricular | Additional mechanical interventions |
| Bridge to destination (BTD) | Right ventricular | LVAD |
| Bridge to transplantation (BTT) | None | Heart ± lung transplantation |

IABP = intraaortic balloon pump; LVAD = left ventricular assist device.

**Table 10.** Potential outcomes of long-term IABP support in chronic heart failure.

terminate hepatic congestion and dysfunction. On the other hand, IABP support improves renal and gastrointestinal blood supply with significant recovery of dysfunctional organs [56]. This strategy can reduce HF symptoms, signs, and laboratory findings (serum total bilirubin and creatinine, plasma BNP levels), especially in the first 48 hours significantly. The most important point is the optimal timing of IABP insertion, which must be earlier as possible, before end-organ dysfunction exceeds the threshold of reversibility, and prophylactic usage must be continued for a minimum of 2 weeks to get effective results. However, long-term IABP support can cause several major complications including acute limb ischemia, severe bleeding, embolic events, infection, and sepsis. When IABP support could not sustain and/or maintain stable hemodynamics, it should be enhanced by implementing more durable devices.

Diagnostic usage is a controversial strategy that could present a significant, favorable alteration in pulmonary arterial pressure and PVR. This improvement could facilitate decisions regarding LVAD implantation or HTx in end-stage HF patients with moderate PVR (6-8 Woods). These patients are not considered to be ideal candidates for HTx according to the guidelines, but they must be investigated whether they could be eligible for initial or postimplant (after LVAD) HTx, or just for destination therapy. More effective left ventricular unloading via IABP also decreases LVEDV, which is the main stimulator for reducing pulmonary venous and consequently pulmonary arterial pressure, and effects a significant reduction in PCWP and CVP initially, as well as in creatinine and total bilirubin concentrations. Two-week application is necessary to see reversibility of PVR, because the positive effect of IABP could be negatively balanced or withdraw after the first week. In this case, PVR will not improve after heart transplant, and mid-term outpatient pharmacologic (sildenafil) and/or mechanical (LVAD) PVR-lowering therapy will be the preferred strategy, with follow-up re-catheterization after 3–6 months to evaluate PVR. Adequate reduction in PVR (<6 Woods) makes these patients potential candidates for HTx. If reduced PVR is sustained, patients will be included in urgent waiting list for HTx (Status 1B) without any additional criteria.

Support with IABP is started after standard maximal pharmacological thresholds (adrenalin or noradrenalin >0.15 μg/kg/min) fail to restore hemodynamic stability. The balloon catheter is usually passed percutaneously into the descending thoracic aorta through the femoral artery, but alternative routes, such as the axillary, the subclavian, or the brachial arteries, can be preferred if the femoral artery is not suitable for usage, as well as the ascending aorta could be preferred surgically [57]. Support with IABP is not a complication-free procedure and the most common complications are peripheral arterial injuries (rupture, perforation, bleeding, dissection, embolism, etc.), which is best avoided by sliding technique under ultrasonographic visulation, or complications of distal tissue malperfusion (extremities' ischemia), which is best prevented by the sheatless application of balloon catheters [58].

As the patient's cardiac performance improves, the IABP support must be removed step by step. First of all, all inotropic medication should be lowered (dobutamine or dopamine dose ≤5 μg/kg/min) parallel to hemodynamic stability, cardiac output, and mixt venous oxygen saturation changes. The next step to reduce balloon augmentation by one of two different methods: decreasing counterpulsation intervals or slow, step-wise deflation. Because a stagnation of the balloon catheter within the blood stream can cause microclots on its surface, decreasing of augmentation levels seems more complication-free. Deflating the balloon catheter simultaneously decreases MCHS; a 50% reduction over 12 to 24 hours is a good indicator of successful weaning, terminating with the removal of the catheter.

### 5.2. Extraaortic counterpulsatile support (EACPS)

*Extraaortic balloon pump (EABP),* C-Pulse, is a new, counterpulsatile, nonblood-contacting device that involves placement of an inflatable cuff with a polyurethane balloon and polyester wrap around the ascending aorta for the management of end-stage HF patients, who remain symptomatic despite IABP therapy with optimum PHS [59]. C-Pulse is designed to provide permanent, long-term, continuous partial MCHS for end-stage HF patients [60]. The cuff inflates inwardly causing thumb-print deflection of the outer curvature of the ascending aorta, which creates a pressure across the aortic wall ranging from 6 to 25 mmHg. Approximately 20–30 mL of ascending aortic blood volume can be displaced per beat, depending on the cuff size and aortic diameter. The implantation is achieved via midline sternotomy, without cardiopulmonary bypass. There is no any deterioration in the aortic valve and aortic regurgitation, no intimal disruption and only minor thickening of the adventitia on microscopy [61].

### 5.3. Paraaortic counterpulsatile circulation support (PACPCS)

*Paraaortic blood pump (PABP)* or *paraaortic circulatory device (PACD)* has been produced to enhance the hemodynamic effect and also to expand the indications of counterpulsation [62]. The first use in humans was disappointing, with large volume (100 mL) and on the ascending aorta implantation. Decreasing the device volume [63] and redesigning it so as to avoid the ascending aorta [64] were successful in decreasing initial systolic hypotensive symptoms and improving hemodynamic success, and for this reason it has been suggested that PABP may be more capable of efficiently supporting end-stage HF patients than IACPS or EACPS approaches. The IACPS systems should have limited dimensions and that is why IABP with limited capacity is preferred mostly in patients with moderate cardiac failure. However, IABP is unsatisfactory in patients with severe LVD, in whom systolic aortic pressure is lower than 70 mmHg. On the other hand, EACPS systems require a disease-free ascending aorta with appropriate length and therefore EABP can be used only in IABP-contraindicated patients with moderate cardiac failure because of nonblood contacting extravascular working principle. However, it needs a midline sternotomy incision and limited capacity related to the size of the ascending aorta could reduce device efficiency. If it is predicted that IABP or EABP may not provide enough stroke volume, blood pressure, and effective support in patients with moderate or more advanced LCOS (CMPs, myocarditis, etc.), PABP may provide better support. Additionally, PABP support must be preferred longer than a couple weeks in patients with severe LVF because it provides higher stroke volume, fewer vascular complications (ischemia, amputation, etc.), allows mobilization, and may be a better bridge to LVAD implantation or HTx [65]. There are several devices to provide PACP, but their usage is limited in special patient population or animal studies [66]. Partial unloading of the failed LV may interrupt the progressive hemodynamic deterioration of HF and improve quality of life in patients with earlier stages of HF. This partial support provided by PACDs may reduce native ventricular workload, augment myocardial blood flow, support positive myocardial remodeling, and prevent RVF [67, 68]. They do not require CBP support during implantation, and a major branch artery is usually the preferred site for in- and outflow graft anastomosis. These devices preserve heart integrity, unload the LV, decrease its energy consumption, enhance native left ventricular functional performance, and retain pulsatility of flow. Recovery occurs usually within the first 3–6 months on mechanical assistance (bridge to recovery). The other philosophy about PACDs is to maintain arterial wall physiology with natural counterpulsatile flow.

## 6. Mechanical circulatory support (MCS)

End-stage HF is usually treated, healed, and stabilized by pharmacologic and/or mechanical hemodynamic support, but advanced HF is characterized by increasing frequency of intervals of decompensation, rehospitalization, and reintervention. If the MHS is insufficient for the recovery of LCOS, MCS is required to maintain CO (**Table 11**). Temporary MCS devices increase arterial blood circulation with or without extracorporeal oxygenation to provide an adequate CO, which acts as a parallel or serial artificial circulation to the physiologic circulation pattern. Permanent mechanical pumps provide a parallel artificial circulation of failed ventricles or entirely assume the pump function of the resected heart. Short-term devices are extracorporeal or paracorporeal pumps located outside the body, whereas durable devices are intracorporeal pumps implanted inside the body. The definitions of circulatory supports are dependent on cardiac chambers and oxygenation (**Table 12**).

| | Counterpulsation | Short-term VAD | Long-term VAD |
|---|---|---|---|
| LVEF | <40% | <30% | <25% |
| LVD | No | Yes/no | Yes |
| Systolic ABP | <90 mmHg | <80 mmHg | <80 mmHg |
| Mean ABP | <60 mmHg | <50 mmHg | <50 mmHg |
| CVP | ≥15 mmHg | ≥18 mmHg | ≥20 mmHg |
| Mean PCWP | ≥15 mmHg | ≥18 mmHg | ≥20 mmHg |
| CI | ≤2.2 L/min/m$^2$ | ≤2 L/min/m$^2$ | <1.8 L/min/m$^2$ |
| SVR | | | >2100 Dynes/cm/sec |
| Inotropic agents with high doses | ≤2 | ≥2 | >2 |
| IABP | No | Yes | Yes |
| Urine output | <0.5 mL/kg/h | <0.5 mL/kg/h | <20 mL/h |
| Metabolic asidosis | Yes/no | Yes/no | Yes |
| HRF | No | Yes/no | Yes/no |
| Application stage | First | Second | Second or last |

ABP = arterial blood pressure; CI = cardiac index; CVP = central venous pressure; HRF = hepatorenal failure; IABP = intraaortic balloon pump; LVD = left ventricular dilatation; LVEF = left ventricular ejection fraction; MCS = mechanical circulatory support; PCWP = pulmonary capillary wedge pressure; SVR = systemic vascular resistance; VAD = ventricular assist device.

**Table 11.** Hemodynamic indication criteria for MCS in patients suffered heart failure.

http://dx.doi.org/10.5772/67455

**Ventricular contribution:** to decrease ventricular unloading and work index

- *Ventricular assist*: ventricular outloading through the left ventricular cavity directly (after mitral valve)
- *Ventricular support*: ventricular unloading through the left atrium (before mitral valve)

**Cardiac relinquishment:** to circulate out-of-heart uni- or biventricularly

- *LV-bypass*: no-loading of the left ventricular
- *RV-bypass*: no-loading of the right ventricle
- *BV-bypass*: no-loading of both ventricles

**With external oxygenator:** to oxygenate blood in the external circulatory circuit

- *va-ECCPS*: veno-arterial circulatory assistance with external oxygenation
- *va-a-ECCPS*: venoatrial-arterial circulatory assistance with external oxygenation
- *aa-ECCPS*: atrio-arterial circulatory assistance with external oxygenation
- *vp-ECCPS*: veno-pulmonary circulatory assistance with external oxygenation

BV = biventricular; ECCPS = extracorporeal cardiopulmonary support; LV = left ventricular; MCS = mechanical circulatory support; RV = right ventricular.

**Table 12.** Definitions of MCS in heart failure.

After full implementation of pharmacological and MHS therapies, most acute failed hearts after cardiogenic shock, interventional coronary revascularization, or surgical or percutaneous cardiac procedures can recover from LCOS within hours (peroperatively) or days (postoperatively). When this primary treatment strategy does not work or fails during a situation of intractable decompensated HF, MCS devices are the only life-saving instruments. These devices can be also used as a bridge to keep patients alive if weaning from CPB is not possible or when intractable LCOS does not recover. Consecutive or combined usage of these devices with or without extracorporeal oxygenation could be also an effective, maybe, an essential preference to get a successful outcome [69].

The working mechanism of MCS devices in HF syndrome is very simple: sucking circulatory blood under negative pressure and ejecting it into the systemic or pulmonary arterial circulation. The inflow cannula (temporary) or inlet tube (permanent) is inserted in the relevant ventricle and the outflow cannula (temporary) or outlet graft (permanent) is connected to the ventricle-associated main artery. These devices have two different action principles: pulsatile or continuous flow. Devices working by pulsatile flow have a blood-compatibility chamber and a moveable diaphragm separating the chamber into the blood and air spaces. The blood space is connected to the aorta or main pulmonary artery through a graft forced with a prosthetic valve. The air space is connected to a compressor-console providing power for counterpulsation through inflation and deflation. Devices working by nonpulsative flow have a blood-compatibility compartment and a frictionless turnable rotor directing input flow to the related circulation.

Pulsatility is the indispensable principle of the native, physiological, durable, regulated, and protective circulation in human. Pulsatile flow has several benefits for maintaining natural life (**Table 13**). The superiority of pulsatility over continuous flow has not yet been definitively demonstrated, but several studies have addressed adverse nonphysiological transformation in the vascular bed, inequable neuroendocrine responses, and device-related complications from mechanical continuous circulation. More complicated extracorporeal devices are required to produce pulsatile flow, while pulsatile intracorporeal devices require more space than centrifugal pumps if used for uni- or biventricular support; however, only total artificial hearts produce the true pulsatile flow as prosthetic HTx.

There are two main types of extracorporeal pumps with different working mechanisms (**Table 14**). Pulsatile pumps are often used in biventricular failure and in pediatric patients [70]. Nonpulsatile pumps are mostly preferred for CPB and MCS. Roller pumps, which generate forward blood flow by roller compression, rate of rotation, and the length of the compression raceway, are useful for

| |
|---|
| Transmission of energy to the microcirculation |
| Reduction critical capillary closing pressure |
| Augmentation of lymphatic flow |
| Improvement of tissue perfusion |
| Amelioration of cellular metabolism |
| Alleviation of vasoconstrictive reflexes |
| Diminution of acidosis |
| Regulation of neuroendocrine responses |

**Table 13.** Physiologic effects of pulsatile flow.

| | | | |
|---|---|---|---|
| **(I)** | Pulsatile flow pumps | | |
| | **1.** | Abiomed | |
| | **2.** | Thoratec paracorporeal ventricular assist device | |
| | **3.** | Excor | |
| **(II)** | Nonpulsatile flow pumps | | |
| | **1.** | Roller pumps | |
| | **2.** | Centrifugal pumps | |
| | | **a.** | Medtronic Bio-Medicus |
| | | **b.** | Maque Rotaflow |
| | | **c.** | Levitronix CentriMag |
| | | **d.** | TandemHeart |
| | **3.** | Axial pumps | |
| | | **a.** | Impella |

MCS = mechanical circulatory support.

**Table 14.** Devices for temporary MCS.

CPB during open heart surgery, but not for circulatory support due to hemolysis and tubing wear. Extracorporeal continuous flow pumps are useful for CBP as well as extended t-MCS with fewer adverse effects than roller pumps. Intracorporeal devices are designed with a smaller structure using two separate pump mechanisms: axial flow pumps have a pump rotor parallel to the blood path, and centrifugal pumps have an impeller rotor perpendicular to the blood path. The rotor is magnetically levitated, and rotation is achieved without friction or wear, thus minimizing blood trauma, mechanical failure, and heat generation. These devices work by an external motor-driven system, direct-drive system, or self-bearing system. In direct-drive system, the impeller becomes the motor rotor supported by a separate levitation system. In self-bearing system, both the drive and the levitation coils share the same stator core [71].

Because the duration of their usage could be limited, the decision for the destination goal should take into hemodynamic, hematologic, and neurologic courses. Even though the gold standard therapy for end-stage HF is HTx, this is possible in only a small number of patients due to limited organ availability. These devices are generally used to maintain adequate organ perfusion for several days, but more time could be required before a final decision is made (**Table 15**). Bridging to curative treatments should be life-saving and any device could be effective, but do not hesitate to change the treatment stages and devices.

Designed to assist the native heart, MCS devices are differentiated by the implant duration [short-term (<10 days), mid-term (10–90 days), long-term (>90 days)], indication [temporary (bridge therapy) versus permanent (destination therapy)], type (cardiopulmonary versus circulatory), approach (percutaneous versus surgical), location (extracorporeal versus intracorporeal), flow characteristic [pulsatile versus continuous), pump mechanism (volume displacement, axial, centrifugal), and the ventricle(s) supported (left, right, biventricular) [72].

### 6.1. Temporary mechanical cardiorespiratory support (t-MCRS)

Acute decompensation of cardiac functions requires emergent circulatory support when pharmacological treatment and/or counterpulsatile support are ineffective or when weaning from CPB fails (**Table 16**). There are several options for t-MCS, which can be applied percutaneously or centrally, but right ventricular and respiratory functions are decision-making factors [73]. Sufficient oxygenation by the lungs suspends usage of external oxygenator, but associated RVF necessitates its usage. Temporary cardiorespiratory support (t-MCRS) devices are designed to rapidly reestablish adequate organ perfusion and oxygenation. Biventricular t-MCRS is the most common approach to maintain adequate CO and oxygenation in the presence of severe RVF; however, univentricular t-MCRS can be the preferred approach in the absence of significant RVF. An ideal device should support adequate flow, maximal hemodynamics, sufficient oxygenation, and avoid need for anticoagulation with its serious related serious complications (**Table 17**). After echocardiography fails to reveal a surgically correctable cause, a temporary mechanical device is considered for MCS according to several hemodynamic data (**Table 11**). Daily follow-up with transthoracic and/or transesophageal echocardiography is mandatory to evaluate biventricular function, regional wall motion abnormalities, valvular mechanics, septal malformations, and extracardiac compression, as well as native heart recovery. On the other hand, the stabilized patient should also undergo daily evaluation for end-organ functions, hematologic and infectious conditions, and neurologic status.

**Bridge to recovery (BTR)**: *Salvage therapy.* Clinical situation consists of either acute developed cardiogenic shock or acutely decompensated Stage-D HF. Acute huge myocardial infarction with or without mechanical complications, acute myocarditis, and postcardiotomy syndrome after cardiac surgery cause acutely developed myocardial dysfunction, which can be refractory to optimal treatment via PHS and counterpulsatile MHS despite viable myocardium. Any reason can worsen and decrease stable Stage-D HF into unstable condition with severe LCOS. The myocardium could be recovered by MCS devices via unloading the left ventricular in a couple of hours or days (<4–7 days), and after that patients should be put into advanced bridging therapies. Daily echocardiographic examinations are guiding and following practices to investigate the reverse remodelling of the failed myocardium. During this period, the main goal is to keep patients alive.

**Bridge to decision (BTD)**: *Rescue therapy.* Acutely cardiac failure subsequent to myocardial infarction or cardiac operations, or acutely decompensation of Stage-D HF requires optimal treatment via MHS and/or MCS devices (1) to keep patients alive, and then (2) to maintain vital functions due to mechanical supported cardiac output, and finally (3) to gain time for decision to the most appropriate curative or egress treatment solution for related patients. Clinicians have a couple of days (<14 days), but not more than one week, to evaluate each patient separately with his/her own cardiac pathology and to decide the next step(s). During this period, the main goal is to let the heart in rest and no-load, and also to keep extracardiac organs in normal functions.

**Bridge to wean (BTW):** *Separation therapy.* Improvement in cardiac functions and healing of acute decompensation of acute or chronic HF improves patient's status and makes it possible to disconnect mechanical devices. After the hemodynamics recover completely in several days or weeks (<30 days), weaning protocol is started via reducing all pharmacological agents to their minimum dosages, improving respiratory functions, and decreasing mechanical support levels. Patients should be followed with daily echocardiography and pulmonary arterial catheterization (wedge pressure, mixt venous oxygen saturation). During this period, the main goal is to keep patients noncardiacly complication-free.

**Bridge to curative surgical and/or percutaneous interventions (BTI)**: *Supportive therapy.* Associated curable cardiac pathologies (CAD, MR, postinfarct VSD, etc.) could be treated to improve cardiac functions and to prevent new decompensations. The hemodynamically stable condition gained by MCS devices enables clinicians (1) to revascularize ischemic myocardium, (2) to repair these structural mechanical complications, (3) to rescue the acute failed heart, (4) to recovery myocardial dysfunction, and (5) to bridge to weaning or advanced treatments. During this period, the main goal is to keep extracardiac organs in normal functions, and also to provide hemodynamic with or without respiratorial support during procedures.

**Bridge to bridge (BTB):** *Exchange therapy.* Short-term mechanical supportive devices cannot provide adequate flow and facilitate further improvement in the clinical status of patients, as the result patients cannot be weaned from MCS. The preferred MCS type should be switched more a failed-oriented type of MCS or more durable approach. Weaning from right ventricular and/or pulmonary support make it possible to disconnected venous cannulas or oxygenator from the circuit (bridge from va-a-ECCPS to aa-ECCS).

**Bridge to candidacy (BTC):** *Preparatory therapy.* Switching from t-MCS to p-MCS due to the necessity of the long-term follow for successful recovery is necessity for the decision (1) to wean from the device, (2) to use the device as the destination therapy, or (3) to take the patients into the transplantation list. The reversibility of the elevated PVR or the prolonged healing of damaged myocardium requires a prolonged treatment-period (>30 days), usually a couple of months, but not more than six months. Long-term predicted recovery should be verified by invasive tests a significant reduction in PVR. During this period, the main goal is to keep patients in their daily lives.

**Bridge to destination (BTD)**: *Continuity therapy.* Long-term mechanical support is a durable treatment alternative to HTx in with Stage-D HF patients, who are not eligible for transplantation due to extracardiac diseases, irreversible elevated PVR, advanced age, or donor inability. Left ventricular assist devices may prolong and improve the quality of life.

**Bridge to transplantation (BTT)**: *Curative therapy.* Irreversible myocardial function is the main indication for HTx in the decompensated or device-dependent Stage-D HF. Progressive lengthening of waiting times on transplantation lists can be an indication for LVAD implantation, but this reason is most pertinent to bridge to destination therapy. On the other hand, there is no widely accepted guideline to show the indication and timing for a mechanical supportive device placement as a bridge treatment. The true indications for this therapy are (1) patients with implanted p-MCS devices with/without complications, (2) unrecoverable patients supported with t-MCS devices, and (3) borderline patients on the bridge to candidacy protocol.

**Table 15.** Bridging from live-saving t-MCS to advanced therapy modalities.

| |
|---|
| Acute myocarditis |
| Acute huge myocardial infarction with/without mechanical complications |
| Cardiogenic shock |
| Cardiopulmonary arrest |
| Postcardiotomy syndrome |
| Acutely decompensation of Stage-D heart failure |
| Intractable decompensation of end-stage cardiomyopathies |
| Intractable ventricular tachycardia in end-stage cardiomyopathies |
| Bridge to destination therapy or heart transplantation |
| Postimplant right ventricular failure |

**Table 16.** Indications of t-MCS for heart failure.

| |
|---|
| Decrease preload |
| Decrease pulmonary capillary wedge pressure |
| Not increase afterload |
| Augment cardiac output |
| Increase coronary perfusion |
| Improve peripheral tissue perfusion |
| Provide adequate oxygen delivery |

**Table 17.** The primary hemodynamic goals of t-MCS.

### 6.1.1. *Cardiopulmonary bypass (CPB)*

The first used life-supportive approach is CBP with a roller or centrifugal pump for circulatory assistance and an oxygenator for respiratory reinforcement during open heart surgery. This shortest extracorporeal circulation has several parts resulting in hemolysis, especially the cardiotomy suction and venous reservoir. Failing to wean from bypass after cardiac procedures enforces to prolong circulatory support via CPB. Because this approach is not suitable for short-term or longer circulatory support, CPB has been used only for ultrashort-term (<1 day) circulatory assistance. The main differences of CBP circuit are the drainage of venous blood, typically by gravity, into venous reservoir of the heart-lung machine, and aspiration of blood from the surgical field into the reservoir. Both of these can cause also inflammatory and humoral responses, thrombosis and bleeding problems. The rest of the supportive mechanism is similar with the other t-MCPS devices: to pump venous blood through an oxygenator for gas exchange, and therefrom into the arterial circulation. This basic extracorporeal perfusion system can be used for partial or total circulatory and respiratory support, or partial support of the LV. Modern membrane oxygenators add up to 470 mL of $O_2$ and remove up to 350 mL of $CO_2$ per minute at

1–7 L of flow with resistances of 12–15 mmHg per liter blood flow. Preferable pumps are centrifugal ones consisting of a vaned impeller or nested smooth plastic cones, which propel blood by centrifugal force when they rotate rapidly. Centrifugal pumps produce forward pressure of up to 900 mmHg, but only half as much of negative pressure, and therefore, less cavitation and fewer gaseous microemboli. Flow rate should be set to maintain mean arterial pressure at ≥70 mmHg at 35 to 37°C, with a hematocrit of 30%. This flow rate provides and maintains adequate body perfusion, with higher mixed venous oxygen saturation >60%.

It is meaningful to use CBP as a mechanical support only in the theater for *ultrashort-term (several hours)* assistance, but advanced technology provides more appropriate devices for short- and long-term MCPS. There are several side effects of CBP that preclude its usage as a short- and long-term cardiopulmonary support. The main problem is left ventricular distention and lack of unloading during CPB support, which will be prevented by insertion of a vent catheter into the LA or LV. The second limitation is the necessity of full dose heparinization to gain an activated clotting time greater than 400 seconds during extracorporeal circulation to prevent thrombo-embolic events, which usually causes bleeding problems. The third possible hazard is massive air embolism due to the integrity of the extracorporeal circuit. The fourth side effect is generalized inflammatory reactions, which result in a number of undesired pathophysiologic cascades. The fifth negative damage is possible lung injury, which is inevitable during CPB support due to increased pulmonary capillary permeability, interstitial lung water, and adverse inflammatory responses.

#### *6.1.2. Extracorporeal life or cardiopulmonary support (ECLS or ECCPS)*

The casually accepted term for these support strategies is ECMO, but the true definition must be extracorporeal cardiopulmonary support (ECCPS) while using for treatment in decompensated Stage-D HF or extracorporeal life support (ECLS) while using for similar support in acute cardiogenic shock. Although the unsuitability of CBP for short- or long-term ECLS has been established, its principles have been applied to never small, durable, practical, integrated, and mobile devices that are practical for providing ECLS in all appropriate circumstances. The principal aim of ECLS is to provide acute temporary ECCPS globally as a bridge to more durable therapy in patients with cardiorespiratory failure refracted to maximal conventional therapy [74]. For extracorporeal membrane oxygenation (ECMO), an oxygenator is inserted in the extracorporeal circuit for gas exchange before returning patient's venous blood to the patient's arterial circulation, which is driven by a centrifugal pump. They are suitable for t-MCS, but single or multiple replacement of the failed oxygenator with a new one can allow prolongation of ECCPS to more than 1 month if myocardial recovery is the desired and expected goal. If pulmonary functions are well or pulmonary recovery occurs during ECCPS, the external oxygenator is not necessary and it must be disconnected from the circuit to provide acute or prolonged temporary extracorporeal circulatory support (ECCS) for the LHF or RHF. Double established ECCSs could be used separately for biventricular HF patients with unimpaired respiratory functions.

The devices designed for short-term ECCPS have a number of advantages in comparison with CPB (lower dose of heparin, a continuous circuit, etc.). A hollow-fiber membrane oxygenator

http://dx.doi.org/10.5772/67455

with an integrated heat-exchange system operated by a centrifugal pump provides circulatory, respiratory, and thermatory supports. These pumps are totally nonocclusive and afterload-dependent, and when myocardial recovery occurs, physiological circulation overtakes artificial circulation, manifesting as reduced device flow. These pumps do not create excessive output pressure (so as not to rupture the circuit) or significant negative input pressure (so as to avoid cavitation and microembolus). Using this system, ECCPS flow is maintained between 4 and 6 L/min by providing a pump speed of between 3000 and 3500 rpm, with higher pump speed risking mechanical trauma to blood cells. The heat exchanger provides normothermia during ECCPS, which is mandatory for physiologic body functions. A biocompatible heparin-coated bypass circuit provides an antithrombotic surface to reduce or eliminate the necessary dose of heparin and inflammatory responses. Because roller pumps cause hemolysis beyond 4 and 5 hours of usage, continuous flow pumps are preferred for ECCPS.

The real problem with ECCPS in end-stage HF patients is how to protect and unload one or both ventricles. Conventional ECLS bypasses both ventricles through the venous drainage and arterial inflow, and physiologically, that will unload the RV without unloading the LV due to the increased afterload. In the borderline depressed LV or during the recovering process of LVF, both a remarkable drop in preload and a certain rise in afterload reduce left ventricular wall stress, produce smaller LVEDV, augment coronary perfusion, and ultimately improve left ventricular contractility. However, if the heart is dilated and/or contracting poorly, a markedly increased afterload handicaps any offset in both LVEDV and LVESV by blocking the opening of the aortic valve. Theoretically, left ventricular wall stress and myocardial oxygen consumption remain increased and inhibit the recovery of the failed LV. The first goal should therefore be to unload the LV using IABP and/or left atrial venting. The second target is to deliver the highly oxygenated blood directly to the coronary and cerebral circulations. Adding an IABP device to support left ventricular systolic function (by reducing afterload) and coronary perfusion (by increasing aortic diastolic pressure) is an integral part of ECLS therapy. Although ECLS balances hemodynamics, the insertion of IABP aggrandizes coronary and cerebral perfusion effects and also maintains aortic valve opening more effectively.

Establishment of ECCPS could be central or peripheral: central approach is superior due to better left ventricular unloading and the avoidance of peripheral vascular complications; however, peripheral cannulation permits later decannulation without reopening the chest. Both approaches are effective for managing cardiorespiratory failure with uni- or biventricular dysfunction associated with respiratory dysfunction (**Table 18**).

*Central ECCPS* is established through cardiac cannulation and is usually preferred for the failure of weaning from the bypass in the theater or postcardiotomy syndrome that develops in the ICU. The preference of central cannulation is based on several physiological hemodynamic requirements that allow shorter myocardial recovery for the acutely decompensated heart: effective biventricular unloading, highly adequate blood flow, sufficient tissue oxygenation, and easy transition from the cardiopulmonary support to left ventricular circulatory support. This approach is superior to peripheral ECCPS due to better coronary, cerebral, and upper extremities perfusion and easy insertion of left atrial vent. Central ECCPS is established via central cannulations used during cardiac surgery for postcardiotomy syndrome, or via full

| ECLS- strategy | Bypass | Type | Establishment between | Approach |
|---|---|---|---|---|
| **A. ECCPS (with ECMO)** | | | | |
| va – ECCPS | *bv-bypass* | *veno-aortic*<br>*veno-arterial* | RA – Ao<br>femoral and/or jugular vein – femoral or subclavian artery | Median sternotomy<br>Peripheral percutaneous |
| va-a-ECCPS | *bv-bypass* | *biatria-aortic*<br>*venoatrio-aortic*<br>*venoatrio-arterial* | (RA + LA) – Ao<br>(femoral vein + LA) – Ao<br>(femoral vein + LA) – femoral or subclavian artery | Median sternotomy<br>Median sternotomy<br>Peripheral percutaneous |
| aa – ECCPS | *lv-bypass* | *atrio-aortic*<br>*atrio-arterial* | LA – Ao<br>LA – femoral/subclavian artery | Median sternotomy<br>Peripheral percutaneous |
| vp – ECCPS | *rv-bypass* | *atrio-pulmonaric*<br>*venopulmonaic* | RA – PA<br>femoral and/or jugular vein – PA | Median sternotomy<br>Peripheral percutaneous |
| **B. ECCS (without ECMO)** | | | | |
| lv – ECCS | *lv-bypass* | *atrio- or ventriculo-aortic*<br>*atrio- or ventriculo-arterial* | LA – or LV – Ao<br>LA – or LV – femoral or subclavian artery | Median sternotomy<br>Mini-thoracotomy |
| rv– ECCS | *rv-bypass* | *atrio-pulmonaric*<br>*veno-pulmonaric* | RA – PA<br>femoral and/or jugular vein – PA | Median sternotomy<br>Mini-thoracotomy |
| bv– ECCS | *bv-bypass* | separately lv- and rv-ECCS | | |

ECCPS = extracorporeal cardiopulmonary support; ECCS = extracorporeal circulatory support; ECLS = extracorporeal life support; ECMO = extracorporeal membranous oxygenation; bv = biventricular; lv = left ventricular; rv = right ventricular; Ao = aorta; LA = left atrium; LV = left ventricle; PA = pulmonary artery; RA = right atrium.

**Table 18.** Temporary ECLS strategies for end-stage HF patients.

or limited sternotomy incision (reverse-T upper hemisternotomy). Both cannulas are taken out from the mediastinum below the xiphoid or through the jugulum. A new design of a biventricular assistance circuit including an oxygenator-bypass line (Kırali circuit) assists and provides the improvement of life-saving HF therapy from the sophisticated immovable t-MCPS circuit to the simplest mobile t-MCS circuit (va-a-ECCPS).

*Peripheral ECCPS* is established through peripheric cannulation and usually preferred as a rescue approach in nonsurgical patients suffered from acute cardiogenic shock or decompensated HF. Any perfusion strategy creating a right to left shunt requires an oxygenator in the circuit. Peripheral ECCPS is generated through the femoral artery (peripheral or upstream) or the axillary artery (periphero-central or downstream). Femoral access is more commonly used in patients requiring urgent ECLS due to rapidity of insertion and avoidance of sternotomy. The most important drawback is the left ventricular afterload mismatch and inadequate left ventricular decompression, which will cause pulmonary edema in patients with very low native CO and severe MR. To assist left ventricular unloading, IABP is used concomitantly to reduce afterload and facilitate aortic valve opening. Failure of aortic valve opening may provoke catastrophic results such as intracardiac thrombosis with or without clot embolism, worsening of LVF, coronary malperfusion, and pulmonary edema. Several percutaneous alternative approaches can be used to unload the LV during peripheral ECCPS: transaortic left ventricular unloading, transseptal left atrial

http://dx.doi.org/10.5772/67455

decompression, atrial septostomy, and transapical left ventricular drainage. On the other hand, coronary and upper body hypoxia can occur if myocardial recovery occurs and lung function remains poor, or as mostly seen, if pump flow is reduced. Peripheral cannulation depends on the arterial structure and size, the presence of any occlusive pathology, and deficiencies in distal perfusion. A distal perfusion cannula is inserted in the selected artery distal to the inflow cannula and connected to the inflow cannula to perfuse distally to prevent extremities from ischemic complications. The same problem may develop in venous system, and a small cannula inserted into distal vein is connected into the outflow cannula to facilitate distal drainage.

Extracorporeal cardiopulmonary support is achieved using an ECMO system as described above. They can be designed according to uni- or biventricular support, and also the system must be prepared for weaning from biventricular and respiratory support step by step (**Figure 3**).

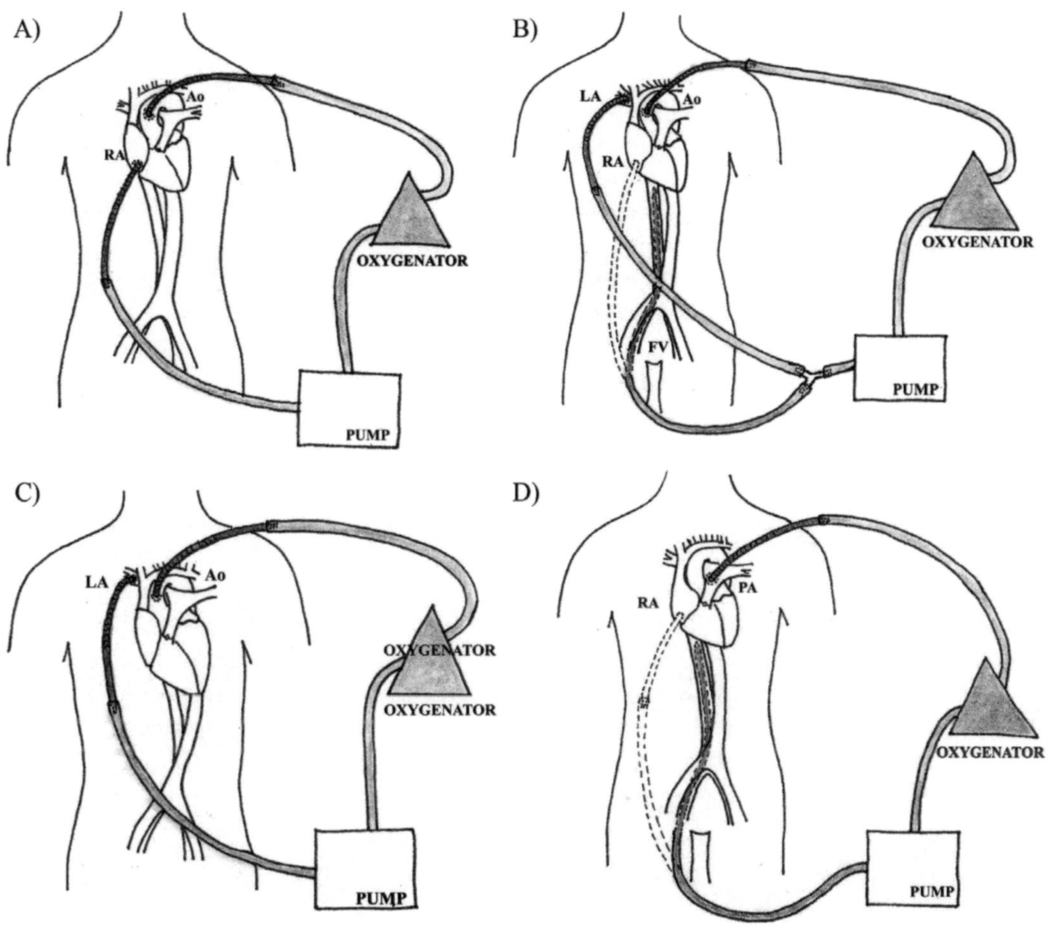


**Figure 3.** ECLS alternatives in Stage-D heart failure treatment. (A) va-ECLS (venoarterial ECMO). (B) va-a-ECLS (venoatrio-arterial ECMO). (C) aa-ECLS (atrio-arterial ECMO). (D) vv-ECLS (veno-venous ECMO). Ao = aorta; FV = femoral vein; LA= left atrium; RA = right atrium.

The ECCPS system can be created with several ways for different indications (**Table 18**).

*va-ECCPS (va-ECMO) (biventricular bypass circuit)* is the conventional ECMO system with biventricular bypass circuit by which a centrifugal pump drives blood from the patient's venous circulation through an externalized membrane oxygenator for gas exchange before returning the blood to the patient's arterial circulation. This approach is usually implemented percutaneously at the bedside in all emergent situations, in order to rescue patients suffering from fatal cardiac failure; however, a final decision about the most beneficial durable strategy should be made within a couple days (<7 days). If weaning does not seem possible, it is more appropriate to convert patients to a longer sustainable ECCPS circuit or to switch to an ECCS design.

*va-a-ECCPS (va-a-ECMO) (biventricular unloading circuit; Kırali circuit)* is a new format of a biventricular assistance circuit including biatrial drainage cannulas and an oxygenator-bypass line (Kırali circuit) assists and provides the improvement of life-saving HF therapy from the sophisticated immovable t-MCPS circuit to the simplest mobile t-MCS circuit (**Figure 4**); particularly it is meaningful in patients with expected RV and respiratory recovery in a couple of weeks (<1 month). This biventricular unloading circuit includes a centrifugal pump that drives blood from the patient's both atria through an externalized membrane oxygenator for gas exchange before returning to the patient's arterial circulation. This circuit has two venous cannulas: the first venous cannula (a multistage venous ECMO 28F cannula) is inserted percutaneously into the femoral vein or directly into the RA for venous drainage, and the second venous cannula (a malleable one-stage venous cannula ranged between 22F and 28F) is placed into the LA at first for left heart venting (drainage), and then for left heart bypassing (unloading). An arterial cannula (an arterial ECMO cannula ranged between 15F and 19F) is inserted into the distal ascending aorta or aortic arch, and the distal end of the cannula is placed distal to cerebral branches. Both left heart cannulas with or without the RA cannula are taken out below the sternal incision and the sternum is closed to prevent bleeding and to allow mobilization. Each outflow line has its own tap that allows blood sampling to follow blood gas and pulmonary recovery, and can be controlled by partial or total clamping to manage adequate blood drainage from each atrium according to the related ventricular dysfunction/recovery cascade. Peripheral venous cannulation is preferred for periods of brief support (<1 week) because decannulation of the percutaneously inserted femoral venous cannula is simple. If RV recovery is expected to take more than a week, then right atrial venous cannulation should be performed centrally or a small drainage cannula is inserted distal to the outflow cannula at the femoral vein to prevent peripheral venous complications. Daily echocardiographic examination introduces RV recovery, and frequently follow-up blood samples from the left atrial inflow line propound the pulmonary recovery. Weaning from the external oxygenator should be completed in ≥4 days, and the external oxygenator should remain in the circuit for the purpose of emergent actuation in case of unexpected respiratory failure during this weaning period.

Weaning from va-a-ECCPS protocol in end-stage HF patients is simpler than others and does not require reopening of the sternum or establish a new circuit and disconnection steps should be made long enough to observe any pulmonary complications or recurrence of respiratory failure (**Table 19**). Decannulation of peripheric venous cannula is very simple when RV

http://dx.doi.org/10.5772/67455

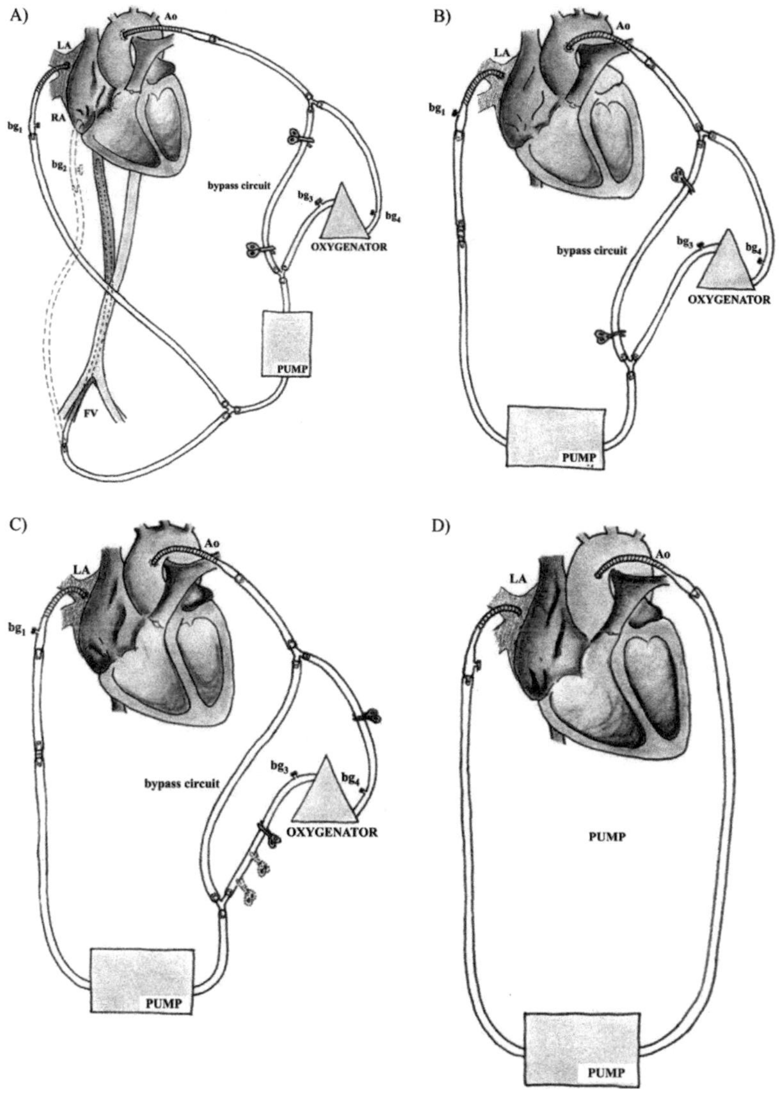


**Figure 4.** Venoatrial-arterial ECLS support (Kırali Circuit for biventricular unloading). (A) The circuit is constituted between both atria and the arterial circulation for right heart, pulmonary, and left heart bypass. Left ventricular unloading is necessary for left heart bypass, right ventricular unloading is necessary for right heart bypass and as well as pulmonary bypass. Blood samples from $bg_1$ (pulmonary gas exchanges) and $bg_2$ (mixt venous) show oxygen saturations in patients, and $bg_3$ (preoxygenator) and $bg_4$ (postoxygenator) gas exchanges; whereas arterial blood sample shows true body oxygenation. (B) After right heart recovery, right heart bypass line is removed from the circuit to get pulmonary and left heart bypass. (C) After pulmonary recovery, oxygenator bypass circuit is actuated to decrease oxygenator support. (D) After pulmonary recovery, oxygenator is removed from the circuit to get isolated left heart bypass. Ao = aorta; bg = blood gas sample; FV = femoral vein; LA= left atrium; RA = right atrium.

recovery is completed, and at this first stage, the circuit is converted to left heart bypass system supported with external oxygenator after removing right ventricular support (aa-ECCPS). After pulmonary recovery, the oxygenator could be removed from the circuit. First, the

| | |
|---|---|
| First step | To convert va-a-ECCPS to aa-ECCPS after sufficiently recovery of the RV. |
| Second step | To reduce the oxygen delivery by respirator (res-$FiO_2$) till 35–40%, while the oxygen delivery by external oxygenator (oxy-$FiO_2$) is stabilized at 40%. |
| Third step | To open the oxygenator bypass line and to direct the left atrial blood flow through both oxygenator inflow lines nonocclusively with a flow ratio 3:1 (bypass line/on line) depending on membrane resistance, after blood samples from the left atrial cannula show effective native pulmonary oxygenation (left atrial oxygen saturation >95%) at least one day. |
| Fourth step | To reduce oxy-$FiO_2$ until the air ratio (21%) or disconnect the external oxygenator from oxygen gas supply, after patient's oxygenation does not collapse at least one day. |
| Fifth step | To begin weaning from mechanical ventilation and to extubate the patient, after arterial oxygen saturation is maintained at a level higher than 95% with res-$FiO_2$ 40% at least one day. |
| Sixth step | To disconnect the external oxygenator from the circuit and to switch aa-ECCPS to aa-ECCS, after arterial oxygenation does not retrogress after extubation at least one day. |

**Table 19.** Disconnection steps from the external oxygenator.

oxygenator bypass line is taken over pump flow step by step, and the full declamping of this line allows approximately three times more blood flow than those passing through the oxygenator due to resistance of membrane. This strategy reduces oxygenator support and enables native lungs to oxygenate most part of the pump blood flow. Finally, oxygenator is switched off and disconnected, and at this stage, the circuit is converted to left heart bypass system without oxygenator (aa-ECCS). The last stage and the simplest LV-ECCS system allows patients to be discharged from the ICU and mobilized at the ward, and provides hemodynamically stable bridging to destination therapies (LVAD or HTx).

This stage of cardiopulmonary circuit used for ECCPS provides several benefits (**Table 20**). This new strategy is independent of recovery durations, and unless any fatal complication occurs, the supportive therapy can be extended for weeks until a destination treatment could be performed, because it is easier to exchange failed oxygenator and/or pump head with a new one in this strategy, converting from "ECCPS to ECCS" or reverse, and from "va-a to aa" or reverse. The presence of the functionally significant MR facilitates left ventricular unloading through the left atrial cannula, but it can increase pulmonary congestion if the pump flow is not increased to sustain and maintain PCWP < 18 mmHg and CVP < 12 mmHg. In this circumstance, wean protocol from LV-ECCS should be started after mitral valve recovery or any percutaneous or transapical mitral valve repair intervention. The presence of the competent mitral valve, which does not facilitate left ventricular unloading due to blocking regurgitant flow, and the increased afterload, which does not enable left ventricular ejection, impair LV recovery. The best solution is provided by arterial pulsation augmenting LV unload via aortic valve opening during all left heart bypass steps.

*aa-ECCPS (aa-ECMO) (left ventricular bypass circuit)* is a univentricular ECMO system in which the left heart bypass circuit uses a centrifugal pump to drive blood from the LA through an external membrane oxygenator for gas exchange before returning to the patient's arterial circulation. This approach is preferred in patients with LVF and respiratorial insufficiency without RVF, who could not be managed with full mechanical ventilation, or can be a part of va-a-ECCPS.

http://dx.doi.org/10.5772/67455

| Stage | Bridging | Established | Converting to | Benefits |
|---|---|---|---|---|
| **Initial** | Bridge to recovery | t-MCS MRS | va-a-ECCPS MRS | Effectively providing of biventricular support and gas exchange through a single pump configuration; Decompression of the left heart, reducing the LV wall stress, better coronary and body perfusion, minimizing oxygen consumption |
| **First** | Bridge to RV recovery | va-a-ECCPS MRS | aa-ECCPS MRS | Decreasing PAP, PCWP, RV afterload; Improvement of the RV; Disconnection of RV support |
| **Second** | Bridge to pulmonary recovery | aa-ECCPS MRS | aa-ECCS MRS | Decreasing LAP, pulmonary unloading; Improvement of gas exchange and adequate oxygenation; Facilitating of pulmonary recovery; disconnection oxygenator |
| **Third** | Bridge to decision | aa-ECCS MRS | aa-ECCS spontaneous ventilation | Significantly decreasing of LVEDV and LVEDP; extubation |
| **Fourth** | Bridge to bridge | aa-ECCS | aa-ECCS | Possibility of weaning, listing for HTX, or candidate for durable therapy; Mobilization in ICU |
| **Fifth** | Bridge to candidacy | aa-ECCS | wean or p-MCS | Mobilization at ward |
| **Sixth** | Bridge to destination therapy | aa-ECCS | LVAD or HTx | Destination treatment |

aa = atrio-aortic; ECCPS = extracorporeal cardiorespiratory support; ECCS = extracorporeal circulatory support; HTx = heart transplantation; ICU = intensive care unit; LAP = left atrial pressure; LV = left ventricular; LVAD = left ventricular assist device; LVEDP = left ventricular end-diastolic pressure; LVEDV = left ventricular end-diastolic volume; p-MCS= permanent mechanical circulatory support; t-MCS = temporary mechanical circulatory support; MRS = mechanical respiratory support; PAP = pulmonary arterial pressure; PCWP = pulmonary capillary wedge pressure; RV = right ventricular; va-a = venoatrio-aortic.

**Table 20.** Bridging effects of va-a-ECCPS in Stage-D HF patients.

*vp-ECCPS (vp-ECMO) (right ventricular bypass circuit)* is a univentricular ECMO system in which the right heart bypass circuit uses a centrifugal pump to drive blood from the patient's vena cava or the RA through an external membrane oxygenator for gas exchange before returning to the patient's pulmonary circulation. This approach is preferred in patients with RVF and respiratorial insufficiency without LVF, who could not be managed with full mechanical ventilation. The more preferred indication can be postimplant RVF accompanied by respiratory failure.

## 6.2. Temporary mechanical circulatory support (t-MCS)

Most patients requiring MCS are candidates for t-MCRS, but there are some conditions that do not require ECMO support. Patients whose pulmonary function is sufficient with spontaneous or mechanical ventilation may be able to avoid or wean from oxygenator use during MCS for decompensated HF. Patients with isolated univentricular failure can mostly be treated with counterpulsatile devices, but if hemodynamic parameters do not improve more aggressively t-MCS should be performed using an ECCS system to assist the failed ventricle. Another alternative is intracorporeal circulation support (ICCS), which can be preferred in cases of cardiogenic shock or left ventricular unloading during va-ECCPS.

*6.2.1. Extracorporeal circulation support (ECCS)*

Isolated left or right heart ECCS is provided by a centrifugal pump; however, an external oxygenator may be implanted in the circuit if any acute respiratory decompensation develops (switch from ECCS to ECCPS). The ECCS is mostly preferred in decompensated CMPs with LVF or refracted LVD to keep patients alive until destination treatments. Another indication for weaning patients from ECCPS-based t-MCPS to ECCS-based t-MCS, by removing the oxygenator from the circuit in patients suffering from acute severe postcardiotomy syndrome. In both situations, moribund patients should be treated and followed very carefully, and HTx should not be considered unless the patients show significant recovery from multisystem organ failure. The ECCS system can be used many weeks to improve clinical status of patients. Limited recovery with appropriate t-MCS could encourage surgeons to implant more permanent LVADs to eliminate external lines and pumps, but t-MCS is also an acceptable treatment modality to maximize patient survival, for mobilize patients, to provide better rehabilitation, and to prepare them for transplantation. Temporary ECCS can be created surgically central for LV support or percutaneously peripheral for RV support (**Table 18**).

*aa-ECCS or left-to-left ECCS (left heart bypass system)* between the LA and aorta (or arterial circulation) is the preferable approach to sustain the end-stage HF patients with irreversible LVF, but preserved right ventricular and pulmonary function. Any of the several types of centrifugal pumps is chosen for long-term left ventricular ECCS (for several weeks), because all of them have similar technologic principles. The inflow cannula is connected to the pump, and the outflow cannula is inserted into the arterial circulation. The inflow cannula is usually inserted in the LA. Left atrial insertion of a malleable venous cannula ranging from 22 to 28F is performed through the left atrial wall just at the interatrial groove, not on the right pulmonary veins like as in left atrial vent insertion, because the drainage cannula is big enough to injury the walls of the pulmonary vein. Similar to standard mitral valve surgery, a limited Sondergaard's plane is dissected approximately 2 cm from the junction of both right pulmonary veins at the left atrial wall. Then, two pledgeted sutures are used to fix the cannula and prevent bleeding. After the removal of the cannula, the dissected tissues support the sutures like a pillow to block bleeding. Left ventricular cannulation is not commonly chosen when the LV is not dilated in postcardiotomy syndrome, or when the left ventricular apex is to be left untouched for permanent LVAD implantation. Two pure-string sutures are placed on the apex, and after the apex is incised. Tubbs dilatators are used to enlarge the vent hole for the venous cannula, and finally the cannula is secured with purse-string sutures. The outflow cannula is inserted into the distal ascending aorta or aortic arch, and a longer ECMO arterial cannula ranging from 15 to 19F is placed. The distal edge of the cannula locates distal to the cerebral arteries in order to avoid cerebral embolic complications. This system is preload-dependent, with an ideal PCWP maintained between 18 and 20 mmHg and CVP between 8 and 12 mmHg, and they should be monitored. Lower dose heparin infusion is necessary (ACT < 200 seconds) to prevent any thromboembolic complication. Absolute contraindications are aortic insufficiency that is any more than mild in degree, or intracardiac septal defects.

*vp-ECCS or right-to-right ECCS (right heart bypass system)* between the RA (or vena cava through the femoral vein) and pulmonary artery is rarely a preferred approach for isolated RVF

http://dx.doi.org/10.5772/67455

because the normally functioning LV can take on most of the right ventricular work. The main indication of right heart bypass systems is acute postimplant RVF after LVAD implantation. Permanent LVADs are increasingly used worldwide, and the most commonly observed cardiac complication is RVF after implantation [75]. Therefore, special attention should be devoted to the evaluation of the right ventricular function when patients are assessed for LVAD implantation. The outflow cannula is inserted either into the RA or in the femoral vein, and the inflow cannula is placed into the pulmonary artery, either directly or through a tubular graft extending outward from the second intercostal space.

*TandemHeart* is approved for ultrashort-term MCS and as a life-saving approach (as aa-ECCS) in the catheterization lab. Percutaneous t-MCS (TandemHeart) could be a more practical alternative due to not reopening the patient's chest. This system could be also used for vp-ECCS, and as well as for ECCPSs. The device consists of a small hydrodynamic centrifugal pump. It is a very versatile system providing easy deployment and discontinuation. For aa-ECCS, the left atrial cannulation is performed through a femoral vein and delivered across the atrial septum, and positioning is facilitated and confirmed by fluoroscopy or TEE guidance. Outflow is directed into the common femoral or axillary artery. Excellent left atrial decompression is obtained as long as the inflow cannula is approximately positioned. The standard percutaneous transseptal approach includes 21F inflow cannula and 17F arterial outflow cannula. However, larger cannulas could be used during surgically implantation and the size of the inflow cannula regulates pump flow between 4 and 8 L/min. Anticoagulation with low dose heparin to keep ACT below 200 s is sufficient while patients are on support. The atrial septum should be repaired when an LVAD is implanted. The most undesirable aspect of this device is that it requires complete immobilization of the patient.

#### 6.2.2. *Intracorporeal circulation support (ICCS)*

Percutaneous t-MCSs are developed to unload the LV for better recovery and to maintain adequate CO in nonsurgical patients suffering from acute decompensated HF (acute cardiogenic shock), especially at bedside in the ICU or immediately in the catheterization laboratory [76]. A second application is short-term support of circulation during high-risk percutaneous or surgical cardiac interventions (coronary revascularization, mitral valve repair, etc.) in very sick patients without HF [77, 78]. The third indication could be transaortic left heart unloading in patients suffering from postcardiotomy syndrome treated with peripheral va-ECMO. The fourth clinical usage area is acute decompensation of end-stage HF to improve end-organ functions and to bridge to advanced HF treatments [79].

*Impella* is an axial-flow pump with three flow options (models 2.5 with flow 2.5 L/min, 5 with flow 5 L/min, CP with flow range between 3 and 4 L/min) and is suggested for t-MCS lasting up to five days [80]. This device is inserted percutaneously into the LV through the aortic valve. Models 2.5 and CP are implemented using 12F or 14F sheaths, respectively; however, model 5 requires surgical cut-down for a 21F catheter. The tip of the device is a pigtail that provides stabilization for the device in the LV. The pigtail connects by a cannula to a pump with a motor housing, intake (below the aortic valve) and output (above the aortic valve) areas, and a pump pressure monitor. The Impella device pumps blood directly from the LV into the proximal aorta, thereby unloading the LV, increasing cardiac output, and improving mean arterial pressure, while reducing LVEDP, myocardial workload, and oxygen consumption [81]. The device is dependent on the left ventricular preload, and hence on satisfactory right ventricular function and adequate CVP (8–12 mmHg).

### 6.3. Permanent mechanical circulatory support (p-MCS)

Use of long-term MCS devices has grown more rapidly than expected in recent years due to disproportionately low number of donor hearts. Advanced technological improvements in permanent MCS, especially LVADs, increase patients' survival and quality of life. Whereas t-MCS devices are implanted as a short-term rescue treatment to keep patients alive as a bridge to more durable long-term MCS devices, p-MCS devices are implanted as a long-term survival and/or bridging treatment to HTx. In the last years, p-MCS has been accepted as a destination therapy for Stage-D HF, and several types of permanent supportive devices could be used for uni- or biventricular assistance. The indication interval has changed in the recent years and will change even more in the future, so that patients in better condition will be referred to LVAD therapy earlier for the purpose of achieving better outcomes. Patients with relative contraindication such as higher PVR, obesity, or tobacco usage may be switched to eligible transplantation candidates over time. Compared with pulsatile flow devices, continuous flow technology has led to notable improvements in survival and reduction of adverse events, as well as in renal and hepatic function as a result of hemodynamic support.

#### *6.3.1. Ventricular assist device (VAD)*

The best technological developments happened in HF therapies, especially surgically. The benefits of different surgical treatment options are depend on underlying causes, and coronary revascularization, valve interventions, or defect repairs can achieve the recovery in early-stage HF. The variety and efficiency of options for surgical intervention decreases with advanced stages, and new surgical strategies must be used to keep patients alive and to provide them with better quality of life. The last step of Stage-D HF surgery is HTx. On the other hand, LVAD implantation has been accepted as a new therapy option for Stage-D HF as destination therapy for older or those who are not otherwise suitable for HTx. Usage of LVAD is promising, will continue to grow, and has become a standard therapy for advanced HF as a bridge to recovery, as a destination therapy, and as a bridge to HTx [82].

A shift from the concept of TAH as heart replacement, toward the development of single-chamber pumps provided the impetus for development of p-MCS devices. In the past decade, ventricular assist device (VAD) systems showed a substantial progress in miniaturization, durability, reliability, and noise emission (**Table 21**) [83]. These devices ensure an adequate and regulable additional blood flow in parallel with the particular ventricle. They can be used either as an isolated LVAD or right ventricular assist device (RVAD) or biventricular VAD. *First generation* VADs were either pneumatically or electrically driven membrane pumps, generating hydrodynamically pulsatile flow with artificial heart valves as the inlet and outlet. *Second generation* VADs with reduced size consists of a rotary pump

http://dx.doi.org/10.5772/67455

| Device type | Name | Assist | Mechanism |
|---|---|---|---|
| 1st generation extracorporeal pulsalite devices | Thoratec PVAD | BV | Pneumatic pump |
| | Excore (Berlin Heart) | BV | Pneumatic pump |
| 1st generation intracorporeal pulsatile devices | Thoratec IVAD | BV | Implantable version of Thoratec pVAD |
| | HeartMate IP, HM VE, XVE | LV | Pneumatic, electric vented pump |
| | Novacor | LV | Pulsatile |
| 2nd generation continuous axial flow devices | EvaHeart LVAS | LV | thromboresistant coating |
| | Micromed DeBakey VAD | LV | Axial flow pump |
| | Jarvik 2000 Flowmarker | LV | Axial flow, intracardiac located small pump |
| | HeartMate II | LV | Axial flow pump |
| 3rd generation continuous centrifugal pumps | Arrow CorAide | LV | |
| | ReliantHeart HeartAssist 5 | LV | Axial, child version is FDA approved. |
| | Incore (Berlin Heart) | LV | Magnetically suspended axial flow |
| | Ventr-assist (Ventracor) | LV | Hydrodynamically suspended rotor |
| | Duraheart | LV | Magnetically suspended centrifugal pump |
| | HeartWare HVAD | BV | Miniature hydromagnetically suspended rotor |
| | HeartMate III | LV | Magnetically suspended centrifugal pump |
| | HeartWare MVAD | BV | development-stage miniature device |
| Total artificial heart | Abiocor | - | Pulsatile, motor driven hydraulic system |
| | CardioWest (Syncardia) | BV | Pulsatile, pneumatic pump, mechanical valves |
| | Carmat | BV | Pulsatile, pneumatic pump, biological valves |

**Table 21.** The characteristics of long-term devices.

(impeller) with axial-flow design electromagnetically generating continuous flow without prosthetic valves, air vents, and compliance chambers. *Third generation* VADs eliminate bearings by using either hydrodynamic or electromagnetic suspension of an impeller. They employ a radial pump with both suspension mechanisms for contact-free rotation of an impeller that centrifugally generates continuous flow to reduce mechanical wear and trauma to blood cells.

Successful long-term outcomes after LVAD implantation are highly dependent on the timing of surgery (**Table 4**) and HF criteria (**Table 11**). If the LVAD is implanted too late, the outcome may worsen due to end-organ damage caused by prolonged HF (e.g. from poor nutritional status, low serum albumin, impaired liver- and renal function, markers of RHF). Long-term survival is best for patients with INTERMACS level 3 to 5, and worse for patients with INTERMACS level 1. With third generation LVADs (HeartWare or HeartMate III), early and mid-term survival has improved (>85% for 6 months and 1 year) with lower complication rates.

Five-year survival is approximately 60% with HeartWare device [84]. Absolute contraindications for LVAD implantation are obstructive or restrictive CMPs, irreversible lung or liver damage, active infection, aortic regurgitation, and severe RVF. Relative contraindications are increased risk of bleeding, cerebral ischemia, irreversible kidney damage, and prior implantation of mechanical aortic valve prosthesis [85].

*6.3.2. Total artificial heart (TAH)*

Total replacement of the biventricular-failed heart with a total prosthetic heart is unlikely to see widespread usage due to the extraordinarily aggressive nature of the surgery. Several complicating factors can constrain the implantation of these devices: patient characteristics, device size, implantation timing and location, and the need for extensive surgery. Implantation of LVAD alone could aid these patients because of its ability to partially right ventricular functions, and this advantage makes the LVAD approach generally preferred over TAH in patients with biventricular failure. The usage of TAH devices is restricted to the patient's in whom LVAD is not feasible due to infiltrative or restrictive CMPs, cardiac malignancies, nonsurgical postinfarction ventricular septal defect, intractable ventricular arrhythmias, and cardiac graft failure [86]. The device has two artificial ventricles lined with polyurethane, and ejects blood via a four-layer, moving diaphragm driven pneumatically or hydraulically [87]. The ventricle cuffs are sutured to patient's atria and outflow grafts to the aorta and pulmonary artery. The device has four mechanical or biological valves maintaining unidirectional flow. The implanted device is powered by a loud and very heavy external compressor. Thrombosis, thromboembolic events, postoperative bleeding, or infections are significant and relatively frequent complications. The other dissuasive structure can be double drivelines tunneled under the skin, but the drive unit can be set inside the patients' body. Both artificial ventricles alternately eject blood to balance left and right heart CO. There are certain sizing criteria for TAH implantation: chest antero-posterior distance $>$10 cm, body surface area $>$1.7 $m^2$, cardiothoracic ratio $>$0.5, and LVEDD $>$66 mm.

## 7. Cardiac transplantation

Heart transplantation is the only curable and durable treatment option for HF, especially with new immunosuppression therapies, improved clinical management, and pharmaceutical development for refractory or end-stage HF. The most common indication is dilated CMP (50%), and the second is ischemic CMP (35%), but retransplantation ratio has not changed (3%) in the last decade. Once patients are approved for HTx, they are listed according to the medical urgency status and severity of the illness (**Table 22**). Worldwide, a steady decline in heart transplantation has been observed over the last 15 years due to a one-third decrease in the availability of donor organs, while the numbers of patients awaiting heart transplant has doubled. About 15–20% of patients listed for transplantation die before a suitable organ becomes available and more than 30% of patients awaiting HTx require an appropriate MCS to bridge to transplant. The median waiting time for HTx in several countries is

http://dx.doi.org/10.5772/67455

| Code status | Description |
|---|---|
| 1A | - Patients in the intensive care unit with inotropic support + mechanical support (ECMO, ECCS) ± respiratorial support + a pulmonary artery catheter for hemodynamic monitoring<br>- LVAD patients with<br>- life-threatening ventricular arrhythmia<br>- right ventricular failure<br>- device malfunction/mechanical failure, thromboembolism, infection<br>- RVAD<br>- LVAD < 30 days<br>- TAH |
| 1B | Patients who are on inotropic support but not meeting 1A criteria<br>Patients have a ventricular assist device longer than 30 days |
| 2 | Patients who are waiting at home on medical therapy |
| 7 | Patients who are on hold because of an intervening medical illness, making them inappropriate candidates for transplantation |

**Table 22.** Transplantation urgency code status.

approximately 6 to 9 months and depends on several factors, including listed status, body weight, blood group, and differences between recipient and donor. Potential transplant recipients can have decompensated HF requiring high-dose pharmacological treatment and/or MCS, symptomatic Stage-D HF under optimal medical therapy, asymptomatic advanced HF with a peak $VO_2$ of less than 15 mL/kg/min, or recurrent arrhythmias despite interventions. Maximal $VO_2$ is the most noninvasively valuable test for better evaluation of potential recipients, and a peak $VO_2$ of less than 12 mL/kg/min indicates a poor prognosis. The most variable relative contraindication among centers is the age limit; however, transplant guidelines extend the eligibility to 70 years of age, leading individual centers to determine their own age cut-off. Malignancy, impaired lung and renal functions can increase morbidity and impair prognosis. Patients with presenting fixed PAH are associated with high early mortality, and should be considered for combined heart-lung transplantation. Nevertheless, it has been shown that a continuous flow LVAD may help to reduce PVR, so that the patient becomes eligible for subsequent cardiac transplantation. The number of HTx recipients on MCS has doubled and reached 45% of total HTx candidates in the last decade (>50% in 2014): LVAD 85.2%, RVAD 7.2%, TAH 3.1%, and ECMO 2.9% [88]. Patients implanted with a LVAD on status 1A because of device complications or a 30-day elective grace period or on Status 1B will be priority to receive the organ unless they are deemed nontransplantation candidate (Status 7). It has been reported that approximately more than 50% patients were in Status 1A, and one-half patients had LVAD with in Status 1A (70%) or 1B (30%) at the time of HTx; whereas one-third of the patients in Status 1A had LVAD, of which 50% had device complications, and one-fifth patients in Status 1B had LVAD [89].

Early (<30 days) mortality ranges from 5% to 10% usually due to primary graft failure (35.3%), multiple organ failure (21.6%), and infection (14.3%); and 1-, 2-, 3-, 4-, 5-, 10-, and 15-year cumulative survival rates are 82, 78, 75, 72.5, 69.5, 52, and 34.4%, respectively [88]. A decline in 1-year overall survival after HTx from 85 to 76% in the EuroTransplant region has been observed, presumably because of increasing donor age and recipient comorbidity [90]. Early mortality and long-term survival rates in recipients assisted by ECMO are worse than those assisted by LVAD: early mortality is 35 versus 5%, and 1-, 2-, 3-, 4-, and 5-year survival rates are 60 versus 89%, 54 versus 86%, 51.5 versus 82%, 51.5 versus 81%, and 51.5 versus 76%, respectively [88]. The one-year survival after HTx is similar in patients with LVAD (89%), but complicated postimplant recipients have worse, 3-year survival than noncomplicated postimplant recipients (78 versus 85%) [89]. Long-term survival is dependent on several factors, but the availability of the donor hearts from younger male donors with shortest ischemic times is identified as the most significant factor improving long-term survival [91]. The median survival is at least 13.5 years for patients who survive the first year. Survival is lower in patients with valvular cardiomyopathy, congenital heart disease, or following retransplantation, and for those requiring pretransplant MCS. Additionally, patients who are sicker prior to transplant have worse survival outcomes [92]. Cardiac allograft vasculopathy is among the primary causes of death after the first year of HTx, and it is the most important limiting factor in long-term survival, along with neoplasms, with an incidence of 8% in the first year, 30% in 5 years, and 50% in 10 years [93].

Heart transplantation surgery is not a complex procedure, and surgical implantation techniques are the easiest part of HTx. The main problem with HTx is cold ischemic time to donor heart transportation, which should be <4 hours without continuous coronary perfusion or >4 hours with coronary perfusion via special equipment. The ideal cold ischemic time is shorter than 2 hours. Second problem is immunosuppression to prevent organ rejection, which is the main risk factor for graft failure preoperatively and early postoperatively (<1 year), and thereafter cardiac allograft vasculopathy is the major problem after the first posttransplant year. Third problem is increased PVR and it should be managed aggressively, because the unprepared donor RV may be unable to overcome this increased afterload. The standard technique is orthotopic HTx. The great arteries are transected at the sinotubular junctions, whereas the LA is insiced along the atrioventricular groove, leaving left atrial cuff for anastomosis. For biatrial technique, the RA is prepared with the same manner; however, for bicaval technique, both vena cavae are transected at their right atrial junctions. Bicaval anastomosis is a more common approach for implantation of the donor heart rather than biatrial technique [94]. The advantages of bicaval technique are reducing the right atrial size, preserving atrial conduction pathways, decreasing the risk of tricuspid regurgitation, and avoiding permanent pacemaker need [95]. Annuloaortic ectasia with the ascending aorta aneurysm could be managed by the replacement of the recipient ascending aorta during HTx [96].

http://dx.doi.org/10.5772/67455

## Author details

Kaan Kırali[1,2]*, Özge Altaş Yerlikhan[1] and Hakan Hançer[1]

*Address all correspondence to: imkbkirali@yahoo.com

1 Department of Cardiac Transplantation and Ventricular Assist Device, Kartal Koşuyolu YIEA Hospital, Istanbul, Turkey

2 Department of Cardiovascular Surgery, Faculty of Medicine, Sakarya University, Sakarya, Turkey

## References

[1] Yancy CW, Jessup M, Bozkurt B, Butler J, Casey DE, Drazner MH, Fonarow GC, Geraci SA, Horwich T, et al. 2013 ACCF/AHA guideline for the management of heart failure. JACC 2013;62(16):e147–239.

[2] Metra M, Ponikowski P, Dickstein K, et al. Advanced chronic heart failure: a position statement from the Study Group on Advanced Heart Failure of the Heart Failure Association of the European Society of Cardiology. Eur J Heart Fail 2007;9:684–94.

[3] Hunt SA, Abraham WT, Chin MH, et al. 2009 Focused update incorporated into the ACC/AHA 2005 guidelines for the diagnosis and management of heart failure in adults: a report of the American College of Cardiology Foundation/American Heart Association Task Force on Practice Guidelines. J Am Coll Cardiol 2009;53:e1–90.

[4] Russell SD, Miller LW, Pagani FD. Advanced heart failure: a call to action. Congest Heart Fail 2008;14:316–21.

[5] Kinugawa K. How to treat stage D heart failure? When to implant left ventricular assist devices in the era of continuous flow pumps? Circ J 2011;75(9):2038–2045.

[6] Stevenson LW, Pagani FD, Young JB, Jessup M, Miller L, Kormos RL, Naftel DC, Ulisney K, Desvigne-Nickens P, Kirklin JK. INTERMACS profiles of advanced heart failure: the current picture. J Heart Lung Transplant 2009;28(6):535–541.

[7] Naegele M, Flammer AJ, Enseleit F, Ruschitzka F. Medical therapy of heart failure with reduced ejection fraction: current evidence and new developments. Swiss Med Ekly 2016;146:w14295.

[8] Mentz RJ, Bakris GL, Waeber B, McMurray JJ, Gheorghiade M, Ruilope LM, Maggioni AP, Swedberg K, Piña IL, Fiuzat M, O'Connor CM, Zannad F, Pitt B. The past, present

and future of renin-angiotensin aldosterone system inhibition. Int J Cardiol 2013;167 (5):1677–1687.

[9] Gradman AH. Evolving understanding of the renin–angiotensin–aldosterone system: pathophysiology and targets for therapeutic intervention. Am Heart J 2009;157:S1–6.

[10] Jhund PS, McMurray JJV. The neprilysin pathway in heart failure: a review and guide on the use of sacubitril/valsartan. Heart 2016;102(17):1342–1347.

[11] Yancy CW, Jessup M, Bozkurt B, Butler J, Casey DE, Colvin MM, Drazner MH, Filippatos G, Fonarow GC, et al. 2016 ACC/AHA/HFSA focused update on new pharmacological therapy for heart failure: an update of the 2013 ACCF/AHA guideline for the management of heart failure. JACC 2016;68(13):1476–1488.

[12] Braunwald E. The Path to an angiotensin receptor antagonist-neprilysin inhibitor in the treatment of heart failure. J Am Coll Cardiol 2015;65(10):1029–1041.

[13] Ambrosy AP, Butler J, Ahmed A, Vaduganathan M, van Veldhuisen DJ, Colucci WS, Gheorghiade M. The use of digoxin in patients with worsening chronic heart failure: reconsidering an old drug to reduce hospital admissions. J Am Coll Cardiol 2014;63 (18):1823–1832.

[14] Konstantinou DM, karvounis H, Giannakoulas G. Digoxin in heart failure with a reduced ejection fraction: a risk factor or a risk marker? Cardiology 2016;134(3):311–319.

[15] Mentz RJ, Broderick S, Shaw LK, Chiswell K, Fiuzat M, O'Connor CM. Persistent angina pectoris in ischaemic cardiomyopathy: increased rehospitalization and major adverse cardiac events. Eur J Heart Fail 2014;16(8):854–860.

[16] De Luca L, Olivari Z, Farina A, Gonzini L, Lucci D, Di Chiara A, Casella G, Chiarella F, Boccanelli A, Di Pasquale G, De Servi S, Bovenzi FM, Gulizia MM, Savonitto S. Temporal trends in the epidemiology, management, and outcome of patients with cardiogenic shock complicating acute coronary syndromes. J Heart Fail 2015;17(11):1124–1132.

[17] Hoebers LP, Claessen BE, Elias J, Dangas GD, Mehran R, Henriques JP. Meta-analysis on the impact of percutaneous coronary intervention of chronic total occlusions on left ventricular function and clinical outcome. Int J Cardiol 2015;187:90–96.

[18] Cardona M, Martín V, Prat-Gonzalez S, Ortiz JT, Perea RJ, de Caralt TM, Masotti M, Pérez-Villa F, Sabaté M. Benefits of chronic total occlusion coronary percutaneous intervention in patients with heart failure and reduced ejection fraction: insights from a cardiovascular magnetic resonance study. J Cardiovasc Magn reson J 2016;18(1):78.

[19] Petrucci E, Balian V, Bocchieri A. Real-time assessment of myocardial viability in the catheterization laboratory using the intracoronary electrograms recorded by the PTCA guidewire in patients with left ventricular dysfunction: comparison with delayed-enhancement magnetic resonance imaging. JACC Cardiovasc Interv 2014;7(9):988–996.

[20] Jolicœur EM, Dunning A, Castelvecchio S, Dabrowski R, Waclawiw MA, Petrie MC, Stewart R, Jhund PS, Desvigne-Nickens P, Panza JA, Bonow RO, Sun B, San TR, Al-

Khalidi HR, Rouleau JL, Velazquez EJ, Cleland JG. Importance of angina in patients with coronary disease, heart failure, and leftventricular systolic dysfunction: insights from STICH. J Am Card Coll 2015;66(19):2092–2100.

[21] Adachi Y, Sakakura K, Wada H, Funayama H, Umemoto T, Fujita H, Momomura S. Determinants of left ventricular systolic function improvement following coronary artery revascularization in heart failure patients with reduced ejection fraction (HFrEF). Int Heart J 2016 Sep 28;57(5):565–72.

[22] King's College, London. Study of efficacy and safety of percutaneous coronary intervention to improve survival in heart failure (REVIVEDBCIS2). 2015. Available at: http://clinicaltrials. gov/show/NCT01920048. Accessed August 30, 2015.

[23] Wrobel K, Stevens SR, Jones RH, Selzman CH, Lamy A, Beaver TM, Djokovic LT, Wang N, Velazquez EJ, Sopko G, Kron IL, DiMaio JM, Michler RE, Lee KL, Yii M, Leng CY, Zembala M, Rouleau JL, Daly RC, Al-Khalidi HR. Influence of baseline characteristics, operative conduct, and postoperative course on 30-day outcomes of coronary artery bypass grafting among patients with left ventricular dysfunction: results from the Surgical Treatment for Ischemic Heart Failure (STICH) Trial. Circulation 2015;132(8):720–730.

[24] Kırali K, Rabus MB, Yakut N, Toker ME, Erdoğan HB, Balkanay M, Alp M, Yakut C. Early- and long-term comparison of the on- and off-pump bypass surgery in patients with left ventricular dysfunction. Heart Surg Forum 2002;5(2):177–181.

[25] Ömeroğlu SN, Kırali K, Güler M, Toker ME, İpek G, Işık Ö, Yakut C. Midterm angiographic assessment of coronary artery bypass grafting without cardiopulmonary bypass. Ann Thorac Surg 2000;70(3):844–849.

[26] Kırali K, Mansuroğlu D, Kayalar N, Güzelmeriç F, Alp M, Yakut C. Markers of myocardial ischemia in the evaluation of the effect of left anterior descending coronary artery lesion and collateral circulation on myocardial injury in 1-vessel off-pump coronary bypass surgery. Heart Surg Forum 2003;6(3):143–148.

[27] Şişmanoğlu M, Sarıkaya S, Onk OA, Adademir T, Aksoy E, Kırali K. Treatment of left anterior descending coronary artery stenosis: stent or surgery. Asian Cardiovasc Thorac Ann 2013;21(5):528–532.

[28] Uyar İ, Mansuroğlı D, Kırali K, Erentuğ V, Bozbuğa NU, Uysal G, Yakut C. Aspartate and glutamate-enriched cardioplegia in left ventricular dysfunction. J Card Surg 2005;20 (4):337–344.

[29] Nishimura RA, Otto CM, Bonow RO, et al. American College of Cardiology/American Heart Association Task Force on Practice Guidelines. 2014 AHA/ACC guideline for the management of patients with valvular heart disease: a report of the American College of Cardiology/American Heart Association Task Force on Practice Guidelines. J Am Coll Cardiol 2014;63(22):e57–185.

[30] Di Salvo TG, Acker MA, Dec GW, Byrne JG. Mitral valve surgery in advanced heart failure. J Am Coll Cardiol 2010;55(4):271–282.

[31] Ramlawi B, Gammie JS. Mitral valve surgery: current minimally invasive and transcatheter options. Methodist Debakey Cardiovasc J 2016;12(1):20–26.

[32] Taramasso M, Kuwata S, Biefer HRC, Nietlispach F, Maisano F. Percutaneous mitral valve repair and replacement: complementary or competitive techniques? EuroIntervention 2016;12:Y97–101.

[33] Chiam PTL, Ruiz CE. Percutaneous transcatheter mitral valve repair: a classification of the technology. J Am Coll Cardiol Intv 2011;4(1):1–13.

[34] Stewart MH, Jenkins JS. The evolving role of percutaneous mitral valve repair. Ochsner J 2016;16(3):270–276.

[35] Neuss M, Schau T, Schoepp M; Seifert M, Hölschermann F, Meyhöfer J, Butter C. Patient selection criteria and midterm clinical outcome for MitraClip therapy in patients with severe mitral regurgitation and severe congestive heart failure. Eur J Heart Fail 2013;15(7):786–795.

[36] Maisano F, Godino C, Giacomini A, Denti P, Buzzatti N, Arendar I, Colombo A, Alfieri O, La Canna G. Patient selection for MitraClip therapy impaired left ventricular systolic function. Minerva Cardioangiol 2011;59(5):455–71.

[37] De Bonis M, Taramasso M, Lapenna E, Denti P, La Canna G, Buzzatti N, Pappalardo F, Di Giannuario G, Cioni M, Giacominni A, Alfieri O. MitraClip therapy and surgical edge-to-edge repair in patients with severe left ventricular dysfunction and secondary mitral regurgitation: mid-term results of a single-centre experience. Eur J Cardiothorac Surg 2016;49(1):255–262.

[38] Philip F, Athappan G, Tuzcu EM, Svensson LG, Kapadia SR. MitraClip for severe symptomatic mitral regurgitation in patients at high surgical risk: a comprehensive systematic review. Catheter Cardiovasc Interv 2014;84(4):581–590.

[39] Lipiecki J, Siminiak T, Sievert H, Müller-Ehmsen J, Deen H, Wu JC, Schandrin C, Kalmucki P, Hofmann I, Reuter D, Goldberg SL, Haude M. Coronary sinus-based percutaneous annuloplasty as treatment for functional mitral regurgitation: the TITAN II trial. Open Heart 2016 Jul 8;3(2):e000411.

[40] Jerzykowska O, Kalmucki P, Woloszyn M, Smuszkiewicz P, Firek L, Sinimiak T. Echocardiographic evaluation of percutaneous valve repair in patients with mitral regurgitation using the CARILLON™ system. Kardiol Pol 2010;68(1):57–63.

[41] Klein N, Pfeiffer D, Goldenberg S, Klein M. Mitral annuloplasty device implantation for non-surgical treatment of mitral regurgitation: clinical experience after the approval studies. J Invasive Cardiol 2016;28(3):115–120.

[42] Schofer J, Siminiak T, Haude M, Herrman JP, Vainer J, Wu JC, Levy WC, Mauri L, Feldman T, Kwong RY, Kaye DM, Duffy SJ, Tübler T, Degen H, Brandt MC, Van Bibber R, Goldberg S, Reuter DG, Hoppe UC. Percutaneous mitral annuloplasty for functional mitral regurgitation results of the CARILLON Mitral Annuloplasty Device European Union Study. Circulation 2009;120(4):326–333.

[43] Seeburger J, Rinaldi M, Nielsen SL, Salizzoni S, Lange R, Schoenburg M, Alfieri O, Borger MA, Mohr FW, Aidietis A. Off-pump transapical implantation of artificial neo-chordae to correct mitral regurgitation: the TACT trial (Transapical Artificial Chordae Tendinae). J am Coll Cardiol 2014;63(9):914–919.

[44] Jensen H, Jensen MO, Waziri F, Honge JL, Sloth E, Gron MF, Nielsen SL. Transapical neochord implantation: is tension of artificial chordae tendineae dependent on the insertion site? J Thorac Cardiovasc Surg 2014;148(1):138–143.

[45] Ståhlberg M, Lund LH, Zabarovskaja S, Gadler F, Braunschweig F, Linde C. Cardiac resynchronization therapy: a breakthrough in heart failure management. J Intern Med 2012;272(4):330–343.

[46] Lu PJ, Lin PY, Yang CFJ, Hung CH, Chan MY, Hsu TC. Hemodynamic and metabolic effects of para- versus intraaortic counterpulsatile circulation supports. ASAIO J 2001;57(1):19–25.

[47] Kontogiannis CD, Malliaras K, Kapelios CJ, Mason JW, Nanas JN. Continuous internal counterpulsation as a bridge to recovery in acute and chronic heart failure. World J Transplant 2016;6(1):115–124.

[48] Parissis H, Graham V, Lampridis S, Lau M, Hooks G, Mhandu PC. IABP: history-evolution-pathophysiology-indications: what we need to know. J Cardiothorac Surg 2016;11 (1):122.

[49] Kırali K, Güler M, Erentuğ V, Dağlar B, Balkanay M, Akıncı E, Ipek G, Işık Ö, Yakut C. Intraaortic balloon pump: 15-years experience with 765 patients. Turkish J Cardiovasc Thorac Surg 1999;7(5):353–357.

[50] Mizuno M, Sato N, Kajimoto K, Sakata Y, Minami Y, Munakata R, Hagiwara N, Takano T. Intra-aortic balloon counterpulsation for acute decompensated heart failure. Int J Cardiol 2014;176(3):1444–1446.

[51] Kapelios CJ, Terrovitis JV, Siskas P, Kontogiannis C, Repasos E, Nanas JN. ounterpulsation: a concept with a remarkable past, an established present and a challenging future. Int J Cardiol 2015;172(2):318–325.

[52] Pilarczyk K, Boening A, Jacob H, Langebartels G, Markewitz A, Haake N, Heringlake M, Trummer G. Preoperative intra-aortic counterpulsation in high-risk patients undergoing cardiac surgery: a meta-analysis of randomized controlled trials. Eur J Cartiothorac Surg 2016;49(1):5–17.

[53] Sá MP, Ferraz PE, Escobar RR, Martins WN, Nunes EO, Vasconcelos FP, Lima RC. Prophylactic intra-aortic balloon pump in high-risk patients undergoing coronary artery bypass surgery: a meta-analysis of randomized controlled trials. Coron Artery Dis 2012;23(7):480–486.

[54] Norkiene I, Ringaitiene D, Rucinskas K, Samalavicius R, Baublys A, Miniauskas S, Sirvydis V. Intra-aortic balloon counterpulsation in decompensated cardiomyopathy

patients: bridge to transplantation or assist device. Interact Cardiovasc Thorac Surg 2007;6(1):66–70.

[55] Imamura T, Kinugawa K, Nitta D, Hatano M, Kinoshita O, Nawata K, Kyo S, Ono M. Prophylactic intra-aortic balloon pump before ventricular assist device implantation reduces perioperative medical expenses and improves postoperative clinical course in INTERMACS profile 2 patients. Circ J 2015;79(9):1963–1969.

[56] Bezerra CG, Adam EL, Baptista ML, Ciambelli GS, Kopel L, Bernoche C, Lopes LNGD, Macatrao-Costa MF, Falcao BAA, Lage SG. Aortic counterpulsation therapy in patients with advanced heart failure: analysis of the TBRIDGE registry. Arq Bras Cardiol 2016;106 (1):26–32.

[57] Sarıkaya S, Adademir T, Özen Y, Aydın E, Başaran EK, Şahin M, Rabuş MB, Kırali K. Alternative non-femoral accesses for intra-aortic balloon pumping. Perfusion 2015;30 (8):629–635.

[58] Erentuğ V, Bozbuğa N, Izgi A, Eren E, Kırali K, Balkanay M, Ipek G, Akıncı E, Alp M, Yakut C. Traumatic vascular complications due to intra-aortic balloon pump support. Ulus Travma Derg 2004;10(1):28–33.

[59] Legget ME, Peters WS, Milsom FP, et al. Extra-aortic balloon counterpulsation: an intraoperative feasibility study. Circulation 2005;112(Supp l):I26–31.

[60] Solanki P. Aortic counterpulsation: C-pulse and other devices for cardiac support. J Cardiovasc Transl Res 2014;7(3):292–300.

[61] Hayward CS, Peters WS, Merry AF, Ruygrok PN, Jansz P, O'Driscoll G, Larbalestier RI, Smith JA, Ho B, Legget ME, Milsom FP. Chronic extra- aortic balloon counterpulsation: first-in-human pilot study in end-stage heart failure. J Heart Lung Transplant 2010;29 (12):1427–1432.

[62] Nanas JN, Lolas CT, Charitos CE, Nanas SN, Margari ZJ, Agapitos EV, et al. A valveless high stroke volume counterpulsation device restores hemodynamics in patients with congestive heart failure and intractable cardiogenic shock awaiting heart transplantation. J Thorac Cardiovasc Surg 1996;111(1):55–61.

[63] Terrovitis JV, Charitos CE, Tsolakis EJ, Dolou P, Pierrakos CN, Siafakas KX, Nanas JN. Superior performance of a paraaortic counterpulsation device compared to the intraaortic balloon pump. World J Surg 2003;27(12):1311–1316.

[64] Shi C, Zhou DD, Liu G, Zhang L, Meng JJ, Geng Y, Liu XG. The left ventricular assist effect and biocompatibility study of a novel para-aortic counterpulsation device. Eur Rev Med Pharmacol Sci 2015;19(10):1869–1865

[65] Zhang JM, Liu XC, Liu ZG, Zhao L, Yang L, Liu TW,He GW. Comparison of effects of extra-thoracic paraaortic counterpulsation to intraaortic balloon pump on circulatory support in acute heart failure. J Cardiothorac Surg 2015;10:173.

[66] Jeevanandam V, Jayakar D, Anderson AS, Martin S, Piccione W Jr, Heroux AL, Wynne J, Stephenson LW, Hsu J, Freed PS, Kantrowitz A. Circulatory assistance with a permanent implantable IABP: initial human experience. Circulation 2002;106(12 Suppl 1):I183–I188.

[67] Marinakis S, Nanas Y, Sarchosi S, Kontogiannis C, Kapelios C, Tachliabouris G, Charitos C, Nanas J, Malliaras K. A novel implantable counterpulsation assist device, the PULVAD, induced superior left ventricular pressure unloading compared to the intraaortic balloon pump in a bovine model of acute heart failure. Eur J Heart Fail 2015;17(Suppl 1):196.

[68] Giridharan GA, Bartoli CR, Spence PA, Dowling RD, Koenig SC. Counterpulsation with symphony prevents retrograde carotid, aortic, and coronary flows observed with intra-aortic balloon pump support. Artif Organs 2012;36(7):600–606.

[69] Mishra S. Upscaling cardiac assist devices in decompensated heart failure: choice of device and its timing. Indian Heart J 2016;68(Suppl 1):S1–4.

[70] Nair PK, Kormos RL, Teuteberg JJ, Mathier MA, Bermudez CA, Toyoda Y, Dew MA, Simon MA. Pulsatile left ventricular assist device support as a bridge to decision in patients with end-stage heart failure complicated by pulmonary hypertension. J Heart Lung Transplant 2010;29(2):201–208.

[71] Loforte A, Montalto A, Ranocchi F, Monica PLD, Casali G, Lappa A, Contento C, Musumeci F. Levitronix CentriMag third-generation magnetically levitated continuous flow pump as bridge to solution. ASAIO J 2011;57(4):247–253.

[72] Sen A, Larson JS, Kashani KB, Libricz SL, Patel BM, Guru PK, Alwardt CM, Pajaro O, Farmer JC. Mechanical circulatory assist devices: a primer for critical care and emergency physicians. Crit Care 2016;20(1):153.

[73] Gilotra NA, Stevens GR. Temporary mechanical circulatory support: a review of the options, indications, and outcomes. Clin Med Insights Cardiol 2014;8(Suppl 1):75–85.

[74] Shekar K, Mullany DV, Thomson B, Ziegenfuss M, Platts DG, Fraser JF. Extracorporeal life support devices and strategies for management of acute cardiorespiratory failure in adult patients: a comprehensive review. Crit Care 2014;18(3):219.

[75] Meineri M, Van Rensburg AE, Vegas A. Right ventricular failure after LVAD implantation: prevention and treatment. Best Pract Res Clin Anaesthesiol 2012;26(2):217–229.

[76] Ergle K, Parto P, Krim SR. Percutaneous ventricular assist devices: a novel approach in the management of patients with acute cardiogenic shock. Ochsner J 2016;16:243–249.

[77] Palacios IF. Left ventricular assistant device Impella 2.5 usage for patients undergoing high-risk PCI. Catheter Cardiovasc Interv 2012;79(7):1135–1137.

[78] Szafron B, Smoczyński RH, Drobiński D, Pawlak A, Wojciechowski D, Liszka IM, Witkowska A, Kaliciński Z, Gil R, Suwalski P. Impella LD microaxial pump supporting

combined mitral and coronary surgery in a patient with dilated cardiomyopathy. A short bridge to recovery? Kardiochir Torakochirurgia Pol 2015;12(1):56–59.

[79] Bansal A, Bhama JK, Patel R, Desai S, Mandras SA, Patel H, Collins T, Reilly JP, Ventura HO, Parrino E. Using the minimally ınvasive Impella 5.0 via the right subclavian artery cutdown for acute on chronic decompensated heart failure as a bridge to decision. Ochsner J 2016;16(3):210–216

[80] Sarkar K, Kini AS. Percutaneous left ventricular support devices. Cardiol Clin 2010;28 (1):169–184.

[81] Rihal CS, Naidu SS, Givertz MM, Szeto WY, Burke JA, Kapur NK, Kern M, Garratt KN, Goldstein JA, Dimas V, Tu T. Society for Cardiovascular Angiography and Interventions (SCAI); Heart Failure Society of America (HFSA); Society of Thoracic Surgeons (STS); American Heart Association (AHA), and American College of Cardiology (ACC). 2015 SCAI/ACC/HFSA/STS clinical expert consensus statement on the use of percutaneous mechanical circulatory support devices in cardiovascular care: endorsed by the American Heart Association, the Cardiological Society of India, and Sociedad Latinoamericana de Cardiolog´ıa Intervencionista; affirmation of value by the Canadian Association of Interventional Cardiology-Association Canadienne de Cardiologie d'Intervention. J Am Coll Cardiol 2015;65(19):e7–26.

[82] Englert JA 3rd, Davis JA, Krim SR. Mechanical circulatory support for the failing heart: continuous-flow left ventricular assist devices. Ochsner J 2016;16(3):263–269.

[83] Prinzing A, Herold U, Berkefeld A, Krane M, Lange R, Voss B. Left ventricular assist devices: current state and perspectives. J Thorac Dis 2016;8(8):E660–666.

[84] Schmitto JD, Zimpfer D, Fiane AE, Larbalestier R, Tsui S, Jansz P, Simon A, Schueler S, Strueber M. Long-term support of patients receiving a left ventricular assist device for advanced heart failure: a follow-up analysis of the Registry to Evaluate the HeartWare Left Ventricular Assist System. Eur J Cardiothorac Surg 2016;50(5):834–838.

[85] Jurkiewicz BS, Szczurek W, Suliga K, Rempega G, Rajwa P. Mechanical circulatory support in heart failure. Kardiochir Torakochirurgia Pol 2016;13(2):130–134.

[86] Samak M, fatullayev J, Sabashnikov A, Zeriouh M, Rahmanian PB, Choi YH, Wippermann J, Wahlers T, Schmack B, Ruhparwar A, Dohmen PM, Karck M, Popov AF, Simon AR, Weymann A. Past and present of total artificial heart therapy: a success story. Med Sci Monit Basic Res 2015;21:183–190.

[87] Gerosa G, Scuri S, Iop L, Torregrossa G. Present and future perspectives on total artificial hearts. Ann Cardiothorac Surg 2014;3(6):595–602.

[88] Lund LH, Edwards LB, Dipchand AI, Goldfarb S, Kucheryavaya AY, Levvey BJ, Meiser B, Rossano JW, Yusen RD, Stehlik J. The Registry of the International Society for Heart and Lung Transplantation: Thirty-third Adult Heart Transplantation Report—2016; focus theme: primary diagnostic indications for transplant. J Heart Lung Transplan 2016;35 (10):1158–1169.

http://dx.doi.org/10.5772/67455

[89] Trivedi JR, Rajagopal K, Schumer EM, Birks EJ, Lenneman A, Cheng A, Slaughter MS. Differences in Status 1A heart transplantation survival in the continuous flow left ventricular assist device era. Ann Thorac Surg 2016;102:1512–1516.

[90] Smits JM. Actual situation in Eurotransplant regarding high urgent heart transplantation. Eur J Cardiothorac Surg 2012;42(4):609–611.

[91] Sareyyüpoğlu B, Kırali K, Göksedef D, Rabuş MB, Tuncer A, Erentuğ V, Mansuroğlu D, Yakut C. Factors associated with long-term survival following cardiac transplantation. Anatol J Cardiol 2008;8(5):360–366.

[92] Katz JN, Waters SB, Hollis IB, Chang PP. Advanced therapies for end-stage heart failure. Curr Cardiol Rev 2015;11(1):63–72.

[93] Lund LH, Edwards LB, Kucheryavaya AY, Dipchand AI, Benden C, Christie JD, Dobbels F, Kirk R, Rahmel AO, Yusen RD, Stehlik J. The Registry of the International Society for Heart and Lung Transplantation: Thirtieth Official Adult Heart Transplant Report—2013; focus theme: age. J Heart Lung Transplant 2013;32(10):951–964.

[94] Kara İ, Mansuroğlu D, Kırali K, Güler M, Ömeroğlu SN, Eren E, Balkanay M, Alp M, İpek G, Işık Ö, Yakut C. Early-term results of bicaval and biatrial techniques in orthotopic heart transplantation. Turk Gogus Kalp Dama 2012;20(2):223–229.

[95] Kara İ, Kırali K, Yakut C. A comparison of the results of the bicaval and biatrial surgical technique in orthotopic heart transplantation: a review and meta-analysis. Turk Gogus Kalp Dama 2012;20(3):672–681.

[96] Kırali K, Eren E, Mataracı İ, Çevirme D. Combined orthotopic heart transplantation and prophylactic ascending aorta replacement in a Marfan patient. Turk Gogus Kalp Dama 2011;19(3):434–436.